CARDIOVASCULAR NUTRITION

Disease Management and Prevention

Jo Ann S. Carson, PhD, RD

Frances M. Burke, MS, RD

Lisa A. Hark, PhD, RD

Editors

Nilo B. Cater, MD
Medical Adviser

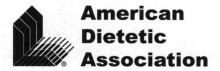

American Dietetic Association

Diana Faulhaber, Publisher
Jason M. Muzinic, Acquisitions Editor
Elizabeth Nishiura, Production Editor

10 9 8 7 6 5 4 3 2 1

Library of Congress Cataloging-in-Publication Data
Cardiovascular nutrition : disease management and prevention / Jo Ann S. Carson, Frances M. Burke, Lisa A. Hark, editors; Nilo B. Cater, medical adviser.
     p. ; cm.
  Includes bibliographical references and index.
  ISBN 0-88091-345-2
  1. Cardiovascular system—Diseases—Nutritional aspects. 2. Cardiovascular system—Diseases—Diet therapy. 3. Cardiovascular system—Diseases—Prevention.
    [DNLM: 1. Cardiovascular Diseases—prevention & control. 2. Complementary Therapies. 3. Nutrition. 4. Risk Factors. WG 120 C26758 2004] I. Carson, Jo Ann S. II. Burke, Frances M. III. Hark, Lisa.

  RC669.C2874 2004
  616.1'0654—dc22

2004013769

CONTENTS

CONTRIBUTORS

Joyce P. Barnett, MS, RD
Department of Clinical Nutrition
The University of Texas Southwestern Medical
*   Center at Dallas*
Dallas, TX

Amy E. Binkoski, RD
Department of Nutritional Sciences
Pennsylvania State University
University Park, PA

Frances M. Burke, MS, RD
Nutrition Education and Prevention Program
University of Pennsylvania School of Medicine
Preventive Cardiology Program
University of Pennsylvania Health System
Philadelphia, PA

Jo Ann S. Carson, PhD, RD
Department of Clinical Nutrition and
Center for Human Nutrition
University of Texas Southwestern Medical Center
*   at Dallas*
Dallas, TX

Aram Chobanian, MD
Boston University School of Medicine
Boston, MA

Maureen E. Conway, MBA, MA, RD
McNeil Nutritionals
Division of McNeil PPC, Inc.
Fort Washington, PA

Ralph B. D'Agostino, PhD
College of Liberal Arts
Boston University
Boston, MA

Darwin D. Deen, MD, MS
Department of Family and Social Medicine
Albert Einstein College of Medicine
Bronx, NY

Gary D. Foster, PhD
Weight and Eating Disorders Program
University of Pennsylvania Health System
Philadelphia, PA

Cindy J. Fuller, PhD, RD
Seattle, WA

Abhimanyu Garg, MD
Center for Human Nutrition and
Department of Internal Medicine
University of Texas Southwestern Medical Center
*   at Dallas*
Dallas, TX

Scott M. Grundy, MD, PhD
Center for Human Nutrition
University of Texas Southwestern Medical Center
*   at Dallas*
Dallas, TX

Wajdi Hamdan, MD
American University of Beirut
Beirut, Lebanon

Lisa A. Hark, PhD, RD
Nutrition Education and Prevention Program
University of Pennsylvania School of Medicine
Philadelphia, PA

William B. Kannel, MD
Department of Preventive Medicine and
*   Epidemiology*
Evans Department of Clinical Research
Boston University School of Medicine
Boston, MA

Wahida Karmally, DrPH, RD, CDE
Irving Center for Clinical Research
Columbia University
New York, NY

Penny M. Kris-Etherton, PhD, RD
Department of Nutritional Sciences
Pennsylvania State University
University Park, PA

Bernadette Latson, MS, RD, CDE
Department of Clinical Nutrition
University of Texas Southwestern Medical Center
*   at Dallas*
Dallas, TX

Gabriela A. Maldonado, MS
Nutrition Education and Prevention Program
University of Pennsylvania School of Medicine
Philadelphia, PA

Emma A. Meagher, MD
Division of Medicine and Pharmacology
University of Pennsylvania School of Medicine
Preventive Cardiology Program
University of Pennsylvania Health System
Philadelphia, PA

Cathy A. Nonas, MS, RD, CDE
Director of Obesity and Diabetes Programs
North General Hospital
New York, NY

Stacey E. Panagotopulos, PhD
Division of Cardiology
Beth Israel Deaconess Medical Center
Boston, MA

Rex Parker, BS
University of Pennsylvania School of Medicine
Philadelphia, PA

F. Xavier Pi-Sunyer, MD, MPH
Division of Endocrinology, Metabolism, and
*   Nutrition*
Columbia University
Obesity Research Center
St Luke's-Roosevelt Hospital
New York, NY

Daniel J. Rader, MD
Division of Medicine and Pathology
University of Pennsylvania School of Medicine
Preventive Cardiology Program
University of Pennsylvania Health System
Philadelphia, PA

Hiba Sarieddine, BS
Nutrition Education and Prevention Program
University of Pennsylvania School of Medicine
Philadelphia, PA

Linda G. Snetselaar, PhD, RD
College of Public Health and College of
*   Medicine*
University of Iowa
Iowa City, IA

Neil Stone, MD
Department of Medicine
Northwestern University Feinberg School of
*   Medicine*
Chicago, IL

Charles Swencionis, PhD
Department of Epidemiology and Population
*   Health*
Albert Einstein College of Medicine
Ferkauf Graduate School of Psychology
Yeshiva University
Bronx, NY

Philippe O. Szapary, MD, FACP
Division of General Internal Medicine
University of Pennsylvania School of Medicine
Preventive Cardiology Program
University of Pennsylvania Health System
Philadelphia, PA

Andrew M. Tershakovec, MD
Clinical Development, U.S. Human Health
Merck and Co., Inc.
Horsham, PA

Thomas J. Thom, BA
Division of Epidemiology and Clinical
*   Applications*
National Heart, Lung, and Blood Institute
Bethesda, MD

Linda Van Horn, PhD, RD
Department of Preventive Medicine
Northwestern University Feinberg School of
*   Medicine*
Chicago, IL

Francine K. Welty, MD, PhD
Division of Medicine
Harvard Medical School
Preventive Cardiology and Nutrition Education
Beth Israel Deaconess Medical Center
Boston, MA

Judith Wylie-Rosett, EdD, RD
Division of Health, Behavior and Nutrition
Department of Epidemiology and Population
*   Health*
Albert Einstein College of Medicine
Bronx, NY

REVIEWERS

Kristen Albani, MS, RD
Dallas, TX

Kristine L. Bach, MS, RD, CDN
Port Jefferson Station, NY

Amy Burris-Burrow, RD
Salado, TX

Cinda S. Chima, MS, RD
Strongsville, OH

Georgia Clark-Albert, MS, RD
Athens, ME

Melanie Douglas, RD, CD
Newton, UT

Marilyn Edwards, PhD, RD
Houston, TX

Catherine V. Hagood, MS, RD, CDE
Jensen Beach, FL

Susan Haines, RD
Minneapolis, MN

Bridget Klawitter, PhD, RD, FADA
Racine, WI

Mikelle McCoin, MPH, RD
San Francisco, CA

Pam Michael, MBA, RD
Chicago, IL

Linda O. Michalsky, PhD, RD
Austin, TX

Elizabeth L. Quintana, MS, RD, CDE, CPT
Morgantown, WV

Nancy J. Reed, RD
Linthicum Height, MD

Julayne Ross, MA, RD, CD
Portland, IN

Geeta Sikand, MA, RD, FADA, CDE
Mission Viejo, CA

Nancy T. Smith, MS, RD, CDE
Tallahassee, FL

Mylissa Trowbride, MS, RD
Union, KY

Gail Underbakke, MS, RD
Madison, WI

Jane V. White, PhD, RD, FADA
Knoxville, TN

ACKNOWLEDGMENTS

As editors we are indebted to many others who have made this book a reality. We express our appreciation to

- Linda Van Horn, PhD, RD, and Penny M. Kris-Etherton, PhD, RD, who encouraged us to accept this responsibility and provided valuable advice and encouragement.
- Nilo B. Cater, MD, our medical adviser, who reviewed content for scientific accuracy and applicability to patient care.
- Marilyn Edwards, PhD, RD, Linda Michalsky, PhD, RD, and Jane White, PhD, RD, who reviewed the book and continuing education examination, thereby helping to qualify the book for Continuing Professional Education credit from the Commission on Dietetic Registration.
- Gail Morrison, MD, vice dean for education at the University of Pennsylvania School of Medicine and Scott Grundy, MD, PhD, director of the Center for Human Nutrition at the University of Texas Southwestern Medical Center at Dallas for supporting our investment of time in this project.
- The authors who generously contributed their time and expertise.
- The dietitians who reviewed the book and provided constructive feedback.
- Our colleagues in Nutrition Academic Award medical schools and the faculty and staff in our home institutions who have nurtured our professional growth.
- Kathryn Fink, RD, who managed many of the details related to references, author releases, and assorted other tasks.
- Jason Muzinic and Elizabeth Nishiura of the American Dietetic Association publishing department, who shepherded each chapter to final publication.
- And last, and perhaps most, our families who graciously shared time, holidays, computers, and conversations related to this book and supported us every step of the way.

FOREWORD

Cardiovascular nutrition is an exciting, evolving field. Fifty years of scientific investigation have established that modification of diet and life habits can make substantial contributions in reducing risk for coronary heart disease (CHD), the leading cause of morbidity and mortality among Americans. Epidemiologic studies have established that dietary intake is an important predictor of cardiovascular risk. Interventional studies have demonstrated that reductions in saturated fat intake, reductions in body weight, and increased physical activity provide overall benefits in reducing cardiovascular risk. Currently, there is increasing interest in the role of dietary adjuncts (eg, soluble fiber and plant stanols and sterols) and newer dietary approaches (eg, Dietary Approaches to Stop Hypertension [DASH] diet) in enhancing the efficacy of diet. The emergence of metabolic syndrome as a major contributor to CHD risk has also underscored the importance of diet and life-habit modification. Clinical management guidelines highlight the role of diet in both the primary and secondary prevention of cardiovascular disease. Approximately 60 million in the US population qualify to receive specific counseling from a health care professional for the diet strategies recommended by the Third Adult Treatment Panel (ATP III) of the National Cholesterol Education Program (NCEP), including the close to 40 million who require LDL cholesterol–lowering drug therapy.

Despite the integral role diet can play in the management of CHD risk factors, some health care professionals may hesitate to address this topic with their patients because they lack confidence in their knowledge about nutrition. This stems in large part from the limited exposure to nutrition that physicians, physician assistants and nurses receive in their medical education. Recent surveys by the Association of American Medical Colleges report that the majority of graduating medical students indicate that coverage of nutrition issues in their medical school education was inadequate. Fortunately, the gap between what students think they need to know about nutrition and what they are being taught is decreasing. Efforts such as the National Institutes of Health's Nutrition Academic Awards are helping to strengthen nutrition within medical curricula in American medical schools.

Cardiovascular Nutrition: Disease Management and Prevention provides clinicians a wealth of up-to-date information on this dynamic topic. For those individuals who are less confident in their knowledge of nutrition issues, this book offers extensive information and points them to resources to use with patients. For others who are more knowledgeable about nutrition, this book provides scholarly and practical summaries of the literature and the guidelines regarding functional foods, dietary supplements, and newer nutrition therapy approaches. The in-depth coverage of the role of nutrition in the prevention and management of CHD provided by this book should prove to be a timely, invaluable resource for all of us dedicated to helping our patients adopt healthful diets and life habits.

Nilo B. Cater, MD, and Scott M. Grundy, MD, PhD
Center for Human Nutrition
University of Texas Southwestern Medical Center at Dallas, Dallas, TX

INTRODUCTION

Nutrition plays a key role in the prevention and treatment of patients with cardiovascular disease (CVD). The underlying principles in *Cardiovascular Nutrition: Disease Management and Prevention* are based on current national guidelines and evidenced-based research on CVD, obesity, and diabetes. Part I describes the prevalence of CVD and reviews the pathophysiology of lipid metabolism and the formation of atherogenic plaque. Part II covers CVD risk assessment, as recommended by the National Cholesterol Education Program's Adult Treatment Panel III, as well as nutrition assessment and counseling strategies for behavior change. Quick nutrition screening tools, such as WAVE and MEDFICTS, are highlighted for the ambulatory setting. This section also includes a chapter on fostering behavior change, which focuses on nutrition and physical activity in the application of these principles.

Part III, Medical Nutrition Therapy and Physical Activity, provides the core information needed to apply medical nutrition therapy to prevent and treat CVD. Chapter 6 addresses dyslipidemias and coronary heart disease. The scientific evidence underlying the Therapeutic Lifestyle Changes (TLC) diet is summarized along with strategies and tools for assisting patients with abnormal serum lipids and individuals with existing heart disease. This chapter also includes an insightful, well-documented discussion of how much dietary fat should be incorporated for different types of patients with various lipid profiles. Chapter 7 covers metabolic syndrome and presents key dietary questions and treatment strategies for use in patients with this disease. Hypertension is the focus of Chapter 8, which includes the discussion of the Dietary Approaches to Stop Hypertension (DASH) diet. Chapter 9 offers guidance specific to individuals with diabetes.

Part IV covers complementary and alternative approaches. We recognize that more patients are looking for nonpharmacologic treatment approaches, such as functional foods and vitamin and mineral supplements. Because obesity has become a major public health problem in the United States, this section also includes a comprehensive review of popular weight-control programs.

To make sure that we address the majority of populations who have or are at risk for CVD, Part V identifies and discusses special issues and intervention strategies for women, children, and selected ethnic and racial groups. Chapter 13 provides extensive information for addressing cardiovascular risk among children, especially those with a strong family history of CVD. Chapter 14 directs attention to issues specific to women, who often underestimate their risk for CVD. Chapter 15 illustrates ways to address cultural influences, with attention to the African-American, Hispanic and Asian-Indian cultures, because race and ethnicity play a role in targeting intervention strategies for CVD prevention.

We have been fortunate to have numerous nationally recognized experts contribute to *Cardiovascular Nutrition: Disease Management and Prevention*. These contributors are nutrition professionals, physicians, and health educators, and we have encouraged physicians and dietitians to coauthor many of the chapters. Readers have the opportunity to learn from this distinguished group of authors. In addition, registered dietitians can gain Continuing Professional Education credit by obtaining and answering the 100 multiple-choice questions that review the content of the book. The test booklet can be purchased from the American Dietetic Association (http://www.eatright.org).

Each of us has brought our own experience to the development of this book. Jo Ann S. Carson, PhD, RD, has blended her experience as an educator with many years of interchange with physicians and lipid researchers working under Scott Grundy, MD, PhD, at the Center for Human Nutrition at the University of Texas Southwestern Medical Center at Dallas. Frances M. Burke, MS, RD, currently works in the Preventive Cardiology and Lipid Clinic at the University of Pennsylvania Health System with Daniel J. Rader, MD, and has been coordinator of the Nutrition Education and Prevention Program in the School of Medicine for 12 years. Having previously edited several editions of a clinical nutrition textbook for medical students and a national leader in nutrition in medical education, Lisa A. Hark, PhD, RD, offers the insights of a seasoned editor in the medical arena. We have all been funded by the Nutrition Academic Award from the National Heart, Lung, and Blood Institute and the National Institute of Diabetes, and Digestive and Kidney Diseases, which has aimed to strengthen nutrition in medical education. Our educational efforts have spanned a variety of students and health care professionals representing dietetics, nursing, medicine and allied health.

Whether you are a dietitian, physician, nurse, or physician assistant working with patients in a lipid or preventive cardiology clinic, in an internal medicine or family medicine practice, or in a public health setting within the community, this book provides valuable reference information and practical tools to help you manage patients who are at risk for or present with CVD. It is our hope that this reference text will provide you with the answers you need, inspiring you to expand your interdisciplinary efforts to manage CVD risk factors, while reducing morbidity, mortality, and health care costs related to CVD.

Jo Ann S. Carson, PhD, RD
Frances M. Burke, MS, RD
Lisa A. Hark, PhD, RD

PART I

Overview

CHAPTER 1

CARDIOVASCULAR DISEASE: PREVALENCE TO PREVENTION

Thomas J. Thom, BA, William B. Kannel, MD, Aram Chobanian, MD, and Ralph B. D'Agostino, PhD

Life expectancy has never been higher in the United States, and its increase in the past 30 years has been largely due to the 50% decline in the death rate for total cardiovascular disease (CVD). The message is clear: cardiovascular disease is not inevitable. Its risk is amenable to preventive and therapeutic management. As death is delayed, however, prevalence will increase in the absence of primary prevention. The circulatory system in the human body works remarkably well, but it is at the mercy of genetics and lifestyle. Control of the modifiable risk factors from an early age and before a cardiovascular event develops is ideal, but it is never too late to improve cardiovascular fitness.

This chapter provides statistics on the prevalence of CVD and risk factors for CVD. In addition, the extent to which approaches to reduce risk factors and manage disease are affecting morbidity and mortality from CVD are presented.

THE RISKS

Everyone faces substantial morbidity and mortality risks from heart disease, stroke, and other blood vessel diseases, that is, CVD. Based on decades of Framingham Heart Study data, the lifetime risk for a 40-year-old developing coronary disease is about 50% for men and 32% for women (1). Once heart disease leads to heart failure, half of the patients die within 5 years (2). The chance of having a stroke before age 70 is 5%; 15% to 30% of stroke survivors become permanently disabled (2). The risks are much greater for persons who have hypertension, a high cholesterol level, or diabetes, or persons who smoke, are overweight, or are physically inactive, especially if more than one of these risk factors are present (3,4). The likelihood of a person eventually having at least one risk factor or developing a cardiovascular disease is extraordinarily high. Overweight, physical inactivity, and high cholesterol levels increase with age. If a person still has normal blood pressure at age 55, the chance of eventually becoming hypertensive is 90% (5).

The risks for CVD begin early in life. Between the ages of 35 and 44 years, the most common cause of death is CVD (6). Heart disease is the leading cause of death in each of the major sex-and-race/ethnicity groups except Asian-American females (7). The black population faces the greatest risk of any group for developing and dying from hypertension, coronary heart disease (CHD), stroke, and heart failure (7-9). Prevalence of self-reported CHD is higher and increasing in blacks compared with whites, and the prevalence of stroke, also highest in blacks, is increasing in all four sex-race groups (refer to Figures 1.1 and 1.2) (7). Men have higher risks than women for most cardiovascular diseases, but after age 65 women are nearly as vulnerable as men (2). The presence of certain risk factors, such as diabetes, in women can attenuate their advantage in CVD risk over men without those risk factors (10).

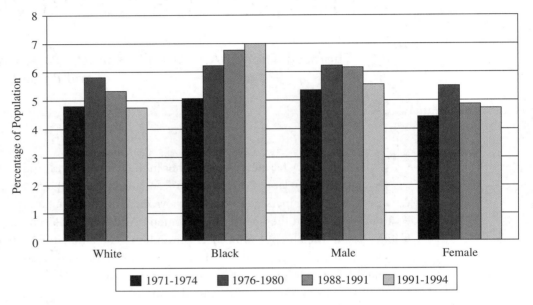

FIGURE 1.1
Prevalence (age-adjusted) of coronary heart disease by race and sex, ages 25 to 74 years, United States, 1971–1974 to 1991–1994. Reprinted from reference 7 (p 28).

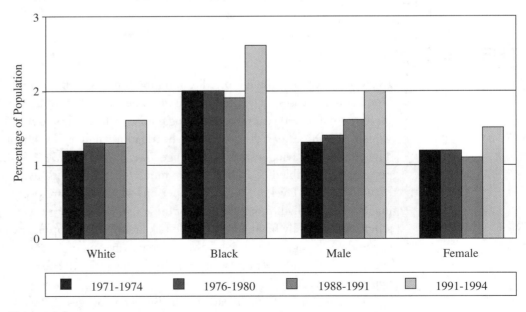

FIGURE 1.2
Prevalence (age-adjusted) of stroke by race and sex, ages 25 to 74 years, United States, 1971–1974 to 1991–1994. Reprinted from reference 7 (p 43).

THE NATIONAL BURDEN

Cardiovascular diseases have long been the cause of more morbidity, mortality, health care use, and economic cost than any other diagnostic group (11,12). An estimated 62 million Americans have CVD, of whom 23 million have heart disease including CHD (13 million), and almost 5 million have cerebrovascular disease (stroke) (refer to Table 1.1) (7,8,13-16). Each year there are more than 1 million heart attacks and 600,000 strokes (7). Based on 2001 data, 922,000 Americans died from CVD, representing 38% of all deaths (13,14).

Hospitalizations and other care services used by patients with CVD are summarized in Table 1.1 (13-16). In 2000, 66 million physician office visits were for CVD, the third most common diagnosis after respiratory and neurologic diseases (16). Essential hypertension is the most common single diagnosis in visits. It is not surprising, therefore, that national health care expenditures for CVD are by far the highest among any diagnostic group, $200 billion in 2002 (12).

TABLE 1.1
The National Cardiovascular Disease Burden

Number of Persons with the Disease*	
Total cardiovascular disease	61,800,000
Total heart disease	23,000,000
Hypertension	50,000,000
Coronary heart disease	12,800,000
Stroke	4,600,000
Heart failure	4,800,000
Atrial fibrillation	2,000,000
Congenital CVD	1,000,000
Annual Number of Attacks	
Heart attack	1,100,000
Stroke	600,000
Heart failure (new attacks only)	550,000
Health Care Utilization Measures, Latest Year	
Hospitalization for CVD	6,226,000
CVD surgical procedures†	6,188,000
ER visits for chest pain	5,669,000
Physician office visits for CVD	65,800,000
Home care visits for CVD	1,777,000
Number of Deaths in 2001	
Total cardiovascular disease	922,000
Coronary heart disease	502,000
Stroke	164,000
Heart failure	57,000
Other CVD	199,000
Health Care Expenditures in 2002 (billion $)	
Total CVD	200
Coronary heart disease	58
Stroke	31
Heart failure	21
Hypertension	34
Other CVD	56

Abbreviations: CVD, cardiovascular disease; ER, emergency room.

*Many persons have more than one CVD.

†More than one type counted in some surgeries.

Source: 2000 to 2002 data are from references 7, 8, and 13–16.

HIGHLY PREVALENT RISK FACTORS

The prevalence of risk factors remains high; not all clinicians routinely assess and follow up their patients' risk factor status, and when they do, compliance by patients is far from optimal (17). An estimated 50 million adult Americans, one in four, have hypertension (defined as systolic blood pressure of 140 mm Hg or higher or diastolic blood pressure of 90 mm Hg or higher or taking antihypertensive medication) (refer to Table 1.2) (7,18). Prevalence of hypertension is highest in the black population, over 40% at ages 20 to 74 years, and it is relatively high in Mexican Americans (refer to Table 1.3) (19). Millions more with a systolic between 120 and 139 mm Hg and/or a diastolic between 80 and 89 mm Hg are considered prehypertensive and are at risk to progress to hypertension (20). Despite appreciable improvement since the 1960s, only 34% of persons with hypertension have it well controlled (blood pressure under 140 mm Hg systolic and 90 mm Hg diastolic), and 41% still do not have medication

TABLE 1.2
Rates of Cardiovascular Disease Risk, 2002 to 2003

Risk Factor	Definition	No. of Individuals Affected
Cholesterol, high	200–239 mg/dL	63,000,000
Cholesterol, very high	≥240 mg/dL	42,000,000
Cigarette smoking	Current smokers	48,700,000
Diabetes	Diagnosed	10,900,000
Diabetes	Undiagnosed	5,700,000
Hypertension	≥140/90 mm Hg or on antihypertension medication	50,000,000
Obese	BMI ≥ 30	61,200,000
Overweight but not obese	BMI 25–29	68,050,000

Abbreviation: BMI, body mass index.

Source: Data compiled from references 7 and 18.

TABLE 1.3
Prevalence* of Hypertension, Overweight, and High Cholesterol for Whites, Blacks, and Hispanics Ages 20–74 Years; United States, 1999 to 2000

	Men, % (SE)	Women, % (SE)
Hypertension[†]		
Non-Hispanic white	29 (2.0)	25 (1.9)
Non-Hispanic black	38 (2.9)	41 (2.4)
Mexican American	31 (2.6)	25 (1.8)
Overweight[‡]		
Non-Hispanic white	67 (2.0)	57 (2.7)
Non-Hispanic black	60 (2.3)	78 (1.9)
Mexican American	74 (2.8)	72 (2.5)
High Cholesterol[§]		
Non-Hispanic white	18 (1.4)	19 (1.7)
Non-Hispanic black	11 (2.1)	17 (2.5)
Mexican American	18 (1.9)	13 (1.3)

*Percentages are age adjusted.

[†]Blood pressure ≥140/90 mm Hg or on antihypertension medication.

[‡]Body mass index ≥25.

[§]Total serum cholesterol ≥240 mg/dL.

Source: Data are from reference 19.

TABLE 1.4
Control of Systolic vs Diastolic Blood Pressure, Framingham Study Subjects, 1990 to 1995

Controlled Blood Pressure	All High Blood Pressure Patients (*N* = 1959)	Patients on Treatment (*N* = 1198)
Systolic blood pressure (<140 mm Hg)	32.7%	49.0%
Diastolic blood pressure (<90 mm Hg)	82.9%	89.7%
Both (<140/90 mm Hg)	29.0%	47.8%

Source: Adapted with permission from Lloyd-Jones DM, Evans JC, Larson MG, ODonnell CJ, Roccella EJ, Levy D. Differential control of systolic and diastolic blood pressure: factors associated with level of blood pressure control in the community. *Hypertension.* 2000;36:594–599, with permission from Lippincott, Williams & Wilkins.

prescribed for their hypertension (20). Although control rates continue to improve, they are relatively low in blacks and Mexican Americans, and nearly 75% of those with diabetes and hypertension did not have blood pressure controlled below 130/85 mm Hg, the recommended level for individuals with diabetes (9). Poor control of hypertension is largely attributable to poor control of elevated systolic blood pressure (refer to Table 1.4) (21).

An estimated 49 million Americans smoke cigarettes, 42 million have total cholesterol values over 240 mg/dL, and 63 million have total cholesterol levels between 200 and 239 mg/dL. Approximately 17 million Americans have diabetes, a diagnosis that increases risk for CHD events comparable to the presence of CHD. (See Chapters 3 and 9 for further discussion of risk of CHD related to diabetes.) About 61 million Americans are classified as obese, and another 68 million, while not obese, are overweight (Table 1.2) (18). The age-adjusted prevalence of overweight shown in Table 1.3 indicates over two thirds of Mexican-American men and women and white men are overweight; slightly fewer white women and black men are overweight (estimated at 60% of black men and 78% of black women ages 20 to 74 years) (19). The prevalence of diabetes in 1998 was 7.7% in non-Hispanic blacks, 6.3% in Hispanics, and 4.9% in non-Hispanic whites, ages 18 years and over (8). Among children 6 to 19 years of age, prevalence of overweight is much greater in blacks and Mexican Americans than in non-Hispanic whites (19).

Recent data indicate that less than half of patients with overt coronary disease receive cholesterol-lowering therapy, and few meet the low-density lipoprotein (LDL) cholesterol goals recommended by the third Adult Treatment Panel of the National Cholesterol Education Program (ATP III) (22,23). Even a smaller fraction of those with severe dyslipidemia, but no CVD, receives such agents. The very high and increasing prevalence of overweight and obesity, in children as well as adults, is of great consequence to CVD, diabetes, and other medical problems, and it shortens life expectancy (24-26). Obesity is a very prevalent disorder in the United States, now reaching epidemic proportions. It is driving an increasing prevalence of diabetes and its atherosclerotic sequelae.

FAVORABLE TRENDS

The national burden of CVD could have been even worse. In the past 30 years, mortality and in-hospital case fatality declined more than 50%. The proportions of persons with the risk factors of smoking, hypertension, or a high cholesterol level have declined 25% to 46% during that time. Cardiovascular health consciousness has flourished, and treatments and access to

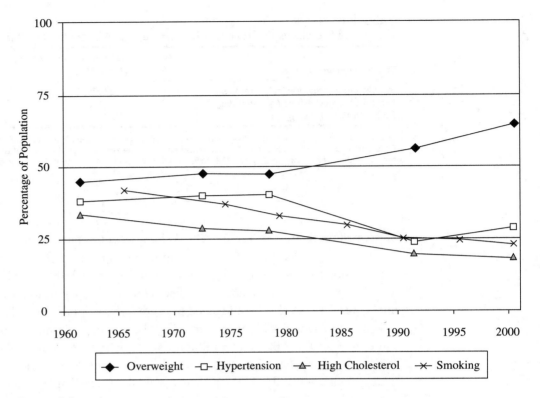

FIGURE 1.3
Prevalence of risk factors, United States 1960–1962 to 1999–2000. Data are from reference 19.

them have substantially improved (7,18,19,27) (refer to Figure 1.3). The precipitous mortality decline for CHD began in the mid 1960s, and the long-term decline for stroke accelerated in the 1970s as more effective pharmaceutical agents became available and a national effort succeeded in improving rates of treatment and control of hypertension (refer to Figure 1.4) (7,19,28). Increased life expectancy during this period was attributed in large part to declines in CVD mortality (29). Improvements in the major modifiable risk factors can account for as much as one half of the decline in CHD mortality (27,30). These favorable trends in mortality and prevalence of elevated cholesterol levels and hypertension would likely have been even more favorable if the large increases in prevalence of overweight and obesity had not occurred (24,25).

These trends are welcome, but the key to reduced prevalence is the reduction in incidence. Available data on incidence rates are conflicting. Whereas CVD mortality rates have clearly declined, reduced incidence rates are less consistently reported. Community- and hospital-based studies report declines in the incidence of CHD prior to about 1988, but indicate mostly flat trends since then (27). Incidence of stroke also does not have a clear direction (31-33). However, the recent decline in national rates of hospitalization for CHD in the 45- to 64-year-old group, and flattening in the rate of hospitalization for stroke, would be consistent with a reduction in incidence (7).

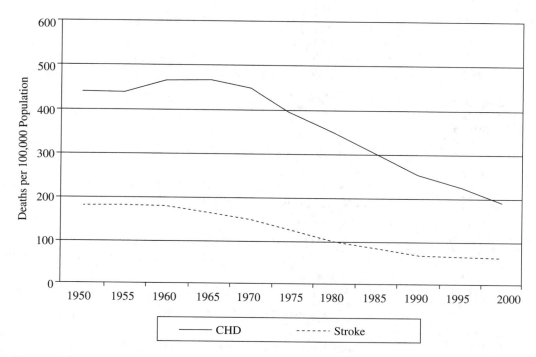

FIGURE 1.4

Age-adjusted death rates for coronary heart disease (CHD) and stroke, United States 1950 to 2000. Data are from reference 19.

POTENTIAL FOR CVD CONTROL

The mortality and risk factor trends for CVD are encouraging, as are some of the reported changes in incidence and hospitalizations. They suggest that this group of diseases can become a much reduced health problem if full potentials for prevention and treatment of CVD are realized. To expect that the national burden can be greatly reduced, it is necessary to anticipate declines in incidence and the potential for primary prevention by reduction in CVD risk factors. Continued success in secondary prevention and treatment to improve case fatality and survival portend well for life expectancy and can improve the outlook for patients with CVD, but the prevalence of clinically significant CVD and health care use would continue to increase. These can decline appreciably only if new cases are prevented. The large prevalence of CVD and its risk factors and aging of the population guarantee a considerable national problem in at least the near future. Successful primary prevention will be required over the long run to substantially reduce the national impact.

Cardiovascular risk profiles composed of the major risk factors predict CHD as efficiently in the elderly as in the young. This, and the fact that the decline in CVD mortality has included the elderly, suggests the potential for prevention in the elderly. It has been suggested that mortality and morbidity risks in future elderly population groups may be moderated by socioeconomic changes that result in better nutrition and higher levels of education (34). Development of CVD in the nation's increasing elderly population can be prevented, reduced, and delayed, but intervention in risk factors in the elderly has limited potential (35,36). For those who already have CVD, the means to prevent recurrences and complications are underused (37-39). This is especially unfortunate because of the health disparities for CVD that exist among socioeconomic groups (40). The potentials exist for prevention and treatment to overcome increased CVD morbidity and mortality as the population ages so that CVD becomes a much smaller health problem, but the greatest potential is in primary prevention.

Prevention

Three basic approaches can contribute to the prevention of CVD:

- The environment can be altered to promote a healthier national diet, engineer physical activity back into daily life, and get rid of cigarettes.
- People can be educated to eat less fat, eat more fruits and vegetables; get more exercise; avoid gaining weight; get their blood pressure, blood lipids, and blood sugar checked periodically; and quit smoking to protect their own health and that of their families.
- High-risk candidates can be sent to their physicians for preventive measures to correct dyslipidemia, hypertension, glucose intolerance, and other risk factors.

It is not clear, however, that the informed public is able and willing to make the changes in lifestyle that are necessary. Nor is it clear that physicians are able to do as much as they could to follow recommended guidelines for controlling risk factors such as dyslipidemia or hypertension.

The greatest impact is likely to come from the population approach designed to shift the distribution of the major modifiable and treatable risk factors down to a more acceptable average level. Manson and coworkers (41) have estimated the potential benefit of reduction of the established major risk factors for myocardial infarction:

- 50% to 70% lower risk in former as compared with current smokers, within 5 years of cessation
- 2% to 3% decline in risk for each reduction of 1% serum cholesterol
- 2% to 3% decline in risk for each reduction of 1 mm Hg in diastolic blood pressure
- 35% to 55% lower risk for those who maintain ideal body weight as compared with those who are at least 20% above desirable weight
- 45% lower risk for those who maintain an active lifestyle compared with a sedentary lifestyle
- 33% lower risk in aspirin users as compared with nonusers.

A 3 mm Hg reduction in blood pressure is estimated to reduce coronary mortality by 8% and stroke deaths by 5% (42). Subsequent to that analysis, some doubt has been cast on the lowered risk in users of postmenopausal estrogen-replacement therapy (43). Given the high attributable risks posed by these factors, the benefits of risk modification would accrue to a large number of people.

Clinical trials have documented the benefits of treating even mild hypertension and dyslipidemia for the prevention of both initial and recurrent cardiovascular events (44-48). Increased use of antihypertensive and cholesterol-lowering drugs in a greater portion of the at-risk population and for longer periods of time should have a major added impact on the course of CVD. However, this approach needs to be combined with the population approach designed to reduce the average level of risk factors. The prevalence of dyslipidemia, cigarette smoking, and untreated hypertension in the population has declined, but the prevalence of obesity and diabetes appear to be on the increase (49). This has ominous implications because insulin resistance appears to be a major contributor to most of the controllable identified atherogenic traits (50).

Although current and projected innovations in the treatment of clinically overt disease have great potential for salvaging individual victims of CVD, their population impact is not likely to be great. The way CVD occurs in the general population indicates that only a preventive approach can make a major impact. Sudden unexpected death is a prominent feature of coronary disease. One in six coronary attacks presents as the first, last, and only symptom (2). About two thirds of coronary deaths occur out of hospital, too precipitously to receive the sophisticated available medical attention (2). One third of myocardial infarctions are either silent or too atypical to be diagnosed, and these carry a serious prognosis. Once they are clinically overt, strokes and heart failure have a serious outlook for disability and mortality. Clearly, a preventive approach is needed. This is now eminently possible by modifying or avoiding already identified and correctable predisposing risk factors well in advance of symptoms. If this can be effectively implemented, a major impact can be expected. Additional risk factors are also under investigation, including elevated serum homocysteine, Lp(a), inflammation measured by C-reactive protein, thrombogenic factors and insulin resistance, and infectious agents, among others (51).

Reduction in Severity

The Atherosclerosis Risk in Communities Study (ARIC) reported no change over time in the incidence of definite and probable cases of coronary heart disease, but studies from the MONICA (Multinational MONitoring of Trends and Determinants in CArdiovascular Disease) Project reported declines in rates of definite cases (52,53). The trend in CHD incidence in ARIC, however, was downward when incident cases were confined to definite cases (54). Because definite cases are likely to be the more severe ones, that decline compared with no decline in CHD incidence as originally defined is consistent with evidence of a decline in severity. The Framingham Study has shown a decline in the severity of strokes, with fewer victims hospitalized in coma or with dense hemiplegia (33).

Overall, age-adjusted mortality for myocardial infarction has declined 3.5% per year (7). The major component of this decline has been in hospital mortality, whereas the declines in mortality rates after discharge have been of lesser magnitude (55). Mortality has also declined substantially more than has incidence in Canada, Australia, and most Western European countries (56-59).

Several studies suggest that there may be a greater decline in patients with Q-wave infarctions (60-63). Furthermore, angiographic investigations suggest that coronary disease may now be less severe. Before thrombolytic therapy was used, prevalence of three-vessel disease was 23% to 50%; it is now only 7% to 20% in the post-thrombolytic trials (64). These trends suggest that coronary disease is being delayed and possibly less severe in its initial presentation. These trends could be related to modification of risk factors for coronary disease and modern innovations in treatment.

Treatment

The medical care now available has been shown by clinical trials to be beneficial in preventing death and other adverse outcomes of coronary disease (50). These treatments include thrombolytics, aspirin, beta-blockers, ACE inhibitors, and coronary revascularization (51). Coronary risk factor control and new treatments, however, apparently do not explain the entire decline in coronary mortality rates.

Further innovations in the diagnosis and treatment of CVD will undoubtedly improve the outlook of patients fortunate enough to survive the initial attack, but this can only have a limited impact on the population burden of CVD because of the unheralded attacks and high initial mortality. It is also evident that we have not realized the full potential benefit of existing therapeutic strategies, and there is a wide variety of new therapeutic opportunities, such as advances in cardiac imaging, molecular genetics, and transgenic techniques (51,55). Therapies of proven efficacy in reducing mortality in patients with myocardial infarctions are seriously underused (64-68).

THE LONG-TERM OUTLOOK

Projections beyond the next 25 or so years are highly speculative, but there is cause for optimism considering the advances occurring in this field. As examples, from the nutrition standpoint, the decision in 1995 to supplement grain products with folic acid to reduce the incidence of neural tube defects appears to have caused significant decreases in blood homocysteine levels since that time (69). The Dietary Approaches to Stop Hypertension (DASH) diet, which emphasizes increased intake of fruits, vegetables, grain products, and low-fat dairy products and reduced intake of saturated and total fat, and which appears to be reasonably well tolerated and practical on a long-term basis, has been shown to cause relatively large reductions in blood pressure in both normotensive and hypertensive individuals (70). More effective and safer drugs to manage hypertension and dyslipidemia are being introduced on a regular basis, and consideration is being given to making available to a broader segment of the population on an over-the-counter basis some of the existing drugs that have a favorable safety profile. New drugs are being introduced to increase insulin sensitivity, and new weight-reducing approaches to decrease appetite, reduce gastrointestinal absorption, or increase thermogenesis are appearing for clinical evaluation. New methods to prevent addiction may prove effective for facilitating smoking cessation. In addition, new potential risk factors for clinically significant disease are being investigated and may become major targets for future interventions. Recent data regarding the association of certain bacteria and viruses (eg, chlamydia, *Helicobacter pylori*, herpes, and cytomegalovirus) with risks for CVD raise the possibility that these infective agents may play a role in the development of CVD in some individuals (71). These potential interventions combined with vigorous public education efforts to enhance personal preventive measures in the population and to increase the proportion of individuals treated for established risk factors should substantially decrease health disparities and prevent CVD. In addition, clinically significant disease can be managed better with new methods for enhancing angiogenesis and organ blood flow, stimulating mycocyte growth and replication, minimizing cardiac and brain injury after interruption of blood flow, and correcting genetic abnormalities by gene therapy.

SUMMARY

Without the favorable national mortality and risk factor trends between 1965 and 1998, today's national problem of CVD would be considerably greater. Yet morbidity, mortality, and use of health care services for these diseases remain high, and, paradoxically, incidence may not have declined appreciably. The improvements resulted in large reductions in the numbers of persons with high levels of risk factors and reductions in the annual increases in CVD deaths that would have otherwise occurred. However, improved CVD mortality and case fatality resulted in increased CVD prevalence, life expectancy, and health care use. The national CVD burden will undoubtedly remain an important health problem during the next 25 years. If the past trends continue and prevention and further treatment potentials are realized, many cases will be less severe, and delay of morbidity and mortality to older ages will continue. Sometime in the 21st century, CVD could become a much-reduced health problem at all but the oldest ages. At older as well as at younger ages, mortality statistics show substantial reduction in CVD as compared with modest declines or increases of non-CVD causes of death. The shift away from CVD as a cause of death portends well for the future of CVD mortality. The key to control of CVD, however, still lies in the better use of proven means of prevention and treatment of the high proportions of persons in the United States who have modifiable CVD risk factors. Focusing on methods that help patients make long-term lifestyle changes (outlined in Chapter 5) can contribute significantly to reducing CVD risk factors.

REFERENCES

1. Lloyd-Jones DM, Larson MG, Levy D. Lifetime risk of developing coronary heart disease. *Lancet.* 1999;353:89-92.
2. Thom TJ, Kannel WB, Silbershatz H, D'Agostino RB. Cardiovascular diseases in the United States and prevention approaches. In: Fuster V, Alexander RW, O'Rourke RA, eds. *Hurst's The Heart.* 10th ed. New York, NY: McGraw-Hill; 2001:3-17.
3. Wilson PWF, Culleton BF. Epidemiology of cardiovascular diseases in the United States. *Am J Kidney Dis.* 1998;32:5(suppl 3):S56-S65.
4. Wilson PWF, D'Agostino RB, Levy D, Belanger AM, Silbershatz H, Kannel WB. Prediction of coronary heart disease using risk factor categories. *Circulation.* 1998;97:1837-1847.
5. Vasan RS, Beiser A, Seshadri S, Larson MG, Kannel B, D'Agostino RB, Levy D. Residual lifetime risk for developing hypertension in middle-aged women and men: the Framingham Heart Study. *JAMA.* 2002;287:1003-1010.
6. Minino AM, Arias E, Kochanek KD, Murphy SL, Smith BS. Deaths: final data for 2000. *Natl Vital Stat Rep.* September 16, 2002;50(15):1-119. Available at: http://www.cdc.gov/nchs/data/nvsr/nvsr50/nvsr50_15.pdf. Accessed July 25, 2003.
7. National Heart, Lung, and Blood Institute. *Morbidity and Mortality: 2002 Chartbook on Cardiovascular, Lung, and Blood Diseases.* Available at: http://www.nhlbi.nih.gov/resources/docs/cht-book.htm. Accessed July 25, 2003.
8. Pleis JR, Coles R. Summary health statistics for U.S. adults: National Health Interview Survey, 1998. *Vital Health Stat.* 2002;10(209). Available at: http://www.cdc.gov/nchs/data/series/sr_10/sr10_209.pdf. Accessed July 25, 2003.
9. Hajjar I, Kotchen TA. Trends in prevalence, awareness, treatment, and control of hypertension in the United States, 1988–2000. *JAMA.* 2003;290:199-206.
10. Kannel WB, Wilson PWF. Risk factors that attenuate the female coronary heart disease advantage. *Arch Intern Med.* 1995;155:57-61.
11. Rice DP, Feldman JJ, White KL. *The Current Burden of Illness in the United States* [occasional paper]. Washington, DC: Institute of Medicine, National Academy of Sciences; 1976:1-35.
12. National Heart, Lung, and Blood Institute. *Fact Book Fiscal Year 2002.* National Institutes of Health, February, 2002. Available at: http://www.nhlbi.nih.gov/about/factpdf.htm. Accessed July 25, 2003.
13. Arias E, Anderson RN, Hsiang-Ching K, Murphy SL, Kochanek KD. Deaths: Final Data for 2001. *Natl Vital Stat Rep.* 2003;52(3):1-113. Available at: http://www.cdc.gov/nchs/data/nvsr/nvsr52/nvsr52_03.pdf. Accessed February 4, 2004.
14. Hall MJ, DeFrances CJ. 2001 National Hospital Discharge Survey. *Adv Data.* April 9, 2003;(332):1-18. Available at: http://www.cdc.gov/nchs/data/ad/ad332.pdf. Accessed July 25, 2003.
15. McCraig LF, Burt CW. National Hospital Ambulatory Medical Care Survey: 2001 Emergency Department Summary. *Adv Data.* June 4, 2003;(335):1-29. Available at: http://www.cdc.gov/nchs/data/ad/ad335.pdf. Accessed July 25, 2003.
16. Cherry DK, Woodwell DA. National Ambulatory Medical Care Survey: 2000 summary. *Adv Data.* June 25, 2002;(328):1-32. Available at: http://www.cdc.gov/nchs/data/ad/ad328.pdf. Accessed July 25, 2003.

17. Greenland P, Grundy S, Pasternak RC, Lenfant C. Problems on the pathway from risk assessment to risk reduction. *Circulation*. 1998;97:1761-1762.

18. American Heart Association. *2003 Heart and Stroke Statistical Update*. Available at: http://www.american heart.org/downloadable/heart/10590179711482003HDSStatsBookREV7-03.pdf. Accessed July 25, 2003.

19. *Health, United States, 2003: With Chartbook on Trends in the Health of Americans*. Hyattsville, Md: National Center for Health Statistics; 2003. DHHS publication 00-1232. Available at: http://www.cdc.gov/ nchs/data/hus/hus02.pdf. Accessed July 25, 2003.

20. Chobanian AV, Bakris GL, Black HR, Cushman WC, Green LA, Izzo, JL, Jones DW, Materson BJ, Oparil S, Wright JT, Roccella EJ. The seventh report of the Joint National Committee on Prevention, Detection, Evaluation, and Treatment of High Blood Pressure: the JNC 7 Report. *JAMA*. 2003;289:2560-2572.

21. Lloyd-Jones DM, Evans JC, Larson MG, O'Donnell CJ, Roccella EJ, Levy D. Differential control of systolic and diastolic blood pressure: factors associated with level of blood pressure control in the community. *Hypertension*. 2000;36:594-599.

22. Smith SC Jr. Lessons from cholesterol-lowering trials. *Am J Med*. 1998;104(suppl):28S-32S.

23. Ford ES, Mokdad AH, Giles WH, Mensah GA. Serum total cholesterol concentrations and awareness, treatment, and control of hypercholesterolemia among US adults: findings from the National Health and Nutrition Examination Survey, 1999 to 2000. *Circulation*. 2003;107:2185-2189.

24. Flegal KM, Carroll MD, Ogden CL, Johnson CL. Prevalence and trends in obesity among US adults, 1999–2000. *JAMA*. 2002;288:1723-1727.

25. Ogden CL, Flegal KM, Carroll MD, Johnson CL. Prevalence and trends in overweight among US children and adolescents, 1999–2000. *JAMA*. 2002;288:1728-1732.

26. Fontaine KR, Redden DT, Wang C, Westfall AO, Allison DB. Years of life lost due to obesity. *JAMA*. 2003;289:187-193.

27. Hunink MG, Goldman L, Tosteson ANA, Mittleman MA, Goldman PA. The recent decline in mortality from coronary heart disease, 1980–1990: the effect of secular trends in risk factors and treatment. *JAMA*. 1997;277:535-542.

28. Burt VL, Cutler JA, Higgins M, Horan MJ, Labarthe D, Whelton P, Brown C, Roccella RJ. Trends in the prevalence, awareness, treatment, and control of hypertension in the adult US population: data from the health examination surveys, 1960 to 1991. *Hypertension*. 1995; 26:60-69.

29. Kochanek KD, Mauer JD, Rosenberg HM. *Causes of Death Contributing to Changes in Life Expectancy: United States 1984–1989*. Hyattsville, Md: National Center for Health Statistics; 1990. Vital Health Statistics series 20, number 23. Available at: http://www.cdc.gov/nchs/data/series/sr_20/sr20_023.pdf. Accessed May 14, 2004.

30. Sytkowski PA, D'Agostino RB, Belanger A, and Kannel WB. Sex and time trends in cardiovascular disease incidence and mortality: the Framingham Study, 1950–1989. *Am J Epidemiol*. 1996;143:338-350.

31. McGovern PG, Shahar E, Sprafka JM, Pankow JS. The role of stroke attack rate and case-fatality in the decline of stroke mortality: The Minnesota Heart Survey. *Ann Epidemiol*. 1993;3:483-487.

32. Brown RD, Whisnant JP, Sicks JD, O'Fallon WM, Wiebers DO. Stroke incidence, prevalence, and survival: secular trends in Rochester, Minnesota, through 1989. *Stroke*. 1996;3:373-380.

33. Wolf PA, D'Agostino RB. Secular trends in stroke in the Framingham Study. *Am J Epidemiol*. 1993;3: 471-475.

34. Institute of Medicine. *Forecasting Survival, Health, and Disability: Workshop Summary. March 9–10, 1993*. Washington, DC: National Academy Press; 1993.

35. Grundy SM, Balady GJ, Criqui MH, Fletcher G, Greenland P, Hiratzka LF, Houston-Miller N, Kris-Etherton P, Krumholz HM, LaRosa J, Ockene IS, Pearson TA, Reed J, Washington R, Smith SC. Primary prevention of coronary heart disease: guidance from Framingham: a statement for health care professionals from the AHA Task Force on Risk Reduction. *Circulation*. 1998;97:1876-1887.

36. Kaplan RM. Imagine no coronary heart disease (editorial). *Circulation*. 1991;83:1452-1455.

37. Krumholz HM, Radford MJ, Wang Y, Chen J, Heiat A, Marciniak TA. National use and effectiveness of beta blockers for the treatment of elderly patients after acute myocardial infarction: national cooperative cardiovascular project. *JAMA*. 1998;280:623-629.

38. Berlowitz DR, Ash AS, Hickey EC, Friedman RH, Glickman M, Kader B, Moskowitz MA. Inadequate management of blood pressure in a hypertensive population. *N Engl J Med*. 1998;339:1957-1963.

39. Gurwitz JH, Goldberg RJ, Chen Z, Gore JM, Alpert JS. Beta-blocker therapy in acute myocardial infarction: evidence for underutilization in the elderly. *Am J Med*. 1992;93:605-610.

40. Cooper R, Cutler J, Desvigne-Nickens P, Fortmann SP, Friedman L, Havlik R, Hogelin G, Marler J, McGovern P, Morosco G, Mosca L, Pearson T, Stamler J, Stryer D, Thom T. Trends and disparities in coronary heart disease, stroke, and other cardiovascular diseases in the United States: findings of the National Conference on Cardiovascular Disease Prevention. *Circulation*. 2000;102:3137-3147.

41. Manson JE, Tosteson H, Ridker PM, Satterfield S, Hebert P, O'Connor GT, Buring JE, Hennekens CH. The primary prevention of myocardial infarction. *N Engl J Med*. 1992;326:1406-1416.

42. Stamler R. Implications of the INTERSALT study. *Hypertension*. 1991;1(suppl):S116-S120.

43. Blumenthal RS, Zacor HA, Reis SE, Post WS. Beyond the null hypothesis—do the HERS results disprove the estrogen/coronary heart disease hypothesis? *Am J Cardiol*. 2000;85:1015-1017.

44. Sacks FM, Pfeffer MA, Moye LA, Rouleau JL, Rutherford JD, Cole TG, Brown L, Warnica JW, Arnold JM, Wun CC, Davis BR, Braunwald E, for the Cholesterol and Recurrent Events Trial investigators. The effect of pravastatin on coronary events after myocardial infarction in patients with average cholesterol levels. N Engl J Med. 1996;335:1001-1009.

45. Shepherd J, Cobbe SM, Ford I, Isles CG, Lorimer AR, MacFarlane PW, McKillop JH, Packard CJ, for the West of Scotland Coronary Prevention Study Group. Prevention of coronary heart disease with pravastatin in men with hypercholesterolemia. N Engl J Med. 1995;333:1301-1307.

46. Scandinavian Simvastatin Survival Study Group. Randomized trial of cholesterol lowering in 4444 patients with coronary heart disease: the Scandinavian Survival Study (4S). Lancet. 1994;19:1383-1389.

47. Joint National Committee on Detection, Evaluation and Treatment of High Blood Pressure. The sixth report of the Joint National Committee on Prevention, Detection, Evaluation and Treatment of High Blood Pressure. Arch Intern Med. 1997;157:2413-2446.

48. Downs JR III, Clearfield M, Weis S, Whitney E, Shapiro DR, Beere PA, Langendorfer A, Stein EA, Kruyer W, Gotto AM Jr, for the AFCAPS/TexCAPS Research Group. Primary prevention of acute coronary events with lovastatin in men and women with average cholesterol levels: results of AFCAPS/TexCAPS. Air Force/Texas Coronary Atherosclerosis Prevention Study. JAMA. 1998;279:1615-1622.

49. Tsevat J, Weinstein MC, Williams LW, Tosteson AN, Goldman L. Expected gains in life expectancy from various coronary heart disease risk factor modifications. Circulation. 1991;83:1194-1201.

50. Reaven GM. Role of insulin resistance in human disease. Banting lecture. Diabetes. 1988;37:1595-1607.

51. Braunwald E. Shattuck Lecture—Cardiovascular medicine at the turn of the millennium: triumphs, concerns, and opportunities. New Engl J Med. 1997;337:1360-1369.

52. Rosamond WD, Chambless LE, Folsom AR, Cooper LS, Conwill DE, Clegg L, Wang CH, Heiss G. Trends in the incidence of myocardial infarction and in mortality due to coronary heart disease, 1987 to 1994. N Eng J Med. 1998;339:861-867.

53. Tunstall-Pedoe H, Kuulasmaa K, Mahonen M, Cepaitis Z, Kuulasmaa K, Keil U, for the MONICA Project. Contributions of trends in survival and coronary-event rates to changes in coronary heart disease mortality: 10-year results from 37 WHO MONICA Project populations. Monitoring trends and determinants in cardiovascular disease. Lancet. 1999;353:1547-1557.

54. Rosamond WD, Chambless LE, Folsom AR. Survival trends, coronary event rates, and the MONICA project. Monitoring trends and determinants in cardiovascular disease. Lancet. 1999;354:864-865.

55. Gersh BJ. The changing late prognosis of acute myocardial infarction. Implications and mechanisms. Eur Heart J. 1995;16(suppl E):S50-S53.

56. Naylor CD, Chen E. Population-wide mortality trends among patients hospitalized for acute myocardial infarction: the Ontario experience, 1981 to 1991. J Am Coll Cardiol. 1994;24:1431-1438.

57. Rouleau JL, Talajic M, Sussex B, Potvin P, Warnica W, Davies RJ, Gardner M, Stewart D, Plante S, Dupuis R, Lauzon C, Mikes E, Balnozan V, Savard P. Myocardial infarction patients in the 1990s—their risk factors, stratification and survival in Canada: the Canadian Assessment of Myocardial Infarction (CAMI) Study. J Am Coll Cardiol. 1996;27:1119-1127.

58. Torp-Pedersen C, Hildebrandt P, Kober L, Nielsen FE, Jensen G, Melchior T, Joen T, Ringsdal V, Nielsen U, Ege M. Improving long-term survival of patients with acute myocardial infarction from 1977–1988 in a region of Denmark. Eur Heart J. 1995;16:14-20.

59. Uemara K, Piza Z. Trends in cardiovascular disease mortality in industrialized countries since 1950. World Health Stat Q. 1988;1155-1178.

60. Edlavitch SA, Crow R, Burke GL, Baxter J. Secular trends in Q wave and non Q wave acute myocardial infarction. The Minnesota Heart Survey. Circulation. 1991;83:492-503.

61. Gheorghiade M, Ruzumna P, Borzak S, Havstad S, Ali A, Goldstein S. Decline in rate of hospital mortality from acute myocardial infarction: impact of changing management strategies. Am Heart J. 1996;131:250-256.

62. Dauerman HL, Lessard D, Yarzebski J, Furman MI, Gore JM, Goldberg RJ. Ten-year trends in the incidence, treatment, and outcome of Q-wave myocardial infarction. Am J Cardiol. 2000;86:730-735.

63. Goff DC Jr, Howard G, Wang CH, Folsom AR, Rosamond WD, Cooper LS, Chambless LE. Trends in severity of hospitalized myocardial infarction: the Atherosclerosis Risk in Communities (ARIC) Study, 1987–1994. Am Heart J. 2000;189:874-880.

64. Topol EJ, Holmes DR, Rogers WJ. Coronary angiography after thrombolytic therapy for acute myocardial infarction. Ann Intern Med. 1991;114:877-885.

65. Ayanian JZ, Hauptman PJ, Guadagnoli E, Antman E, Pashos CL, McNeil BJ. Knowledge and practices of generalist and specialist physicians regarding drug therapy for acute myocardial infarction. N Engl J Med. 1994;331:1136-1142.

66. Rogers WJ, Babb JD, Baim DS, Chesebro JH, Gore JM, Roberts R, Williams DO, Frederick M, Passamani ER, Braunwald E, for TIMI II investigators. Selective versus routine predischarge coronary arteriography after therapy with recombinant tissue-type plasminogen activator, heparin and aspirin for acute myocardial infarction. J Am Coll Cardiol. 1991;17:1007-1016.

67. Lamas GA, Pfeffer MA, Hamm P, Wertheimer J, Rouleau JL, Braunwald E, for the SAVE investigators. Do the results of randomized clinical trials of cardiovascular drugs influence medical practice? N Engl J Med. 1992;327:241-247.

68. Yim JM, Hoon TJ, Bittar N, Bauman JL, Brown EJ, Celestin C, Phillips BG, Vlasses PH. Angiotensin-converting enzyme inhibitor use in survivors of acute myocardial infarction. *Am J Cardiol.* 1995;75:1184-1186.

69. Jacques PF, Selhub J, Bostom AG, Wilson PWF, Rosenberg IH. The effect of folic acid fortification on plasma folate and total homosysteine concentrations. *N Engl J Med.* 1999;340:1449-1454.

70. Appel LJ, Moore TJ, Obarzanek E, Vollmer WM, Svetkey LP, Sacks FM, Bray GA, Vogt TM, Cutler JA, Windhauser MM, Lin PH, Karanja N. The effect of dietary patterns on blood pressure: Results from the Dietary Approaches to Stop Hypertension (DASH) trial. *N Engl J Med.* 1997;376:1117-1124.

71. Libby P, Egan D, Skarlatos S. Role of infectious agents in atherosclerosis and restenosis: an assessment of the evidence and need for further research. *Circulation.* 1997;96:4095-4103.

CHAPTER 2

LIPOPROTEIN METABOLISM

Daniel J. Rader, MD

This chapter focuses on the role of lipids and lipoproteins in the development of atherosclerotic lesions. Detailed reviews of lipoproteins and atherosclerosis are beyond the scope of this chapter, but several excellent reviews are available (1-5).

PATHOPHYSIOLOGY OF ATHEROSCLEROSIS

Despite a rapidly growing base of knowledge on the cell and molecular biology of the vessel wall, plasma lipids and lipoproteins still occupy a central role in atherogenesis. A brief overview of lipoprotein transport is provided to set the stage for a review of atherogenesis.

Lipid Transport

Plasma cholesterol and triglycerides are transported through the plasma in the core of lipoprotein particles (see Figure 2.1 and Table 2.1) (6,7). These serum lipids are composed of free and esterified cholesterol, triglycerides, and phospholipids. As shown in Figure 2.1, hydrophobic neutral lipids, triglycerides, and cholesteryl esters are in the core of the spherical particle, whereas amphipathic components, such as phospholipids and apolipoproteins, compose the surface.

As shown in Figure 2.2 (5), lipoproteins are synthesized, transported, and catabolized through a series of interrelated steps:

1. Chylomicrons, which are assembled in the small intestine, carry dietary triglycerides and cholesterol.
2. Very-low-density lipoproteins (VLDL), which are assembled in the liver, transport mainly endogenously derived core lipids.
3. Chylomicrons and VLDL can exchange their core triglyceride for core cholesteryl ester from high-density lipoproteins (HDL) (8).

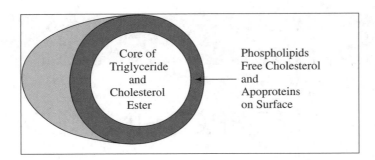

FIGURE 2.1
Basic structure of a lipoprotein.

TABLE 2.1
Chemical Characteristics of the Major Lipoprotein Classes

| Lipoprotein | Lipid (%)* | | |
	Triglyceride	Cholesterol	Phospholipid
Chylomicrons	80–95	2–7	3–9
VLDL	55–80	5–10	10–20
IDL	20–50	20–40	15–25
LDL	5–15	40–50	20–25
HDL	5–10	15–25	20–30

Abbreviations: HDL, high-density lipoprotein; IDL, intermediate density lipoprotein; LDL, low-density lipoprotein; VLDL, very-low-density lipoprotein.

*Percent composition of lipids; apolipoproteins make up the rest.

4. Or in the plasma, chylomicrons and VLDL lose their triglycerides after interacting with lipoprotein lipase (LPL) at the vessel wall; they become, respectively, chylomicron remnants and VLDL remnants (the latter are also called intermediate-density lipoproteins).
5. VLDL remnants can also be cleared by the liver or they can be converted to low-density lipoproteins (LDL) (9).
6. Chylomicron remnants are removed from plasma by the liver.
7. LDL is removed from plasma largely by LDL receptors in the liver (10,11).
8. Cholesterol from peripheral cells is picked up by HDL.
9. HDL returns cholesterol to the liver.

The protein portions of lipoproteins are named alphabetically as apolipoproteins; they are listed in Table 2.2 (4). Apolipoprotein B (apo B) is the major apolipoprotein on chylomicrons, VLDL, their remnants, and LDL (12). The liver makes a full-length version called apo B-100 that is necessary for both the initial secretion of VLDL into the bloodstream and the removal of LDL via the LDL receptor. The intestine makes a shortened version of the protein called apo B-48. Although still required for chylomicron secretion into the circulation, this shortened version lacks the receptor-binding domain present in full-length apo B. All of the apo B–containing lipoproteins are potentially atherogenic if their metabolism is not regulated properly. Because there is one apo B for each LDL particle, laboratory measurement of the quantity of apo B can indicate whether an individual has the more atherogenic, small dense LDL or the less atherogenic, large buoyant LDL (13).

Apo B–containing lipoproteins transport exogenously and endogenously derived lipids to peripheral tissues: triglycerides for energy use or storage and cholesterol for synthesis of steroids and cell membrane structural integrity. To carry out their role, lipoproteins must be able to

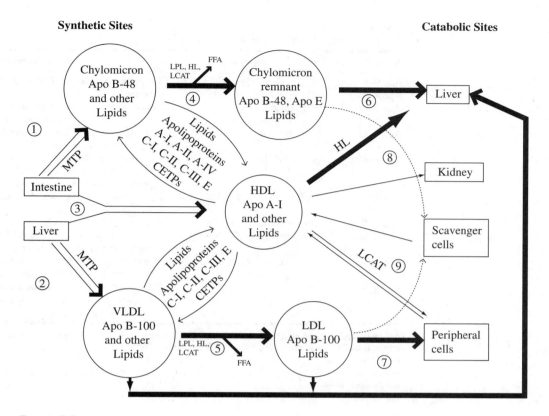

FIGURE 2.2
Lipoprotein synthesis, transport, and catabolism. CETP, cholesterol ester transfer protein; FFA, free fatty acid; HDL, high-density lipoprotein; HL, hepatic lipase; LCAT, lecithin cholesterol acyl tranferase; LDL, low-density lipoprotein; LPL, lipoprotein lipase; MTP, microsomal transfer protein; VLDL, very-low-density lipoprotein. Adapted from Schaefer EJ. Lipoproteins, nutrition, and heart disease. *Am J Clin Nutr.* 2002;75:191–212. Adapted with permission by the *American Journal of Clinical Nutrition.* © Am J Clin Nutr. American Society for Clinical Nutrition.

cross the endothelial barrier in blood vessels and reach the extracellular space. LDL are the predominant lipoproteins passing through the endothelial layer, but both chylomicron and VLDL remnants can do so as well. Much of this movement across the endothelial barrier occurs in the capillaries, but some occurs in all vessels, including the large arteries. The passage of lipoproteins into the subendothelial space of larger arteries is viewed as one of the first critical steps in atherogenesis.

Lipid Infiltration in Atherogenesis

An early step in atherogenesis is modification of apo B–containing lipoproteins (1,3,14,15). A typical modification is oxidation of phospholipids in an LDL molecule. Once modified, apo B–containing lipoproteins may more likely aggregate or stick to extracellular matrix molecules in the subendothelial space of arteries. Alternatively, unmodified apo B lipoproteins may be modified after adhering to matrix molecules in the subendothelial space. In either scheme, greater numbers of circulating lipoproteins are associated with entry of more apo B–containing lipoproteins into the central wall.

After modification and retention of apo B–containing lipoproteins, a series of events leads to the development of foam cells (16-19). Endothelial cells are signaled to synthesize factors that foster accumulation of cells within the artery wall: cell-adhesion molecules,

TABLE 2.2
Characteristics of the Major Apolipoproteins

Apolipoprotein	Lipoproteins	Metabolic Functions
Apo A-I	HDL, chylomicrons	Structural component of HDL; LCAT activator
Apo A-II	HDL, chylomicrons	Unknown
Apo A-IV	HDL, chylomicrons	Unknown; possibly facilitates transfer of apolipoproteins between HDL and chylomicrons
Apo B-48	Chylomicrons	Necessary for assembly and secretion of chylomicrons from the small intestine
Apo B-100	VLDL, IDL, LDL	Necessary for the assembly and secretion of VLDL from the liver; structural protein of VLDL, IDL and LDL; ligand for the LDL receptor
Apo C-I	Chylomicrons, VLDL, IDL, HDL	May inhibit hepatic uptake of chylomicrons VLDL remnants
Apo C-II	Chylomicrons, VLDL, IDL, HDL	Activator of lipoprotein lipase
Apo C-III	Chylomicrons, VLDL, IDL, HDL	Inhibitor of lipoprotein lipase; inhibits hepatic uptake of chylomicron and VLDL remnants
Apo E	Chylomicrons, VLDL, IDL, HDL	Ligand for binding of several lipoproteins to the LDL receptor, LRP, and proteoglycans
Apo(a)	Lp(a)	Composed of LDL apo B linked covalently to apo(a); function unknown but is an independent predictor of coronary artery disease

Abbreviations: HDL, high-density lipoprotein; IDL, intermediate-density lipoprotein; LCAT, lecithin cholesterol acyl tranferase; LDL, low-density lipoprotein; LRP, low-density lipoprotein receptor-related protein; VLDL, very-low-density lipoprotein.

Source: Reprinted with permission from Ginsberg HN. Cardiovascular disease in diabetes: the lipid connection. *On the Cutting Edge.* 2002;23:12.

monocyte chemotactic proteins (MCP), and monocyte-colony stimulating factor. Together, these molecules stimulate circulating monocytes to accumulate at the initial site of retained subendothelial lipoproteins (16). After monocytes enter the subendothelial space, they are activated and transformed into macrophages. These macrophages take up the modified lipoproteins and develop into foam cells (17). They also secrete factors that can stimulate smooth muscle cell proliferation and migration. At this point, all of the components of the advanced lesion are in place and atherogenesis is well under way. In Figure 2.3 (17) monocytes, the major precursor for foam cells in the fatty streak, are shown adhering to the endothelium and then penetrating to the subendothelial space. Oxidized LDL can directly stimulate this; minimally modified LDL (MM-LDL) can stimulate indirectly by increasing the release of MCP-1 from endothelial cells. As a ligand for the scavenger receptor that is expressed as the monocyte differentiates to a macrophage, oxidized LDL enters the macrophage (20). As LDL enters the cell, lipids accumulate in the developing foam cells. This monocyte-macrophage differentiation can be facilitated by the release of macrophage-colony stimulating factor (M-CSF) from endothelial cells under the influence of MM-LDL. Finally, oxidized LDL can induce endothelial damage, fostering atherogenesis by allowing entry of elements from the blood and adherence of platelets (17,19).

HDL contains apo A-I as its major protein and appears to protect against atherosclerosis (21-24). Animal studies have shown that apo A-I reduces progression and in some instances promotes regression of atherosclerosis (25-27). HDL transports cholesterol from tissues throughout the body back to the liver; this is known as "reverse cholesterol transport" (23,24). HDL begins to accumulate cholesterol from cells as lipid-poor apo A-I promotes the efflux of free cholesterol and phospholipids from cells via the cellular lipid transporter adenosine triphosphate–binding cassette protein (ABCA1) (27). Nascent HDL particles enriched in free cholesterol can then be

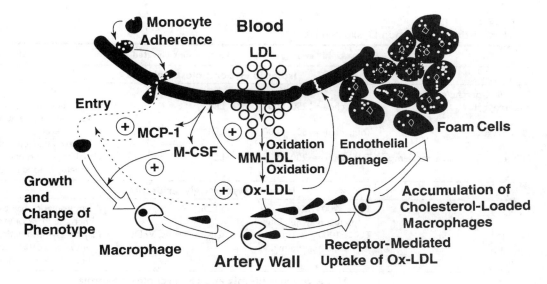

FIGURE 2.3

A schematic outline of the oxidative modification hypothesis showing the several ways in which Ox-LDL is potentially more atherogenic than native LDL. LDL, low-density lipoprotein; MCP-1, monocyte chemoattractant protein-1; M-CSF, macrophage-colony stimulating factor; MM, minimally modified; Ox, oxidized. Reprinted from Steinberg D. Antioxidants and atherosclerosis: a current assessment. *Circulation.* 1991;84:1420–1425, with permission from Lippincott Williams & Wilkins.

modified by the enzyme lecithin cholesterol acyl transferase (LCAT), which transfers a fatty acid from phospholipid to free cholesterol, forming cholesteryl ester. The cholesteryl ester moves from the surface of the lipoprotein to the core (because it is hydrophobic), allowing more free cholesterol to be adsorbed onto the surface and enlarging the particle. As HDL becomes enriched in cholesterol ester, it becomes larger and more buoyant. HDL delivers cholesteryl esters to the liver for conversion to bile acids or excretion as biliary cholesterol. This final step in the reverse cholesterol transport pathway is achieved through at least two different pathways: (*a*) delivery of the cholesteryl esters directly to the liver via selective uptake mediated by scavenger receptor class B type I (SR-BI) (28,29), or (*b*) transferal of the cholesteryl esters to triglyceride-rich VLDLs or chylomicrons via the cholesterol ester transfer proteins (CETP) (30), followed by uptake of the chylomicron or VLDL remnant by the liver. In addition to promoting reverse cholesterol transport, HDL has antioxidant, anti-inflammatory, and antiaggregant properties that may contribute to its antiatherogenic effects (18).

PATHOPHYSIOLOGY OF DYSLIPIDEMIA

Despite the complexity of the atherosclerotic process and the multicomponent nature of advanced lesions, the root of the problem is simple: increased quantities of atherogenic lipoproteins are present in the blood and are retained and modified in the subendothelial space. It is, therefore, important to understand the pathophysiology of the various dyslipidemias. The following discussion presents some details of the genetic and molecular basis of various dyslipidemias grouped by clinical relevance (Table 2.3):

- Hypercholesterolemia
- Hypertriglyceridemia

TABLE 2.3

Characteristics of Common Dyslipidemias

Type	Plasma Lipid Levels (mg/dL)	Lipoproteins Elevated	Clinical Signs
Isolated Hypercholesterolemia			
Familial Hypercholesterolemia			
Heterozygotes	Total chol = 250–500	LDL	Usually develop xanthomas in adulthood and vascular disease at 30-50 years
Homozygotes	Total chol = 500–1000	LDL	Usually develop xanthomas and vascular disease in childhood
Polygenic hypercholesterolemia	Total chol = 200–300	LDL	Usually asymptomatic until vascular disease develops; no xanthomas
Isolated Hypertriglyceridemia			
Mild	TG = 200–1000 (plasma may be cloudy)	VLDL	Asymptomatic; may be associated with increased risk of vascular disease
Severe	TG > 1000 (plasma may be milky)	Chylomicrons, VLDL	May be asymptomatic; may be associated with pancreatitis, abdominal pain, hepatosplenomegaly
Hypertriglyceridemia and Hypercholesterolemia			
Combined hyperlipidemia	TG = 200–1000 Total chol = 200–400	VLDL, LDL	Usually asymptomatic until vascular disease develops; familial form may also be present as isolated high TG or as isolated high LDL cholesterol
Dysbetalipoproteinemia	TG = 200–600 Total chol = 250–500	VLDL, IDL (LDL normal)	Usually asymptomatic until vascular disease develops; may have palmar or tuboeruptive xanthoma

Abbreviations: Chol, cholesterol; IDL, intermediate-density lipoprotein; LDL, low-density lipoprotein; TG, triglyceride; VLDL, very-low-density lipoprotein.

- Hypertriglyceridemia with hypercholesterolemia (combined hyperlipidemia)
- Reduced HDL cholesterol

Hypercholesterolemia

Elevated concentrations of plasma total cholesterol in a fasting state are usually associated with increased concentrations of plasma LDL cholesterol because LDL carries about 65% to 75% of total plasma cholesterol. If plasma triglyceride concentrations are markedly increased, however, VLDL cholesterol, which is usually 5% to 10% of total plasma cholesterol, may be high enough to elevate total plasma cholesterol concentrations even when LDL cholesterol concentrations are normal. VLDL cholesterol may also be a major component of total cholesterol in dysbetalipoproteinemic subjects (with the apo E2/2 phenotype). The patient with significantly elevated HDL cholesterol levels may also appear to have moderately increased total plasma cholesterol.

Elevations of LDL cholesterol can result from single-gene defects, polygenic disorders, and environmental effects, such as diet, on lipoprotein metabolism. Familial hypercholesterolemia, which occurs in the heterozygous form in approximately one of 500 individuals, is associated with mutations in the gene for the LDL receptor (10). In people with familial hypercholesterolemia, plasma total cholesterol and LDL cholesterol levels are increased at birth and remain so throughout life. Adults heterozygous for familial hypercholesterolemia have total cholesterol levels that range from 250 to 500 mg/dL when untreated. Both tendon xanthomas and premature atherosclerosis with coronary heart disease (CHD) are common.

Plasma triglyceride concentrations are usually normal, whereas HDL cholesterol levels may be normal or reduced. Metabolic studies showed decreased fractional clearance of LDL apo B in subjects with familial hypercholesterolemia, consistent with reduced numbers of LDL receptors. Markedly elevated levels of LDL cholesterol are the hallmark of familial hypercholesterolemia and are associated with the increased risk for CHD in these patients. The homozygous form of familial hypercholesterolemia occurs in 1 in 1 million individuals and is associated with plasma cholesterol levels greater than 500 mg/dL, tendon and planar xanthomas, and very premature CHD in childhood and adolescence (31).

A second single-gene disorder causing significant LDL cholesterol elevations involves a mutation in apo B in the region of the protein associated with binding to the LDL receptor. This disorder, called familial defective apo B, has been linked to defective catabolism of LDL in vivo and to an autosomal dominant hypercholesterolemia (32). Isolated elevations of LDL cholesterol also have been found in subjects from families with familial combined hyperlipidemia (FCHL) (33).

Polygenic causes of hypercholesterolemia, which are likely to interact with environmental effects on lipoprotein metabolism, are much more common than familial hypercholesterolemia. Most evidence indicates that both overproduction and reduced fractional catabolism of LDL play significant roles in this disorder. Production and fractional catabolism are probably affected by dietary saturated fat and cholesterol consumption, age, and level of physical activity. Plasma total cholesterol values are in the range of 200 to 300 mg/dL, plasma triglyceride and HDL cholesterol values are usually normal, and tendon xanthomas are not present. As genes related to regulation of cholesterol metabolism are identified, some of the "polygenic" forms of hypercholesterolemia probably will be found to result from the interaction of two or three specific genes.

Hypertriglyceridemia

Elevated levels of fasting plasma triglycerides in the range of 200 to 1,000 mg/dL are generally associated with increased concentrations of VLDL triglycerides. When fasting triglycerides exceed 1,000 mg/dL, chylomicrons are almost always also present. Elevations in VLDL triglycerides most often are associated with the synthesis and secretion of excessive quantities of VLDL triglyceride by the liver (33). Hepatic triglyceride synthesis is regulated by substrate flow (particularly the availability of free fatty acids), energy status (particularly the glycogen stores in the liver), and hormonal status (particularly the balance between insulin and glucagon). Obesity, excessive consumption of simple sugars and saturated fats, inactivity, alcohol consumption, and glucose intolerance or diabetes mellitus have been commonly associated with hypertriglyceridemia (34,35).

Although no single-gene disorder associated with increased hepatic synthesis of triglycerides has been identified, some recent studies have suggested a link between abnormal bile acid metabolism and overproduction of triglycerides in some subjects with hypertriglyceridemia (36). It is believed that in this group of disorders, sometimes referred to as "primary hypertriglyceridemia," only triglyceride synthesis is increased and the liver secretes a normal number of large, triglyceride-enriched VLDL particles. The secretion of a normal number of VLDL particles limits the rate of production of LDL particles, and these subjects may not be at increased risk for coincident elevations of LDL cholesterol. However, subjects from families with FCHL can present with isolated hypertriglyceridemia.

The degree of hypertriglyceridemia present in any individual also depends on the quantity and activity of LPL. Most data suggest that LPL activity is normal in most subjects with moderate hypertriglyceridemia (200 to 500 mg/dL) but may be reduced in more severely affected individuals (having levels greater than 500 mg/dL). However, several studies suggested that heterozygosity for LPL deficiency, as a result of specific mutations, can occur in approximately 5% to 10% of the hypertriglyceridemic population (37-39). When fasting triglyceride concentrations are markedly elevated (greater than 1,000 mg/dL), otherwise normal LPL may be either saturated or actually consumed, so that the patient is relatively deficient in the enzyme during the postprandial period. If LPL is totally deficient, plasma triglyceride concentrations greater than 2,000 mg/dL are common, with both chylomicrons and VLDL significantly contributing to the hyperlipidemia.

Hypertriglyceridemia with Hypercholesterolemia

Hypertriglyceridemia can also occur in two phenotypes in association with hypercholesterolemia. In the first, called "combined hyperlipidemia," both total plasma triglycerides and LDL cholesterol levels are elevated compared with age- and sex-matched controls (33). Although it is likely that a variety of combinations of regulatory defects in lipid metabolism account for a significant number of individuals with this phenotype, FCHL has been identified in which patients may have combined hyperlipidemia, only hypertriglyceridemia, or only elevated LDL cholesterol levels. In the familial disorder, which appears to be transmitted as an autosomal dominant gene (40,41), the diagnosis must rest on the presentation of combined hyperlipidemia or the presence of various lipid phenotypes in first-degree family members along with either isolated hypertriglyceridemia or isolated LDL cholesterol elevation in the patient.

Familial Combined Hyperlipidemia

FCHL appears to be associated with secretion of increased numbers of VLDL particles (42,43). Therefore, individuals with FCHL are predisposed to high levels of plasma VLDL triglycerides if they synthesize triglycerides at an increased rate. Once these individuals assemble and secrete increased numbers of large, triglyceride-rich VLDL particles, their plasma triglyceride concentrations depend on their ability to hydrolyze VLDL triglycerides. The ability to hydrolyze VLDL triglycerides also regulates the generation of LDL in plasma. Thus, subjects with FCHL who had very high VLDL triglyceride concentrations (and were not able to efficiently catabolize VLDL) might have normal or reduced numbers of LDL particles in the circulation and thus a normal LDL cholesterol level. If these same individuals were able to efficiently catabolize the increased numbers of VLDL particles that were entering their plasma, they would generate increased numbers of LDL particles and have both hypertriglyceridemia and a high LDL cholesterol level. Individuals with FCHL who synthesized only normal quantities of triglycerides and secreted increased numbers of VLDL particles carrying normal triglyceride loads would generate increased numbers of LDL particles and have elevated plasma LDL cholesterol levels only.

FCHL may occur in as many as 1 in 100 Americans and is the most common familial lipid disorder found in survivors of myocardial infarction (33). A link exists between combined hyperlipidemia and insulin resistance (44,45). The pathophysiologic basis for this link has not been elucidated, although increased free fatty acid flux to the liver, which is common in individuals with insulin resistance, could stimulate the secretion of VLDL.

Familial Dysbetalipoproteinemia

The second disorder in which elevations of both plasma triglycerides and cholesterol can occur is dysbetalipoproteinemia. In this disorder affecting 1 in 10,000 people, genetic variation in the gene for apo E results in the synthesis of defective forms of this apolipoprotein. Because apo E plays a crucial role in the catabolism of chylomicron and VLDL remnants (46), subjects with defective apo E accumulate these cholesteryl ester–enriched remnant lipoproteins in their plasma. Hence, both VLDL triglyceride and VLDL cholesterol levels are elevated, and chylomicron remnants are present in fasting plasma from dysbetalipoproteinemic subjects. LDL cholesterol levels are not elevated in this disorder. One in 100 people are homozygous for the apo E2 isoform, the most common cause of familial dysbetalipoproteinemia. Interestingly, 99% of these homozygous subjects have normal plasma triglyceride and cholesterol concentrations. Thus, a second factor influencing lipoprotein metabolism must be present in the 1 in 10,000 individuals with the clinically relevant entity, familial dysbetalipoproteinemia.

Primary Hypoalphalipoproteinemia (Reduced HDL Cholesterol)

Low concentrations of HDL cholesterol are most often seen in patients with coexistent hypertriglyceridemia, although primary hypoalphalipoproteinemia has been identified in both individuals and families (47). The pathophysiologic basis of reduced HDL cholesterol levels is not well defined and is probably complex (30,48). The relationship between hypertriglyceridemia and low HDL cholesterol concentrations probably results from the transfer of cholesteryl ester from the core of HDL to VLDL mediated by CETP; the shift of surface components, particularly phospholipids and apolipoproteins C-II and C-III, from HDL to VLDL; and the increased fractional catabolism of the cholesteryl ester-poor, surface-poor HDL that results from the first two processes. The complexity of the situation is highlighted by the failure of HDL cholesterol levels to normalize when fasting plasma triglycerides are significantly reduced in most patients who present initially with hypertriglyceridemia and low HDL cholesterol levels.

Primary hypoalphalipoproteinemia refers to the state when HDL cholesterol levels are markedly reduced but plasma triglyceride levels are normal. Although this disorder certainly exists, many individuals who present with this phenotype have had hypertriglyceridemia in the past or have an older (or more obese) first-degree relative who has both low HDL cholesterol and increased triglyceride levels. Therefore, carefully conducted family studies and long-term follow-up may be necessary to identify individuals who truly have primary reductions in HDL cholesterol levels. The basis for such reductions is unknown except for extremely rare situations in which genetic mutations in the area of the apo A-I gene have been described (49,50). HDL cholesterol is severely reduced in the rare Tangier disease (owing to mutations in ABCA1) and LCAT deficiency.

SUMMARY

Atherosclerotic cardiovascular disease is the number one cause of death in Western nations and is rapidly becoming a prominent cause of death in economically underdeveloped countries as well. In this review, the abnormalities of lipoprotein transport have been linked to the atherogenic process and common lipid phenotypes have been used as examples of atherogenic disorders of lipoprotein metabolism.

Many of the key genes that either alone or, more commonly, in combination result in abnormalities of lipid transport and increased risk of atherosclerosis will be identified in the next several years. These new findings should allow for better dietary and pharmacologic approaches to lipid disorders, leading in turn to further reductions in morbidity and mortality from cardiovascular disease.

REFERENCES

1. Ginsberg HN. Lipoprotein physiology. In: Hoeg J, ed. *Endocrinology and Metabolism Clinics of North America*. Philadelphia, Pa: WB Saunders Co; 1998:503-519.
2. Ross R. Cell biology of atherosclerosis. *Annu Rev Physiol*. 1995;57:791-804.
3. Berliner JA, Navab M, Fogelman AM, Frank JS, Demer LL, Edwards PA, Watson AD, Louis AJ. Atherosclerosis: basic mechanisms. Oxidation, inflammation, and genetics. *Circulation*. 1995;91:1488-1496.
4. Ginsberg HN. Cardiovascular disease in diabetes: the lipid connection. *On the Cutting Edge*. 2002;23:11-14.
5. Schaefer EJ. Lipoproteins, nutrition, and heart disease. *Am J Clin Nutr*. 2002;75:191-212.
6. Gotto AM Jr, Pownall JH, Havel RJ. Introduction to the plasma lipoproteins. *Methods Enzymol*. 1986;128:3-41.
7. Ginsberg HN. Lipoprotein physiology and its relationship to atherogenesis. *Endocrinol Metab Clin North Am*. 1990;19:211-228.
8. Tall AR. Plasma lipid transfer proteins. *J Lipid Res*. 1986;27:361-367.
9. Ginsberg HN. Lipoprotein metabolism and its relationship to atherosclerosis. *Med Clin North Am*. 1994;78:1-20.
10. Brown MS, Goldstein JL. How LDL receptors influence cholesterol and atherosclerosis. *Sci Am*. 1984;251:58-66.
11. Brown MS, Herz J, Kowal RC, Goldstein JL. The low-density lipoprotein receptor-related protein: double agent or decoy? *Curr Opin Lipidol*. 1991;2:65-72.
12. Young SG. Recent progress in understanding apolipoprotein B. *Circulation*. 1990;82:1574-1594.
13. Williams K, Sniderman AD, Sattar N, D'Agostino R Jr, Wagenknecht LE, Haffner SM. Comparison of the associations of apolipoprotein B and low-density lipoprotein cholesterol with other cardiovascular risk factors in the Insulin Resistance Atherosclerosis Study (IRAS). *Circulation*. 2003;108:2312-2316.
14. Parthasarathy S, Steinberg D, Witztum JL. The role of oxidized low-density lipoproteins in the pathogenesis of atherosclerosis. *Annu Rev Med*. 1992;43:219-225.
15. Steinberg D. Modified forms of low-density lipoprotein and atherosclerosis. *J Intern Med*. 1993;233:227-232.
16. Cybulsky MI, Gimbrone MA Jr. Endothelial expression of a mononuclear leukocyte adhesion molecule during atherogenesis. *Science*. 1991;251:788-791.
17. Steinberg D. Antioxidants and atherosclerosis: a current assessment. *Circulation*. 1991;84:1420-1425.
18. Chisolm GM, Steinberg D. The oxidative modification hypothesis of atherogenesis: an overview. *Free Radic Biol Med*. 2000;28:1815-1826.
19. Vainio S, Ikonen E. Macrophage cholesterol transport: a critical player in foam cell formation. *Ann Med*. 2003;35:146-155.
20. Boullier A, Bird DA, Chang MK, Dennis EA, Friedman P, Gillotre-Taylor K, Horkko S, Palinski W, Quehenberger O, Shaw P, Steinberg D, Terpstra V, Witztum JL. Scavenger receptors, oxidized LDL, and atherosclerosis. *Ann N Y Acad Sci*. 2001;947:214-222.
21. Rader DJ. High-density lipoproteins and atherosclerosis. *Am J Cardiol*. 2002;90:62i-70i.
22. Reichl D, Miller NE. Pathophysiology of reverse cholesterol transport: insights from inherited disorders of lipoprotein metabolism. *Arteriosclerosis*. 1989;9:785-797.
23. Phillips MC, Gillotte KL, Haynes MP, Johnson WJ, Lund-Katz S, Rothblat GH. Mechanisms of high density lipoprotein-mediated efflux of cholesterol from cell plasma membranes. *Atherosclerosis*. 1998;137(suppl):S13-S17.
24. Zhang Y, Zanotti I, Reilly M, Glick JM, Rothblat GH, and Rader DJ. Overexpression of apo A-I promotes reverse transport of cholesterol from macrophages to feces in vivo. *Circulation*. 2003;108:661-663.
25. Tangirala RK, Tsukamoto K, Chun SH, Usher D, Puré E, Rader DJ. Regression of atherosclerosis induced by liver-directed gene transfer of apolipoprotein A-I in mice. *Circulation*. 1999;100:1816-1822.
26. Duverger N, Kruth H, Emmanuel F, Caillaud J, Viglietta C, Castro G, Tailleux A, Fievet C, Fruchart J, Houdebine LM, Denefle P. Inhibition of atherosclerosis development in cholesterol-fed human apolipoprotein A-I-Transgenic rabbits. *Circulation*. 1996;94:713-717.
27. Vaisman BL, Lambert G, Amar M, Joyce C, Ito T, Shamburek RD, Cain WJ, Fruchart-Najib J, Neufeld ED, Remaley AT, Brewer HB Jr, Santamarina-Fojo S. ABCA1 overexpression leads to hyperalphalipoproteinemia and increased biliary cholesterol excretion in transgenic mice. *J Clin Invest*. 2001;108:303-309.
28. Pitmann RC, Knecht TP, Rosenbaum MS, Taylor CA Jr. A non-endocytic mechanism for the selective uptake of high density lipoprotein-associated cholesterol esters. *J Biol Chem*. 1987;262:2443-2451.
29. Trigatti B, Rigotti A, Krieger M. The role of the high-density lipoprotein receptor SR-BI in cholesterol metabolism. *Curr Opin Lipidol*. 2000;11:123-131.
30. Tall AR. Plasma high density lipoproteins. Metabolism and relationship to atherogenesis. *J Clin Invest*. 1990;86:379-384.
31. Rader DJ, Cohen J, Hobbs HH. Monogenic hypercholesterolemia: new insights in pathogenesis and treatment. *J Clin Invest*. 2003;111:1795-1803.
32. Innerarity TL, Mahley RW, Weisgraber KH, Bersot TP, Krauss RM, Vega GL, Grundy SM, Friedl W, Davignon J, McCarthy BJ. Familial defective apolipoprotein B-100: a mutation of apolipoprotein B that causes hypercholesterolemia. *J Lipid Res*. 1990;31:1337-1349.

33. Goldstein JL, Schrott HG, Hazzard WR, Bierman EL, Motulsky AG. Hyperlipidemia in coronary heart disease: II. Genetic analysis in 176 families and delineation of a new inherited disorder, combined hyperlipidemia. *J Clin Invest.* 1973;52:1544-1568.

34. Ginsberg HN. Very low density lipoprotein metabolism in diabetes mellitus. *Diabetes Metab Rev.* 1987;3:571-589.

35. Expert Panel on Detection, Evaluation, and Treatment of High Blood Cholesterol in Adults. Executive summary of the Third Report of the National Cholesterol Education Program (NCEP) Expert Panel on Detection, Evaluation, and Treatment of High Blood Cholesterol in Adults (Adult Treatment Panel III). *JAMA.* 2001;285:2486-2497. Full report: National Institutes of Health. *Third Report of the National Cholesterol Education Program Expert Panel on Detection, Evaluation, and Treatment of High Blood Cholesterol in Adults (Adult Treatment Panel III).* Bethesda, Md: National Institutes of Health; 2001. NIH Publication 01-3670. Available at: http://www.nhlbi.nih.gov/guidelines/cholesterol/atp3_rpt.htm. Accessed March 29, 2004.

36. Duane WC. Abnormal bile acid absorption in familial hypertriglyceridemia. *J Lipid Res.* 1995;36:96-107.

37. Reymer PW, Gagne E, Groenemeyer BE, Zhang H, Forsyth I, Jansen H, Seidell JC, Kromhout D, Lie KE, Kastelein J, et al. A lipoprotein lipase mutation (Asn291Ser) is associated with reduced HDL cholesterol levels in premature atherosclerosis. *Nat Genet.* 1995;10:28-34.

38. Henderson HE, Kastelein JJ, Zwinderman AH, Gagne E, Jukema JW, Reymer PW, Groenemeyer BE, Lie KI, Bruschke AV, Hayden MR, Jansen H. Lipoprotein lipase activity is decreased in a large cohort of patients with coronary artery disease and is associated with changes in lipids and lipoproteins. *J Lipid Res.* 1999;40:735-743.

39. Minnich A, Kessling A, Roy M, Giry C, DeLangavant G, Lavigne J, Lussier-Cacan S, Davignon J. Prevalence of alleles encoding defective lipoprotein lipase in hypertriglyceridemic patients of French Canadian descent. *J Lipid Res.* 1995;36:117-124.

40. Austin MA. Genetic and environmental influences on LDL subclass phenotypes. *Clin Genet.* 1994;46:64-70.

41. Jarvik GP, Brunzell JD, Austin MA, Krauss RM, Motulsky AG, Wijsman E. Genetic predictors of FCHL in four large pedigrees. Influence of apo B level major locus predicted genotype and LDL subclass phenotype. *Arterioscler Thromb.* 1994;14:1687-1694.

42. Teng B, Sniderman AD, Soutar AK, Thompson GR. Metabolic basis of hyperapobetalipoproteinemia: turnover of apolipoprotein B in low density lipoprotein and its precursors and subfractions compared with normal and familial hypercholesterolemia. *J Clin Invest.* 1986;77:663-672.

43. Arad Y, Ramakrishnan R, Ginsberg HN. Lovastatin therapy reduces low density lipoprotein apo B levels in subjects with combined hyperlipidemia by reducing the production of apo B–containing lipoproteins: implications for the pathophysiology of apo B production. *J Lipid Res.* 1990;31:567-582.

44. Reaven GM. Role of insulin resistance in human disease. *Diabetes.* 1988;37:1595-1607.

45. Reaven GM. Syndrome X: 6 years later. *J Intern Med.* 1994;736:13-22.

46. Mahley RW. Apolipoprotein E: cholesterol transport protein with expanding role in cell biology. *Science.* 1988;240:622-630.

47. Ginsberg HN, Ngai C, Wang X, Ramakrishnan R. Increased production rates of low density lipoproteins are common in individuals with low plasma levels of high density lipoprotein cholesterol, independent of plasma triglyceride concentrations. *Arterioscler Thromb Vasc Biol.* 1993;13:842-851.

48. Horowitz BS, Goldberg IJ, Merab J, Vanni T, Ramakrishnan R, Ginsberg HN. Increased plasma and renal clearance of an exchangeable pool of apolipoprotein A-I in subjects with low levels of high density lipoprotein cholesterol. *J Clin Invest.* 1993;91:1743-1752.

49. Norum RA, Forte TM, Alaupovic P, Ginsberg HN. Clinical syndrome and lipid metabolism in hereditary deficiency of apolipoproteins A-I and C-III, variant I. In: Angel A, Frohlich J, eds. *Lipoprotein Deficiency Syndromes.* New York, NY: Plenum Publishing; 1986:137-149.

50. Norum RA, Lakier JB, Goldstein S, Angel A, Goldberg RB, Block WD, Noffze DK, Dolphin PJ, Edelglass J, Bogorad DD, Alaupovic P. Familial deficiency of apolipoproteins A-I and C-III and precocious coronary-artery disease. *N Engl J Med.* 1982;306:1513-1519.

PART II

Assessment

CHAPTER 3

RISK FACTOR ASSESSMENT FOR CARDIOVASCULAR DISEASE

Stacey E. Panagotopulos, PhD, and Francine K. Welty, MD, PhD

INTRODUCTION

Risk factors are characteristics that are associated with an increased likelihood of developing a disease. Risk factors may be laboratory measurements, such as serum low-density lipoprotein (LDL) cholesterol or high-density lipoprotein (HDL) cholesterol, or physical exam measurements, such as blood pressure, or habits such as cigarette smoking. Risk factors for cardiovascular disease (CVD) are classified as either modifiable, which means they are amenable to modification, or nonmodifiable (refer to Table 3.1 [1]). For example, high blood pressure and LDL cholesterol can be treated with medication, whereas age and family history cannot be changed. This chapter presents the scientific evidence that supports the major risk factors for CVD as identified by the third Adult Treatment Panel of the National Cholesterol Education Program (ATP III) (1). First, the evidence for the LDL cholesterol goal is presented, followed by evidence related to the five major risk factors used for determining the LDL cholesterol goal. Next, the scientific evidence supporting CVD risk equivalents is discussed. The evidence supporting emerging risk factors is then presented in an attempt to clearly define when certain tests are appropriate. The chapter closes with the steps to evaluate patients and establish treatment plans and goals.

PATHOPHYSIOLOGY OF ATHEROSCLEROSIS AS RELATED TO RISK FACTORS

When examining risk factors for coronary heart disease (CHD), it is important to understand the atherosclerotic process because each risk factor contributes to plaque formation. Theories for the pathophysiology of atherosclerosis include vascular injury, monoclonal response, and viral or bacterial infection, but the most widely accepted is the lipid infiltration hypothesis. As described in Chapter 2, excess LDL can become oxidized and taken up in various tissues by scavenger receptors, which recognize modified forms of cholesterol and are not regulated by

TABLE 3.1
Modifiable and Nonmodifiable Coronary Heart Disease (CHD) Risk Factors

Modifiable Factors	Nonmodifiable Factors
Cigarette smoking	Increasing age (men ≥45 years; women ≥55 years)
Hypertension (blood pressure ≥140/90 mm Hg or on antihypertensive medication)	Family history of premature CHD (male first-degree relative <55 years; female first-degree relative <65 years)
Dyslipidemia	
Diabetes mellitus	
Obesity	
Physical inactivity	

Source: Adapted from reference 1 (table II.41, p II-14).

the presence of cholesterol. This contrasts with the LDL receptor uptake of unmodified LDL cholesterol, which can be down-regulated in the presence of cholesterol (2). Many enzymes that function in normal cell processes produce free radicals that can oxidize LDL. Such enzymes include NADPH oxidase, 15-lipoxygenase, myeloperoxidase, and the mitochondrial electron transport system. All of these enzymes are active during normal cell metabolism. During an inflammatory response, as occurs in the atherosclerotic lesion, even more free radicals are produced (3). Environmental factors, such as cigarette smoking, increase the amount of free radicals in the circulation and increase the risk of oxidation. Genetic conditions, such as high homocysteine levels due to inefficient methionine metabolism, can also cause oxidative damage to LDL. In addition, the increase in glycation products in diabetes leads to LDL modification such that it is recognized by scavenger receptors (4).

Monocytes or macrophages in the arterial wall can take up oxidized or otherwise modified cholesterol in an uncontrolled manner via class A scavenger receptors, which are not regulated by the presence of cholesterol (3,4). When the macrophages in the arteries take up excess amounts of cholesterol, they take on a foamy appearance and release cytokines that cause the recruitment of more monocytes as well as lymphocytes, thus provoking an inflammatory response in the artery (4). In addition, the oxidized LDL itself attracts more monocytes to the inflamed area and inhibits the mobility of the macrophages that are already present (3). Meanwhile, the endothelial cells begin expressing adhesion molecules, which causes the entry of more monocytes and leukocytes into the subendothelial space, in this case the intima of the artery. The escalating inflammatory response recruits more macrophages, which in turn increases the number of foam cells and lipid (4). The incoming cholesterol is also more likely to become oxidized because of the free radicals generated during the inflammatory response (4). These interactions induce and propagate the fatty streak, which progresses to the arterial lesions characteristic of heart disease (3).

Fatty lesions are characterized by a fibrous cap, which is a by-product of the inflammatory response, and the recruitment of smooth muscle cells from the media (their normal location) to the intima (5). T lymphocytes and macrophages secrete cytokines that recruit smooth muscle cells and cause them to grow. The smooth muscle cells lay down a matrix, which includes collagen, elastic fibers, and proteoglycans. This matrix forms the fibrous cap, which can become thicker and undergo calcification as the disease progresses. The ongoing inflammation within the fibrous cap, including lipid deposition and cell death, forms a necrotic core. Rupture of this fibrous cap can be caused by high shear stress from blood flowing through the narrowing artery. Plaque rupture can also be caused by matrix breakdown due to infection or matrix metalloproteinases (MMP) that break down the collagen and elastic matrix. A high-fat diet increases the amount of MMP released, thus increasing risk of rupture (6). When the plaque ruptures, tissue factor is released, which causes thrombus formation, which in turn causes heart attacks and strokes.

Risk factors for atherosclerosis include smoking, high blood pressure, and diabetes, all of which can damage the arterial wall and increase production of free radicals (5). In addition, genetic factors such as defects in the LDL receptor, presence of apolipoprotein B or E, and presence of lipoprotein lipase increase the risk for atherosclerosis because these deficiencies cause a great increase in plasma LDL cholesterol. A diet high in saturated fat and a sedentary lifestyle also increase plasma LDL cholesterol and the risk for atherosclerosis.

The risk for coronary artery disease can be reduced with a low-fat diet and regular exercise, both of which are known to reduce plasma LDL cholesterol levels (5). In addition, regular consumption of foods containing vitamins with antioxidant properties can reduce the amount of free radicals available to oxidize LDL (3). Adding fiber to the diet can increase loss of cholesterol through the intestine and help maintain cholesterol homeostasis in the body. Finally, high levels of HDL cholesterol are inversely correlated with the risk for heart disease (7). HDL has been shown to be protective in several ways. It may have antioxidant properties and, thus, prevent oxidation of LDL. In addition, it has been shown to reduce the growth and migration of smooth muscle cells and inhibit adhesion of monocytes to endothelial cells (8). Finally, HDL is the major lipoprotein involved in the process of reverse cholesterol transport, where cholesterol is removed from peripheral cells (the arterial intima in this case) and returned to the liver for catabolism, thus preventing an overaccumulation of cholesterol in the tissues (9).

LDL AS THE PRIMARY RISK FACTOR

ATP III defines LDL as the major risk factor in heart disease and LDL cholesterol level as the treatment goal (1). LDL cholesterol contributes at all levels of plaque development, from the formation of the fatty streak to the stability of the plaque (10).

Evidence for LDL cholesterol as the main contributor to CHD spans genetic, epidemiologic, animal, cell, and biochemical studies, as well as human population studies and clinical trials. An early example was the genetic mutation of the LDL receptor that causes familial hypercholesterolemia, a condition that causes accelerated atherosclerosis in humans (11,12). In addition, animal models in which the LDL receptor is defective show the development of atherosclerosis in animals that do not normally develop coronary lesions (13,14).

Population studies, such as the Framingham Heart Study (15), Multiple Risk Factor Intervention Trial (MRFIT) (16), and the Lipid Research Clinics Study (LRC) (17,18), have shown a direct relationship between LDL cholesterol level (or total cholesterol) and new onset CHD in both men and women initially free of CHD. In the MRFIT trial of 12,866 high-risk men, subjects randomized to clinical intervention had a 7.5% decrease in total cholesterol and a 15% decrease in CHD incidence compared with subjects randomized to usual care after a 6-year follow-up (19). Therefore, a 1% reduction in serum cholesterol level yielded a 2% reduction in the risk of CHD.

Populations with higher LDL cholesterol levels have more atherosclerosis than populations with lower LDL cholesterol levels (20). To determine whether diet or genetics is a more important predictor in populations, Japanese men living in three locations were compared in the Ni-Hon-San Study (21). Dietary saturated fat intake was 7% in Japanese men living in

Japan, 12% in Japanese men living in Hawaii, and 14% in Japanese men living in San Francisco. Serum cholesterol correlated with saturated fat intake with the lowest levels in Japan and highest levels in San Francisco. Death rates from CHD were 1.7 times higher in Hawaii and 2.8 times greater in San Francisco than in Japan. Therefore, diet appears to be a more important factor than genetics.

Recent studies have shown that high cholesterol levels in early youth can predict the development of CHD later in life (22). Long-term follow-up in three prospective studies showed that increased cholesterol levels in early adulthood were associated with increased risk for CHD in middle age (22-24). In contrast, populations with total cholesterol levels less than 150 mg/dL or LDL cholesterol levels less than 100 mg/dL throughout life have almost no clinical CHD (25-27). Therefore, starting intervention for high LDL cholesterol early in life is important for prevention.

A review of numerous statin trials (3-hydroxy-3-methylglutaryl coenzyme A [HMG-CoA] reductase inhibitors) (28-30) showed that CHD mortality and total mortality were reduced with LDL cholesterol reduction. Several of these studies showed favorable changes in lesion architecture through coronary angiography with LDL cholesterol lowering. Statins were associated with reduction of CHD in both elderly and younger subjects, men and women, individuals with and without heart disease, individuals with and without diabetes, hypertensives and normotensives, and at most cholesterol levels (31).

GLOBAL RISK

In addition to LDL cholesterol level, ATP III has defined five other major risk factors to assess absolute or global risk of CHD and determine the individual's LDL cholesterol goal: cigarette smoking; hypertension (blood pressure ≥ 140/90 mm Hg or on antihypertensive medication); family history of premature CHD (male < 55 years, female < 65 years); age (men ≥ 45 years, women ≥ 55 years); and low HDL cholesterol levels (less than 40 mg/dL) (1). The evidence supporting the use of these five major risk factors to set the LDL cholesterol goal is described in the following sections.

Cigarette Smoking

Cigarette smoking is a potent contributor to risk for CHD and other forms of CVD. Estimates suggest that smokers have double or triple the risk of myocardial infarction (MI) or fatal CHD as compared with nonsmokers (32-34). The risk increases with number of cigarettes smoked each day (32). For instance, heavy smokers have six times the risk of MI or fatal CHD as compared with nonsmokers (32-34). Smoking decreases HDL cholesterol levels and increases lipid oxidation, which, in turn, leads to uptake of excess cholesterol into the arteries by scavenger receptors (35). Observational data suggest cardiovascular benefits occur within months of quitting (36). Randomized clinical trials of smoking cessation have also shown substantial reduction in risk for cardiac events in those who quit (37-39). Within 2 years of quitting, women who smoked reduced their CHD risk to levels of women who never smoked (34,40).

Hypertension

For individuals aged 40 to 70 years, the risk of CVD doubles with each increase in blood pressure of 20/10 mm Hg across blood pressure ranges from 115/75 to 185/115 mm Hg (41). A continuous relationship exists between blood pressure and risk of CVD—the higher the blood pressure, the higher the risk of MI, stroke, heart failure, and kidney disease.

The Framingham Heart Study has shown that subjects with blood pressure of 130/80 to 139/89 mm Hg are twice as likely to progress to hypertension than those with lower values (42). High normal blood pressure is associated with increased risk for CHD (43-46). On the basis of these studies, the latest Joint National Committee on Prevention, Detection, Evaluation, and Treatment of High Blood Pressure guidelines (JNC 7) introduced a new classification of prehypertension as systolic blood pressure of 120 to 139 mm Hg or diastolic blood pressure of 80 to 89 mm Hg (47). Subjects with prehypertension should be counseled on lifestyle modifications to prevent CVD. Stage 1 hypertension is defined as systolic blood pressure of 140 to 159 mm Hg or diastolic blood pressure of 90 to 99 mm Hg. Stages 2 and 3 hypertension from JNC 6 have been combined into one category in the JNC 7 report: systolic blood pressure equal to or greater than 160 mm Hg or diastolic blood pressure equal to or greater than 100 mm Hg (47).

Clinical trial evidence that blood pressure reduction decreases CHD endpoints provides further support of hypertension as a major risk factor (48-50). Antihypertensive therapy in clinical trials has been associated with a 20% to 25% reduction in MI, 35% to 40% reduction in stroke, and more than 50% reduction in heart failure (51). Estimates predict that achieving a 12-mm Hg reduction in systolic blood pressure for 10 years in patients with stage 1 hypertension will prevent one death for every 11 patients treated (52). Use of lifestyle modification and medications for control of hypertension is discussed in Chapter 8.

Family History of Premature CHD

In prospective cohort and case-control studies, family history of premature CHD is a major independent risk factor associated with increased CHD risk (53,54). CHD in a first-degree relative increases relative risk of CHD 2 to 12 times (55-57). Risk further increases with number of primary relatives affected and with younger age at onset (58,59). In contrast, the Framingham Heart Study found that family history analysis does not demonstrate sufficient incremental risk to be included in risk assessment equations (60). Many modifiable risk factors are also seen in people with premature CHD and with first-degree relatives with CHD, a finding suggesting that lifestyle factors are also important (61,62).

ATP III states that a positive family history for CHD in a first-degree relative is a major risk factor for CHD and is associated with high prevalence of modifiable risk factors. The report states that risk for CHD is higher the younger the age of onset of CHD and the greater the number of first-degree relatives with CHD. It is recommended that the presence and age of onset of CHD in all first-degree relatives be assessed. ATP III defines a positive family history as CHD or sudden death in a first-degree male relative younger than 55 years or first-degree female relative younger than 65 years (1).

HDL Cholesterol

Based on epidemiologic studies, low HDL cholesterol ($\leq$ 40 mg/dL) is an independent risk factor for CHD after adjustment for other risk variables in multivariate analysis (63,64). Conversely, high HDL cholesterol is associated with decreased risk for CHD (15,65,66). These studies have shown that a 1% decrease in HDL cholesterol yields a 2% to 3% increase in CHD risk. Some genetic forms of HDL deficiency increase the risk of CHD, whereas others do not (67-71). Genetic causes account for approximately 50% of variation in HDL cholesterol levels.

For certain populations, HDL cholesterol levels may be a better predictor for CVD than LDL cholesterol levels. For example, compared with an LDL cholesterol level less than 140 mg/dL, an LDL cholesterol level greater than 160 mg/dL is a weaker predictor of CHD risk in women age 65 years or older than in men (72). In contrast, compared with an HDL cholesterol greater than 60 mg/dL, an HDL cholesterol level less than 50 doubled the risk of death from CHD in women younger than 65 years. In addition, HDL cholesterol was the strongest predictor of CHD risk in four large epidemiologic studies (65,73-76). Furthermore, in men and women older than age 85, HDL cholesterol levels predict CHD mortality better than LDL cholesterol levels, which may be because subjects with high LDL cholesterol levels had already died from CHD (77).

Studies of mechanisms for the protective effect of HDL in genetically manipulated animals and cell culture of foam cells have shown that HDL is directly antiatherogenic by removing excess cholesterol from the arterial wall via the adenine triphosphate–binding cassette A1 transporter (ABCA1) (78-81). HDL has also been shown to have antioxidant and anti-inflammatory properties (82,83).

Low levels of HDL cholesterol are associated with other atherogenic lipid factors, such as high triglyceride levels, remnant lipoproteins, and small dense LDL. The combination is known as the lipid triad and is discussed later in this chapter. Low levels of HDL cholesterol can also be associated with insulin resistance and metabolic syndrome (see Chapter 7).

Several trials have shown that statins have more benefit in subjects with low levels of HDL cholesterol compared with subjects with higher levels of HDL cholesterol. Because statin drugs lower LDL cholesterol 30% to 50% and raise HDL cholesterol 6% to 7%, the independent clinical benefit from raising HDL cholesterol levels is difficult to determine; however, retrospective analysis of all the statin trials has shown that, among individuals on statin therapy, subjects with lower levels of HDL cholesterol had higher rates of coronary events than individuals with higher levels of HDL cholesterol. In the Lipoprotein and Coronary Atherosclerosis Study, compared with placebo, individuals on fluvastatin with HDL cholesterol levels less than 35 mg/dL had a greater reduction in angiographically measured CHD progression and more prolonged event-free survival than subjects with HDL cholesterol levels greater than 35 mg/dL (84). The Air Force Coronary Atherosclerosis Prevention Study (AFCAPS) found groups of subjects with HDL cholesterol levels below 34 mg/dL and between 35 and 39 mg/dL had approximately 45% reduction in CHD events, compared with only a 15% event-rate reduction in subjects with HDL cholesterol levels greater than 40 mg/dL (85). On the basis of these results, ATP III raised the cut point for low HDL cholesterol from less than 35 mg/dL for both men and women to less than 40 mg/dL in men and less than 50 mg/dL in women (1). If HDL cholesterol level is equal to or greater than 60 mg/dL, one risk factor is subtracted from the total number of risk factors in calculating LDL cholesterol goal. Because it is unknown whether the benefit resulting from raising HDL cholesterol occurs independently of lowering LDL cholesterol, ATP III does not define an HDL cholesterol target goal for therapy.

Age

On average, older people have more coronary atherosclerosis than younger people (15). Men develop CHD on average about 10 years younger than women; this difference is probably explained by the protective effect of estrogen in premenopausal women (86,87). Rates of CHD increase in women after menopause (whether surgical or natural). For these reasons, ATP III defines advancing age as a major independent risk factor and recommends that age 45 years or older in men and 55 years or older in women should count as a risk factor in determining an LDL cholesterol goal in primary prevention (1).

Subgroup analyses by age (using cut points of 65 or 55 years) in statin trials have shown that the benefits for older subjects of LDL cholesterol levels are equivalent to the benefits for younger adults (85,88-93). The Prospective Study of Pravastatin in the Elderly at Risk (PROSPER) trial was the first statin trial to examine exclusively subjects between the ages of 70 and 82 years. In this study, 2,804 men and 3,000 women were randomized to pravastatin 40 mg/day or placebo (89). Established vascular disease was present in 44.2% of the subjects, whereas 55.8% had no known disease but had risk factors of smoking, hypertension, or diabetes. At an average follow-up of 3.2 years, men taking pravastatin had a 23% decrease in the combined endpoint of coronary death, nonfatal MI, and fatal or nonfatal stroke, whereas women taking pravastatin had no benefit (89). Subjects with established vascular disease who took pravastatin had a 24% reduction in events, whereas there was no benefit in primary prevention from taking the medication. Of note, new diagnoses of cancer were 25% higher in subjects on pravastatin than in subjects taking a placebo ($P = .02$). This raises the question of whether older adults may be more susceptible to the immunosuppressive effects of statin drugs in terms of cancer development and highlights the need for more trials in older subjects. For subjects older than 85 years, a recent study by Weverling et al (77) showed that low HDL cholesterol level was a better predictor of CVD death than LDL cholesterol levels. Low HDL cholesterol levels were associated with a two- to threefold increased risk of death from CVD in male and female subjects older than age 85 years with low HDL cholesterol levels (32 to 40 mg/dL). These findings raise the question of whether efforts to lower LDL cholesterol are appropriate for this age group.

Other Modifiable Risk Factors

Overweight, sedentary lifestyle, and atherogenic diet are all modifiable risk factors. Although they do not count as major risk factors in determining an individual's LDL cholesterol goal, they can contribute to the presence and severity of the five major risk factors.

Overweight and Obesity

Obesity is defined as a body mass index (BMI) of 30 or higher, and overweight is defined as a BMI of 25 to 29.9. Both of these conditions predispose patients to CHD, stroke, and greater all-cause mortality. Being overweight or obese causes high levels of other CHD risk factors, such as dyslipidemia (94,95), type 2 diabetes (96,97), low HDL cholesterol (98), and hypertension (99). The risk for CVD is especially high when abdominal obesity is present (waist circumference > 102 cm [40 in] in men or 88 cm [35 in] in women) (100,101). Abdominal obesity and its related risk factors are now recognized as part of metabolic syndrome.

Sedentary Lifestyle

Physical inactivity has been shown to increase risk for CHD, whereas physical activity favorably modifies LDL cholesterol levels, triglyceride levels, and HDL cholesterol levels and improves blood pressure and insulin sensitivity (102-105). Sedentary lifestyles lead to decreased energy expenditure, which causes obesity, which, in turn, is associated with other CVD risk factors, such as hypertension, low HDL cholesterol levels, and insulin resistance. Although most evidence that physical activity reduces risk comes from observational studies (106-111), the recent randomized Diabetes Prevention Program (DPP) supports the hypothesis that increased physical activity decreases the risk for type 2 diabetes (112). In this trial, subjects were randomized to placebo, metformin (850 mg/day), or lifestyle modification which included an average of 150 minutes of physical activity per week and an average of 7% weight loss. After an average follow-up of 2.8 years, the incidence of type 2 diabetes, a major risk factor for CVD, was decreased 58% in those randomized to lifestyle changes and 31% those randomized to metformin as compared with placebo (112).

ATP III defines physical inactivity as a major modifiable risk factor for CHD but does not include it as a risk factor for determining an individual's LDL cholesterol goal because inactivity is collinear with many risk factors and therefore is not an independent predictor. ATP III defines activity as the major intervention for sedentary lifestyle (1).

Atherogenic Diet

A dietary pattern that includes fruits, vegetables, and lean meats is associated with reduced CHD risk (113,114). Intake of *trans* fatty acids in baked goods and foods fried in partially hydrogenated oils is associated with increased CHD risk (115). When the most atherogenic components of the diet are defined by their LDL-raising abilities, saturated and *trans* fatty acids are identified as the dietary villains (1). (See Chapter 6.) Recent research into beneficial compounds has produced a number of functional foods (see Chapter 10).

CHD RISK EQUIVALENTS

ATP III enumerates CHD risk equivalents, factors that confer a risk of CHD events similar to that in persons with established coronary artery disease, which is 2% per year. In autopsy studies, atherosclerosis in one arterial region predicts atherosclerosis in other regions. Risk factors are similar for atherosclerosis in the coronary, peripheral, and carotid arteries. Risk equivalents include other clinical atherosclerotic disease (symptomatic carotid disease, peripheral vascular disease [PVD], or abdominal aortic aneurysm [AAA]), diabetes mellitus, and multiple risk factors that confer greater than 20% risk of heart disease within 10 years (as assessed by the Framingham risk assessment criteria). The LDL cholesterol goal for these risk equivalents is identical to that for clinical CHD: less than 100 mg/dL. The LDL cholesterol level at which drug therapy is started is also similar for CHD: greater than 130 mg/dL (1). The evidence supporting these risk equivalents follows.

Diabetes

ATP III defines diabetes (a fasting glucose ≥ of 126 mg/dL) as a risk equivalent for CHD (1). Several lines of evidence support this concept. First, both persons with type 1 and those with type 2 diabetes have a high risk of new CHD within 10 years, which approximates the risk in patients with known CHD but no diabetes (116-118). The relative risk (but not absolute risk) in women with diabetes exceeds that in men with diabetes (118).

Second, absolute risk for first major coronary events in persons with type 2 diabetes is similar to that for recurrent MI in persons without diabetes but with a prior MI. In Finland, the 7-year incidence of MI in persons with type 2 diabetes with no known CHD (20.2%) approximated that for recurrent MI in nondiabetic subjects with prior MI (18.8%) (119). Thus, in persons with type 2 diabetes without prior CHD, the risk for MI is as great as it is for persons without diabetes with prior MI (119). In the Organization to Assess Strategies for Ischemic Syndromes registry, the rates of CHD events in persons with type 2 diabetes were similar to those of persons with established CHD (120). Furthermore, in the Heart Outcomes Prevention Evaluation Study, subjects with type 2 diabetes without prior CVD, but with one additional risk factor, had a 2.5% annual event rate for CHD (equivalent to a 10-year risk of 25%) (121). In the United Kingdom Prospective Diabetes Study (UKPDS) of subjects with type 2 diabetes, the absolute 10-year risk for hard CHD was 15% to 20% (122-124). These subjects were less obese on average than individuals with type 2 diabetes in the United States. When

TABLE 3.2
Benefits of Lowering LDL Cholesterol among Individuals with Diabetes

Study	Results Comparing Statin with Placebo
Primary Prevention	
AFCAPS (85)	43% reduction in CHD risk
Secondary Prevention	
4 S (137)	55% reduction in CHD risk
CARE (93)	25% decrease in CHD risk
Heart Protection Study (146)	20% reduction coronary mortality
	30% reduction in major vascular events for those without occlusive disease and LDL <116 mg/dL

Abbreviations: CHD, coronary heart disease; LDL, low-density lipoprotein.

UKPDS considered individuals with BMIs greater than 30, 10-year risk exceeded 20%. These trial results support the concept that people with diabetes without clinical CHD have a CHD risk equivalent to people with known CHD.

Third, CHD mortality rates after MI are higher in patients with type 2 diabetes than in patients without diabetes (66,125,126). Fourth, overall prognosis for survival is much worse for persons with type 2 diabetes once they develop CHD than in patients with known CHD but without diabetes (119,127-132).

Subjects with type 1 diabetes have an increased risk for CHD (133,134); however, no study has reported whether subjects with type 1 diabetes have a CHD risk similar to that for age- and sex-matched nondiabetic subjects with clinical CHD. Such a study would be difficult to perform because subjects often develop type 1 diabetes at an early age when their contemporaries have no CHD. ATP III recommends that recent-onset type 1 diabetes is not a CHD risk equivalent and reduction of LDL cholesterol to less than 130 mg/dL is sufficient. However, an LDL cholesterol goal less than 100 mg/dL should be considered as duration of type 1 diabetes increases (1).

Part of the increased risk for CHD in diabetes results from the major risk factors (116,135). Management of these risk factors (blood pressure, cholesterol, and triglyceride lowering) has been shown to reduce the risk of a coronary event in patients with diabetes (85,91,124,136-141). The risk attributed to hyperglycemia is independent of being obese or overweight. Some studies have shown a strong association between glycemia and CHD in type 2 diabetes (142), whereas others have shown a weak association (143) or no association (144). A trend toward benefit of controlling glucose has been shown but is not yet definitive (122,123,145).

Classification of diabetes as a CHD risk equivalent implies that benefit should be achieved by lowering LDL cholesterol levels. AFCAPS, a primary prevention trial, showed a 43% reduction in CHD risk in patients with diabetes on statin compared with placebo (85). Secondary prevention trials of statin drugs have also shown benefit in diabetes. Results are summarized in Table 3.2 (85,93,137,146).

Clinical Forms of Noncoronary Atherosclerosis

In addition to risk factors associated with atherosclerosis, ATP III enumerates clinical atherosclerotic diseases that confer a CHD risk equivalent. These include peripheral arterial disease (PAD), symptomatic carotid artery disease, and AAA.

Peripheral Arterial Disease

The conclusion that atherosclerosis in peripheral arteries, carotids, and abdominal aorta represents a CHD risk equivalent is based on prospective studies. At least five studies of persons with PAD have provided data on CHD mortality rates based on the ankle-brachial blood pressure index (ABI) measured at baseline. ABI is an inexpensive, noninvasive, measurement of systolic blood pressure measured by Doppler probe in brachial, posterior tibial, and dorsalis pedis arteries. An ABI of 0.9 or less in either leg is considered PAD. Findings from prospective studies of those with an ABI less than 0.85 to 0.9 include the following: CHD event rates per year were 2.4% in a 5-year follow-up in the Edinburgh study (147), 2.9% in women without baseline CHD and 3.0% in women with baseline CHD during the 4-year follow-up in the Multicenter Study of Osteoporotic Fracture (148), and 6% during 3-year follow-up in another study (149). In a 10-year follow-up of subjects without baseline CHD in the LRC San Diego cohort, annual CHD mortality rates were 2.5% in men with PVD compared with 0.4% in men without PVD (150). In contrast, rates in women with PVD were 0.4% compared with 0.2% in women without PVD, a finding opposite that observed in the Edinburgh study. Poulias et al (151) observed a 2.4% annual CHD mortality rate at an average follow-up of 8 years following aortofemoral bypass. These studies support an annual risk of CHD of at least 2% in those with PVD. ABI can be considered a diagnostic test to identify people with a CHD risk equivalent of at least 2% per year, which equates to a 10-year risk of at least 20% and, thus, would support an LDL cholesterol goal less than 100 mg/dL.

Carotid Artery Disease

Carotid disease can be symptomatic (transient ischemic attack or stroke of carotid origin) or asymptomatic (stenosis > 50%). In a cohort of 1,415 symptomatic patients randomized to carotid endarterectomy, 10-year CHD death rate was 19% (152). Because coronary mortality is usually two to three times that of major coronary events, 10-year CHD event rates could be estimated at 38% to 57%. Therefore, the high CHD mortality rate in this trial is indicative of a CHD risk equivalent. In the European Carotid Surgery Trial (ECST), symptomatic patients had a 10-year CHD death rate estimated at 30% regardless of the baseline percentage carotid artery stenosis (153).

High CHD event rates have been observed in asymptomatic patients with carotid bruits and a carotid stenosis greater than 50%. In the Asymptomatic Carotid Atherosclerosis Study (ACAS) of 1,662 patients randomized to carotid surgery or medical management (154), 10-year CHD mortality was 19% if stenosis was equal to or greater than 60%. Asymptomatic stenosis equal to or greater than 50% was associated with a 10-year CHD mortality of 51% in the Veterans Affairs Cooperative Study Group of 444 men (155). In the Carotid Artery Stenosis with Asymptomatic Narrowing: Operation Versus Aspirin study of 410 patients with asymptomatic stenosis equal to or greater than 50%, 10-year CHD mortality was 35% (156). In the Mayo Asymptomatic Carotid Endarterectomy Study of 158 patients, the 10-year CHD event rate was 30% (157). The high CHD event and mortality rates in these trials provide support for identifying symptomatic carotid disease and asymptomatic carotid disease with a greater than 50% stenosis as a CHD risk equivalent.

Abdominal Aortic Aneurysm

Hertzer (158) separated 343 persons undergoing AAA resection into four groups on the basis of preoperative history of coronary disease. At average follow-up of 6 to 11 years, annual CHD mortality rates were 1.9% in those with no CHD at baseline and 3.9% in those with prior MI.

Because the CHD event rate is at least twice that of CHD mortality rates, even those without CHD at AAA resection would be in the category of CHD risk equivalent.

EMERGING RISK FACTORS

The major risk factors account for about half of the variability in CHD risk in the United States (1); therefore, research to identify new risk factors is important. The discussion below evaluates emerging risk factors against the following criteria: (*a*) predictive power independent of other major risk factors; (*b*) high prevalence in the population; (*c*) widely available, standardized, inexpensive laboratory or clinical measurement with accepted population values and biological stability; and (*d*) reduction in risk through modification of the risk factor in clinical trials. Emerging risk factors could become major risk factors in the future, and this search for new risk factors will enhance the power to predict CHD.

Emerging Lipid Risk Factors

Triglycerides

Atherogenic triglyceride-rich lipoproteins are small very-low-density lipoprotein (VLDL) and intermediate-density lipoprotein remnant particles. These particles are the main triglyceride carriers in plasma and have been shown to be atherogenic in animal models (159,160) and in human beings (161). Clinical studies specifically identifying remnants showed that when remnants accumulate, CHD is produced (161-169). People with no major risk factors tend to have serum triglyceride less than 100 mg/dL (170), and as major risk factors develop, triglyceride levels rise to 150 mg/dL or above.

Prospective epidemiologic studies have shown a positive relationship between triglyceride levels and CHD. In a meta-analysis of 11 studies, the relative risk for the development of CVD with an 88.5 mg/dL (1 mmol/liter) increase in triglycerides was 1.12 for males and 1.37 for females after adjustment for HDL cholesterol levels (171). The Prospective Cardiovascular Munster Study showed that, in 4,849 middle-aged men followed up for 8 years, triglycerides were an independent risk factor for CHD, autonomous from LDL or HDL cholesterol levels (172). In a 10-year follow-up of the Atherosclerosis Risk in Communities Study, elevated triglycerides significantly increased the risk of CHD 29% in women after adjusting for age, race, LDL cholesterol level, and HDL cholesterol level; however, triglyceride levels were not an independent predictor in men (173). Hypertriglyceridemia is rarely seen in isolation but is associated with low HDL cholesterol levels, an increase in small dense LDL particles, abdominal obesity, hypertension, insulin resistance, elevated apo B, and the prothrombotic state, all of which increase risk for CHD, and all of which are components of metabolic syndrome (161).

Small Dense LDL Particles

LDL particles are divided into seven classes based on size and density. The larger sized LDL particles, class 1 (1.019 to 1.033 g/mL, 26 to 28.5 nm) and classes 2 and 3 (1.033 to 1.038 g/mL, 25.5 to 26.4 nm) are associated with a healthy lipid profile (174-176). Small LDL particles are classes 4 and 5 (1.038 to 1.050 g/mL, 24.2 to 25.5 nm) and classes 6 and 7 (1.050 to 1.063 g/mL, 22 to 24.1 nm) and have been identified as part of atherogenic dyslipidemia. They are usually formed in response to high levels of triglycerides. Their presence is associated with increased risk for CHD, but their ability to predict independently of other risk factors is unknown, primarily because of their strong correlation with triglyceride levels (177). In addition, there are no inexpensive methods for measurement. Therefore, ATP III does not recommend measurement of small LDL particles in routine practice. Triglyceride level is the best predictor of small dense LDL particles (176).

Atherogenic Dyslipidemia

The combination of elevated triglycerides, small LDL particles, and reduced HDL cholesterol levels is called "atherogenic dyslipidemia" and is common in people with premature CHD (178). Many people with type 2 diabetes have this type of dyslipidemia (179-181). There is a strong trend toward reduction in risk of CHD with treatment of atherogenic dyslipidemia. Most therapies that lower triglyceride levels or raise HDL cholesterol levels modify all components of the dyslipidemia. Weight reduction (100,101), physical activity (182), fibrates, and nicotinic acid specifically improve all components of atherogenic dyslipidemia (183-186). Both primary and secondary prevention trials with fibric acid derivatives, niacin, or both have shown a reduction in CHD risk (90,187-190). Three trials of fibrate therapy have shown coronary atherosclerosis, as assessed by angiography, to be reduced without reducing LDL cholesterol (191-193). Two trials of combined drug therapy have looked at changes in lumen diameter, one targeting LDL and one targeting atherogenic dyslipidemia, and both produced favorable changes (194-196). ATP III recommends lifestyle modification, weight control, and increased physical activity for treatment of atherogenic dyslipidemia. For higher risk patients, ATP III recommends treatment with specific drug therapy such as fibrates and nicotinic acid. ATP III does not recommend triglyceride levels as a direct target for therapy because of their high fluctuation (1).

Metabolic Syndrome

The simultaneous presence of high triglyceride levels, low HDL cholesterol levels, diabetes, obesity, and hypertension was first noted in the late 1960s (197). The combination of these risk factors was designated metabolic syndrome, and the association with atherosclerosis was first described in 1977 (198,199). The diagnosis of metabolic syndrome is becoming increasingly more important and more common. Individuals with metabolic syndrome are usually overweight or obese, particularly in the abdominal area (200-202). The borderline high (150 to 199 mg/dL) and high ($\geq$ 200 mg/dL) triglyceride levels seen in metabolic syndrome are highly correlated with abdominal obesity. The elevated triglyceride levels are in turn accompanied by low HDL cholesterol levels ($<$ 40 mg/dL) (203). Low HDL cholesterol levels are commonly found in men with insulin resistance, and a marginal reduction of HDL cholesterol is also found in women with insulin resistance (204). A strong association exists between insulin resistance and hypertension or high normal blood pressure. Fasting serum glucose levels of 100 to 125 mg/dL have been defined as indicative of impaired glucose tolerance (205). Such levels usually indicate insulin resistance and are usually accompanied by other metabolic risk factors (206,207). Metabolic syndrome is also associated with a prothrombotic state and proinflammatory state and closely associated with insulin resistance, abdominal obesity, and a genetic predisposition (200,201,208-213).

The recent identification of monogenic forms of insulin resistance has provided important insight into the mechanisms of metabolic syndrome. Peroxisome proliferator-activated receptor (PPAR)-gamma is a member of the nuclear hormone receptor superfamily that is expressed at high levels in adipose tissue, monocytes or macrophages, and colon. By regulating the transcription of target genes in response to a variety of naturally occurring lipid-based molecules (polyunsaturated fatty acids, 13-[S]-hydroxyoctadecadienoic acid [HODE] and 9-HODE), PPAR-gamma regulates adipose tissue function, the differentiation of preadipocytes to mature fat cells, glucose metabolism, and blood pressure in human beings. Rare mutations in PPAR-gamma are associated with the features of metabolic syndrome including insulin resistance, dyslipidemia, and hypertension (214,215). With defective PPAR-gamma, adipo-cytes overproduce the cytokines, tumor necrosis factor alpha (TNF-α), and interleukin-1 (IL-1), which leads to insulin resistance. Angiotensin, the most potent vasoconstrictor known, is also produced by adipocytes and can lead to hypertension. Increased plasminogen activator inhibitor (PAI-1) production by the adipocyte leads to thrombus formation. Free fatty acids from the diet provide fuel to these cells and increase production of the aforementioned products.

Human autosomal dominant familial partial lipodystrophy (FPLD), which is characterized by insulin resistance, dyslipidemia, and hypertension, occurs with nuclear lamin A/C mutations (216) and is associated with premature atherosclerosis (217) and elevated levels of C-reactive protein (CRP) and free fatty acids (218). PPAR-gamma mutations have also been associated with FPLD (219,220). Future research on the genetic causes of metabolic syndrome may provide further important information on the pathophysiology and mechanisms of the syndrome.

Recent prospective studies demonstrate a high mortality risk in metabolic syndrome. During 11.4-year follow-up of a population-based, prospective cohort study of 1,209 Finnish men aged 42 to 60 years and without CVD at baseline, those with metabolic syndrome were almost three times more likely to die of CHD after adjustment for cardiovascular risk factors (221). Metabolic syndrome is considered equal to cigarette smoking as a contributor to premature heart disease (15,100,101,220-224). In addition, the insulin resistance found with metabolic syndrome is one of the underlying causes of type 2 diabetes, which is a CHD risk equivalent.

Metabolic syndrome may affect the prevalence of CHD in patients with diabetes. In a recent analysis of the Third National Health and Nutrition Examination Survey data (NHANES III) (225), 44% of adults older than 50 years had metabolic syndrome. Although diabetes is present without metabolic syndrome in only 13% of this population, the absence of metabolic syndrome may offer some protection against CHD. As shown below in Table 3.3 (225), the presence of metabolic syndrome is associated with greater CHD in individuals with diabetes and in those without.

ATP III indicates that the presence of metabolic syndrome accentuates risk accompanying elevated LDL cholesterol levels and appears to be mediated through multiple risk factors (major and emerging). ATP III defines metabolic syndrome as three or more of the following:

TABLE 3.3
Prevalence of Coronary Heart Disease Related to Metabolic Syndrome and Diabetes

	Without Diabetes	With Diabetes
Without metabolic syndrome	8.7%	7.5%
With metabolic syndrome	13.9%	19.2%

Source: Data are from reference 225.

- Abdominal obesity (waist circumference ≥ 40 inches [> 102 cm] for men, ≥ 35 inches [> 88 cm] for women)
- Triglyceride level equal to or greater than 150 mg/dL
- HDL less than 40 mg/dL in men (atherogenic dyslipidemia), less than 50 mg/dL in women
- Blood pressure of 130/85 mm Hg or higher
- Elevated fasting glucose (> 110 mg/dL in ATP III, but now defined as > 100 mg/dL) (1,205).

These criteria are also outlined in Table 7.1 in Chapter 7. ATP III suggests two approaches to treatment: (a) modification of the root causes by encouraging weight reduction and increased physical activity, both of which lower insulin resistance and indirectly lower metabolic risk factors, and (b) direct treatment of metabolic factors (atherogenic dyslipidemia, hypertension, prothrombotic state, insulin resistance) with pharmacologic modification of associated risk factors. Support for increased physical activity in decreasing conversion of impaired glucose tolerance to diabetes comes from the DPP discussed earlier in this chapter (112) and the Finnish Diabetes Prevention Study (226). Clinical trials also show that modifying the three major components (atherogenic dyslipidemia, hypertension, and prothrombotic state) reduces risk for CHD (47). See Chapter 7 for further discussion of metabolic syndrome in the clinical setting.

Non-HDL Cholesterol

Non-HDL cholesterol is defined as the sum of VLDL cholesterol and LDL cholesterol and is calculated as total cholesterol minus HDL cholesterol. It includes all apo B–containing lipoproteins, and, as a result, non-HDL cholesterol is highly correlated with total apo B and can function as an acceptable surrogate marker for apo B (227,228). When serum triglycerides are high, non-HDL cholesterol may predict risk better than LDL cholesterol alone because non-HDL cholesterol includes VLDL, the main triglyceride carrier in circulation, which is likely elevated in such a case. VLDL may be a marker for CHD because triglyceride-rich VLDL lipoprotein remnants are atherogenic particles. Frost et al (229) have suggested that the use of non-HDL cholesterol is superior to LDL cholesterol in assessment of CHD risk. A recent article from a follow-up of the Lipid Research Clinic cohort showed a stronger correlation between non-HDL cholesterol and coronary mortality than between LDL cholesterol and coronary mortality (230). When triglyceride levels are greater than 1,000 mg/dL, chylomicrons are elevated and non-HDL cholesterol is less of a predictor of CHD (227,228). No lipid-lowering trials have randomized hypertriglyceridemic patients on the basis of non-HDL cholesterol levels; therefore, the reduction of risk from lowering of non-HDL cholesterol is unknown. ATP III identifies non-HDL cholesterol as a secondary target for therapy if triglyceride levels are greater than 200 mg/dL after LDL cholesterol goal is reached (1).

Lipoprotein (a)

Lipoprotein (a) [Lp(a)] is an additional protein found on LDL in some people. Several studies have found a strong association of Lp(a) and CHD (231-234), whereas other prospective studies have not shown an independent prediction (235,236). In the Familial Atherosclerosis Treatment Study, 146 men with coronary artery disease (CAD) were randomized to the combination of lovastatin, colestipol, and niacin vs placebo for 2.5 years (237). In 40 patients with

Lp(a) level at or above the 90th percentile, those with an LDL cholesterol reduction greater than 10% had an event rate of 9%, compared with 36% in those with LDL cholesterol reduction less than 10%. The best correlate of baseline CAD severity was the Lp(a) level. Estrogen and niacin are the only two drugs that lower levels of Lp(a) (238-240). Estrogen may be harmful, and niacin is not well tolerated. In addition, issues related to measurement have not been resolved. The immunologic assay is standardized in only a few laboratories and is not established in hospital clinical chemistry labs, so samples must be sent to specialized laboratories. Therefore, until results of randomized trials lowering Lp(a) levels are available, the best course of treatment is lowering LDL cholesterol to goal in patients with CHD. ATP III suggests that a high Lp(a) may justify a lower LDL cholesterol goal and that Lp(a) measurement be limited to people with family history of premature CHD or genetic causes of hypercholesterolemia (1). At the Beth Israel Deaconess Lipid Clinic, Lp(a) is measured in subjects with CHD who have no other risk factors.

Emerging Nonlipid Risk Factors

Homocysteine

People with inherited forms of homocysteinemia have premature vascular injury and atherosclerosis (241). In observational studies, elevations of homocysteine have been shown to be positively correlated with CHD risk (241-248). Randomized trials to determine whether lowering homocysteine levels with folic acid lowers risk of CHD are under way. A randomized double blind placebo-controlled trial of 553 subjects assigned to a combined treatment ($n = 272$) of folic acid (1 mg/day), vitamin B-12 (cyanocobalamin, 400 μg/day), and vitamin B-6 (pyridoxine hydrochloride, 10 mg/day), or placebo ($n = 281$) for 6 months after percutaneous transluminal coronary angioplasty (PTCA) showed that adverse cardiovascular endpoints were significantly reduced in subjects on folic acid (249). In an open-label trial, 593 patients with CHD were randomized to 0.5 mg folic acid or control; all subjects were on statins (250). At mean follow-up of 24 months, homocysteine levels were lowered 18% (from 12 to 9.4 mg/dL); however, all-cause mortality and a composite of vascular events were not significantly different in subjects on folic acid compared with the control group (10.3% vs 9.6%, respectively; relative risk: 1.05; 95% confidence interval: 0.63 to 1.75).

The American Heart Association recommends supplemental folic acid to patients with high homocysteine levels (242). ATP III does not recommend routine measurement of homocysteine as part of assessment to modify LDL cholesterol levels because of uncertainty about the strength of relation with CHD (1). Measurement is an option for cases with a strong family history of premature CHD. If a person is otherwise at low risk, ATP III recommends treating with B vitamins and folic acid because treatment is safe and inexpensive. Breakfast cereals, broccoli, oranges, flour, and multivitamins have high amounts of folic acid. Issues related to folate and homocysteine levels are also discussed in Chapters 6 and 11.

Thrombogenic and Hemostatic Factors

Platelets and coagulation factors are involved in the thrombotic process that can lead to MI. Aspirin and antiplatelet therapy reduce risk and show that hyperaggregability can predispose to CHD (251-253). Also, fibrinogen has been associated with increased risk independent of cholesterol level because low fibrinogen indicates reduced risk even with high total cholesterol levels. Other prothrombotic factors that have been associated with CHD include von Willebrand factor, factor V Leiden, protein C, and antithrombin III. Some of these factors are elevated with metabolic syndrome; therefore, lifestyle changes may reverse metabolic syndrome and reduce serum levels of prothrombotic factors.

ATP III does not recommend measurement of prothrombotic factors as routine measurement of CHD risk because the strength of association has not been defined and specific intervention, other than aspirin, is not available (1). Clinical trials targeting specific factors have not been conducted. In addition, the laboratory measurements for these factors are not standardized.

Inflammatory Markers: CRP

Because atherosclerosis is a chronic inflammatory process, it makes sense that inflammatory markers would be increased in subjects with atherosclerosis. Recent articles indicate that serum levels of CRP are predictive of coronary events (254-259). Smoking is associated with increased CRP levels. Obesity and metabolic syndrome are also commonly accompanied by increases in CRP, so there is likely a relationship between metabolic factors and inflammation.

High-sensitivity (hs)-CRP may have independent predictive power beyond lipid risk factors (258). A randomized trial is currently under way to determine whether lowering CRP with rosuvastatin decreases CHD events in primary prevention. Statin drugs and aspirin lower CRP, and in secondary prevention both should be prescribed; therefore, measurement of CRP is not indicated. Indications for measurement of CRP in primary prediction will be clearer when the results of the randomized trial are available.

Impaired Fasting Glucose

Some investigators view impaired fasting glucose as an independent risk factor (260,261), but the strong association between impaired fasting glucose, insulin resistance, and other risk factors of metabolic syndrome lends doubt to its independent predictive power (262-264). The Framingham Heart Study showed that the association between plasma glucose and CHD risk is a continuous variable (260). As a result, ATP III defines impaired fasting glucose as one component of metabolic syndrome that signifies need for lifestyle therapies (weight loss and physical activity) (1).

ASSESSING THE PATIENT AND LABORATORY MEASUREMENTS

ATP III (1) outlines ten steps to assess CHD risk in patients, determine their LDL cholesterol goals, and establish treatment and follow-up plans.

Step 1: Lipid Measurements

ATP III guidelines recommend that a 9- to 12-hour fasting complete lipid profile be determined in adults age 20 and older every 5 years. This profile should include total cholesterol, HDL, and triglyceride levels. When the triglyceride level is less than 400 mg/dL, LDL cholesterol can be calculated using the Friedewald equation: **LDL cholesterol = Total cholesterol – HDL cholesterol – (triglyceride/5)**. When the triglyceride level is greater than 400 mg/dL, the level of LDL cholesterol must be measured directly. Glucose levels should also be measured to assess for the presence of diabetes or metabolic syndrome. In patients with hyperlipidemia, it is important to rule out secondary causes of high cholesterol because such causes may necessitate treatment other than lipid-lowering drugs. Major causes include hypothyroidism, diabetes, multiple myeloma, and obstructive liver disease. Laboratory values that are important in assessing these secondary causes include thyroid stimulating hormone, fasting glucose, serum

TABLE 3.4
Treatment According to Risk Category

Risk Category	LDL Cholesterol Goal	LDL Cholesterol Level at Which to Initiate TLC	LDL Cholesterol Level at Which to Consider Drug Therapy	
			ATP III	Update
CHD or CHD risk equivalents (10-year risk >20%)	<100 mg/dL*	≥100 mg/dL	≥130 mg/dL	≥100 mg/dL[†]
2+ risk factors (10-year risk 10%–20%)	<130 mg/dL	≥130 mg/dL	≥130 mg/dL	≥130 mg/dL[‡]
2+ risk factors (10-year risk <10%)	<130 mg/dL	≥130 mg/dL	≥160 mg/dL	≥160 mg/dL
0–1 risk factor	<160 mg/dL	≥160 mg/dL	≥190 mg/dL	≥190 mg/dL

Abbreviations: CHD, coronary heart disease; LDL, low-density lipoprotein; TLC, Therapeutic Lifestyle Changes.

*As this book went to press, a July 2004 update to ATP III (265) recommended an optimal goal of lowering LDL cholesterol to less than 70 mg/dL in high-risk patients.

[†]Consider drug options at <100 mg/dL.

[‡]Consider drug options at 100 to 129 mg/dL.

Source: Adapted from references 1 and 265.

and urine protein electrophoresis, aspartate aminotransferase (AST), alanine aminotransferase (ALT), and alkaline phosphatase.

Step 2: Identify Clinical CHD or Risk Equivalent

Taking a careful history for the presence of angina pectoris, history of MI, diabetes, transient ischemic attack, or pain in the calves or thighs with exercise (claudication) is most important in determining whether clinical atherosclerosis is present. If any of these are present, the LDL cholesterol goal is less than 100 mg/dL (refer to Table 3.4) (1).

Step 3: Determine Presence of Major Risk Factors (Other than LDL Cholesterol)

When determining a patient's LDL cholesterol goal, the number of major risk factors—cigarette smoking, hypertension, low HDL cholesterol level, family history of premature CHD, and age—should be counted (refer to Table 3.4 [1,265]). Smoking, family history, and age can be obtained from the history. If HDL cholesterol is greater than 60 mg/dL (measured as in step 1 above), one risk factor is subtracted. During the physical exam, blood pressure, height, weight, and waist circumference should be measured and BMI calculated.

Blood pressure should be measured using the auscultatory method with a properly calibrated and validated cuff that encircles at least 80% of the arm (266). Patients should be seated quietly in a chair (rather than on an exam table) for at least 5 minutes with feet on the floor and arm supported at heart level. At least two measurements should be made. Systolic blood pressure is the point at which the first of two or more sounds is heard (phase 1). Diastolic blood pressure is the point before disappearance of sounds (phase 5).

Routine laboratory tests recommended for the evaluation of hypertension include urinalysis, blood glucose, hematocrit, serum potassium, creatinine (or estimated glomerular filtration rate), calcium, and electrocardiogram. The JNC 7 guidelines state that urinary albumin excretion is optional; however, it should be performed in patients with diabetes (47). Ninety percent of cases of hypertension result from essential hypertension where no identifiable cause is apparent. If blood pressure control is not achieved, identifiable causes of hypertension should be considered. Causes include sleep apnea, drugs (nonsteroidal anti-inflammatory drugs, cyclooxygenase 2 inhibitors, cocaine, amphetamines, decongestants, anorectics, oral contraceptives, cyclosporine and tacrolimus, erythropoietin, licorice, and over-the-counter dietary supplements [ephedra, ma haung, and bitter orange]), chronic kidney disease, primary aldosteronism, renovascular disease, chronic steroid therapy or Cushing syndrome, pheochromocytoma, aortic coarctation, and thyroid or parathyroid disease.

Metabolic syndrome should also be assessed at the initial visit. Initial treatment is implementing Therapeutic Lifestyle Changes (TLC) as described in ATP III (1). Because weight loss can take time, it is important to counsel the patient as early as possible to increase physical activity and change diet in an attempt to lose weight. Small, realistic weight loss goals are important. Weight loss of 5% to 10% of body weight has been shown to be beneficial (112). Because the presence of abdominal obesity is more highly correlated with high triglycerides, low HDL cholesterol levels, increased blood pressure, and elevated fasting glucose than is BMI (200), ATP III recommends use of waist circumference measurement to identify the body weight component of metabolic syndrome (1).

Steps 4 and 5: Determine Risk Category and Establish LDL Cholesterol Goal

Determining a patient's CHD risk category is necessary to identify the LDL cholesterol goal (see Table 3.4) (1). Calculation of a 10-year CHD risk using the Framingham risk scores (refer to Table 3.5) allows more precise differentiation of an appropriate LDL cholesterol goal (1).

- For people with low risk (<2 risk factors), the 10-year risk assessment is not needed.
- For people with two or more risk factors, the 10-year risk assessment yields one of three levels of 10-year risk: (a) less than 10%; (b) 10% to 20%; or (c) greater than 20%.

For a 10-year risk less than 10%, the LDL cholesterol threshold at which to start drug therapy is greater than 160 mg/dL. For a 10-year risk of 10% to 20%, ATP III indicates drug therapy when LDL cholesterol is greater than 130 mg/dL. However, a July 2004 update to ATP III (265) includes drug therapy as an option for LDL cholesterol between 100 and 129 mg/dL. Those with a risk greater than 20% are placed in the same category as subjects with established CHD, and the LDL cholesterol goal is less than 100 mg/dL according to ATP III (1) and less than 70 mg/dL according to the ATP III update (265).

Step 6: Initiate TLC if LDL Cholesterol Is Above Goal

Once a patient's risk category is determined and the LDL cholesterol goal is established, the need for TLC or drug consideration is assessed. If the patient's current LDL cholesterol level is above the goal level, then TLC therapy is initiated. The TLC diet consists of less than 7% of energy from saturated fat and less than 200 mg of cholesterol per day, increased soluble (viscous) fiber (10 to 25 g/day), and plant stanol or sterols (2 g/day) to enhance LDL lowering (1). Weight management is encouraged both through diet and increased physical activity. (See Chapter 6 for further discussion of TLC.)

Step 7: Consider Adding Drug Therapy If LDL Cholesterol Exceeds Threshold Levels

Drug therapy is often started simultaneously with TLC for patients with CHD, diabetes, and CHD risk equivalents. After at least 3 months of TLC, if LDL cholesterol does not reach the level indicated in Table 3.4, consider adding drug therapy to TLC. TLC therapy should complement drug therapy and should be continually encouraged. Common drug classes are the statins, bile acid sequestrants, nicotinic acid, and fibric acids. One class may be sufficient, but

TABLE 3.5
Estimate of 10-Year CHD Risk (Framingham Point Scores)

Women

Age, y	Points
20–34	−7
35–39	−3
40–44	0
45–49	3
50–54	6
55–59	8
60–64	10
65–69	12
70–74	14
75–79	16

	Points				
Total Cholesterol, mg/dL	Age 20–39 y	Age 40–49 y	Age 50–59 y	Age 60–69 y	Age 70–79 y
<160	0	0	0	0	0
160–199	4	3	2	1	1
200–239	8	6	4	2	1
240–279	11	8	5	3	2
≥280	13	10	7	4	2

	Points				
	Age 20–39 y	Age 40–49 y	Age 50–59 y	Age 60–69 y	Age 70–79 y
Nonsmoker	0	0	0	0	0
Smoker	9	7	4	2	1

HDL, mg/dL	Points
≥60	−1
50–59	0
40–49	1
<40	2

Systolic BP, mm Hg	If Untreated	If Treated
<120	0	0
120–129	1	3
130–139	2	4
140–159	3	5
≥160	4	6

Point Total	10-Year Risk, %
<9	<1
9	1
10	1
11	1
12	1
13	2
14	2
15	3
16	4
17	5
18	6
19	8
20	11
21	14
22	17
23	22
24	27
≥25	≥30

(continues)

TABLE 3.5 (*continued*)
Estimate of 10-Year CHD Risk (Framingham Point Scores)

Men Age, y	Points
20–34	−9
35–39	−4
40–44	0
45–49	3
50–54	6
55–59	8
60–64	10
65–69	11
70–74	12
75–79	13

Total Cholesterol, mg/dL	Points				
	Age 20–39 y	Age 40–49 y	Age 50–59 y	Age 60–69 y	Age 70–79 y
<160	0	0	0	0	0
160–199	4	3	2	1	0
200–239	7	5	3	1	0
240–279	9	6	4	2	1
≥280	11	8	5	3	1

	Points				
	Age 20–39 y	Age 40–49 y	Age 50–59 y	Age 60–69 y	Age 70–79 y
Nonsmoker	0	0	0	0	0
Smoker	8	5	3	1	1

HDL, mg/dL	Points
≥60	−1
50–59	0
40–49	1
<40	2

Systolic BP, mm Hg	If Untreated	If Treated
<120	0	0
120–129	0	1
130–139	1	2
140–159	1	2
≥160	2	3

Point Total	10-Year Risk, %
<0	<1
0	1
1	1
2	1
3	1
4	1
5	2
6	2
7	3
8	4
9	5
10	6
11	8
12	10
13	12
14	16
15	20
16	25
≥17	≥30

Abbreviations: BP, blood pressure; HDL, high-density lipoprotein.

Source: Reprinted from reference 1.

drugs can be combined if necessary to reach goal. (See Table 6.11 in Chapter 6 for additional information on medications.)

Step 8: Identify Metabolic Syndrome and Treat, If Present, After 3 Months of TLC

Identifying and treating metabolic syndrome is important because this condition can lead to diabetes. The underlying causes of metabolic syndrome (obesity, physical inactivity, and insulin resistance) are most simply and effectively treated by intensifying weight management and increasing physical activity (112,226,267-270).

After 3 months of TLC, the lipid and nonlipid risk factors should also be treated if they persist despite the lifestyle therapies. Hypertension should be treated with antihypertensives (47), the prothrombotic state should be treated with aspirin (251), and elevated triglyceride or low HDL cholesterol levels should be treated as shown in steps 9 and 10.

Step 9: Treat Elevated Triglyceride Levels

Causes of elevated triglyceride levels include being overweight or obese, physical inactivity, cigarette smoking, excess alcohol intake, very high (> 60%) carbohydrate diets, other diseases (type 2 diabetes, chronic renal failure, nephrotic syndrome), some drugs (corticosteroids, protease inhibitors for human immunodeficiency virus, beta-adrenergic blocking agents, estrogen), and genetic factors. Weight management can be intensified and physical activity increased to lower triglyceride levels.

If triglyceride levels are still 200 mg/dL or higher after the LDL cholesterol goal is met, the secondary goal for non-HDL cholesterol (total cholesterol minus HDL cholesterol) is set 30 mg/dL higher than the LDL cholesterol goal. If triglyceride levels are 200 to 499 mg/dL after the LDL cholesterol goal is reached, intensify therapy with an LDL cholesterol–lowering drug or add nicotinic acid or fibrate to lower VLDL. Improving blood glucose management in patients with elevated glucose can also improve triglyceride levels.

If triglyceride levels are 500 mg/dL or higher, triglycerides are lowered first to prevent pancreatitis. The patient should be put on a very-low-fat diet (≤ 15% of energy from fat) and should be advised on weight management and physical activity and to abstain from alcohol ingestion. Fibrate or nicotinic acid may be necessary. When triglycerides are less than 500 mg/dL, consider whether LDL cholesterol–lowering therapy is necessary.

Step 10: Treat Low HDL Cholesterol Levels (< 40 mg/dL)

First, reach the LDL cholesterol goal. Once the LDL cholesterol goal is reached, if the HDL cholesterol level is less than 40 mg/dL, weight management and physical activity should be increased. Potentially reversible causes of low HDL cholesterol levels include high triglyceride levels, cigarette smoking, type 2 diabetes, being overweight or obese, physical inactivity, very high carbohydrate intake (> 60%), and drugs such as beta-blockers, anabolic steroids, and progestational agents. Hygienic measures to raise HDL cholesterol levels include modifying the underlying cause through diet and weight loss in the overweight and obese, increased physical activity in the sedentary, and smoking cessation. These measures should be instituted first to raise HDL cholesterol levels in both primary and secondary prevention.

If the triglyceride level is 200 to 499 mg/dL, achieve the non-HDL cholesterol goal. If the triglyceride levels are less than 200 mg/dL (isolated low HDL cholesterol) in CHD or CHD equivalent, nicotinic acid or fibrate should be considered.

CONCLUSION

A number of risk factors contribute to the development of CHD. Identifying both modifiable and nonmodifiable risk factors using ATP III criteria allows one to assess risk for CHD, determine whether intervention is prudent, and then proceed with treatment to prevent development or acceleration of CHD. In addition to high LDL cholesterol levels, ATP III identifies the major risk factors to be cigarette smoking, hypertension, a low HDL cholesterol level, family history of premature CHD, and age. Regardless of risk factors, the presence of clinical atherosclerotic disease or diabetes points to the need for intervention. A number of other emerging risk factors, such as Lp(a), hyperhomocysteinemia, and CRP, may be considered in patients at high risk, while further research clarifies their roles in CHD. Once patients are identified for intervention, methods are needed to assess current diet and lifestyle habits and then to assist patients in making long-term behavior changes consistent with principles for their specific problems, such as hypertension, metabolic syndrome, and diabetes. These issues are covered in the chapters that follow.

REFERENCES

1. Expert Panel on Detection, Evaluation, and Treatment of High Blood Cholesterol in Adults. Executive summary of the Third Report of the National Cholesterol Education Program (NCEP) Expert Panel on Detection, Evaluation, and Treatment of High Blood Cholesterol in Adults (Adult Treatment Panel III). *JAMA.* 2001;285:2486-2497. Full report: National Institutes of Health. *Third Report of the National Cholesterol Education Program Expert Panel on Detection, Evaluation, and Treatment of High Blood Cholesterol in Adults (Adult Treatment Panel III).* Bethesda, Md: National Institutes of Health; 2001. NIH Publication 01-3670. Available at: http://www.nhlbi.nih.gov/guidelines/cholesterol/atp3_rpt.htm. Accessed March 29, 2004.
2. Brown MS, Goldstein JL. Lipoprotein metabolism in the macrophage: implications for cholesterol deposition in atherosclerosis. *Annu Rev Biochem.* 1983;52:223-261.
3. Steinberg D. Low density lipoprotein oxidation and its pathobiological significance. *J Biol Chem.* 1997;272:20963-20966.
4. Ross R. Atherosclerosis—an inflammatory disease. *N Engl J Med.* 1999;340:115-126.
5. Lusis AJ. Atherosclerosis. *Nature.* 2000;407:233-241.
6. Aikawa M, Rabkin E, Okada Y, Voglic SJ, Clinton SK, Brinckerhoff CE, Sukhova GK, Libby P. Lipid lowering by diet reduces matrix metalloproteinase activity and increases collagen content of rabbit atheroma: a potential mechanism of lesion stabilization. *Circulation.* 1998;97:2433-2444.
7. Wilson PW, Abbott RD, Castelli WP. High density lipoprotein cholesterol and mortality. The Framingham Heart Study. *Arteriosclerosis.* 1988;8:737-741.
8. Barter PJ, Rye KA. High density lipoproteins and coronary heart disease. *Atherosclerosis.* 1996;121:1-12.
9. Fielding CJ. Reverse cholesterol transport. *Curr Opin Lipidol.* 1991;2:376-378.
10. Libby P, Schoenbeck U, Mach F, Selwyn AP, Gantz P. Current concepts in cardiovascular pathology: the role of LDL cholesterol in plaque rupture and stabilization. *Am J Med.* 1998;104:14S-18S.
11. Brown MS, Goldstein JL. A receptor-mediated pathway for cholesterol homeostasis. *Science.* 1986;232 34-37.
12. Russell DW, Lehrman MA, Sudhof TC, Yamamoto T, Davis CG, Hobbs HH, Brown MS, Goldstein JL. The LDL receptor in familial hypercholesterolemia: use of human mutations to dissect a membrane protein. *Cold Spring Harbor Symposia on Quantitative Biology.* 1986;51:811-819.
13. Buja LM, Clubb FJ Jr, Bilheimer DW, Willerson JT. Pathobiology of human familial hypercholesterolaemia and a related animal model, the Watanabe heritable hyperlipidaemic rabbit. *Eur Heart J.* 1990;11:41-52.
14. Kowala MC, Recce R, Beyer S, Gu C, Valentine M. Characterization of atherosclerosis in LDL receptor knockout mice: macrophage accumulation correlates with rapid and sustained expression of aortic MCP-1/JE. *Atherosclerosis.* 2000;149:323-330.
15. Wilson PWF, D'Agostino RB, Levy D, Belanger AM, Silbershatz H, Kannel WB. Prediction of coronary heart disease using risk factor categories. *Circulation.* 1998;97:1837-1847.
16. Stamler J, Wentworth D, Neaton JD, for the MRFIT Research Group. Is relationship between serum cholesterol and risk of premature death from coronary heart disease continuous and graded? Findings in 356,222 primary screenees of the Multiple Risk Factor Intervention Trial (MRFIT). *JAMA.* 1986;256:2823-2828.
17. Lipid Research Clinics Program. The Lipid Research Clinics Coronary Primary Prevention Trial results. I: Reduction in the incidence of coronary heart disease. *JAMA.* 1984;251:351-364.

18. Lipid Research Clinics Program. The Lipid Research Clinics Coronary Primary Prevention Trial results. II: The relationship of reduction in incidence of coronary heart disease to cholesterol lowering. *JAMA.* 1984;251:365-374.

19. Rosborough TK, Bank CH, Cummings MK, Phillips PP, Pierach CA. MRFIT after 10.5 years [letter]. *JAMA.* 1990;264:1534-1535.

20. Keys A, Menotti A, Aravanis C, Blackburn H, Djordjevic BS, Buzina R, Dontas AS, Fidanza F, Karvonen MJ, Kimura N, Mohacek I, Nedeljkovic S, Puddu V, Punsar S, Taylor HL, Conti S, Kromhout D, Toshima H. The Seven Countries Study: 2,289 deaths in 15 years. *Prev Med.* 1984;13:141-154.

21. Kagan A, Harris BR, Winkelstein W Jr, Johnson KG, Kato H, Syme SL, Rhoads GG, Gay ML, Nichaman MZ, Hamilton HB, Tillotson J. Epidemiologic studies of coronary heart disease and stroke in Japanese men living in Japan, Hawaii, and California: demographic, physical, dietary and biochemical characteristics. *J Chron Dis.* 1974;27:345-364.

22. Stamler J, Daviglus ML, Garside DB, Dyer AR, Greenland P, Neaton JD. Relationship of baseline serum cholesterol levels in 3 large cohorts of younger men to long-term coronary, cardiovascular, and all-cause mortality and to longevity. *JAMA.* 2000;284:311-318.

23. Anderson KM, Castelli WP, Levy D. Cholesterol and mortality: 30 years of follow-up from the Framingham Study. *JAMA.* 1987;257:2176-2180.

24. Klag MJ, Ford DE, Mead LA, He J, Whelton PK, Liang K-Y, Levine DM. Serum cholesterol in young men and subsequent cardiovascular disease. *N Engl J Med.* 1993;328:313-318.

25. Law MR, Wald NJ, Thompson SG. By how much and how quickly does reduction in serum cholesterol concentration lower risk of ischaemic heart disease? *BMJ.* 1994;308:367-372.

26. Law MR. Lowering heart disease risk with cholesterol reduction: evidence from observational studies and clinical trials. *Eur Heart J.* 1999;1(suppl S):S3-S8.

27. Grundy SM, Wilhelmsen L, Rose G, Campbell RWF, Assmann G. Coronary heart disease in high-risk populations: lessons from Finland. *Eur Heart J.* 1990;11:462-471.

28. Grundy SM. Cholesterol-lowering trials: a historical perspective. In: Grundy SM, ed. *Cholesterol Lowering Therapy: Evaluation of Clinical Trial Evidence.* New York, NY: Marcel Dekker Inc; 2000:1-44.

29. Gordon DJ. Cholesterol lowering reduces mortality: the statins. In: Grundy SM, ed. *Cholesterol-Lowering Therapy: Evaluation of Clinical Trial Evidence.* New York, NY: Marcel Dekker Inc; 2000:299-311.

30. Holmes CL, Schulzer M, Mancini GB. Angiographic results of lipid-lowering trials: a systematic review and meta-analysis. In: Grundy SM, ed. *Cholesterol-Lowering Therapy: Evaluation of Clinical Trial Evidence.* New York, NY: Marcel Dekker Inc; 2000:191-220.

31. Sacks FM, Tonkin AM, Shepherd J, Braunwald E, Cobbe S, Hawkins CM, Keech A, Packard C, Simes J, Byington R, Furberg CD, for the Prospective Pravastatin Pooling Project Investigators Group. Effect of pravastatin on coronary disease events in subgroups defined by coronary risk factors: the Prospective Pravastatin Pooling Project. *Circulation.* 2000;102:1893-1900.

32. Hansen EF, Anderson LT, Von Eyben FE. Cigarette smoking and age at first acute myocardial infarction, and influence of gender and extent of smoking. *Am J Cardiol.* 1993;71:1439-1442.

33. Nyboe J, Jensen G, Appelyard M, Schnohr P. Smoking and the risk of first acute myocardial infarction. *Am Heart J.* 1991;122:438-447.

34. Willett WC, Green A, Stampfer MJ, Speizer FE, Colditz GA, Rosner B, Monson RR, Stason W, Hennekens CH. Relative and absolute excess risks of coronary heart disease among women who smoke cigarettes. *N Engl J Med.* 1987;317:1303-1309.

35. Valkonen M, Kuusi T. Passive smoking induces atherogenic changes in low-density lipoprotein. *Circulation.* 1998;97,2012-2016.

36. US Department of Health and Human Services. *The Health Benefits of Smoking Cessation: A Report of the Surgeon General.* Washington, DC: US Department of Health and Human Services; 1990. DHHS (CDC) publication 90-8416. Available at: http://profiles.nlm.nih.gov/NN/B/B/C/T/_/nnbbct.pdf. Accessed May 14, 2004.

37. Hjermann I, Holme I, Velve BK, Leren P. Effect of diet and smoking intervention on the incidence of coronary heart disease: report from the Oslo Study Group of a randomised trial in healthy men. *Lancet.* 1981;2:1303-1310.

38. Rose G, Hamilton PJS, Colwell L, Shipley MJ. A randomised controlled trial of anti-smoking advice: 10-year results. *J Epidemiol Community Health.* 1982;36:102-108.

39. Multiple Risk Factor Intervention Trial Research Group. Multiple Risk Factor Intervention Trial: risk factor changes and mortality results. *JAMA.* 1982;248:1465-1477.

40. Kawachi I, Colditz GA, Stampfer MJ, Manson JE, Rosner B, Hunter DJ, Hennekens CH, Speizer FE. Smoking cessation in relation to total mortality rates in women. A prospective cohort study. *Ann Intern Med.* 1993;119:992-1000.

41. Lewington S, Clarke R, Qizilbash N, Peto R, Collins R. Age-specific relevance of usual blood pressure to vascular mortality. *Lancet.* 2002;360:1903-1913.

42. Vasan RS, Larson MG, Leip EP, Kannel WB, Levy D. Assessment of frequency of progression to hypertension in nonhypertensive participants in the Framingham Heart Study. *Lancet.* 2001;358:1682-1686.

43. Franklin SS, Khan SA, Wong ND, Larson MG, Levy D. Is pulse pressure useful in predicting risk for coronary heart disease? The Framingham Heart Study. *Circulation.* 1999;100:354-360.

44. van den Hoogen PCW, Feskens EJM, Nagelkerke NJD, Menotti A, Nissinen A, Kromhout D, for the Seven Countries Research Group. The relation between blood pressure and mortality due to coronary heart disease among men in different parts of the world. *N Engl J Med.* 2000;342:1-8.

45. Rodgers A, MacMahon S. Blood pressure and the global burden of cardiovascular disease. *Clin Exp Hypertens.* 1999;21:543-552.

46. Vasan RS, Larson MG, Evans JC, O'Donnell CJ, Levy D. High normal blood pressure and risk of cardiovascular disease: the Framingham Heart Study. *Circulation.* 1999;100(18 suppl 1):34.

47. Chobanian AV, Bakris GL, Black HR, Cushman WC, Green LA, Izzo JL Jr, Jones DW, Materson BJ, Oparil S, Wright JT Jr, Roccella EJ, and the National High Blood Pressure Education Program Coordinating Committee. The Seventh Report of the Joint National Committee on Prevention, Detection, Evaluation, and Treatment of High Blood Pressure: the JNC 7 report. *JAMA.* 2003;289:2560-2572.

48. Cutler JA, Psaty BM, MacMahon S, Furberg CD. Public health issues in hypertension control: what has been learned from clinical trials. In: Laragh JH, Brenner BM eds. *Hypertension: Pathophysiology, Diagnosis, and Management.* 2nd ed. New York, NY: Raven Press; 1995:253-270.

49. SHEP Cooperative Research Group. Prevention of stroke by antihypertensive drug treatment in older persons with isolated systolic hypertension: final results of the Systolic Hypertension in the Elderly Program (SHEP). *JAMA.* 1991;265:3255-3264.

50. Staessen JA, Fagard R, Thijs L, Celis H, Arabidze GG, Birkenhäger WH, Bulpitt CJ, de Leeuw PW, Dollery CT, Fletcher AE, Forette F, Leonetti G, Nachev C, O'Brien ET, Rosenfeld J, Rodicio JL, Tuomilehto J, Zanchetti A, for the Systolic Hypertension in Europe (Syst-Eur) Trial Investigators. Randomised double-blind comparison of placebo and active treatment for older persons with isolated systolic hypertension. *Lancet.* 1997;1:757-764.

51. Neal B, MacMahon S, Chapman N. Effects of ACE inhibitors, calcium antagonists, and other blood-pressure-lowering drugs. *Lancet.* 2000;356:1955-1964.

52. Ogden LG, He J, Lydick E, Whelton PK. Long-term absolute benefit of lowering blood pressure in hypertensive patients according to the JNC VI risk stratification. *Hypertension.* 2000;35:539-543.

53. Li R, Bensen JT, Hutchinson RG, Province MA, Hertz-Picciotto I, Sprafka JM, Tyroler HA. Family risk score of coronary heart disease (CHD) as a predictor of CHD: the Atherosclerosis Risk in Communities (ARIC) Study and the NHLBI Family Heart Study. *Genet Epidemiol.* 2000;18:236-250.

54. Williams RR, Hunt SC, Heiss G, Province MA, Bensen JT, Higgins M, Chamberlain RM, Ware J, Hopkins PN. Usefulness of cardiovascular family history data for population-based preventive medicine and medical research (the Health Family Tree Study and the NHLBI Family Heart Study). *Am J Cardiol.* 2001;87:129-135.

55. Slack J. Risks of ischaemic heart-disease in familial hyperlipoproteinaemic states. *Lancet.* 1969;2:1380-1382.

56. Phillips RL, Lilienfeld AM, Diamond EL, Kagan A. Frequency of coronary heart disease and cerebrovascular accidents in parents and sons of coronary heart disease index cases and controls. *Am J Epidemiol.* 1974;100:87-100.

57. Rissanen AM. Familial aggregation of coronary heart disease in a high incidence area (North Karelia, Finland). *Br Heart J.* 1979;42:294-303.

58. Pohjola-Sintonen S, Rissanen A, Liskola P, Luomanmaki K. Family history as a risk factor of coronary heart disease in patients under 60 years of age. *Eur Heart J.* 1998;19:235-239.

59. Rissanen AM, Nikkilä E. Coronary artery disease and its risk factors in families of young men with angina pectoris and in controls. *Br Heart J.* 1977;39:875-883.

60. Snowden CB, McNamara PM, Garrison RJ, Feinleib M, Kannel WB, Epstein FH. Predicting coronary heart disease in siblings—a multivariate assessment: the Framingham Heart Study. *Am J Epidemiol.* 1982;115:217-222.

61. Becker DM, Becker LC, Pearson TA, Fintel DJ, Levine DM, Kwiterovich PO. Risk factors in siblings of people with premature coronary heart disease. *J Am Coll Cardiol.* 1988;12:1273-1280.

62. Becker DM, Raqueno JV, Yook RM, Kral BG, Blumenthal RS, Moy TF, Bezirdjian PJ, Becker LC. Nurse-mediated cholesterol management compared with enhanced primary care in siblings of individuals with premature coronary disease. *Arch Intern Med.* 1998;158:1533-1539.

63. Wilson PW, Garrison RJ, Castelli WP, Feinleib M, McNamara PM, Kannel WB. Prevalence of coronary heart disease in the Framingham Offspring Study: role of lipoprotein cholesterols. *Am J Cardiol.* 1980;46:649-654.

64. Assmann G, Schulte H, von Eckardstein A, Huang Y. High-density lipoprotein cholesterol as a predictor of coronary heart disease risk: the PROCAM experience and pathophysiological implications for reverse cholesterol transport. *Atherosclerosis.* 1996;124(suppl 6):S11-S20.

65. Gordon DJ, Probstfield JL, Garrison RJ, Neaton JD, Castelli WP, Knoke JD, Jacobs DR Jr, Bangdiwala S, Tyroler HA. High-density lipoprotein cholesterol and cardiovascular disease: four prospective American studies. *Circulation.* 1989;79:8-15.

66. Abbott RD, Donahue RP, Kannel WB, Wilson PW. The impact of diabetes on survival following myocardial infarction in men vs women: the Framingham Study. *JAMA.* 1988;260:3456-3460.

67. Ng DS, Vezina C, Wolever TS, Kuksis A, Hegele RA, Connelly PW. Apolipoprotein A-I deficiency: biochemical and metabolic characteristics. *Arterioscler Thromb Vasc Biol.* 1995;15:2157-2164.

68. Miller M, Aiello D, Pritchard H, Friel G, Zeller K. Apolipoprotein A-I$_{Zavalla}$ (Leu$_{159}$ → Pro): HDL choles-

terol deficiency in a kindred associated with premature coronary artery disease. *Arterioscler Thromb Vasc Biol.* 1998;18:1242-1247.

69. Römling R, von Eckardstein A, Funke H, Motti C, Fragiacomo GC, Noseda G, Assmann G. A nonsense mutation in the apolipoprotein A-I gene is associated with high-density lipoprotein deficiency and periorbital xanthelasmas. *Arterioscler Thromb.* 1994;14:1915-1922.

70. Takata K, Saku K, Ohta T, Takata M, Bai H, Jimi S, Liu R, Sato H, Kajiyama G, Arakawa K. A new case of Apo A-I deficiency showing codon 8 nonsense mutation of the Apo A-I gene without evidence of coronary heart disease. *Arterioscler Thromb Vasc Biol.* 1995;15:1866-1874.

71. Miccoli R, Bertolotto A, Navalesi R, Odoguardi L, Boni A, Wessling J, Funke H, Wiebusch H, von Eckardstein A, Assmann G. Compound heterozygosity for a structural apolipoprotein A-I variant, apo A-I (L141R)$_{Pisa}$, and an apolipoprotein A-I null allele in patients with absence of HDL cholesterol, corneal opacifications, and coronary heart disease. *Circulation.* 1996;94:1622-1628.

72. Manolio TA, Pearson TA, Wenger NK, Barrett-Connor E, Payne GH, Harlan WR. Cholesterol and heart disease in older persons and women: review of an NHLBI workshop. *Ann Epidemiol.* 1992;2:161-176.

73. Corti M-C, Guralnik JM, Salive ME, Harris T, Field TS, Wallace RB, Berkman LF, Seeman TE, Glynn RJ, Hennekens CH, Havlik RJ. HDL cholesterol predicts coronary heart disease mortality in older persons. *JAMA.* 1995;274:539-544.

74. Bass KM, Newschaffer CJ, Koag MJ, Bush TL. Plasma lipoprotein levels as predictors of cardiovascular death in women. *Arch Intern Med.* 1993;153:2209-2216.

75. Castelli WP, Garrison RJ, Wilson PWF, Abbott RD, Kalousdian S, Kannel WB. Incidence of coronary heart disease and lipoprotein cholesterol levels: the Framingham Study. *JAMA.* 1986;256:2835-2838.

76. Brunner D, Weisbort J, Meshulam N, Schwartz S, Gross J, Saltz-Rennert H, Altman S, Loebl K. Relation of serum total cholesterol and high density lipoprotein cholesterol percentage to the incidence of definite coronary events: twenty-year follow-up of the Donolo-Tel Aviv Prospective Coronary Artery Disease Study. *Am J Cardiol.* 1987;59:1271-1276.

77. Weverling-Rijnsburger AW, Jonkers IJ, van Exel E, Gussekloo J, Westendorp RG. High-density vs low-density lipoprotein cholesterol as the risk factor for coronary artery disease and stroke in old age. *Arch Intern Med.* 2003;163:1549-1554.

78. Rubin EM, Krauss RM, Spangler EA, Verstuyft JG, Clift SM. Inhibition of early atherogenesis in transgenic mice by human apolipoprotein AI. *Nature.* 1991;353:265-267.

79. Plump AS, Scott CJ, Breslow JL. Human apolipoprotein A-I gene expression increases high density lipoprotein and suppresses atherosclerosis in apolipoprotein E-deficient mouse. *Proc Natl Acad Sci U S A.* 1994;91:9607-9611.

80. Tangirala RK, Tsukamoto K, Chun SH, Usher D, Puré E, Rader DJ. Regression of atherosclerosis induced by liver-directed gene transfer of apolipoprotein A-I in mice. *Circulation.* 1999;100:1816-1822.

81. Tall AR. An overview of reverse cholesterol transport. *Eur Heart J.* 1998;19(suppl A):A31-A35.

82. Navab M, Hama SY, Anantharamaiah GM, Hassan K, Hough GP, Watson AD, Reddy ST, Sevanian A, Fonarow GC, Fogelman AM. Normal high density lipoprotein inhibits three steps in the formation of mildly oxidized low density lipoprotein: steps 2 and 3. *J Lipid Res.* 2000;41:1495-1508.

83. Navab M, Hama SY, Cooke CJ, Anantharamaiah GM, Chaddha M, Jin L, Subbanagounder G, Faull KF, Reddy ST, Miller NE, Fogelman AM. Normal high density lipoprotein inhibits three steps in the formation of mildly oxidized low density lipoprotein: step 1. *J Lipid Res.* 2000;41:1481-1494.

84. Ballantyne CM, Herd JA, Ferlic LL, Dunn JK, Farmer JA, Jones PH, Schein JR, Gotto AM Jr. Influence of low HDL on progression of coronary artery disease and response to fluvastatin therapy. *Circulation.* 1999;99:736-743.

85. Downs JR, Clearfield M, Weis S, Whitney E, Shapiro DR, Beere PA, Langendorfer A, Stein EA, Kruyer W, Gotto AM Jr, for the AFCAPS/TexCAPS Research Group. Primary prevention of acute coronary events with lovastatin in men and women with average cholesterol levels: results of AFCAPS/TexCAPS. *JAMA.* 1998;279:1615-1622.

86. Kannel WB, Wilson PW. Risk factors that attenuate the female coronary disease advantage. *Arch Intern Med.* 1995;155:57-61.

87. Lerner DJ, Kannel WB. Patterns of coronary heart disease morbidity and mortality in the sexes: a 26-year follow-up of the Framingham population. *Am Heart J.* 1986;111:383-390.

88. Heart Protection Study Collaborative Group. MRC/BHF Heart Protection Study of cholesterol lowering with simvastatin in 20,536 high-risk individuals: a randomized placebo-controlled trial. *Lancet.* 2002;360:7-22.

89. Shepherd J, Blauw GJ, Murphy MB, Bollen EL, Buckley BM, Cobbe SM, Ford I, Gaw A, Hyland M, Jukema JW, Kamper AM, Macfarlane PW, Meinders AE, Norrie J, Packard CJ, Perry IJ, Stott DJ, Sweeney BJ, Twomey C, Westendorp RG, for the PROSPER study group. Prospective Study of Pravastatin in the Elderly at Risk. Pravastatin in elderly individuals at risk of vascular disease (PROSPER): a randomised controlled trial. *Lancet.* 2002;360:1623-1630.

90. Rubins HB, Robins SJ, Collins D, Fye CL, Anderson JW, Elam MB, Faas FH, Linares E, Schaefer EJ, Schectman G, Wilt TJ, Wittes J, for the Veterans Affairs High-Density Lipoprotein Cholesterol Intervention Trial Study Group. Gemfibrozil for the secondary prevention of coronary heart disease in men with low levels of high-density lipoprotein cholesterol. *N Engl J Med.* 1999;341:410-418.

91. Long-Term Intervention with Pravastatin in Ischaemic Disease (LIPID) Study Group. Prevention of cardiovascular events and death with pravastatin in patients with coronary heart disease and a broad range of initial cholesterol levels. *N Engl J Med*. 1998;339:1349-1357.

92. Waters D, Higginson L, Gladstsone P, Kimball B, Le May M, Boccuzzi SJ, Lespérance J. Effects of monotherapy with an HMG-CoA reductase inhibitor on the progression of coronary atherosclerosis as assessed by serial quantitative arteriography: the Canadian Coronary Atherosclerosis Intervention Trial. *Circulation*. 1994;89:959-968.

93. Sacks FM, Pfeffer MA, Moye LA, Rouleau JL, Rutherford JD, Cole TG, Brown L, Warnica JW, Arnold JMO, Wun C-C, Davis BR, Braunwald E, for the Cholesterol and Recurrent Events Trial Investigators. The effect of pravastatin on coronary events after myocardial infarction in patients with average cholesterol levels. *N Engl J Med*. 1996;335:1001-1009.

94. Denke MA, Sempos CT, Grundy SM. Excess body weight: an underrecognized contributor to high blood cholesterol levels in white American men. *Arch Intern Med*. 1993;153:1093-1103.

95. Denke MA, Sempos CT, Grundy SM. Excess body weight: an under-recognized contributor to dyslipidemia in white American women. *Arch Intern Med*. 1994;154:401-410.

96. Hartz AJ, Rupley DC, Kalkhoff RD, Rimm AA. Relationship of obesity to diabetes: influence of obesity level and body fat distribution. *Prev Med*. 1983;12:351-357.

97. Stern MP, Haffner SM. Body fat distribution and hyperinsulinemia as risk factors for diabetes and cardiovascular disease. *Arteriosclerosis*. 1986;6:123-130.

98. Berchtold P, Berger M, Jorgens V, Daweke C, Chantelau E, Gries FA, Zimmermann H. Cardiovascular risk factors and HDL-cholesterol levels in obesity. *Int J Obes*. 1981;5:1-10.

99. Blair D, Habicht J-P, Sims EAH, Sylwester D, Abraham S. Evidence for an increased risk for hypertension with centrally located body fat and the effect of race and sex on this risk. *Am J Epidemiol*. 1984;119:526-540.

100. National Institutes of Health. Clinical guidelines on the identification, evaluation, and treatment of overweight and obesity in adults—the evidence report. Bethesda, Md: National Heart, Lung and Blood Institute; 1998. NIH publication 98-4083. Available at: www.nhlbi.nih.gov/guidelines/obesity/ob_home.htm. Accessed March 29, 2004.

101. National Institutes of Health. Clinical guidelines on the identification, evaluation, and treatment of overweight and obesity in adults—the evidence report. *Obesity Res*. 1998;6(suppl 2):51S-209S.

102. Blair SN, Cooper KH, Gibbons LW, Gettman LR, Lewis S, Goodyear N. Changes in coronary heart disease risk factors associated with increased treadmill time in 753 men. *Am J Epidemiol*. 1983;118:352-359.

103. King H, Kriska AM. Prevention of type II diabetes by physical training: epidemiological considerations and study methods. *Diabetes Care*. 1992;15(suppl 4):1794-1799.

104. Helmrich SP, Ragland DR, Leung RW, Paffenbarger RS Jr. Physical activity and reduced occurrence of non-insulin-dependent diabetes mellitus. *N Engl J Med*. 1991;325:147-152.

105. Haskell WL, Alderman EL, Fair JM, Maron DJ, Mackey SF, Superko HR, Williams PT, Johnstone IM, Champagne MA, Krauss RM, Farquhar JW. Effects of intensive multiple risk factor reduction on coronary atherosclerosis and clinical cardiac events in men and women with coronary artery disease: the Stanford Coronary Risk Intervention Project (SCRIP). *Circulation*. 1994;89:975-990.

106. Leon AS, Connett J. Physical activity and 10.5 year mortality in the Multiple Risk Factor Intervention Trial. *Int J Epidemiol*. 1991;20:690-697.

107. Ekelund LG, Haskell WL, Johnson JL, Whaley FS, Criqui MH, Sheps DS. Physical fitness as a predictor of cardiovascular mortality in asymptomatic North American men: the Lipid Research Clinics Mortality Follow-up Study. *N Engl J Med*. 1988;319:1379-1384.

108. Blair SN, Jackson AS. Physical fitness and activity as separate heart disease risk factors: a meta-analysis. *Med Sci Sports Exerc*. 2001;33:762-764.

109. Morris JN, Clayton DG, Everitt MG, Semmence AM, Burgess EH. Exercise in leisure time: coronary attack and death rates. *Br Heart J*. 1990;63:325-334.

110. Sandvik L, Erikssen J, Thaulow E, Erikssen G, Mundal R, Rodahl K. Physical fitness as a predictor of mortality among healthy, middle-aged Norwegian men. *N Engl J Med*. 1993;328:533-537.

111. Paffenbarger RS Jr, Hyde RT, Wing AL, Lee I-M, Jung DL, Kampert JB. The association of changes in physical-activity level and other lifestyle characteristics with mortality among men. *N Engl J Med*. 1993;328:538-545.

112. Diabetes Prevention Program Research Group. Reduction in the incidence of type 2 diabetes with lifestyle intervention or metformin. *N Engl J Med*. 2002;346:393-403.

113. Bazzano LA, He J, Ogden LG, Loria CM, Vupputuri S, Myers L, Whelton PK. Fruit and vegetable intake and risk of cardiovascular disease in US adults: the first National Health and Nutrition Examination Survey Epidemiologic Follow-up Study. *Am J Clin Nutr*. 2002;76:93-99.

114. Van Dam RM, Giervink L, Ocke MC, Feskens EJM. Patterns of food consumption and risk factors for cardiovascular disease in the general Dutch population. *Am J Clin Nutr*. 2003;77:1156-1163.

115. Oomen CM, Ocke MC, Feskens EJM, van Erp-Baart MAJ, Kok FJ, Kromhout D. Association between trans fatty acid intake and 10-year risk of coronary heart disease in the Zutphen Elderly Study: a prospective population-based study. *Lancet*. 2001;357:746-751.

116. Kannel WB, McGee DL. Diabetes and glucose tolerance as risk factors for cardiovascular disease: the Framingham Study. *Diabetes Care*. 1979;2:120-126.

117. Wingard DL, Barrett-Connor E. Heart disease and diabetes. In: Harris MI, Cowie CC, Stern MP, Boyko EJ, Reiber GE, Bennett PH eds. *Diabetes in America.* 2nd ed. Bethesda, Md: US Department of Health and Human Services; 1995:429-448.

118. Pyörälä K, Laakso M, Uusitupa M. Diabetes and atherosclerosis: an epidemiologic view. *Diabetes Metab Rev.* 1987;3:463-524.

119. Haffner SM, Lehto S, Rönnemaa T, Pyörälä K, Laakso M. Mortality from coronary heart disease in subjects with type 2 diabetes and in nondiabetic subjects with and without prior myocardial infarction. *N Engl J Med.* 1998;339:229-234.

120. Malmberg K, Yusuf S, Gerstein HC, Brown J, Zhao F, Hunt D, Piegas L, Calvin J, Keltai M, Budaj A, for the OASIS Registry Investigators. Impact of diabetes on long-term prognosis in patients with unstable angina and non-Q-wave myocardial infarction: results of the OASIS (Organization to Assess Strategies for Ischemic Syndromes) Registry. *Circulation.* 2000;102:1014-1019.

121. Heart Outcomes Prevention Evaluation Study Investigators. Effects of an angiotensin-converting-enzyme inhibitor, ramipril, on cardiovascular events in high-risk patients. *N Engl J Med.* 2000;342:145-153.

122. UK Prospective Diabetes Study (UKPDS) Group. Effect of intensive blood-glucose control with metformin on complications in overweight patients with type 2 diabetes (UKPDS 34). *Lancet.* 1998;352:854-865.

123. UK Prospective Diabetes Study (UKPDS) Group. Intensive blood-glucose control with sulphonylureas or insulin compared with conventional treatment and risk of complications in patients with type 2 diabetes (UKPDS 33). *Lancet.* 1998;352:837-853.

124. UK Prospective Diabetes Study Group. Tight blood pressure control and risk of macrovascular and microvascular complications in type 2 diabetes: UKPDS 38. *BMJ.* 1998;317:703-713.

125. Herlitz J, Karlson BW, Edrardsson N, Emanuelsson H, Hjalmarson A. Prognosis in diabetics with chest pain or other symptoms suggestive of acute myocardial infarction. *Cardiology.* 1992;80:237-245.

126. Miettinen H, Lehto S, Salomaa V, Mähönen M, Niemelä M, Haffner SM, Pyörälä K, Tuomilehto J, for the FINMONICA Myocardial Infarction Register Study group. Impact of diabetes on mortality after the first myocardial infarction. *Diabetes Care.* 1998;21:69-75.

127. Behar S, Boyko V, Reicher-Reiss H, Goldbourt U, for the Sprint Study Group. Ten-year survival after acute myocardial infarction: comparison of patients with and without diabetes. *Am Heart J.* 1997;133:290-296.

128. Benderly M, Behar S, Reicher-Reiss H, Boyko V, Goldbourt U, for the Sprint Study Group. Long-term prognosis of women after myocardial infarction. *Am J Epidemiol.* 1997;146:153-160.

129. Karlson BW, Wiklund O, Hallgren P, Sjölin M, Lindqvist J, Herlitz J. Ten-year mortality amongst patients with a very small or unconfirmed acute myocardial infarction in relation to clinical history, metabolic screening and signs of myocardial ischaemia. *J Intern Med.* 2000;247:449-456.

130. Gustafsson I, Hildebrandt P, Seibaek M, Melchior T, Torp-Pedersen C, Kober L, Kaiser-Nielsen P, and the TRACE Study Group. Long-term prognosis of diabetic patients with myocardial infarction: relation to antidiabetic treatment regimen. *Eur Heart J.* 2000;21:1937-1943.

131. Thourani VH, Weintraub WS, Stein B, Gebhart SSP, Craver JM, Jones EL, Guyton RA. Influence of diabetes mellitus on early and late outcome after coronary artery bypass grafting. *Ann Thorac Surg.* 1999;67:1045-1052.

132. Herlitz J, Wognsen GB, Karlson BW, Sjöland H, Karlsson T, Caidahl K, Hartford M, Haglid M. Mortality, mode of death and risk indicators for death during 5 years after coronary artery bypass grafting among patients with and without a history of diabetes mellitus. *Coron Artery Dis.* 2000;11:339-346.

133. Jensen T, Borch-Johnsen K, Kofoed-Enevoldsen A, Deckert T. Coronary heart disease in young type 1 (insulin-dependent) diabetic patients with and without diabetic nephropathy: incidence and risk factors. *Diabetologia.* 1987;30:144-148.

134. Krolewski AS, Kosinksi EJ, Warram JH, Leland OS, Busick EJ, Asmal AC, Rand LI, Christlieb AR, Bradley RF, Kahn CR. Magnitude and determinants of coronary artery disease in juvenile-onset, insulin dependent diabetes mellitus. *Am J Cardiol.* 1987;59:750-755.

135. Bierman EL. George Lyman Duff Memorial Lecture. Atherogenesis in diabetes. *Arterioscler Thromb.* 1992;12:647-656.

136. UK Prospective Diabetes Study Group. Efficacy of atenolol and captopril in reducing risk of macrovascular and microvascular complications in type 2 diabetes: UKPDS 39. *BMJ.* 1998;317:713-720.

137. Pyörälä K, Pedersen TR, Kjekshus J, Faergeman O, Olsson AG, Thorgeirsson G, the Scandinavian Simvastatin Survival Study (4S) Group. Cholesterol lowering with simvastatin improves prognosis of diabetic patients with coronary heart disease: a subgroup analysis of the Scandinavian Simvastatin Survival Study (4S). *Diabetes Care.* 1997;20:614-620.

138. Haffner SM, Alexander CM, Cook TJ, Boccuzzi SJ, Musliner TA, Pedersen TR, Kjekshus J, Pyörälä K, for the Scandinavian Simvastatin Survival Study Group. Reduced coronary events in simvastatin-treated patients with coronary heart disease and diabetes or impaired fasting glucose levels: subgroup analyses from the Scandinavian Simvastatin Survival Study. *Arch Intern Med.* 1999;159:2661-2667.

139. Goldberg RB, Mellies MJ, Sacks FM, Moyé LA, Howard BV, Howard WJ, Davis BR, Cole TG, Pfeffer MA, Braunwald E, for the CARE Investigators. Cardiovascular events and their reduction with pravastatin in diabetic and glucose-intolerant myocardial infarction survivors with average cholesterol levels: subgroup analyses in the Cholesterol and Recurrent Events (CARE) trial. *Circulation.* 1998;98:2513-2519.

140. Hoogwerf BJ, Waness A, Cressman M, Canner J, Campeau L, Domanski M, Geller N, Herd A, Hickey A, Hunninghake DB, Knatterud GL, White C. Effects of aggressive cholesterol lowering and low-dose anticoagulation on clinical and angiographic outcomes in patients with diabetes: the Post Coronary Artery Bypass Graft trial. *Diabetes.* 1999;48:1289-1294.

141. Koskinen P, Mänttäri M, Manninen V, Huttunen JK, Heinonen OP, Frick MH. Coronary heart disease incidence in NIDDM patients in the Helsinki Heart Study. *Diabetes Care.* 1992;15:820-825.

142. Kuusisto J, Mykkänen L, Pyörälä K, Laakso M. NIDDM and its metabolic control predict coronary heart disease in elderly subjects. *Diabetes.* 1994;43:960-967.

143. Klein R. Kelly West Lecture 1994: hyperglycemia and microvascular and macrovascular disease in diabetes. *Diabetes Care.* 1995;18:258-268.

144. West KM, Ahuja MMS, Bennett PH, Czyzyk A, DeAcosta OM, Fuller JH, Grab B, Bragauskas V, Jarrett RJ, Kosaka K. The role of circulating glucose and triglyceride concentrations and their interactions with other "risk factors" as determinants of arterial disease in nine diabetic population samples from the WHO Multinational Study. *Diabetes Care.* 1983;6:361-369.

145. Diabetes Control and Complications Trial Research Group. The effect of intensive treatment of diabetes on the development and progression of long-term complications in insulin-dependent diabetes mellitus. *N Engl J Med.* 1993;329:977-986.

146. Heart Protection Study Collaborative Group. MRC/BHF Heart Protection Study of cholesterol-lowering with simvastatin in 5963 people with diabetes: a randomized placebo-controlled trial. *Lancet.* 2003;361:2005-2016.

147. Leng GC, Fowkes FGR, Lee AJ, Dunbar J, Housley E, Ruckley CV. Use of ankle brachial pressure index to predict cardiovascular events and death: a cohort study. *BMJ.* 1996;313:1440-1443.

148. Vogt MT, Cauley JA, Newman AB, Kuller LH, Hulley SB. Decreased ankle/arm blood pressure index and mortality in elderly women. *JAMA.* 1993;270:465-469.

149. McKenna M, Wolfson S, Kuller L. The ratio of ankle and arm arterial pressure as an independent predictor of mortality. *Atherosclerosis.* 1991;87:119-128.

150. Criqui MH, Langer RD, Fronek A, Feigelson HS, Klauber MR, McCann TJ, Browner D. Mortality over a period of 10 years in patients with peripheral arterial disease. *N Engl J Med.* 1992;326:381-386.

151. Poulias GE, Doundoulakis N, Prombonas E, Haddad H, Papaioannou K, Lymberiades D, Savopoulos G. Aorto-femoral bypass and determinants of early success and late favourable outcome: experience with 1,000 consecutive cases. *J Cardiovasc Surg.* 1992;33:664-678.

152. Ferguson GC, Eliasziw M, Barr HWK, Clagett GP, Barnes RW, Wallace C, Taylor DW, Haynes RB, Finan JW, Hachinski VC, Barnett HJM, for the North American Symptomatic Carotid Endarterectomy Trial (NASCET) Collaborators. The North American Symptomatic Carotid Endarterectomy Trial: surgical results in 1415 patients. *Stroke.* 1999;30:1751-1758.

153. Barnett HJ, Taylor DW, Eliasziw M, Fox AJ, Ferguson GG, Haynes RB, Rankin RN, Clagett GP, Hachinski VC, Sackett DL, Thorpe KE, Meldrum HE, for the North American Symptomatic Carotid Endarterectomy Trial Collaborators. Benefit of carotid endarterectomy in patients with symptomatic moderate or severe stenosis. *N Engl J Med.* 1998;339:1415-1425.

154. Executive Committee for the Asymptomatic Carotid Atherosclerosis Study. Endarterectomy for Asymptomatic Carotid Artery Stenosis. *JAMA.* 1995;273:1421-1428.

155. Hobson RW II, Weiss DG, Fields WS, Goldstone J, Moore WS, Towne JB, Wright CB, for the Veterans Affairs Cooperative Study Group. Efficacy of carotid endarterectomy for asymptomatic carotid stenosis. *N Engl J Med.* 1993;328:221-227.

156. CASANOVA Study Group. Carotid surgery versus medical therapy in asymptomatic carotid stenosis. *Stroke.* 1991;22:1229-1235.

157. Mayo Asymptomatic Carotid Endarterectomy Study Group. Results of a randomized controlled trial of carotid endarterectomy for asymptomatic carotid stenosis. *Mayo Clin Proc.* 1992;67:513-518.

158. Hertzer NR. Fatal myocardial infarction following abdominal aortic aneurysm resection: three hundred forty-three patients followed 6–11 years postoperatively. *Ann Surg.* 1980;192:667-673.

159. Nordestgaard BG, Lewis B. Intermediate density lipoprotein levels are strong predictors of the extent of aortic atherosclerosis in the St. Thomas's Hospital rabbit strain. *Atherosclerosis.* 1991;87:39-46.

160. Breslow JL. Mouse models of atherosclerosis. *Science.* 1996;272:685-688.

161. Grundy SM. Hypertriglyceridemia, atherogenic dyslipidemia, and the metabolic syndrome. *Am J Cardiol.* 1998;81:18B-25B.

162. Krauss RM. Atherogenicity of triglyceride-rich lipoproteins. *Am J Cardiol.* 1998;81:13B-17B.

163. Phillips NR, Waters D, Havel RJ. Plasma lipoproteins and progression of coronary artery disease evaluated by angiography and clinical events. *Circulation.* 1993;88:2762-2770.

164. Tornvall P, Bavenholm P, Landou C, de Faire U, Hamsten A. Relation of plasma levels and composition of apolipoprotein B-containing lipoproteins to angiographically defined coronary artery disease in young patients with myocardial infarction. *Circulation.* 1993;88:2180-2189.

165. Koren E, Corder C, Mueller G, Centurion H, Hallum G, Fesmire J, McConathy WD, Alaupovic P. Triglyceride enriched lipoprotein particles correlate with the severity of coronary artery disease. *Atherosclerosis.* 1996;122:105-115.

166. Karpe F, Boquist S, Tang R, Bond GM, de Faire U, Hamsten A. Remnant lipoproteins are related to intima-

media thickness of the carotid artery independently of LDL cholesterol and plasma triglycerides. *J Lipid Res.* 2001;42:17-21.

167. Takeichi S, Yukawa N, Nakajima Y, Osawa M, Saito T, Seto Y, Nakano T, Saniabadi AR, Adachi M, Wang T, Nakajima K. Association of plasma triglyceride-rich lipoprotein remnants with coronary atherosclerosis in cases of sudden cardiac death. *Atherosclerosis.* 1999;142:309-315.

168. Thompson GR. Angiographic evidence for the role of triglyceride-rich lipoproteins in progression of coronary artery disease. *Eur Heart J.* 1998;19(suppl H):H31-H36.

169. Sacks FM, Alaupovic P, Moye LA, Cole TG, Sussex B, Stampfer MJ, Pfeffer MA, Braunwald E. VLDL, apolipoproteins B, CIII, and E, and risk of recurrent coronary events in the Cholesterol and Recurrent Events (CARE) trial. *Circulation.* 2000;102:1886-1892.

170. Heiss G, Tamir I, Davis CE, Tyroler HA, Rifkind BM, Schonfeld G, Jacobs D, Frantz ID Jr. Lipoprotein-cholesterol distributions in selected North American populations: the Lipid Research Clinics Program Prevalence Study. *Circulation.* 1980;61:302-315.

171. Abdel-Maksoud MF, Hokanson JE. The complex role of triglycerides in cardiovascular disease. *Semin Vasc Med.* 2002;2:325-333.

172. Assmann G, Schulte H, Funke H, von Eckardstein A. The emergence of triglycerides as a significant independent risk factor in coronary artery disease. *Eur Heart J.* 1998;19(suppl M):M8-M14.

173. Sharrett AR, Ballantyne CM, Coady SA, Heiss G, Sorlie PD, Catellier D, Patsch W. Coronary heart disease prediction from lipoprotein cholesterol levels, triglycerides, lipoprotein(a), apolipoproteins A-I and B, and HDL density subfractions: the Atherosclerosis Risk in Communities (ARIC) Study. *Circulation.* 2001;104:1108-1113.

174. Austin MA, Breslow JL, Hennekens CH, Buring JE, Willett WC, Krauss RM. Low-density lipoprotein subclass patterns and risk of myocardial infarction. *JAMA.* 1988;260:1917-1921.

175. Swinkels DW, Demacker P, Hendriks J, Brenninkmeijer BJ, Stuyt P. The relevance of a protein-enriched low density lipoprotein as a risk factor for coronary heart disease in relation to other known risk factors. *Atherosclerosis.* 1989;77:59-67.

176. Campos H, Genest J, Blijlevens E, McNamara JR, Jenner JL, Ordovas JM, Wilson PWF, Schaefer EJ. Low density lipoprotein particle size and coronary artery disease. *Arterioscler Thromb.* 1992;12:187-195.

177. Mykkänen L, Kuusisto J, Haffner SM, Laakso M, Austin MA. LDL size and risk of coronary heart disease in elderly men and women. *Arterioscler Thromb Vasc Biol.* 1999;19:2742-2748.

178. Austin MA, King M-C, Vranizan KM, Krauss RM. Atherogenic lipoprotein phenotype: a proposed genetic marker for coronary heart disease risk. *Circulation.* 1990;82:495-506.

179. Verges BL. Dyslipidaemia in diabetes mellitus: review of the main lipoprotein abnormalities and their consequences on the development of atherogenesis. *Diabetes Metab.* 1999;25(suppl 3):32-40.

180. Durrington PN. Diabetic dyslipidaemia. *Baillière's Clin Endocrinol Metab.* 1999;13:265-278.

181. Kreisberg RA. Diabetic dyslipidemia. *Am J Cardiol.* 1998;82:67U-73U.

182. Kokkinos PF, Fernhall B. Physical activity and high density lipoprotein cholesterol levels: what is the relationship? *Sports Med.* 1999;28:307-314.

183. Vega GL, Grundy SM. Lipoprotein responses to treatment with lovastatin, gemfibrozil, and nicotinic acid in normolipidemic patients with hypoalphalipoproteinemia. *Arch Intern Med.* 1994;154:73-82.

184. Martin-Jadraque R, Tato F, Mostaza JM, Vega GL, Grundy SM. Effectiveness of low-dose crystalline nicotinic acid in men with low high-density lipoprotein cholesterol levels. *Arch Intern Med.* 1996;156:1081-1088.

185. Guyton JR, Blazing MA, Hagar J, Kashyap ML, Knopp RH, McKenney JM, Nash DT, Nash SD, for the Niaspan-Gemfibrozil Study Group. Extended-release niacin vs. gemfibrozil for the treatment of low levels of high-density lipoprotein cholesterol. *Arch Intern Med.* 2000;160:1177-1184.

186. Zema MJ. Gemfibrozil, nicotinic acid and combination therapy in patients with isolated hypoalphalipoproteinemia: a randomized, open-label, crossover study. *J Am Coll Cardiol.* 2000;35:640-646.

187. Committee of Principal Investigators. A co-operative trial in the primary prevention of ischemic heart disease using clofibrate: Report from the Committee of Principal Investigators. *Br Heart J.* 1978;40:1069-1118.

188. Frick MH, Elo MO, Haapa K, Heinonen OP, Heinsalmi P, Helo P, Huttunen JK, Kaitaniemi P, Koskinen P, Manninen V, Mäenpää H, Mälkönen M, Mänttäri M, Norola S, Pasternack A, Pikkarainen J, Romo M, Sjoblom T, Nikkila EA. Helsinki Heart Study: primary-prevention trial with gemfibrozil in middle-aged men with dyslipidemia: safety of treatment, changes in risk factors, and incidence of coronary heart disease. *N Engl J Med.* 1987;317:1237-1245.

189. Carlson LA, Rosenhamer G. Reduction of mortality in the Stockholm Ischaemic Heart Disease Secondary Prevention Study by combined treatment with clofibrate and nicotinic acid. *Acta Med Scand.* 1988;223:405-418.

190. Bezafibrate Infarction Prevention (BIP) Study Group. Secondary prevention by raising HDL cholesterol and reducing triglycerides in patients with coronary artery disease. *Circulation.* 2000;102:21-27.

191. Ericsson C-G, Hamsten A, Nilsson J, Grip L, Svane B, de Faire U. Angiographic assessment of effects of bezafibrate on progression of coronary artery disease in young male postinfarction patients. *Lancet.* 1996;347:849-853.

192. Frick MH, Syvänne M, Nieminen MS, Kauma H, Majahalme S, Virtanen V, Kesäniemi YA, Pasternack A, Taskinen M-R, for the Lopid Coronary Angiography Trial (LOCAT) Study Group. Prevention of the angiographic progression of coronary and vein-graft atherosclerosis by gemfibrozil after coronary bypass surgery in men with low levels of HDL cholesterol. *Circulation.* 1997;96:2137-2143.

193. Diabetes Atherosclerosis Intervention Study Investigators. Effect of fenofibrate on progression of coronary-artery disease in type 2 diabetes: the Diabetes Atherosclerosis Intervention Study, a randomised study. *Lancet.* 2001;357:905-910.

194. Blankenhorn DH, Nessim SA, Johnson RL, Sanmarco ME, Azen SP, Cashin-Hemphill L. Beneficial effects of combined colestipol-niacin therapy on coronary atherosclerosis and coronary venous bypass grafts. *JAMA.* 1987;257:3233-3240.

195. Brown G, Albers JJ, Fisher LD, Schaefer SM, Lin J-T, Kaplan C, Zhao X-Q, Bisson BD, Fitzpatrick VF, Dodge HT. Regression of coronary artery disease as a result of intensive lipid-lowering therapy in men with high levels of apolipoprotein B. *N Engl J Med.* 1990;323:1289-1298.

196. Brown BG, Zhao XQ, Chait A, Fisher LD, Cheung MC, Morse JS, Dowdy AA, Marino EK, Bolson EL, Alaupovic P, Frohlich J, Albers JJ. Simvastatin and niacin, antioxidant vitamins, or the combination for the prevention of coronary disease. *N Engl J Med.* 2001;345:1583-1592.

197. Avogaro P, Crepaldi G, Enzi G, Tiengo A. Associazione di iperlipidemia, diabete mellito e obesità di medio grado. *Acta Diabetol Lat.* 1967;4:36-41.

198. Haller H. Epidemiology and associated risk factors of hyperlipoproteinemia. *Z Gesamte Inn Med.* 1977;32:124-128.

199. Singer P. Diagnosis of primary hyperlipoproteinemias. *Z Gesamte Inn Med.* 1977;32:129-133.

200. Després J-P. Abdominal obesity as important component of insulin-resistance syndrome. *Nutrition.* 1993;9:452-459.

201. Bjorntorp P. Body fat distribution, insulin resistance, and metabolic diseases. *Nutrition.* 1997;13:795-803.

202. Okosun IS, Liao Y, Rotimi CN, Prewitt TE, Cooper RS. Abdominal adiposity and clustering of multiple metabolic syndrome in white, black and Hispanic Americans. *Ann Epidemiol.* 2000;10:263-270.

203. Schaefer EJ, McNamara JR, Genest J Jr, Ordovas JM. Clinical significance of hypertriglyceridemia. *Semin Thromb Hemost.* 1988;14:143-148.

204. Karhapää P, Malkki M, Laakso M. Isolated low HDL cholesterol: an insulin-resistant state. *Diabetes.* 1994;43:411-417.

205. The Expert Committee on the Diagnosis and Classification of Diabetes Mellitus. Follow-up report on the diagnosis of diabetes mellitus. *Diabetes Care.* 2003;26:3160-3167.

206. Tripathy D, Carlsson M, Almgren P, Isomaa B, Taskinen M-R, Tuomi T, Groop LC. Insulin secretion and insulin sensitivity in relation to glucose tolerance: lessons from the Botnia Study. *Diabetes.* 2000;49:975-980.

207. Haffner SM, Miettinen H, Gaskill SP, Stern MP. Decreased insulin action and insulin secretion predict the development of impaired glucose tolerance. *Diabetologia.* 1996;39:1201-1207.

208. Reaven GM. Pathophysiology of insulin resistance in human disease. *Physiol Rev.* 1995;75:473-486.

209. Grundy SM. Hypertriglyceridemia, insulin resistance, and the metabolic syndrome. *Am J Cardiol.* 1999;83:25F-29F.

210. Meigs JB. Invited commentary: insulin resistance syndrome? Syndrome X? Multiple metabolic syndrome? A syndrome at all? Factor analysis reveals patterns in the fabric of correlated metabolic risk factors. *Am J Epidemiol.* 2000;152:908-911.

211. Zimmet P, Boyko EJ, Collier GR, de Courten M. Etiology of the metabolic syndrome: potential role of insulin resistance, leptin resistance, and other players. *Ann NY Acad Sci.* 1999;892:25-44.

212. Haffner SM. Epidemiology of insulin resistance and its relation to coronary artery disease. *Am J Cardiol.* 1999;84:11J-14J.

213. Després J-P. The insulin resistance-dyslipidemic syndrome of visceral obesity: effect on patients' risk. *Obes Res.* 1998;6(suppl 1):8S-17S.

214. Savage DB, Tan GD, Acerini CL, Jebb SA, Agostini M, Gurnell M, Williams RL, Umpleby AM, Thomas EL, Bell JD, Dixon AK, Dunne F, Boiani R, Cinti S, Vidal-Puig A, Karpe F, Chatterjee V, Krishna K, O'Rahilly S. Human metabolic syndrome resulting from dominant-negative mutations in the nuclear receptor peroxisome proliferator-activated receptor-(gamma). *Diabetes.* 2003;52:910-917.

215. Barroso I, Gurnell M, Crowley VE, Agostini M, Schwabe JW, Soos MA, Maslen GL, Williams TD, Lewis H, Schafer AJ, Chatterjee VK, O'Rahilly S. Dominant negative mutations in human PPAR gamma associated with severe insulin resistance, diabetes mellitus and hypertension. *Nature.* 1999;402:880-883.

216. Hegele RA, Anderson CM, Wang J, Jones DC, Cao H. Association between nuclear lamin A/C R482Q mutation and partial lipodystrophy with hyperinsulinemia, dyslipidemia, hypertension and diabetes. *Genome Research.* 2000;10:652-658.

217. Hegele RA. Premature atherosclerosis associated with monogenic insulin resistance. *Circulation.* 2001;103:2225-2229.

218. Hegele RA, Kraw ME, Ban MR, Miskie BA, Huff MW, Cao H. Elevated serum C-reactive protein and free fatty acids among nondiabetic carriers of missense mutations in the gene encoding lamin A/C (LMNA) with partial lipodystrophy. *Arterioscler Thromb Vasc Biol.* 2003;23:111-116.

219. Hegele RA, Cao H, Frankowski C, Mathews ST, Leff T. PPARG F388L, a transactivation-deficient mutant, in familial partial lipodystrophy. *Diabetes.* 2002;51:3586-3590.

220. Agarwal AK, Garg A. A novel heterozygous mutation in peroxisome proliferator-activated receptor-gamma gene in a patient with familial partial lipodystrophy. *J Clin Endocrinol Metab.* 2002;87:408-411.

221. Lakka HM, Laaksonen DE, Lakka TA, Niskanen LK, Kumpusalo E, Tuomilehto J, Salonen JT. The metabolic syndrome and total and cardiovascular disease mortality in middle-aged men. *JAMA.* 2002;288:2709-2716.

222. US Department of Health and Human Services. Physical activity and health: a Report of the Surgeon General. Atlanta, Ga: US Department of Health and Human Services, Centers for Disease Control and Prevention, National Center for Chronic Disease Prevention and Health Promotion; 1996.

223. Assmann G, Cullen P, Schulte H. The Münster Heart Study (PROCAM): results of follow-up at 8 years. *Eur Heart J.* 1998;19(suppl A):A2-A11.

224. Eckel RH, Krauss RM, for the AHA Nutrition Committee. American Heart Association call to action: obesity as a major risk factor for coronary heart disease. *Circulation.* 1998;97:2099-2100.

225. Alexander CM, Landsman PB, Teutsch SM, Haffner SM. 2NCEP-defined metabolic syndrome, diabetes, and prevalence of coronary heart disease among NHANES III participants age 50 years and older. *Diabetes.* 2003;52:1210-1214.

226. Tuomilehto J, Lindstrom J, Eriksson JG, Valle TT, Hamalainen H, Ilanne-Parikka P, Keinanen-Kiukaanniemi S, Laakso M, Louheranta A, Rastas M, Salminen V, Uusitupa M, Finnish Diabetes Prevention Study Group. Prevention of type 2 diabetes mellitus by changes in lifestyle among subjects with impaired glucose tolerance. *N Engl J Med.* 2001;344:1343-1350.

227. Vega GL, Grundy SM. Does measurement of apolipoprotein B have a place in cholesterol management? *Arteriosclerosis.* 1990;10:668-671.

228. Abate N, Vega GL, Grundy SM. Variability in cholesterol content and physical properties of lipoproteins containing apolipoprotein B-100. *Atherosclerosis.* 1993;104:159-171.

229. Frost PH, Havel RJ. Rationale for use of non-high-density lipoprotein cholesterol rather than low-density lipoprotein cholesterol as a tool for lipoprotein cholesterol screening and assessment of risk and therapy. *Am J Cardiol.* 1998;81:26B-31B.

230. Cui Y, Blumenthal RS, Flaws JA, Whiteman MK, Langenberg P, Bachorik PS, Bush TL. Non-high-density lipoprotein cholesterol level as a predictor of cardiovascular disease mortality. *Arch Intern Med.* 2001;161:1413-1419.

231. Stubbs P, Seed M, Lane D, Collinson P, Kendall F, Noble M. Lipoprotein(a) as a risk predictor for cardiac mortality in patients with acute coronary syndromes. *Eur Heart J.* 1998;19:1355-1364.

232. Budde T, Fechtrup C, Bosenberg E, Vielhauer C, Enbergs A, Schulte H, Assmann G, Breithardt G. Plasma Lp(a) levels correlate with number, severity, and length-extension of coronary lesions in male patients undergoing coronary arteriography for clinically suspected coronary atherosclerosis. *Arterioscler Thromb.* 1994;14:1730-1736.

233. Seman LJ, DeLuca C, Jenner JL, Cupples LA, McNamara JR, Wilson PWF, Castelli WP, Ordovas JM, Schaefer EJ. Lipoprotein(a)-cholesterol and coronary heart disease in the Framingham Heart Study. *Clin Chem.* 1999;45:1039-1046.

234. Danesh J, Collins R, Peto R. Lipoprotein(a) and coronary heart disease: meta-analysis of prospective studies. *Circulation.* 2000;102:1082-1085.

235. Moliterno DJ, Jokinen EV, Miserez AR, Lange RA, Willard JE, Boerwinkle E, Hillis LD, Hobbs HH. No association between plasma lipoprotein(a) concentrations and the presence or absence of coronary atherosclerosis in African Americans. *Arterioscler Thromb Vasc Biol.* 1995;15:850-855.

236. Nishino M, Malloy MJ, Naya-Vigne J, Russell J, Kane JP, Redberg RF. Lack of association of lipoprotein(a) levels with coronary calcium deposits in asymptomatic postmenopausal women. *J Am Coll Cardiol.* 2000;35:314-320.

237. Maher VM, Brown BG, Marcovina SM, Hillger LA, Zhao XQ, Albers JJ. Effects of lowering elevated LDL cholesterol on the cardiovascular risk of lipoprotein (a). *JAMA.* 1995;274:1771-1774.

238. Carlson LA, Hamsten A, Asplund A. Pronounced lowering of serum levels of lipoprotein Lp(a) in hyperlipidaemic subjects treated with nicotinic acid. *J Intern Med.* 1989;226:271-276.

239. Angelin B. Therapy for lowering lipoprotein(a) levels. *Curr Opin Lipidol.* 1997;8:337-341.

240. Su W, Campos H, Judge H, Walsh BW, Sacks FM. Metabolism of Apo(a) and Apo B-100 of lipoprotein(a) in women: effect of postmenopausal estrogen replacement. *J Clin Endocrinol Metab.* 1998;83:3267-3276.

241. Kang SS, Wong PWK, Malinow MR. Hyperhomocyst(e)inemia as a risk factor for occlusive vascular disease. *Ann Rev Nutr.* 1992;12:279-298.

242. Malinow MR, Bostom AG, Krauss RM. Homocyst(e)ine, diet, and cardiovascular diseases: a statement for healthcare professionals from the Nutrition Committee, American Heart Association. *Circulation.* 1999;99:178-182.

243. Stehouwer CDA, Weijenberg MP, van den Berg M., Jakobs C, Feskens EJM, Kromhout D. Serum homocysteine and risk of coronary heart disease and cerebrovascular disease in elderly men: a 10-year follow-up. *Arterioscler Thromb Vasc Biol.* 1998;18:1895-1901.

244. Folsom AR, Nieto FJ, McGovern PG, Tsai MY, Malinow MR, Eckfeldt JH, Hess DL, Davis CE. Prospective study of coronary heart disease incidence in relation to fasting total homocysteine, related genetic polymorphisms, and B vitamins: the Atherosclerosis Risk in Communities (ARIC) Study. *Circulation.* 1998;98:204-210.

245. Whincup PH, Refsum H, Perry IJ, Morris R, Walker M, Lennon L, Thomson A, Ueland PM, Ebrahim SBJ. Serum total homocysteine and coronary heart disease: prospective study in middle aged men. *Heart.* 1999;82:448-454.

246. Bostom AG, Rosenberg IH, Silbershatz H, Jacques PF, Selhub J, D'Agostino RB, Wilson PWF, Wolf PA. Nonfasting plasma total homocysteine levels and stroke incidence in elderly persons: the Framingham Study. *Ann Intern Med.* 1999;131:352-355.

247. Giles WH, Croft JB, Greenlund KJ, Ford ES, Kittner SJ. Association between total homocyst(e)ine and the likelihood for a history of acute myocardial infarction by race and ethnicity: results from the Third National Health and Nutrition Examination Survey. *Am Heart J.* 2000;139:446-453.

248. Eikelboom JW, Lonn E, Genst J Jr, Hankey G, Yusuf S. Homocysteine and cardiovascular disease: a critical review of the epidemiologic evidence. *Ann Intern Med.* 1999;131:363-375.

249. Schnyder G, Roffi M, Flammer Y, Pin R, Hess OM. Effect of homocysteine-lowering therapy with folic acid, vitamin B12, and vitamin B6 on clinical outcome after percutaneous coronary intervention: the Swiss Heart Study: a randomized controlled trial. *JAMA.* 2002;288:973-979.

250. Liem A, Reynierse-Buitenwerf GH, Zwinderman AH, Jukema JW, van Veldhuisen DJ. Secondary prevention with folic acid: effects on clinical outcomes. *J Am Coll Cardiol.* 2003;41:2105-2113.

251. Hennekens CH, Dyken ML, Fuster V. Aspirin as a therapeutic agent in cardiovascular disease: a statement for healthcare professionals from the American Heart Association. *Circulation.* 1997;96:2751-2753.

252. Creager MA. Results of the CAPRIE trial: efficacy and safety of clopidogrel. *Vasc Med.* 1998;3:257-260.

253. Hansson L, Zanchetti A, Carruthers SG, Dahlöf B, Elmfeldt D, Julius S, Ménard J, Rahn KH, Wedel H, Westerling S, for the HOT Study Group. Effects of intensive blood-pressure lowering and low-dose aspirin in patients with hypertension: principal results of the Hypertension Optimal Treatment (HOT) randomised trial. *Lancet.* 1998;351:1755-1762.

254. Tracy RP, Lemaitre RN, Psaty BM, Ives DG, Evans RW, Cushman M, Meilahn EN, Kuller LH. Relationship of C-reactive protein to risk of cardiovascular disease in the elderly: results from the Cardiovascular Health Study and the Rural Health Promotion Project. *Arterioscler Thromb Vasc Biol.* 1997;17:1121-1127.

255. Ridker PM, Buring JE, Shih J, Matias M, Hennekens CH. Prospective study of C-reactive protein and the risk of future cardiovascular events among apparently healthy women. *Circulation.* 1998;98:731-733.

256. Ridker PM, Glynn RJ, Hennekens CH. C-reactive protein adds to the predictive value of total and HDL cholesterol in determining risk of first myocardial infarction. *Circulation.* 1998;97:2007-2011.

257. Ridker PM, Rifai N, Pfeffer MA, Sacks F, Braunwald E, for the Cholesterol and Recurrent Events (CARE) Investigators. Long-term effects of pravastatin on plasma concentration of C-reactive protein. *Circulation.* 1999;100:230-235.

258. Ridker PM, Hennekens CH, Buring JE, Rifai N. C-reactive protein and other markers of inflammation in the prediction of cardiovascular disease in women. *N Engl J Med.* 2000;342:836-843.

259. Koenig W, Sund M, Fröhlich M, Fischer H-G, Löwel H, Döring A, Hutchinson WL, Pepys MB. C-reactive protein, a sensitive marker of inflammation, predicts future risk of coronary heart disease in initially healthy middle-aged men: results from the MONICA (Monitoring Trends and Determinants in Cardiovascular Disease) Augsburg Cohort Study, 1984 to 1992. *Circulation.* 1999;99:237-242.

260. Meigs JB, Nathan DM, Wilson PWF, Cupples LA, Singer DE. Metabolic risk factors worsen continuously across the spectrum of nondiabetic glucose tolerance: the Framingham Offspring Study. *Ann Intern Med.* 1998;128:524-533.

261. Meigs JB, Mittleman MA, Nathan DM, Tofler GH, Singer DE, Murphy-Sheehy PM, Lipinska I, D'Agostino RB, Wilson PWF. Hyperinsulinemia, hyperglycemia, and impaired hemostasis: the Framingham Offspring Study. *JAMA.* 2000;283:221-228.

262. Haffner SM. Impaired glucose tolerance: is it relevant for cardiovascular disease? *Diabetologia.* 1997;40(suppl):S138-S140.

263. Laakso M, Lehto S. Epidemiology of risk factors for cardiovascular disease in diabetes and impaired glucose tolerance. *Atherosclerosis.* 1998;137(suppl):S65-S73.

264. Gerstein HC, Pais P, Pogue J, Yusuf S. Relationship of glucose and insulin levels to the risk of myocardial infarction: a case-control study. *J Am Coll Cardiol.* 1999;33:612-619.

265. Grundy SM, Cleeman JI, Merz CNB, Brewer HB, Clark LT, Hunninghake DB, Pasternak RC, Smith SC, Stone NJ, for the Coordinating Committee of the National Cholesterol Education Program. Implications of recent clinical trials for the National Cholesterol Education Program Adult Treatment Panel III guidelines. *Circulation.* 2004;110:227-239.

266. World Hypertension League. Measuring your blood pressure. Available at: http://www.mco.edu/org/whl/bloodpre.html. Accessed March 29, 2004.

267. Dengel DR, Galecki AT, Hagberg JM, Pratley RE. The independent and combined effects of weight loss and aerobic exercise on blood pressure and oral glucose tolerance in older men. *Am J Hypertens.* 1998;11:1405-1412.

268. Su H-Y, Sheu WH, Chin H-M, Jeng C-Y, Chen Y-D, Reaven GM. Effect of weight loss on blood pressure and insulin resistance in normotensive and hypertensive obese individuals. *Am J Hypertens.* 1995;8:1067-1071.

269. Hu FB, Stampfer MJ, Solomon C, Liu S, Colditz GA, Speizer FE, Willett WC, Manson JE. Physical activity and risk for cardiovascular events in diabetic women. *Ann Intern Med.* 2001;134:96-105.

270. Farrell SW, Kampert JB, Kohl HW III, Barlow CE, Macera CA, Paffenbarger RS Jr, Gibbons LW, Blair SN. Influences of cardiorespiratory fitness levels and other predictors on cardiovascular disease mortality in men. *Med Sci Sports Exerc.* 1998;30:899-905.

CHAPTER 4

NUTRITION ASSESSMENT FOR CARDIOVASCULAR DISEASE

Judith Wylie-Rosett, EdD, RD, and Lisa A. Hark, PhD, RD

PURPOSE OF NUTRITION ASSESSMENT

Nutrition assessment is the evaluation of an individual's nutritional status based on the interpretation of clinical information obtained from the medical history, diet history, review of systems, physical examination, and laboratory data. In relation to cardiovascular disease (CVD) risk, the nutrition assessment is used to evaluate an individual's dietary intake and nutritional status to formulate a plan for implementing medical nutrition therapy (MNT). The effects of MNT on CVD risk factors and related metabolic parameters should be monitored and reevaluated periodically. The assessment focuses on lifestyle factors (dietary intake and physical activity) relative to measures associated with increased cardiovascular risk, such as diabetes, hypertension, and dyslipidemia.

This chapter discusses the CVD-related nutrition assessment including the primary as well as secondary and tertiary prevention of CVD. As a result, the risk and age continuum are broad. Nutrition assessment is an important tool for patients with CVD because weight, blood pressure, glucose, lipids, and other parameters, as well as lifestyle variables, must be monitored to address the emerging obesity epidemic and the concomitant rise in indices associated with CVD risk.

Past Medical History

The past medical history provides an overview of CVD-related risk and usually focuses on hospitalizations, surgeries, major injuries, and specific diagnoses such as hypertension, diabetes, established (coronary, peripheral, or cerebral) artery disease, and congestive heart failure. Other relevant information includes patterns of health care, as well as chronic illnesses and significant acute illnesses that may have nutritional implications. Detailed information should be obtained about current or recent prescription medications with emphasis on those used to treat CVD risk factors. High-risk patients may be prescribed multiple medications in an effort to achieve normal blood pressure, lipid values, and glucose levels. For high–CVD risk patients, the standards of medical care include aspirin therapy and influenza and pneumonia immunization. Other components in the assessment include use of vitamins, minerals, laxatives, topical medications, over-the-counter medications, and products such as nutritional or herbal supplements that patients frequently do not recognize as medications. Nutritional supplements include any products that patients use to increase their energy, vitamin, or protein intake. It is also important to query the patient about any identified food allergies or intolerances.

Family History

Familial occurrences of disease and health status of parents, siblings, children, and partners should be part of a comprehensive medical evaluation. Respective ages of family members and cause of death of those deceased should be included. Family history of diabetes, heart disease, obesity, or hypertension provides valuable insights for intervention. Patterns of weight gain from childhood to adulthood among family members and questions about distribution of body fat should be addressed to assess the genetic vs environmental factors in weight gain.

Reviewing Laboratory Tests, Medications, and CVD Risk Assessment

Review of laboratory tests needs to be integrated into the nutrition assessment related to CVD risk. However, the specific tests and goals for intervention vary by risk status. The American Heart Association's guidelines for the primary prevention of CVD and stroke recommend that routine risk factor assessment begin at 20 years of age. The blood specimens for risk assessment should be obtained at least every 5 years or at least every 2 years if risk factors are present to evaluate serum lipoproteins or total and high-density lipoprotein (HDL) cholesterol and fasting glucose levels (1). The National Cholesterol Education Program's Adult Treatment Panel III (ATP III) guidelines for risk assessment (2) are discussed in Chapter 3.

Evidenced-based guidelines for evaluating and monitoring CVD risk status have been developed as a key component for primary, secondary, and tertiary prevention of CVD. Much of the effort for primary prevention focused on early detection and prevention of the associated metabolic abnormalities that increase CVD risk. As a result, the focus at the population level emphasizes promoting a healthier lifestyle, especially in youth, to reduce the risk of developing obesity, diabetes, and hypertension. The emphasis of secondary prevention is detection and treatment of cardiovascular risk factors such as hypertension, diabetes, and dyslipidemia for patients with clinical evidence of heart disease. For example, risk reduction after a myocardial infarction is essential to prevent a future event. ATP III has established the criteria for lipid profile and for treatment strata based on risk factors including metabolic syndrome (3). (See Chapters 3 and 7.) Tertiary prevention focuses on the population with existing disease to minimize end organ damage.

MNT is based on integrating nutrition into the overall treatment plan. Therefore, the nutrition assessment involves evaluating the wide array of medications that are used to reduce CVD risk, as well as dietary intake. For patients with multiple risk factors or with existing disease, nutrition counseling involves addressing how lifestyle changes can be integrated with the patient's treatment regimen.

Social History

Pertinent nonmedical information recorded in the social history includes the patient's occupation, daily exercise pattern, and marital and family status. Information is also solicited regarding the patient's education, economic status, residence, emotional response, adjustment to illness, and any other information that might influence the patient's understanding of his or her illness and adherence to a nutrition program. Details concerning the duration and frequency of the patient's use of substances such as alcohol, tobacco, illicit drugs, and caffeine are also recorded in the social history. These data can be extremely useful when formulating the nutrition plan. Economic limitations that influence access to an adequate diet, difficulties shopping for or preparing food, and participation in feeding programs (eg, Special Supplemental Nutrition Program for Women, Infants, and Children [WIC], Meals on Wheels) are relevant to nutrition assessment. Economic insecurity questions include the following: Have you run out of money to buy food? Do you worry about running out of money to buy food? Individuals who face food insecurities have higher rates of obesity. More research is needed to determine whether this relation is due to binge eating or other forms of overeating because of fears of not having enough food (4).

Methods for Obtaining Information about Dietary Intake

There are several methods for obtaining information about food intake (see Table 4.1), and each method has advantages and disadvantages. Using multiple methods is time consuming but can overcome the inherent limitations of the various techniques. As the ethnic and age diversity of the target population increases, the need for open-ended questions and obtaining data by interview also increases. The basic methods for collecting dietary intake data include 24-hour recall, food record or diary, food frequency questionnaire (FFQ), dietary history, and quick screeners (5-12).

Twenty-four-Hour Recall

The 24-hour recall is widely used in clinical practice and for national food surveys. A recall of food intake can be for any length of time, but usually covers a 24-hour period. The recall can be self-administered or obtained by interview. Although one 24-hour recall does not accurately represent a person's usual or habitual intake, it can provide a clinically useful overview of the diet if the day is typical. If intake on the previous day was atypical, the participant can be asked to recall or to record an earlier typical day or describe in what manner the day was different from usual.

Large food intakes are frequently underestimated by the recall method, and small intakes are often overestimated. An analysis of almost 12,000 recalls reported by participants in the National Health and Nutrition Examination Survey II suggested that 31% of respondents significantly underestimated 24-hour food recalls (13).

The United States Department of Agriculture (USDA) has developed a five-step multiple pass interview to reduce the risk of underreporting food intake (14). These steps are as follows:

1. *Quick food list*: the respondent reports an uninterrupted listing of all food and beverages consumed during the day (to cover a 24-hour period) before the interview.

TABLE 4.1

Tailoring Dietary Assessment Tools for Cardiovascular Disease Risk Factors

Assessment Tool Methodology	Diabetes (see also Obesity)	Hypertension	Dyslipidemia	Obesity	Heart Disease
24-hour recall	Assess day-to-day variability in intake to address food intake in relation to glycemic control.	Assess compared with the DASH recommendations.	Assess sources of saturated fat and cholesterol if LDL cholesterol is elevated and alcohol if triglycerides are elevated.	Assess for sources of excess calories, skipped meals, binge eating behavior, and night eating syndrome.	Evaluate intake in relation to MNT goals. If heart failure is present, assess intake of fluids and sodium.
Food record or food diary	Focus self-monitoring on carbohydrate intake for glycemic control and calories and fat, if weight loss is a treatment goal.	Focus on dietary pattern based on DASH if self-monitoring.	Monitor intake of saturated fat and cholesterol as noted above. If weight loss is treatment goal, energy intake may be more important because dyslipidemia is responsive to weight loss.	Monitor cues for eating and times when food is eaten, as well as sources of excess calories.	Monitor as above based on MNT goals.
Food frequency questionnaire	FFQs cannot be used to assess for matching medication and dietary intake.	FFQs can provide an overview of the overall dietary pattern but may lack sensitivity to assess sodium intake.	FFQs can be useful for assessing fatty acid and cholesterol intake, but weight issues may also need to be addressed as noted above.	Use FFQ to examine excess energy, but behavioral monitoring also needs to be addressed.	May not be sensitive enough to evaluate goals for MNT.
Dietary history	Focus on how various insulin action times match eating times, if on sulfonylureas or insulin. Assess complications and the treatment goals for blood pressure, lipids, and glucose. Examine postprandial glucose in relation to meal carbohydrate content.	Assess knowledge and attitudes as well as behavior in relation to all of the recommended dietary goals: weight loss, exercise, and elements in the DASH combined dietary program.	Assess carbohydrate, weight, activity, and alcohol in relation to triglyceride and HDL cholesterol levels. Assess *trans* and saturated fat and cholesterol in relation to LDL cholesterol focusing on knowledge and attitude as well as behavior.	Assess past experience with weight loss, if any. Focus on attitudes, skills, and motivation before focusing on behaviors.	Assess education in relation to managing heart disease or congestive heart failure. Focus on sodium and fluid retention in congestive heart failure. Address behavior in relation to risk factors.
Brief dietary scanners	May not be very useful to address medical nutrition therapy matching medical action to dietary habits.	Can be useful to evaluate DASH dietary pattern.	Can monitor key nutrients as above.	Screen for food insecurity as well as sources of excess energy and key eating behaviors.	Monitor using a brief screener of key behavioral-related MNT goals may be useful.

Abbreviations: DASH, Dietary Approaches to Stop Hypertension; FFQ, food frequency questionnaire; HDL, high-density lipoprotein; LDL, low-density lipoprotein; MNT, medical nutrition therapy.

Source: Developed by Judith Wylie-Rosett, EdD, RD, Albert Einstein College of Medicine. Copyright 2004. Used with permission of the author.

2. *Forgotten food list:* the interviewer asks about foods that the respondent may have forgotten in nine food categories (nonalcoholic beverages, alcoholic beverages, sweets, savory snacks, fruits and vegetables, cheese, breads and rolls, and any other foods).
3. *Time and occasion:* the interviewer asks about the time the respondent began eating or drinking each item reported and what the respondent can recall about each eating occasion.

4. *Detail cycle:* the interviewer asks standardized questions developed by the USDA about how to probe for information about the foods eaten, preparation methods, ingredients, and so on. The detail cycle also includes a review of eating occasions and time between occasions.

5. *Final review and probe:* the interviewer asks about anything else consumed while trying to help the respondent remember any forgotten items.

A recent study found that both normal weight and obese women provided estimates of macronutrient and energy intake that were within 10% of actual intake when telephone interviewers used the USDA five-step multiple pass method to question them (14). The obese women were more accurate in their estimations of energy intake than the normal weight women. However, the USDA five-step process requires 20 to 30 minutes and visual aids to facilitate portion size estimation. Dietitians in clinical practice can use some of the probing techniques developed by the USDA to elicit more details about target nutrient intake in their interviews with patients, but they may not find routine use of multiple passes practical. Other health professionals seldom have more than a few minutes to obtain a food recall. A brief interview focusing questions on the patient's risk factor profile can identify key behavioral and food patterns associated with target nutrient excess or inadequacy.

Food Record or Food Diary

Food records and diaries involve writing down food items soon after they are eaten for a specified period of time (15). Self-monitoring diaries that combine several methods can be used over extended periods of time (16). Computerized devices may also be used to reduce the burden of self-monitoring, but the database of foods needs to include items consumed by the users (17).

A food record that includes weighing foods before they are eaten for several days can provide a detailed and valid assessment of macronutrient and micronutrient intake (9). However, the act of recording can alter intake and thus limit the potential for accurately reflecting typical intake. The accuracy of food records is increased by training clients to measure or estimate portion sizes and to provide a more detailed description of foods eaten. The burden of recording food intake is substantial and can be intimidating to patients with a limited education level. When food records are used in research, an interview is used to clarify portion sizes and preparation methods as well as to elicit food items that may have been forgotten. As the number of days of food recording increase, the ability to characterize the nutrient intake of an individual improves. A few days are needed to estimate macronutrient intake and energy intake, which tend to be relatively consistent from day to day. For nutrients that are concentrated in relatively few foods (such as beta carotene), the number of days required to accurately assess intake increases.

Food Frequency Questionnaire

FFQs are usually self-administered instruments that list common foods by food groups. The response frame is designed to elicit how frequently listed items are consumed. The response options usually include columns for daily, weekly, monthly, or yearly times the food was eaten. An FFQ designed for use in identifying dietary changes needed to improve serum lipids is Medficts (see Figure 4.1) (2). FFQs may include an open format to add items that may be frequently consumed by a relatively small subset of those completing the questionnaire. This approach facilitates tailoring the use of FFQs for ethnically diverse populations. However, staff assistance

Sample Dietary Assessment Questionnaire
MEDFICTS*

In each food category for both Group 1 and Group 2 foods check one box from the "Weekly Consumption" column (number of servings eaten per week) and then check one box from the "Serving Size" column. If you check Rarely/Never, do not check a serving size box. See next page for score.

Food Category	Weekly Consumption			Serving Size			Score
	Rarely/never	3 or less	4 or more	Small <5 oz/d 1 pt	Average 5 oz/d 2 pts	Large >5 oz/d 3 pts	

Meats

- Recommended amount per day: ≤5 oz (equal in size to 2 decks of playing cards).
- Base your estimate on the food you consume most often.
- Beef and lamb selections are trimmed to 1/8" fat.

	Weekly Consumption			Serving Size			Score
Group 1. 10g or more total fat in 3 oz cooked portion **Beef –** Ground beef, Ribs, Steak (T-bone, Flank, Porterhouse, Tenderloin), Chuck blade roast, Brisket, Meatloaf (w/ground beef), Corned beef **Processed meats –** 1/4 lb burger or lg. sandwich, Bacon, Lunch meat, Sausage/knockwurst, Hot dogs, Ham (bone-end), Ground turkey **Other meats, Poultry, Seafood –** Pork chops (center loin), Pork roast (Blade, Boston, Sirloin), Pork spareribs, Ground pork, Lamb chops, Lamb (ribs), Organ meats[†], Chicken w/skin, Eel, Mackerel, Pompano	☐	☐ 3 pts	☐ 7pts	x ☐ 1 pt	☐ 2 pts	☐ 3 pts	___
Group 2. Less than 10g total fat in 3 oz cooked portion **Lean beef –** Round steak (Eye of round, Top round), Sirloin[‡], Tip & bottom round[‡], Chuck arm pot roast[‡], Top Loin[‡] **Low-fat processed meats –** Low-fat lunch meat, Canadian bacon, "Lean" fast food sandwich, Boneless ham **Other meats, Poultry, Seafood –** Chicken, Turkey (w/o skin)[§], most Seafood[†], Lamb leg shank, Pork tenderloin, Sirloin top loin, Veal cutlets, Sirloin, Shoulder, Ground veal, Venison, Veal chops and ribs[‡], Lamb (whole leg, loin, fore-shank, sirloin)[‡]	☐	☐	☐	x		☐¥ 6 pts	___

Eggs – Weekly consumption is the number of times you eat eggs each week ⟶ Check the number of eggs eaten each time

	Weekly Consumption			≤1	2	≥3	Score
Group 1. Whole eggs, Yolks	☐	☐ 3 pts	☐ 7pts	x ☐ 1 pt	☐ 2 pts	☐ 3 pts	___
Group 2. Egg whites, Egg substitutes (1/2 cup)	☐	☐	☐	☐	☐	☐	___

Dairy

	Weekly Consumption			Serving Size			Score
Milk – Average serving 1 cup **Group 1.** Whole milk, 2% milk, 2% buttermilk, Yogurt (whole milk)	☐	☐ 3 pts	☐ 7pts	x ☐ 1 pt	☐ 2 pts	☐ 3 pts	___
Group 2. Fat-free milk, 1% milk, Fat-free buttermilk, Yogurt (Fat-free, 1% low fat)	☐	☐	☐	☐	☐	☐	___
Cheese – Average serving 1 oz **Group 1.** Cream cheese, Cheddar, Monterey Jack, Colby, Swiss, American processed, Blue cheese, Regular cottage cheese (1/2 cup), and Ricotta (1/4 cup)	☐	☐ 3 pts	☐ 7pts	x ☐ 1 pt	☐ 2 pts	☐ 3 pts	___
Group 2. Low-fat & fat-free cheeses, Fat-free milk mozzarella, String cheese, Low-fat, Fat-free milk & Fat-free cottage cheese (1/2 cup) and Ricotta (1/4 cup)	☐	☐	☐	☐	☐	☐	___
Frozen Desserts – Average serving 1/2 cup **Group 1.** Ice cream, Milk shakes	☐	☐ 3 pts	☐ 7pts	☐ 1 pt	☐ 2 pts	☐ 3 pts	___
Group 2. Low-fat ice cream, Frozen yogurt	☐	☐	☐	x ☐	☐	☐	___

FIG MEDFICTS assessment tool.
* MEDFICTS was orginally developed for and printed in ATP II[1-2]

FIGURE 4.1
Medficts. Reprinted from Appendix A in reference 2.
Available at: http://www.nhlbi.nih.gov/guidelines/cholesterol/atp3full.pdf. Accessed May 14, 2004.

may be needed to elicit these items. FFQs may also include listings of nutrient and herbal supplements. Typically, FFQs underestimate energy intake but may overestimate micronutrient intake. Software for analyzing the National Cancer Institute (NCI) FFQ is available free of charge, but other FFQs are proprietary. Subar et al (18) compared the validity of the NCI, Block, and Willett FFQs. The Block and the NCI FFQs have higher correlations with the 24-

Sample Dietary Assessment Questionnaire (Continued)
MEDFICTS*

Food Category	Weekly Consumption			Serving Size			Score
	Rarely/ never	3 or less	4 or more	Small <5 oz/d 1 pt	Average 5 oz/d 2 pts	Large >5 oz/d 3 pts	

Frying Foods – Average servings: see below. This section refers to method of preparation for vegetables and meat.

Group 1. French fries, Fried vegetables (1/2 cup), Fried chicken, fish, meat (3 oz)	☐	☐ 3 pts	☐ 7 pts	x ☐ 1 pt	☐ 2 pts	☐ 3 pts	_____
Group 2. Vegetables, not deep fried (1/2 cup), Meat, poultry, or fish—prepared by baking, broiling, grilling, poaching, roasting, stewing: (3 oz)	☐	☐	☐	☐	☐	☐	

In Baked Goods – 1 Average serving

Group 1. Doughnuts, Biscuits, Butter rolls, Muffins, Croissants, Sweet rolls, Danish, Cakes, Pies, Coffee cakes, Cookies	☐	☐ 3 pts	☐ 7 pts	x ☐ 1 pt	☐ 2 pts	☐ 3 pts	_____
Group 2. Fruit bars, Low-fat cookies/cakes/pastries, Angel food cake, Homemade baked goods with vegetable oils, breads, bagels	☐	☐	☐	☐	☐	☐	

Convenience Foods

Group 1. Canned, Packaged, or Frozen dinners: e.g., Pizza (1 slice), Macaroni & cheese (1 cup), Pot pie (1), Cream soups (1 cup), Potato, rice & pasta dishes with cream/cheese sauces (1/2 cup)	☐	☐ 3 pts	☐ 7 pts	x ☐ 1 pt	☐ 2 pts	☐ 3 pts	_____
Group 2. Diet/Reduced calorie or reduced fat dinners (1), Potato, rice & pasta dishes without cream/cheese sauces (1/2 cup)	☐	☐	☐	☐	☐	☐	_____
Table Fats – Average serving: 1 Tbsp **Group 1.** Butter, Stick margarine, Regular salad dressing, Mayonnaise, Sour cream (2 Tbsp)	☐	☐ 3 pts	☐ 7 pts	x ☐ 1 pt	☐ 2 pts	☐ 3 pts	_____
Group 2. Diet and tub margarine, Low-fat & fat-free salad dressing, Low-fat & fat-free mayonnaise	☐	☐	☐	☐	☐	☐	

Snacks

Group 1. Chips (potato, corn, taco), Cheese puffs, Snack mix, Nuts (1 oz), Regular crackers (1/2 oz), Candy (milk chocolate, caramel, coconut) (about 1 1/2 oz), Regular popcorn (3 cups)	☐	☐ 3 pts	☐ 7 pts	x ☐ 1 pt	☐ 2 pts	☐ 3 pts	_____
Group 2. Pretzels, Fat-free chips (1 oz), Low-fat crackers (1/2 oz), Fruit, Fruit rolls, Licorice, Hard candy (1 med piece), Bread sticks (1–2 pcs), Air-popped or low-fat popcorn (3 cups)	☐	☐	☐	☐	☐	☐	_____

† Organ meats, shrimp, abalone, and squid are low in fat but high in cholesterol.
‡ Only lean cuts with all visible fat trimmed. If not trimmed of all visible fat, score as if in Group 1.
¥ Score 6 pts if this box is checked.
§ All parts not listed in group 1 have <10g total fat.

Total from page 1 _____

Total from page 2 _____

Final Score _____

To Score: For each food category, multiply points in weekly consumption box by points in serving size box and record total in score column. If Group 2 foods checked, no points are scored (except for Group 2 meats, large serving = 6 pts).

Example:

☐	☐ 3 pts	☑ 7 pts	x ☐ 1 pt	☐ 2 pts	☑ 3 pts	21 pts

Add score on page 1 and page 2 to get final score.

Key:
≥70   Need to make some dietary changes
40–70 Heart-Healthy Diet
<40   TLC Diet

FIG. MEDFICTS assessment tool.
* MEDFICTS was orginally developed for and printed in ATP II[1,2]

FIGURE 4.1 (continued)
Medfics. Reprinted from Appendix A in reference 2.
Available at: http://www.nhlbi.nih.gov/guidelines/cholesterol/atp3full.pdf. Accessed May 14, 2004.

hour recall data for total energy and macronutrients. After adjusting for energy intake, all three FFQs were comparable for nutrients.

Diet History

Diet history refers to any dietary assessment that requires patients to report their normal daily food intake pattern, including amounts of foods consumed. Dietary histories range from questionnaires that use questions from major national government surveys to FFQs. Historically, a dietary history would use a triangulation of methods combining a 3-day food record, an FFQ, a 24-hour recall, and questions about typical food intake. More recently, economic concerns have focused on food insecurity and worries about having enough money to purchase food. Ironically, food insecurity needs to be assessed as an integral component of a cardiovascular dietary history because of its link to obesity (4).

Brief Dietary Scanners

Many of the dietary assessment methods used in clinical practice require too much time to be used in a community setting or large managed care organization. Table 4.2 lists screeners developed to identify key behaviors associated with increased CVD risk. They may assess adherence to a set of recommendations such as the ATP III guidelines or screen for key behaviors such as weight, activity, variety, and excess (WAVE), as shown in the WAVE tool in Figure 4.2 (19). Some are self-administered and others can be obtained in a brief interview (see Table 4.2) (12,20,21).

Disordered eating associated with obesity also needs to be assessed. Criteria for assessing binge eating have been available for some time. Stunkard and Allison (22) suggest that obese patients need to be screened to differentiate night eating syndrome (NES) from binge eating. A recent review of these conditions indicates an inconsistent finding with regard to the effects of appetite suppressants and antidepressants on the frequency of binge eating with high rates of relapse with discontinuation of therapy (22). If NES is accompanied by insomnia, antidepressants help restore a more normal sleep and eating pattern. Therefore, taking a careful history can provide valuable insights for the treatment approach.

Review of Systems

The review of systems is a subjective reexamination of the patient's history organized by body systems. It differs from the past medical history by concentrating on symptoms, not diagnoses, and by emphasizing current more than past information. The review of systems for CVD risk can yield information about the circulatory system such as fluid retention. The most complex system review is endocrine function because, by definition, hormones released by an organ in one area of the body have effects elsewhere in the body. Identification of proteins and peptides released from adipose tissue has resulted in redefining the role of body fat to focus on its endocrine functions. Fat is now considered to be endocrine tissue rather than merely a vehicle for energy storage because newly identified protein and peptides secreted from adipose tissue affect energy metabolism in the liver and elsewhere. Although historically a review of body fat would be beyond the scope of the review of systems, its role in health warrants a reexamination of body fat in the review of systems. Questions about patterns of body fat distribution during weight gain and loss are becoming increasingly important.

Other examples within the review of systems that may have nutritional implications (and their significance) include the following: weakness and fatigue (anemia); clothes tighter or looser (weight gain or loss); vomiting, nausea, diarrhea (poor nutrition intake, lactose intolerance); dehydration, constipation (low fiber or fluid intake); and amenorrhea (anorexia nervosa).

Physical Examination

The physical examination begins with the patient's vital signs (blood pressure, heart rate, respiration rate, and temperature), height, weight, body mass index (BMI), waist circumference,

Assessment

W eight

Assess patient's Body Mass Index*
Patient is overweight if BMI > 25

Height	Body Weight (lbs.)	Height	Body Weight (lbs.)
4' 10"	> 119	5' 8"	> 164
4' 11"	> 124	5' 9"	> 169
5' 0"	> 128	5' 10"	> 174
5' 1"	> 132	5' 11"	> 179
5' 2"	> 136	6' 0"	> 184
5' 3"	> 141	6' 1"	> 189
5' 4"	> 145	6' 2"	> 194
5' 5"	> 150	6' 3"	> 200
5' 6"	> 155	6' 4"	> 205
5' 7"	> 159		

*Certain patients may require assessment for underweight and/or unintentional weight loss

A ctivity

Ask patient about any physical activity in the past week: walking briskly, jogging, gardening, swimming, biking, dancing, golf, etc.

1. Does patient do **30 minutes** of moderate activity on **most days/week?**
2. Does patient do "lifestyle" activity like taking the stairs instead of elevators, etc?
3. Does patient usually watch **less than 2 hours TV or videos/day?**

If patient answers NO to above questions, assess whether patient is willing to increase physical activity.

V ariety

Is patient eating a variety of foods from important sections of the food pyramid? Determine **Variety** and **Excess** using one (or a combination) of the following methods:

- Compare foods eaten with Food Pyramid recommendations: "Think about what you usually eat for each food group and indicate the number of servings of each pyramid section."
- Perform a quick one-day recall: "Briefly describe everything you eat or drink in a typical day, beginning with the first thing eaten after waking up."
- Ask patient to complete a self-administered eating habits questionnaire.

E xcess

Look at the patient's typical intake. Is patient eating too much:

Fat? Saturated fat?

Sugar? Calories?

Salt?

Alcohol?

- Ask about serving/portion sizes, preparation methods and added fats, like butter, mayonnaise, sour cream, salad dressing, etc.
- Does patient eat 4 or more meals from sit-down or take-out restaurants/week?
- Is patient's weekend eating much different from weekday eating?

Discuss with the patient:
- "How do you think what you eat and how you exercise affect your health?"
- "What do you think is positive/negative about the way you eat?"
- If patient needs to improve eating and/or activity habits, assess willingness to make changes.

(continued)

FIGURE 4.2

Weight, activity, variety, and excess (WAVE) assessment and recommendations. Developed through National Heart, Lung, and Blood Institute–funded Nutrition Academic Awards. (See references 12 and 20.)

Recommendations

Weight	**A**ctivity
If patient is overweight:	**Examples of moderate amounts of physical activity:**

1. State concern for the patient, e.g., "I am concerned your weight is affecting your health."
 2. Give the patient specific advice, i.e.,
    a) Make 1 or 2 changes in eating habits to reduce calorie intake as identified by food intake assessment.
    b) Gradually increase activity/decrease inactivity.
    c) Enroll in a weight management program or
    d) Consult a dietitian
 3. If patient is ready to make behavior changes, **jointly set goals** for a plan of action and arrange for follow-up.
 4. Give patient education materials/resources.
	• Walking 2 miles in 30 minutes
	 • Stairwalking for 15 minutes
	 • Washing and waxing a car for 45-60 minutes
	 • Washing windows or floors for 45-60 minutes
	 • Gardening for 30-45 minutes
	 • Pushing a stroller for 1 1/2 miles in 30 minutes
	 • Raking leaves for 30 minutes
	 • Shoveling snow for 15 minutes
	
	 1. If patient is ready to increase physical activity, jointly set specific activity goals and arrange for follow-up.
	 2. Give patient education materials/resources.

Variety	**E**xcess

What is a serving?
 Grains (6-11 servings)
   1 slice bread, 1 oz. Ready-to eat cereal, 1/2 cup cooked cereal, rice or pasta, 1 tortilla
   Is patient eating whole grains?
 Fruits (2-4 servings)
   1 medium fresh fruit, 1/2 cup chopped or canned fruit, 3/4 cup fruit juice
 Vegetables (3-5 servings)
   1 cup raw leafy vegetables, 1/2 cup cooked or chopped raw vegetables, 3/4 cup vegetable juice
 Protein (2-3 servings)
   2-3 oz. poultry, fish, or lean meat, 1-1/2 cup cooked dry beans, 1 egg equals 1 oz. meat, 4 oz. or 1/2 cup tofu
 Dairy (2-3 servings)
   1 cup milk or yogurt, 1-1/2 oz. cheese
 	
 See instructions 1-4 under Excess
	How much is too much?
	 Too much fat, saturated fat, calories
	 • > 6 oz/day of meat
	 • Ice cream, high-fat dairy products
	 • Fried foods
	 • High-fat snacks and desserts
	 • Eating out > 4 meals/week
	 Too much sugar, calories
	 • High sugar beverages
	 • Sugary snacks/desserts
	 Too much salt
	 • Processed meats, canned/frozen meals, salty snacks
	 Too much alcohol
	 • More than one drink/day for women and two drinks/day for men
	
	 1. Discuss pros and cons of patient's eating pattern keeping in mind Variety and Excess.
	 2. If patient is ready, jointly set specific dietary goals and arrange for follow-up.
	 3. Give patient education materials/resources.
	 4. Consider referral to a dietitian for more extensive counseling and support.

FIGURE 4.2 (*continued*)
Weight, activity, variety, and excess (WAVE) assessment and recommendations. Developed through National Heart, Lung, and Blood Institute–funded Nutrition Academic Awards.

TABLE 4.2

Rapid Eating and Activity Assessment for Patients (REAP) and Weight, Activity, Variety, and Excess (WAVE): Clinical Tools for Integrating a Brief Nutrition Dialogue into Primary Care

Instrument*	Description	Administration	Comments
WAVE	Four-letter acronym helps to facilitate brief provider-patient dialogue about the patient's current status related to weight, activity, variety, and excess (12,20). The WAVE pocket guide has questions in four assessment quadrants on one side. The recommendations side provides Food Guide Pyramid food choices and service sizes. The card also includes counseling tips for practitioners.	WAVE can be incorporated into a patient interview with the addition of 5–10 minutes. Information about dietary intake can be obtained by 24-hour recall or brief screener.	Additional WAVE materials include techniques for tailoring the assessment and recommendations based on cardiovascular risk factors (11). A self-administered quick WAVE screener (21) has also been developed and formatively evaluated. The pediatric version includes 10 items and the adolescent-adult version includes 15 items or 17 items with food insecurity screening.
REAP	REAP has been designed to assess diet related to the Food Pyramid Guide and the 2000 US dietary guidelines. Questions assess intake of whole grains; calcium-rich foods; fruits and vegetables; fat, saturated fat, and cholesterol; sugar-sweetened beverages and foods; high sodium foods; alcoholic beverages; and physical activity.	REAP is designed to be a self-administered questionnaire at the 5th-grade reading level. Completion requires approximately 10 minutes. The time will be longer if administered by interview or reading level is low.	An accompanying physicians key includes section on patient at risk, further evaluation, and treatment as well as counseling points and further information for each of the major dietary areas. The validity of REAP was assessed on the basis of correlation with healthy eating index scores. Instrument reliability has also been established (12).

*The template for the WAVE Pocket Card and REAP materials can be downloaded from the Internet at http://biomedical.brown.edu/courses/nutrition/naa/resources.html. A Palm Pilot version is available at http://med2mercer.edu/ncvd/default.htm.

and general appearance. For example, "On examination, she is a well-developed, overweight woman." When terms such as obese, overweight, undernourished, thin, well-nourished, well-developed, or cachectic (profound, marked state of ill health and undernutrition) are used, they should be supported by findings in the physical exam and noted in the problem list. Nutrition-oriented aspects of the physical exam focus on the skin, head, hair, eyes, mouth, nails, extremities, abdomen, skeletal muscle, and fat stores. Areas that provide signs of CVD risk status include abdominal accumulation of body fat, which is associated with insulin resistance, and fluid retention, which may be indicative of hypertension or congestive heart failure or occur as a side effect of calcium channel blocker therapy. Body weight measurements are not valid for assessing obesity-related CVD risks in patients with congestive heart failure. Therefore, examination of the ankles for edema and the face for temporal wasting can help determine the patient's overall nutritional status.

Dyslipidemia can result in lipid deposition or xanthomas on the skin or on tendons. Various clinical forms of xanthomas, such as planar, eruptive, and tendinous, can be important physical signs of underlying metabolic disorders. The specific disorders range from genetic lipoprotein diseases to conditions such as diabetes, obstructive liver disease, thyroid disease, renal disease, and pancreatitis that in turn lead to lipoproteinemia (23,24). Eruptive xanthomas, which may be mistaken for a skin rash, are often linked to hypertriglyceridemia. Medications that increase insulin resistance and triglyceride levels, such as psychotropic drugs, can also cause eruptive xanthomas. Hypercholesterolemia is often associated with xanthomas on or below the eyelids or as a corneal arch. However, individuals who manifest these skin lesions may have normal lipid levels. Acanthosis nigricans (also referred to as "pseudoacanthosis nigricans") is a skin lesion closely linked to insulin resistance. Local growth factors may be the link between insulin resistance and the development of velvety skin with dark striations in skin folds in the neck, underarms, and groin region. Acanthosis nigricans can develop before 10 years of age in hyperinsulinemic obese children. Although many individuals with insulin resistance may not develop acanthosis nigricans, the appearance of this skin lesion is an indication that circulating insulin levels are likely to be elevated (25).

Subcutaneous fat stores should be examined for losses due to a sudden decrease in weight or for excess accumulation that commonly occurs in obesity. At the present time, obesity is the most commonly encountered nutrition problem seen in clinical practices in the United States and many other developed countries.

CVD Risk Assessment

A wide variety of physiological parameters have been linked to CVD. The most widely recognized risk markers are those included in the Framingham risk equation, which is a regression equation used to predict CVD risk over a period of time, usually 10 years. Risk factors in the Framingham equation include systolic blood pressure, total cholesterol, HDL cholesterol, smoking, and age with consideration of gender. Although not specifically included in the Framingham equation, the following risk factors should also be considered: low-density lipoprotein (LDL) cholesterol, serum triglyceride levels, family history, and presence of diabetes. Additional novel markers, which are increasingly the focus of research studies, include lipoprotein (a), C-reactive protein, fibrinogen, and homocysteine. A recent evidence-based review of 373 published studies related to these novel markers concluded that little data exist regarding the additive yield of screening for these factors (26). Clinicians who measure these markers in high-risk patients should focus on interventions known to reduce risk measured by more traditional markers. Chapter 3 provides an in-depth discussion of CVD risk factors.

ASSESSING OBESITY AND OVERWEIGHT AS NATIONAL PRIORITY CVD RISK FACTORS

Obesity is associated with a 50% to 100% increased risk of premature death from all causes compared with normal weight individuals, as well as a dramatic increase in CVD risk. However, there has been confusion with regard to whether excess body weight should be considered an independent cardiovascular risk factor. Nonetheless, the National Heart, Lung, and Blood Institute (NHLBI) states that "next to smoking, obesity is the second leading cause of preventable death in the US today" (27). Overweight and obese individuals have an increased risk of diabetes, coronary heart disease, hyperlipidemia, hypertension, stroke, gallbladder disease, sleep apnea, osteoarthritis, respiratory problems, and certain types of cancers (endometrium, breast, prostate, and colon), all of which increase their risk of mortality (see Figure 4.3) (28).

Strong evidence confirms that a 10% decrease in body weight results in a reduction of blood pressure, fasting glucose, and lipid levels. Therefore, assessment of obesity in relation to cardiovascular risk is vitally important. Treatment for obese individuals with three or more of the following risk factors should be aggressive: cigarette smoking, hypertension, high LDL cholesterol levels, low HDL cholesterol levels, elevated fasting glucose levels,

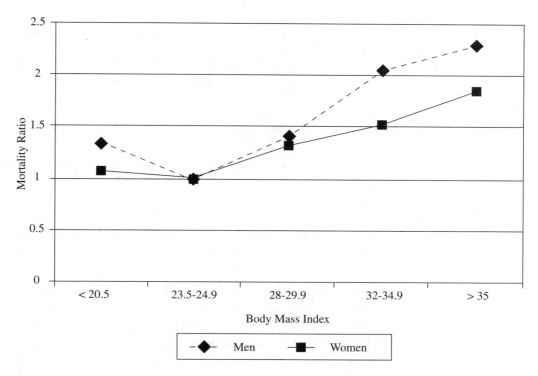

FIGURE 4.3
Obesity and mortality risk. Data are from reference 28.

family history of coronary heart disease, and age above 45 in men and 55 years in women (see Chapter 6).

The *Healthy People 2010* objectives address nutrition assessment for the United States, with individual chapters devoted to diabetes, nutrition and overweight, physical activity and fitness, food safety, and heart, kidney, and pulmonary diseases. One goal of *Healthy People 2010* is to promote health and reduce chronic diseases associated with diet and overweight. The objectives to reach these goals are related to weight status and growth, food and nutrient consumption, iron deficiency and anemia, and access issues related to food (often referred to as "food security") and preventive health care. Progress is monitored with data derived from schools, work sites, and communities as well as data about more traditional nutrition counseling (medical nutrition therapy) (29).

Body Mass Index

Overweight and obesity are now defined using BMI, which can be determined with the calculator on the NHLBI "Calculate Your Body Mass Index" Web site (http://www.nhlbisupport.com/bmi) or derived from the following formula (19):

$$BMI = \frac{Weight\ (kg)}{Height^2\ (m^2)}$$

According to the NHLBI's Clinical Guidelines (19), BMI provides a more accurate measure of total body fat than body weight alone. There are also a number of other accurate

TABLE 4.3
Classification of Overweight and Obesity by Body Mass Index

Weight Classification	Body Mass Index
Underweight	<18.5
Normal weight	18.5–24.9
Overweight	25–29.9
Obesity (class 1)	30–34.9
Obesity (class 2)	35–39.9
Extreme obesity (class 3)	≥40

Source: Adapted from Table ES-2 in reference 19.

methods for measuring body fat, including bioelectric impedance, which is now increasingly available at a lower cost and could be an adjunct tool in the clinical setting (19). The BMI value is more accurate than the ideal height-weight tables that were based on a homogeneous population, primarily white, with higher than average socioeconomic status. These values did not accurately reflect body fat content in the general population. In addition, these values were gender specific, whereas the BMI uses a direct calculation comparing weight relative to height, regardless of gender. BMI can therefore be used, along with waist circumference and other risk factors, to assess an individual's CVD risk. However, there are some limitations: BMI may overestimate body fat in very muscular people and underestimate body fat in some underweight people who have lost lean tissue, such as older adults.

The NHLBI clinical guidelines classify BMI as shown in Table 4.3 (19). Because many people with a BMI of 25 or higher begin to experience health problems associated with obesity, such as elevated LDL cholesterol and total cholesterol levels, high blood pressure, and glucose intolerance, the guidelines define overweight individuals as those with a BMI of 25 to 29.9 and obese individuals as those with a BMI of 30 and above. CVD risk usually increases as the severity of obesity increases.

Waist Circumference

Because the location of body fat is predictive of CVD risk, measuring waist circumference is recommended (ATP III). Excess fat located in the abdominal area (termed "visceral adipose tissue") is an independent measure of risk in normal weight, as well as in overweight and obese individuals. Waist circumference is an independent predictor of morbidity and is considered an independent risk factor for diabetes, dyslipidemia, hypertension, and CVD, even when BMI is not markedly increased, although this may differ among ethnic groups. In patients with a BMI greater than 35, there is little additional risk from elevated waist circumference, as severe risk is already present. Therefore, measuring waist circumference is recommended in patients with a BMI less than 35. The waist circumference measurement may be particularly important for patients who are overweight (BMI 25 to 29.9) and have a family history of diabetes.

To obtain an accurate waist circumference measurement, patients should be standing in only their underwear. A horizontal mark should be drawn just above the uppermost lateral border of the right iliac crest, which should then be crossed with a vertical mark in the mid-axillary line. The measuring tape is placed in a horizontal plane around the abdomen at the level of this marked point on the right side of the trunk. The plane of the tape should be parallel to the floor, and the tape should be snug but not tight. The patient should be advised to breathe normally when the measurement is taken. Waist circumference values greater than 102 cm (40 inches) in men and greater than 88 cm (35 inches) in women are considered indicators of increased risk. These values also represent one of the diagnostic criteria of metabolic syndrome (see Chapter 7). Tracking waist circumference over time in individuals attempting to lose weight is recommended.

Having a waist circumference greater than 35 inches in women and greater than 40 inches in men is associated with visceral fat accumulation, which is also a hallmark characteristic of insulin resistance. Waist measurements are less precise than imaging techniques such as magnetic resonance imaging (MRI) and computerized tomography (CT) scans, which permit visualization of fat in the visceral compartment. Nonetheless, waist measurement is the most practical measure and has become the recommended technique for clinical practice. The waist-hip ratio was recommended in the past as a measure, but data from the World Health Organization from 19 population groups indicate that the waist measurement alone is the preferred measurement in monitoring trends and determining CVD risk (30).

DIETARY ASSESSMENT AND COUNSELING OF DIVERSE POPULATIONS

Working with diverse populations is extremely challenging (see Chapter 15). The concept of cultural competence has been advanced to help health care professionals identify those skills required to respectfully treat patients from other cultures. If one accepts the biopsychosocial model of health and attempts to provide care that nurtures individuals and respects their relationships with others, then one must consider the importance of cultural dietary patterns when recommending dietary change. The patient-centered method provides the practitioner with an easy mechanism for developing cultural competence. Rather than presenting diet information as if the dietitian is "right" and the patient is "wrong," the patient-centered method recognizes patients as the experts regarding their own culture and environment. The dietitian then plays the role of consultant, gathering information and reframing it into a treatment paradigm that makes sense to patients by acknowledging their unique situations (culture, family, community). The goal is to seek common ground where a negotiated treatment plan acknowledges the importance of cultural eating patterns (when present), the degree of acculturation, and the potential health effects of each of these influences.

Although there had been an overall decline in CVD mortality, this has been primarily due to the reduction in CVD mortality in whites (31). Rates of obesity, diabetes, and CVD risk factors are increasing, especially in low-income African-American and Hispanic women. As individuals from non-Western societies and indigenous subpopulations in the United States adapt to a Western or American diet, the adaptations may have a deleterious impact on heart health.

Maintaining healthful traditional dietary habits, such as eating fresh fruits and vegetables in youth, is often linked to the role of social sphere and family in instilling the importance of a traditional diet (32). Dietary recommendations increasingly emphasize the importance of risk-factor reduction based on individual risk patterns.

African Americans

The traditional dietary pattern of individuals of African ancestry can vary widely. The dietary pattern may reflect a geographic region within the United States, such as Southern soul food, or reflect a country or region of origin, such as Great Britain or the Caribbean. Typically, Southern cooking for individuals of all racial groups includes greater use of fried foods, high-fat meats (fried poultry, fatty pork) (33), and lower intake of fats from dairy foods. Other sources of fats include biscuits and ham hocks or fat back cooked with vegetables. Intervention studies indicate that dietary fat can be lowered for the Southern population by purchasing low-fat cuts of meat and by "oven frying" breaded meats using a nonstick spray (34). Caribbean populations tend to prefer fat reduction strategies that include eating fresh fruits and vegetables and baking, roasting, or stewing rather than frying foods (35). Several studies have suggested that a reduced physical activity level that begins during adolescence may contribute to a rise in obesity that is most dramatically observed in African-American women (36,37).

Hispanic Americans

In the United States, a Hispanic individual may have come from Mexico, Cuba, Puerto Rico, the Dominican Republic, or another Central or South American country. The Hispanic population is quite diverse with respect to eating preferences. One approach is to focus on acculturation in Hispanic dietary habits and to examine food choices on a continuum from the typical food of the country of origin to what might be considered as typical American food (38). However, what is often considered to be Mexican food may be Tex-Mex or Cal-Mex rather than a reflection of historical dietary patterns from any region of Mexico. Data from the National Nutrition Survey and the Hispanic Health and Nutrition Examination Survey suggest that Mexican Americans have a higher total fat and cholesterol intake than Puerto Ricans or Cuban Americans (39,40). Traditional eating patterns tend to revolve around rice and beans for Puerto Ricans, meat fritters and turnovers for Cuban Americans, and a greater use of corn (eg, tortillas) for Mexican Americans. Fat for all groups comes from pastries and fried foods. Acculturation may be accompanied by increased intake of sources of saturated fat, such as meat, and increased milk intake, which is likely to be whole, canned evaporated, or condensed milk. Conserving dietary fat (eg, using chicken fat or bacon grease) in food preparation becomes a health issue as food intake becomes more plentiful. Traditional sources of fruits and vegetables may be expensive, of poor quality, or unavailable.

Asian Americans

The Asian-American population is heterogeneous, and there is great variation in dietary intake by age, culture, gender, and years in the United States. Korean foods include rice, kimchi, garlic, green onions, and traditionally prepared Korean soup (41). Eating patterns among Japanese Americans tend to vary with succeeding generations from the traditional fare to a diet containing many complementary and accessory foods that are higher in fat, sugar, and energy (42). Sources of fat for Asians from the Indian subcontinent are primarily ghee (clarified butter) and fried foods (43). Sources of fat for Chinese immigrants who adopt Western dietary practices include milk, cheese, and snack foods (44).

CONCLUSION

It is essential to integrate nutrition-related information into the history and physical examination to obtain a comprehensive assessment of the patient seeking CVD management and treatment. Effectively communicating a summary of the patient's current dietary intake pattern and recommended dietary goals to the physician can promote efficient and effective health care for the prevention and management of CVD.

REFERENCES

1. Pearson TA, Blair SN, Daniels SR, Eckel RH, Fair JM, Fortmann SP, Franklin BA, Goldstein LB, Greenland P, Grundy SM, Hong Y, Miller NH, Lauer RM, Ockene IS, Sacco RL, Sallis JF Jr, Smith SC Jr, Stone NJ, Taubert KA. AHA Guidelines for Primary Prevention of Cardiovascular Disease and Stroke: 2002 Update: Consensus Panel Guide to Comprehensive Risk Reduction for Adult Patients without Coronary or Other Atherosclerotic Vascular Diseases. American Heart Association Science Advisory and Coordinating Committee. *Circulation*. 2002;106:388-131.

2. Expert Panel on Detection, Evaluation, and Treatment of High Blood Cholesterol in Adults. Executive summary of the Third Report of the National Cholesterol Education Program (NCEP) Expert Panel on Detection, Evaluation, and Treatment of High Blood Cholesterol in Adults (Adult Treatment Panel III). *JAMA*. 2001;285:2486-2497. Full report available at: http://www.nhlbi.nih.gov/guidelines/cholesterol/atp3_rpt.htm. Accessed May 14, 2004.

3. Linton MF, Faxio S, for the National Cholesterol Education Program Adult Treatment Panel III. A practical approach to risk assessment to prevent coronary artery disease and its complications. *Am J Cardiol*. 2004;92(1A):19i-26i.

4. Centers for Disease Control and Prevention. Self-reported concern about food security associated with obesity—Washington, 1995–1999. *MMWR Morb Mortal Wkly Rep*. 2003;52:840-842.

5. Murphy SP. Collection and analysis of intake data from the integrated survey. *J Nutr*. 2003;133(suppl):585S-589S.

6. Subar AF, Ziegler RG, Thompson FE, Johnson CC, Weissfeld JL, Reding D, Kavounis KH, Hayes RB. Is shorter always better? Relative importance of questionnaire length and cognitive ease on response rates and data quality for two dietary questionnaires. *Am J Epidemiol*. 2001;153:404-409.

7. Rockett HR, Berkey CS, Colditz GA. Evaluation of dietary assessment instruments in adolescents. *Curr Opin Clin Nutr Metab Care*. 2003;6:557-562.

8. Bingham SA, Luben R, Welch A, Wareham N, Khaw KT, Day N. Are imprecise methods obscuring a relation between fat and breast cancer? *Lancet*. 2003;362:212-214.

9. Solomons NW. Methods for the measurement of nutrition impact and adaptation of laboratory methods into field settings to enhance and support community-based nutrition research. *Nutr Rev*. 2002;60(suppl):S126-131.

10. Biro G, Hulshof KF, Ovesen L, Amorim Cruz JA; EFCOSUM Group. Selection of methodology to assess food intake. *Eur J Clin Nutr*. 2002;56(suppl 2):S25-S32.

11. Wylie-Rosett J, Mossavar-Rahmani Y, Gans K. Recent dietary guidelines to prevent and treat cardiovascular disease, diabetes, and obesity. *Heart Dis*. 2002;4:220-230.

12. Gans KM, Ross E, Barner CW, Wylie-Rosett J, McMurray J, Eaton C. REAP and WAVE: new tools to rapidly assess/discuss nutrition with patients. *J Nutr*. 2003;133(suppl):556S-562S.

13. Klesges RC, Eck LH, Ray JW. Who underreports dietary intake in a dietary recall? Evidence from the second National Health and Nutrition Examination Survey. *J Consult Clin Psychol*. 1995;63:438-444.

14. Conway JM, Ingwersen LA, Vinaard, BT, Moshfegh AJ. Effectiveness of the US Department of Agriculture 5-step multiple-pass method in assessing food intake in obese and nonobese women. *Am J Clin Nutr*. 2003;77:1171-1178.

15. Prentice RL. Dietary assessment and the reliability of nutritional epidemiology reports. *Lancet*. 2003;362:182-183.

16. Heetderks-Cox MJ, Alford BB, Bednar CM, Heiss CJ, Tauai LA, Edgren KK. CD-ROM nutrient analysis database assists self-monitoring behavior of active duty Air Force personnel receiving nutrition counseling for weight loss. *J Am Diet Assoc*. 2001;101:1041-1046.

17. Rafferty AP, Anderson JV, McGee HB, Miller CE. A healthy diet indicator: quantifying compliance with the dietary guidelines using the BRFSS. *Prev Med*. 2002;35:9-15.

18. Subar AF, Thompson FE, Kipnis V, Midthune D, Hurwitz P, McNutt S, McIntosh A, Rosenfeld S. Comparative validation of the Block, Willett, and National Cancer Institute food frequency questionnaires: the Eating at America's Table Study. *Am J Epidemiol*. 2001;154:1089-1099.

19. National Heart, Lung and Blood Institute, Obesity Education Initiative Expert Panel. *Clinical Guidelines on the Identification, Evaluation, and Treatment of Overweight and Obesity in Adults, The Evidence Report.* Bethesda, Md: US Department of Health and Human Services; 1998. NIH publication 98-4038.

20. Barner CW, Wylie-Rosett J, Gans K. WAVE: a pocket guide for a brief nutrition dialogue in primary care. *Diabetes Educ.* 2001;27:352-362.

21. Soroudi N, Wylie-Rosett J, Mogul D. Self-administered quick WAVE screener. *Diabetes Educ.* 2004;30 (in press). Available at: http://www.aecom.yu.edu/nutrition/instrume.htm. Accessed April 16, 2004.

22. Stunkard AJ, Allison KC. Two forms of disordered eating in obesity: binge eating and night eating. *Int J Obes Relat Metab Disord.* 2003;27:1-12.

23. Parker F. Xanthomas and hyperlipidemias. *J Am Acad Dermatol.* 1985;13:1-30.

24. Cruz, PD Jr, East C, Bergstresser PR. Dermal, subcutaneous, and tendon xanthomas: diagnostic markers for specific lipoprotein disorders. *J Am Acad Dermatol.* 1988;19:95-101.

25. Stuart CA, Driscoll MS, Lundquist KF, Gilkison CR, Shaheb S, Smith MM. Acanthosis nigricans. *J Basic Clin Physiol Pharmacol.* 1998;9:407-418.

26. Hachkam DG, Anand SS. Emerging risk factors for atherosclerotic vascular disease. *JAMA.* 2003;290:932-940.

27. Moksdad AH, Marks JS, Stroup DF, Gerberding JL. Actual causes of death in the United States, 2000. *JAMA.* 2004;291:1238-1245.

28. Calle EE, Thun MJ, Petrelli JM, Rodriguez C, Heath CW Jr. Body mass index and mortality in a prospective cohort of US adults. *N Engl J Med.* 1999;341:1097-1105.

29. Healthy People 2010: Understanding and Improving Health. 2nd ed. Available at: http://www.healthy people.gov. Accessed June 4, 2004.

30. Molarius A, Seidell JC, Sans S, Tuomilehto J, Kuulasmaa K. Waist and hip circumferences, and waist-hip ratio in 19 population groups of the WHO MONICA Project. *Int J Obes Relat Metab Disord.* 1999;23:116-125.

31. Cooper RS, Cutler J, Desvigne-Nickens P, Fortmann SP, Friedman L, Havlik R, Hogelin G, Marler J, McGovern P, Morosco G, Mosca L, Pearson T, Stamler J, Stryer D, Thom T. Trends and disparities in coronary heart disease stroke, and other cardiovascular diseases in the United States: findings of the National Conference on Cardiovascular Disease Prevention. *Circulation.* 2000;102:3137-3147.

32. Devine CM, Wolfe WS, Frongillo EA Jr, Bisogni CA. Life-course events and experiences: association with fruit and vegetable consumption in 3 ethnic groups. *J Am Diet Assoc.* 1999;99:309-314.

33. Smit E, Nieto FJ, Crespo CJ, Mitchell P. Estimates of animal and plant protein intakes in US adults; results from the Third National Health and Nutrition Examination Survey, 1988–2001. *J Am Diet Assoc.* 1999;99:813-820.

34. Kristal AR, Shattuck AL, Patterson RE: Differences in fat-related dietary patterns between black, Hispanic, and white women: results from the Women's Health Trial Feasibility Study in Minority Populations. *Public Health Nutr.* 1999;2:253-262.

35. Greenberg MR, Schneider D, Northridge ME, Ganz ML. Region of birth and black diets: the Harlem Household Survey. *Am J Public Health.* 1998;88:1199-1202.

36. Rotimi CN, Cooper RS, Okosun IS, Olatunbosun ST, Bella AF, Wilks R, Bennett F, Cruickshank JK, Forrester TE. Prevalence of diabetes and impaired glucose tolerance Nigerians, Jamaicans and US blacks. *Ethn Dis.* 1999;9:1909-2000.

37. Kimm SY, Barton BA, Obarzanek E, McMahon RP, Kronsberg SS, Waclawiw MA, Morrison JA, Schreiber GB, Sabry ZI, Daniels SR, for the NHLBI Growth and Health Study. Obesity development during adolescence in a biracial cohort: the NHLBI Growth and Health Study. *Pediatrics.* 2002;110:e54.

38. Garcia RA, Taren D, Teufel NI. Factors associated with the reproducibility of specific food items from the Southwest Food Frequency Questionnaire. *Ecol Food Nutr.* 2000;38:549-556.

39. Sundquist J, Winkelby MA, Pudaric S. Cardiovascular disease risk factors among older black, Mexican-American, and white women and men: an analysis of NHANES III, 1988–1994. Third National Health and Nutrition Examination Survey. *J Am Geriatr Soc.* 2001;49:109-116.

40. Loria CM, Bush TL, Carroll MD, Looker AC, McDowell MA, Johnson CL, Sempos CT. Macronutrient intakes among adult Hispanics: a comparison of Mexican Americans, Cuban Americans, and mainland Puerto Ricans. *Am J Public Health.* 1995;85:684-689.

41. Lee SK, Sobal J, Frongillo EA. Acculturation and dietary practices among Korean Americans. *J Am Diet Assoc.* 1999;99:1084-1089.

42. Kudo Y, Falciglia GA, Couch SC. Evolution of meal patterns and food choices of Japanese-American females born in the United States. *Eur J Clin Nutr.* 2000;54:665-670.

43. Ahmed S. Coronary heart disease: the Indian Asian diet. *Nutr Stand.* 1999;13:45-47.

44. Satia JA, Patterson RE, Kristal AR, Hislop TG, Yasui Y, Taylor VM. Development of scales to measure dietary acculturation among Chinese-Americans and Chinese-Canadians. *J Am Diet Assoc.* 2001;101:548-553.

CHAPTER 5

LIFESTYLE COUNSELING STRATEGIES FOR BEHAVIOR CHANGE

Darwin D. Deen, MD, MS, and Charles Swencionis, PhD;
case study by Bernadette Latson, MS, RD, CDE

One of the challenges in providing nutrition care to patients is that simply explaining the relationship between their diagnosis and their diet is only the beginning of the process of helping them to change their behavior. In addition, dietary change should be viewed as one aspect of improving health, which should also include avoiding cigarette or other toxic exposure and getting adequate amounts of exercise and sleep. The sum of these lifestyle behaviors have been shown to be alterable according to certain identified principles. This chapter reviews the process of behavior change as it applies particularly to nutrition advice for patients with cardiovascular disease and, in addition, helps dietitians to help clients create and achieve exercise goals. Topics covered include agenda setting for the visit, interview strategies that promote lifestyle changes (emphasizing diet and exercise behaviors), and methods to enhance dietitians' success in helping patients change behaviors.

The following questions are addressed:

- What is motivational interviewing and how can it help dietitians to motivate their patients?
- What is the stages of change model and how does it apply to the way dietitians care for patients?
- What is the health beliefs model (HBM) and how does it influence working with patients at various stages?
- How can the stages of change model be combined with motivational interviewing and the HBM to maximize long-term behavior change?
- How can other current models contribute to our understanding of how patients change and improve our effectiveness at facilitating change?
- What are appropriate goals for physical activity and how can the behavior change models described be used to help patients achieve these goals?

THE INITIAL INTERVIEW

Objectives

Dietitians assess dietary intake as an integral component of providing medical nutrition therapy (MNT) to prevent or control a patient's cardiovascular disease (CVD) risk. The importance of MNT in reducing risk is reinforced when other members of the health care team also address dietary issues as part of their assessments. Thus, brief assessments of dietary intake and lifestyle should be considered key components of the medical and social history for physicians, physician assistants, and nurses, as well as dietitians. The behavior change strategies outlined in this chapter are similarly useful to all practitioners working to help patients change behaviors.

It is imperative at the earliest stages of an initial interview to determine the patient's expectations for the session, his or her understanding of the illness, and the reason for the consultation. This provides the practitioner and the patient with a common language to use in determining what changes need to be made and provide a starting point for the process of making changes (setting both short- and long-term goals).

For example, a patient may be referred for nutrition counseling to help reduce his or her serum cholesterol level. Patients may know their "good" and "bad" cholesterol levels, but the specific diet prescription may vary depending upon weight, triglyceride level, or blood pressure. Thus, the dietitian must make a judgment about how to proceed with dietary changes that patients are not in a position to understand. On the other hand, patients may have specific ideas about their personal food preferences. A successful intervention occurs only when the patient and the dietitian agree on what problems need to be addressed and how they should be addressed.

Dialogue for Dietary Assessment

Typically a physician begins the medical assessment by querying a patient about his or her chief complaint or the reason for the medical visit. Likewise a dietitian should begin dietary assessments by querying patients about their understanding of how their dietary intake and lifestyle are related to specific medical problems and what their treatment goals are. Such a query can provide valuable insights for addressing readiness to make dietary changes. The transtheoretical model (see Table 5.1[1]) of behavior change is well suited to assessing a patient's motivation and readiness to make lifestyle changes to reduce obesity, diabetes, and cardiovascular-related risks (1-5). According to the transtheoretical model, individuals go through the following stages: precontemplation (not considering making a change in the target behavior), contemplation (considering the pros and cons of making a behavior change), preparation (planning steps to make changes), action (actually changing the targeted behavior), maintenance (making the changed behavior habitual), and relapse (when a formerly altered behavior pattern returns).

An assessment of readiness to change can be obtained with a self-administered questionnaire or in an interview (3):

1. Have you *ever* changed or tried to change the way you eat to lose weight or improve your health?
   If "no," skip to question 4.
   If "yes," proceed to question 2.
2. Are you currently following a dietary plan to lose weight or for other health-related reasons?

TABLE 5.1
Stages of Change and Counseling Actions

Client Stage	Counselor's Motivational Actions
Precontemplation	Give information, ask troubling questions about the client's perceptions of risks and difficulties with problem behavior.
Contemplation	Help the client provide reasons to move from con change to pro change. Prop up self-efficacy.
Determination	Help the client think up and choose among possible strategies for change.
Action	Support the client's choices and help develop new ones if needed.
Maintenance	Help the client develop, choose, rehearse, and employ strategies to prevent relapse.
Relapse	Support the client to start the process again without becoming demoralized or stuck.

Source: Data are from reference 1.

If "no," skip to question 4.

If "yes," proceed to question 3.

3. How long have you been following this plan?

If less than a month, the patient is in *action* stage.

If longer than 6 months, the patient is in *maintenance* stage.

4. During the past month, have you thought about dietary changes you could make to lose weight or improve your health?

If "yes," the patient is in *contemplation* stage. If plan is specific and to be implemented within a month, the patient is in *preparation* stage.

If no, the patient is in *precontemplation* stage.

For example, discussing past attempts to lose weight and the dietary therapies used can be helpful in opening the dialogue. This information provides a foundation for assessing a patient's current stage of behavior change. The stage of behavioral readiness is fluid—for example, life stressors can easily move a person from maintenance to precontemplation. The risk of relapse is greater for the veteran dieter, who may be quite knowledgeable about food composition compared with the novice who may be ready for change but needs food composition information. Making dietary changes is often fraught with ambivalence and conflict over the commitment to behave differently in certain eating situations and to change food choices. Therefore, an assessment of the patient's readiness to change behavior and level of motivation helps determine how to proceed.

MOTIVATIONAL INTERVIEWING TO HELP PATIENTS MAKE CHANGES

Objectives

Motivation varies from one moment to the next. Motivational interviewing can effectively help patients modify addictive behaviors. To some degree, habitual behavior patterns, such as unhealthy eating and a sedentary lifestyle, are like addictive behaviors and, therefore, motivational interviewing, which was developed for drug addiction, is increasingly being applied to lifestyle problems (6). The goal of motivational interviewing is to understand what the motivational state of the client is at that point in time and to act appropriately. The process of motivational interviewing has been described as moving from "doing to" to "being with" patients (7).

Motivational interviewing elicits motivation from the client, instead of trying to impose it from the outside. It has been defined as a directive, client-centered counseling style for eliciting behavior change by helping clients to explore and resolve ambivalence (8). Resolving ambivalence is the key to motivational interviewing. When people move into the contemplation stage, when they are thinking about changing vs not changing, balancing out the pros and cons, they are more susceptible to real change. However, a professional who inadvertently starts pushing behavior change at the client at this stage often meets resistance.

It is the client's task, not the counselor's, to identify and resolve his or her ambivalence. What clients need at this point is help listing pros and cons and a health professional willing to listen. Clients determine whether their current behavior is consistent with their goals and then make choices to move toward these goals. Direct persuasion is not an effective method to resolve ambivalence. If a counselor lists positive arguments for change, clients may respond with arguments against change. The counselor must allow clients to identify both positive and negative factors for themselves. The counseling style is generally a quiet and supportive one. In this setting, effective patient education requires the counselor listen more and talk less. Readiness to change is not a client trait but a fluctuating product of interpersonal interaction. The therapeutic relationship should be a partnership, not a hierarchy directed by an expert. Patient motivation requires establishing a therapeutic relationship from which motivation can grow.

Motivation as a Behavioral Probability

The counselor can never really know what clients are thinking and feeling. Health care professionals can infer thoughts and feelings from what clients say, the emotions they show, and what they do. Thus, "motivation can be defined as the probability that a person will enter into, continue, and adhere to a specific change strategy" (9). This definition shifts the emphasis from "motivated" as a passive adjective to the active verb "motivate," which is the counselor's responsibility. The counselor does not just give advice, but motivates, increasing the likelihood that clients understand and perform all the necessary steps to achieve change. Instead of blaming patients for lacking motivation, counselors need to provide the appropriate pieces at each stage of the process. Motivation becomes an integral component of the professional's job.

Components of Motivational Interviewing

The goals of a motivational interviewing session are achieved when:

- The patient's self-esteem is maintained or enhanced.
- The practitioner uses active listening.
- The interview focuses on specific behaviors that are steps to an overall goal.
- Incremental goals are set that create progress toward an overall outcome.

For example, if clients usually drink several cups of coffee with half-and-half each day and a goal is to cut down on dietary saturated fat, then they must first recognize that half-and-half is a significant source of saturated fat and that changing to whole or low-fat milk would reduce their saturated fat intake (see Table 5.2). Next they can evaluate how important half-and-half is to them. Then clients must consider how best to institute that change. Some clients may decide to make a change to use whole milk for use at home, but continue to buy half-and half when ordering coffee at a restaurant. This would be a first step toward reducing their taste preference for half-and-half.

TABLE 5.2
Amount of Fat in Milk or Creamer

Product	Total Energy (kcal)	Percentage of Energy from Fat
Half-and-half cream, 1 Tbsp (15 g)	40	90
Whole milk, ¼ cup	38	72
Reduced-fat milk, ¼ cup	30	45
Low-fat milk, ¼ cup	26	27
Nonfat milk, ¼ cup	22	0

Active Listening

Active listening is a technique that increases the bond between the practitioner and the patient. It is an important step in creating an environment conducive to behavior change. The techniques of active listening include the following (10):

- Observing the patient
- Remaining quiet to let the patient talk
- Listening to the words the patient uses that indicate an understanding of what the problem is
- Listening to how the patient describes each problem and noting discrepancies between what the patient says and how the patient says it
- Listening for the patient's interpretation of what is happening

Assessment to Identify Ambivalence

Developing and maintaining motivation is key to achieving lasting dietary behavior change. The motivational interviewing assessment proceeds by identifying and resolving the internal ambivalence about giving up unhealthy habits associated with increased cardiovascular risk, such as smoking, physical inactivity, or poor eating habits. The probing questions listed below can be used to identify sources of ambivalence and help enhance the motivation for dietary change.

Probing Questions on Benefits of Current Unhealthy Practices

- What do you like about the way you eat now? (*Consider convenience, flavor, feelings, and so on.*)
- What changes do you feel are necessary in the way you currently eat? (*Which behaviors is the patient most ready to change at the present time?*)
- What benefits do you gain from the way you eat? (*Visualize eating situations and feelings after eating.*)
- How does your eating pattern change depending on various situations or stressors? (*Examine coping style for various stressors and how that relates to eating.*)
- How does your eating pattern change to reflect certain feelings? (*Consider anger, frustration, anxiety, stress, and so on.*)
- What would your life be like if you changed the way you eat? (*Visualize lifestyle changes and explore potential feeling of loss, concerns about feeling hunger.*)
- What foods that you *like* do you think you would have to give up or be "told" to eat less frequently? (*Consider favorite foods, foods at social events, snacking pattern.*)

- What foods that you dislike do you think you "should" or will be "told to" eat? (*Explore "Diet food" perceptions, food groups not currently eaten, such as vegetables, and so on.*)

Probing Questions on Benefits of Changing Eating Pattern

- What benefits do you think you might gain from changing the way you eat? (*Brainstorm range of potential benefits—eg, fit into clothes, feel better, keep family from nagging.*)
- How does your eating (or lifestyle) pattern relate to chronic health problems, for example, high cholesterol, diabetes, hypertension? (*Explore patient's perception of how MNT may affect CVD risk factors, and medication dosage and side effects—for example, myopathies, sexual function, and so on.*)
- How could changing your lifestyle improve your long-term health and ability to function? (*Explore future important personal events.*)
- How could lifestyle changes improve the way you currently function? (*Explore fatigue, energy level, ability to concentrate, stamina, and so on.*)
- What food or lifestyle changes do you think you may like? (*Explore potential misperceptions of restrictions, or how some of the dislikes may be addressed—for example, feeling hungry.*)
- How do you think you could change your lifestyle to gain the potential benefits without feeling deprived? (*List some of the reasons given for not changing dietary intake.*)

Although readiness to lose weight may be fairly common, the stage of readiness for changing specific food items or behaviors may vary widely. For two different individuals who want to lose weight, one may be ready to substitute lower fat or nonfat milk for whole milk, but the other individual may be reluctant to make the same substitution. However, these individuals may switch roles on another food behavior such as reducing red meat portion sizes. Thus, assessing why a change may be difficult can facilitate the development of the solution. At a precontemplation or contemplation stage, open-ended questions can provide valuable information about how the patient views dietary advice. Thus, the interviewer asks "why" questions about eating rather than the "what" questions that are used to quantify food intake. Much of the dialogue focuses on the ambivalence elicited regarding the perceived pros and cons of making dietary changes. At the preparation or action stage, "what" questions can identify specific food items that can be targeted for behavior change. At the maintenance stage, "when" questions can be used to identify situations producing risk of relapse (for example, "How will you handle it when . . . ?).

Factors That Facilitate Change

Considerable research supports Rogers's view (11) that the therapeutic relationship is the most important factor in the counseling process. In a client-centered helping relationship, the client feels safe enough to explore change. The counselor is not directive, problem solving, or analytic. The counselor must provide empathy, warmth, and genuineness.

Empathy

Empathy is different than sympathy. It involves active listening and acceptance: restating what the client has said in a way that clarifies the counselor's understanding of what the client has said. An empathic counselor provides the opportunity for clients to have their experiences fully understood. It is demonstrated in the following formula. "You *feel* . . . [name the correct emotion expressed by the client] . . . *because* or *when* . . . [indicate the correct experiences and behaviors that give rise to the feelings] . . ." (12). This is a tool that helps one learn to understand and perform the expression of empathy. When counselors nonjudgmentally state their understanding of patients' emotional conditions, they take the risk of being wrong. Clients are given the opportunity to agree that this is an accurate depiction of their feelings or to correct their counselors. When a client is fully understood, the chances for progress to action are increased.

Warmth

Warmth is the second factor that strengthens a therapeutic relationship. Clients must feel that the counselor accepts and respects them. A counselor can maintain a sense of professionalism while exhibiting a warm and caring attitude. The client senses if the counselor is cold or indifferent. A few clients are difficult to work with in an atmosphere of warmth and caring. If a counselor cannot work with a patient, a referral should be made to another professional. The same client may work very well with a counselor who has a different personality.

Genuineness

Genuineness is the third essential element of the therapeutic alliance. The counselor must tell the client what he or she thinks and feels about what the client says and does. This does not mean brutal honesty at all times. It means telling clients as much as they are ready to hear at that moment in words they will understand. This statement may seem to be a mixed message. It is—genuineness is difficult but essential. To be too honest may bruise emotions, but not conveying enough truth may impede a client's progress.

Overcoming Barriers to Change

Being judgmental, talking too much, and not listening enough are severe barriers to change that diminish the effectiveness of some helping professionals. Five basic principles suggested by Miller and Rollnick (13) can help the professional work around client-imposed communication barriers.

1. *Express empathy.* Start by using the empathy formula if needed, but work up to expressing empathy without the formula. Counselors should make it clear that the patient is being understood and accepted. Acceptance does not mean that the therapist agrees with the client or approves of the client's behavior. It means that the counselor accepts and understands the client's perspective without judging it. Paradoxically, this acceptance of people as they are frees them to become something else.

2. *Develop discrepancy.* The goal of motivational interviewing is not to have clients accept themselves completely as they are and not change. Neither is motivational interviewing directly confrontational. Rather, the goal is to have the client present the reasons for change, rather than the counselor. People persuade themselves better than any other person can. In discussion, point out discrepancies between what clients say they want and the consequences of their behavior. In particular, point out when a client has identified such a discrepancy. Discrepancies between current behavior and goals are motivational.

3. *Avoid argument.* Counselors should avoid direct confrontations. When counselors argue that clients have problems and need to change, the clients feel defensive, which may

cause them to take the other side of the argument. The purpose of motivational interviewing is to get the client to become aware of problems and the need to change. Gentle persuasion or "soft confrontation" is indicated. Resistance is a signal to counselors to change their approach.

4. *Roll with resistance.* Certain martial arts teach that a smaller, weaker fighter may overcome a larger, stronger opponent by moving toward or turning with a blow and magnifying it, thus causing the attacker to fall. In a similar way, a counselor should not impose new viewpoints or goals, but rather encourage clients to consider new information and offer new perspectives. "Take what you want and leave the rest" is the permissive kind of advice that is embodied in the motivational interviewing approach. The counselor exaggerates the client's point of view, or turns a question or problem back to the client, directing resistance back to the client, and asking the client to find solutions.

5. *Support self-efficacy.* Self-efficacy is a person's belief that he or she can carry out a change or a task (14). The counselor must take any opportunity to convey messages that the counselor has confidence in the client's ability to carry out change tasks. One method is to tell stories of others who have changed. If the client has made some changes, build on these early successes. If the client has experienced setbacks, emphasize that there are many paths to the goal and the best approach for the client has simply not yet been discovered.

The Importance of Self-Efficacy

Self-efficacy predicts when knowledge will determine behavior (15). Self-efficacy is the client's perception of a personal ability to exert control. Once knowledge gaps have been identified and addressed, addressing self-efficacy may be the most effective method of promoting behavior change. Self-efficacy is assessed by asking clients about who they feel is most in control of their diets (or exercise patterns), who was responsible for any past failures, and how they have responded to obstacles in the past. If clients do not feel in control of their behavior, helping them to identify those areas where they can gain control makes behavior change more likely. If patients blame themselves for past failures (low self-efficacy), they need a plan that addresses how to make things different this time. If patients feel that external factors were responsible for past failures, ask them to describe what has changed in the environment that will prevent this from happening again. To address self-efficacy, clients must be asked to make a realistic appraisal of their abilities. There are four main sources of self-efficacy:

1. Verbal persuasion (including self-talk)
2. Performance accomplishment
3. Vicarious performance
4. Physiologic arousal

Activities that have been shown to influence self-efficacy include the following:

1. Modeling behavior (such as cooking classes)
2. Reflection on past accomplishments (positive reinforcement)
3. Role playing (practicing potential difficult situations)
4. Emphasizing effective benefit (short-term benefits)

For example, rather than concentrating on the long-term health benefits of a new dietary regimen, advise patients to think instead about how good they will feel about accomplishing a goal that they set for themselves.

Perceived Severity	Perceived Susceptibility
Outcome Efficacy	Cost vs Benefit

FIGURE 5.1
Health beliefs model. Data are from reference 16.

USING THE HEALTH BELIEFS MODEL TO EXPLAIN WHY PEOPLE CHANGE

The HBM seeks to explain what motivates patients to change health behaviors (16). Patients vary greatly in their interest in health and in their willingness to change personal habits in the pursuit of improved health. The HBM shown in Figure 5.1 (16) considers perceived susceptibility, perceived severity, outcome efficacy, and cost vs benefit in explaining why people choose to change.

Perceived susceptibility means that the client considers himself or herself to be at risk from his or her current behavior. For example, many patients discount the health risks associated with saturated fat consumption. They are not willing to reduce saturated fat in their diet because they believe that carbohydrate intake is the real problem or because they do not acknowledge that dietary saturated fat leads to increases in serum cholesterol and low-density lipoprotein (LDL) cholesterol levels.

Perceived severity reflects the extent to which the client believes the outcome is bad enough to warrant action to prevent it. For example, if overweight patients feel that being overweight is acceptable, they will not be interested in making dietary and lifestyle changes in an effort to control body weight.

Outcome efficacy reflects the relationship between the behavior to be changed and the expected outcome. Very often clients say, "I've been eating this way for my whole life, how much difference will it make if I change now?" Unfortunately, no one can say for sure what the outcome of any specific dietary change will be. Patients should be offered the benefit of the professional's experience and the assurances that stem from the existing scientific literature.

Cost vs benefit may be the hardest aspect to address for specific individuals. It reflects the internalization of the belief that the outcome of an effort to change will be worth the effort expended. All change is difficult, and some changes are more difficult than others. The routine changes expected may seem small to the health professional, but they may represent a real challenge for the patient, especially because food is more than just a vehicle for sustenance. Dealing with the impact of dietary modifications on holiday meals, parties and other special occasions, eating with friends, and so on can present a real challenge for the individual.

THE TRANSTHEORETICAL MODEL: STAGES OF CHANGE

The transtheoretical model was developed by Prochaska and DiClemente to describe a unifying theory of how people with addictions change behavior (17). Prochaska initially reviewed existing psychological treatment modalities in an effort to find common themes. These themes were then tested with patients trying to quit smoking, and the six distinct stages they advance through on the path to successful behavior change were identified (18). (See Table 5.1.)

Prochaska and DiClemente developed a treatment model based on identifying the stage the patient was in and recommended using stage-appropriate interventions. Their research has documented the effectiveness of this approach in tobacco cessation, alcohol dependency, and other drug addictions. Application of the model for diet and exercise behavior change is still in its infancy, but studies continue to show positive results. It is important to recognize that behavior change is not always a linear process whereby patients move smoothly from one stage to the next. Patients often relapse back to old habits and are unable to move forward again until they successfully address whatever barriers are interfering with their continued progress.

Precontemplation

At this stage in the model, patients have no plans to make any changes in their current behavior. Although many people know a lot about the relationship between diet, exercise, and health, a particular patient may have significant misinformation. Presumably, if patients are referred to a dietitian for counseling, the referring physician has told them that their health could be improved by changing diet and lifestyle. Alternatively, if patients take it upon themselves to seek the advice of a dietitian, they should be aware of the relationship between what they eat and their health conditions or risks. But are these correct assumptions? Can someone who comes to your office self-referred or having been referred by a physician really be in the precontemplation stage? Although we would like to think otherwise, an appropriate use of the stages of change model begins with taking nothing for granted. Ask patients what they know about their current health problems or medical conditions and what, if anything, they have considered doing to address the issues. This line of questioning helps the counselor to assess whether the patient has indeed moved beyond the precontemplation stage. Knowing the link between behavior and risk for a specific disease outcome is an important first step in recognizing the need to make behavior changes. This interaction allows the dietitian to correct clients' misunderstandings and to reinforce the causal link between their lifestyle and their CVD risk.

Contemplation

The second step in the model describes a stage when the patient has at least begun to think about making changes. Ideally, patients referred for nutrition counseling are aware of their medical condition or risks and have been thinking about making a change in their diet. (Although researchers usually restrict the definition of contemplation to planning a change within the next 6 months, in counseling sessions it can be viewed as a time when the patient is ready to make a change and is seeking help to determine which changes to make.) Effective users of this model do not presume patients are ready to change; instead, they engage patients in a discussion of what the patients think they need to change and why, as well as what they hope to accomplish when the change has been made.

Given the media coverage about diet and health, most people are somewhat aware that what they eat is an important determinant of their health risk. Many patients believe that the scientific evidence is contradictory or confusing and conclude that everything is bad for them, so they just do not try to make changes. For a client stuck in this futile cycle, these beliefs must be addressed before any significant progress can be made. Although headline news tends to sensationalize each new study result, health professionals need to place these results in the context of scientific inquiry. There is much that we do not know, but we do know how to build an enjoyable diet that improves cardiovascular risk, lowers blood sugar and lipid levels, and reduces the risk of a variety of cancers. This is the good news. Patients need to hear that they can make changes and reap health benefits.

Preparation

In the preparation stage, a patient intends to take action within the next 30 days and may begin to take some behavioral steps to get ready for action. The psychological task at this stage is to ensure that patients come to the conclusion that they have the ability and knowledge necessary to make a change. Selecting one change among a set of options is also part of preparation. For example, a client in the preparation stage may learn to modify recipes and then go shopping for the ingredients to prepare those recipes. Although these are also actions, they are actions without an intended result, until the new meal is prepared and eaten. Preparation may be the most important stage to predict success. If the tasks associated with preparation for change are accomplished, then successful change is much more likely. For example, if a client does not like any vegetables and the counselor negotiates with him or her that the first dietary change should be to increase fruit and vegetable intake, success is unlikely. On the other hand, if the first task is to try one new vegetable per week for 4 weeks, the client has a much better chance at success. Even if the client does not like any of the four new recipes tried during the month, he or she should be congratulated for the effort and reminded that he or she is well on the way to eventually identifying some vegetables to eat regularly. This positive reinforcement is a key motivational strategy.

Action

Action is the stage toward which all the others build. In this stage, clients have determined that they need to make a change, and, with help, they have selected a small step that will produce real progress toward the ultimate goal. Clients may already have done many small preparatory steps, but they have not become accustomed to the new behavior pattern. Researchers have determined that any change that has not persisted for at least 6 months should still be considered transient and characterized as part of the action stage. Action can refer to an overarching goal, such as keeping carbohydrate intake to less than 45 g per meal, or it can be a smaller element of that goal such as recognizing and recording 15-g carbohydrate portion sizes. Recording is an action in itself and a significant predictor of successful behavior change. Another example would be the series of steps necessary to ensure less than 30% of energy comes from fat: using low-fat dairy, removing the skin from chicken, using fat-free salad dressings, and using less or no spread on breads (19). Each of these is a series of knowledge and decision points that collectively create an achievable goal.

Maintenance

A patient reaches the maintenance phase when the attempted behavior change has been sustained for more than 6 months. It is rare that patients last this long on a diet, which may be the best argument for discouraging patients from dieting at all. If efforts are framed as lifestyle behavior changes, then relapse is less likely and it is not necessary to focus on new skills or different behaviors to transition from action to maintenance. Many weight-loss diets include the expectation that patients will eventually return to some other form of eating pattern, not that they will stay on the diet for the rest of their life. Much evidence demonstrates that this transition to some other form of eating results in weight regain for most people. It is one of the things that all dieters fear—"what will I do when the diet ends?" Many diet books now include both induction and maintenance phase programs so that patients know before they start what will eventually be expected of them. Research indicates that just making the effort to lose weight may provide health benefits such as lowered blood pressure and improved insulin resistance, even without actual weight loss (20).

Relapse

One of the most important aspects of the transtheoretical model of behavior change is the recognition that relapse is a part of the process and not something to be avoided or feared. A potential destructive aspect of a therapeutic relationship is the guilt associated with relapse. Clients neglect to tell counselors that they have not been able to keep to their goals because they do not want to disappoint or they fear recrimination. They avoid coming for follow-up or fail to keep or bring in their food diaries in an effort to avoid the expected admonishment of their clinicians. Although this pattern is true of addictive behaviors, it may be even more prominent in dietary change, which has to be applied repetitively to be successful (eating one healthful meal does not change one's health, only making consistently healthful choices is effective).

COMBINING STAGES OF CHANGE WITH MOTIVATIONAL INTERVIEWING

Objectives

The same client may be at different stages with respect to different behaviors. A patient with hypertension may need to restrict sodium, increase exercise, and lose weight by reducing dietary fat intake, portion sizes, or simple sugar intake. This person may be at the stage of pre-contemplation when it comes to exercise because he or she does not appreciate the relationship between exercise habits and blood pressure, but at a different stage regarding sodium intake. For example, the patient may have already stopped adding salt at the table and may be reading food labels in an effort to replace products high in sodium. The goals of motivational interviewing with these clients are to determine the stage relative to each potential change and to help them progress to the next stage in one or more of these areas.

Patient Example

JM is a 58-year-old male with a 16-year history of diabetes and hyperlipidemia. Ten years ago he participated in the Weight Watchers program and lost 45 lbs during an 8-month period. Unfortunately, his diet at that time was extremely strict, and at the end of this period he became frustrated and stopped dieting. During the next 2 years, he gained back all of his lost weight. He eats most of his meals out and prefers Italian restaurants, where he orders a pasta entree and usually finishes all of his food. He is unwilling to discuss any dietary change such as reducing his portion sizes, replacing some pasta with broiled meat or fish, or eating at home more frequently.

This patient has relapsed from a very successful action phase and is currently resistant to any further efforts to change his behavior. When this occurs, understanding the source of resistance is critical. DiClemente identifies four types of resistance: reluctance, rebellion, resignation, and rationalization (18). In this case the patient has developed rebellious resistance. Food is his one refuge in what he increasingly perceives as a disappointing life. His rebelliousness stems from this unhappiness.

The place to begin with this patient is his desire to make more global changes in his life. How he feels about his life and the role that diet plays for him must be addressed before he can commit to dietary and lifestyle change again. The dietitian allows JM to express his disappointments with his life. Using reflective listening techniques, the dietitian can help JM understand that his diet and exercise habits are under his control and that mastering these can help him feel positive about other areas of his life. JM gradually overcomes his refusal to address his diet once he understands that his attitudes are standing in the way of his progress (he identifies his ambivalence).

OTHER METHODS FOR PROMOTING BEHAVIOR CHANGE

Although the stages of change model is an effective method for helping identify which interventions are likely to succeed with a given patient at a given time, it is by no means the only method of working with patients on behavior change issues. Other methods can be just as effective and may be easier to learn and apply.

Using a Decision Balance Tool

A decision balance tool helps practitioners gauge their patient's level of commitment to make change while helping patients clarify their goals and feelings (21). This tool provides a simplified form of some of the staging questions discussed in the section of this chapter on motivational interviewing and can be a helpful way to rapidly identify sources of resistance. Patients are asked to list both positive and negative attributes of changing and of staying the same. A decision balance is then constructed, which can be a helpful guidepost for both nutritionist and patient. Figure 5.2 (21) shows a model decision balance. Substitute whichever change is under consideration for the word "changing" when asking the questions—for example, "what would be good about eating smaller portions?" If resistance is high to certain specific behavior changes but low to others, it may be a good idea to select a small change with little resistance as the first step and work up to more difficult ones.

Choices and Changes

Keller and White have described the choices and changes model for practitioners seeking to influence health behaviors (22). It is designed as an adjunct to the transtheoretical model. It proposes that patients change when they have both conviction and confidence (and fail to change when they lack either). Conviction reflects the patient's belief that making a certain change influences his or her health. Confidence reflects the patient's belief that he or she has the ability to make a given change (see Figure 5.3). The practitioner uses the therapeutic relationship to help identify patients' levels of conviction and confidence and provides counseling to move them toward being more convinced and more confident regarding a specific

Reason Not to Change (Resistance)	Reason to Change (Motivation)
Benefits of Not Changing	Concerns about Not Changing
Concerns about Changing	Benefits of Changing

FIGURE 5.2
Decision balance. Data are from reference 21.

SUCCESS

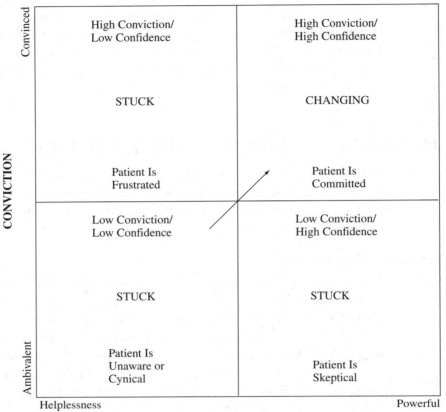

FIGURE 5.3

Choices and changes model. Reproduced from Keller VF, White MK. Choices and changes: a new model for influencing patient health behavior. *J Clin Outcomes Manage.* 1997;4:33–36. Reprinted with permission from Maysel Kemp White.

behavior change. The therapeutic relationship is established by eliciting the patient's experiences with open-ended questions and using reflective listening and empathy (providing acceptance for the patient's perspectives).

Practitioners can determine levels of conviction using questions such as "How important do you think this change is to your health?" or "How committed are you to making this change?" When the practitioner identifies a patient who has conviction ("I know this is important") but lacks confidence, counseling proceeds in an effort to identify the source of this helplessness and addresses ways to improve confidence. Confidence may grow by reviewing past accomplishments in other areas, by presenting change as a choice rather than a mandate, and by setting smaller realistic goals. Exploring ambivalence is important at this point ("What are the benefits or problems associated with changing? What are the benefits or problems with not changing?"). For example, remembering to buy apples at the supermarket may be considered as a goal in itself, although it is really only one step leading to the larger goal of eating more fruit and vegetables.

Practitioners can determine patients' level of confidence by asking "How confident are you that you can make this change? How important is it for you to make this change?" Patients who feel confident in their ability to make change ("I know that I can do this") but lack the conviction about a specific change benefit from discussions focused on their ambivalence and any discrepancies between the outcome they desire and current behavior (eg, "it will be very difficult to lower your cholesterol level if you continue to eat hot dogs or cheeseburgers for lunch every day"). Help patients to clarify what is most important to them and whether their current behavior is consistent with their goals.

Patients who lack both conviction and confidence may benefit from new information. They may not be ready for change at this time, and they need for their practitioner to accept them without judgment while offering support for the potential for change at some later date. Patients are ready to change when both confidence and conviction are high. Discussions with these patients can focus on barriers and situations that may cause setbacks.

The Five A Model

Another method for helping patients to change behavior, the five A model, was developed by the National Cancer Institute (23) to help physicians provide smoking cessation counseling to their patients. The model has since been refined and can be applied to any health behavior change. The As stand for assess, advise, agree, assist, and arrange. The following is a brief description of the recommended content for each step.

Assess

Assess specifics of the patient's current behavior, identifying health risk factors, level of knowledge, level of interest and commitment to change, and social supports that influence the change process.

Advise

Advise the patient by reviewing specific primary and secondary goals for behavior change, such as increasing soluble fiber intake or reducing the use of *trans* fatty acid–containing foods, and the expected long- and short-term health outcomes that might result.

Agree

Negotiate an agreement with the client to follow a plan that makes sense to both parties and facilitates behavior change.

Assist

Assist the patient in identifying methods to accomplish change, identifying available resources, and shepherding the client through the process of change. This includes monitoring the plan and modifying specific aspects as needed.

Arrange

Arrange for follow-up, acknowledging that behavior change does not occur immediately and requires time to translate into new habits. Ensuring adequate follow-up with patients, whether by repeat visits or other contact (telephone reminders, letters, or e-mail), is an important part of most successful behavior change strategies.

Choices and changes and the five A method are easily understood behavior change models that can be used as alternatives or in conjunction with the transtheoretical model and motivational interviewing. At an individual visit, practitioners may find it useful to think in terms of which stage of change the patient is in (regarding a specific behavior) and where he or she falls on the conviction and confidence scales. The counselor can then use this information to determine how to proceed with counseling. All counseling should employ motivational interviewing methods. For the overall behavior change plan, select an appropriate A to be the focus of each visit.

CHANGING PHYSICAL ACTIVITY BEHAVIOR

Just as changes in dietary behavior require a blend of psychological principles and specific, science-based advice, similar intervention is needed to assist patients in achieving healthy physical activity goals. When several health care team members are knowledgeable and reinforce concepts, achievement of change is more likely.

Benefits of Regular Physical Activity

Regular physical activity increases cardiac output and improves the ability of skeletal and heart muscle to extract oxygen from the blood. Benefits occur in hemodynamic, hormonal, metabolic, neurologic, and respiratory function. The exercise-trained heart demands less oxygen for the same level of work. Exercise training improves lipid and carbohydrate metabolism. Exercise develops endurance, joint flexibility, and muscle strength and has been shown to reduce anxiety and depression (24).

Sedentary Behavior as a Risk Factor

Research has consistently found an inverse association between physical activity and incidence of coronary heart disease (CHD) (25). Physical fitness predicted cardiovascular mortality in the Lipid Research Clinics Mortality Follow-up Study and among men in Norway (26,27). Physical fitness is also associated with reduced frequency of CHD events (28). Starting to exercise is associated with lower rates of death from all causes among middle-aged and older men (29). Physical activity was associated with lower mortality from CHD in the Multiple Risk Factor Intervention Trial (30). Exercise is essential for the treatment of hyperlipidemia, hypertension, impaired glucose tolerance, and diabetes mellitus.

Types of Exercise: How Much, What Type, and for How Long

Frequency, intensity, and time spent (referred to as FIT) are the basic parameters of exercise. Most studies of exercise and its effects on chronic disease use a standard exercise program with a single level of physical activity. One study performed several randomized crossover interventions to determine the dose-response relationship between exercise training and blood pressure (31). The intensity and duration of exercise bouts were constant, but their frequency varied. Standard bouts consisted of 30 minutes of bicycling at 60% to 70% of maximum work capacity. The exercise was either performed three or seven times per week, and the level was maintained for 1 month. In sedentary normal subjects, three bouts per week for a total of 90 minutes lowered systolic blood pressure by 10 mm Hg and diastolic blood pressure by 7 mm Hg. Seven bouts per week lowered blood pressure only slightly more than three bouts per week, with reductions of 12 mm Hg systolic and 7 mm Hg diastolic. Similar results were obtained in hypertensive patients.

Paffenbarger (32) studied 16,936 Harvard male alumni and found that those whose energy expenditure from exercise was less than 2,000 kcal per week were at 64% higher risk for disease than classmates who exercised more. Two thousand kilocalories per week is the equivalent of 30 minutes of moderately intense aerobic exercise 7 days per week, or 60 minutes, 3 or 4 days per week. The STRRIDE study (33) was a randomized controlled intervention examining the impact of exercise of different durations and intensities on serum lipid levels. To avoid the impact of dietary change, the patients were asked to maintain their baseline dietary intake. All exercising patients lost small amounts of weight and body fat, with the greatest fat loss in the group that exercised the most (both intensity and amount). Cardiovascular fitness (measured by peak oxygen consumption) was greatest in subjects whose exercise intensity was greatest regardless of duration of exercise. Exercise training was found to have no overall effect on total cholesterol or LDL cholesterol levels, but LDL subfractions were significantly altered. Although low-intensity and low-duration exercise had some nonsignificant beneficial effects, only the high-intensity and high-amount group had a significant increase in LDL size, with a reduction in the number of small dense LDL and intermediate-density lipoprotein (IDL) particles. In addition, subjects in this high-intensity and high-amount group had significantly increased high-density lipoprotein (HDL) levels, thus markedly improving their cardiovascular risk profiles. In this study, the low-amount of exercise was equivalent to jogging 12 miles per week, whereas the high amount was about 20 miles of jogging per week. Low intensity was 50% to 60% peak oxygen consumption, whereas high intensity was 65% to 80%. Although many studies have demonstrated that moderate exercise can have a significant effect on cardiovascular mortality (34), STRRIDE helped identify the amount and intensity of exercise required to provide specific benefit to patients (33).

The American Heart Association Scientific Council Statement on Exercise (24) recommends "30 minutes or more of moderate-intensity physical activity on most (preferably all) days of the week." However, the Institute of Medicine states that "30 minutes per day of regular activity is insufficient to maintain body weight in adults" and recommends 60 minutes daily (35). The American College of Sports Medicine (34) makes recommendations that are specific for the type of activity: 3 to 5 days per week; 55%–65% to 90% of maximum heart rate, with minimum values for people most unfit; 20 to 60 minutes of continuous or intermittent (minimum of 10-minute bouts accumulated throughout the day) aerobic activity. Duration is dependent on the type of activity; therefore, lower intensity exercises should be carried out for longer time periods. In addition, the American College of Sports Medicine recommends resistance training to maintain fat-free mass and flexibility training to maintain range of motion. Resistance training should be progressive, individualized, and stimulate all the major muscle groups. One set of 8 to 10 exercises for all muscle groups 2 to 3 days per week is recommended. Multiple sets provide greater benefits if time allows. Most people should perform 8 to 12 repetitions of each exercise, but individuals older than 50 years may prefer to do 10 to 15 repetitions using lower resistance levels (less weight). Flexibility training should be a part of the overall exercise program. These exercises should stretch the major muscle groups and be performed at least 2 to 3 days per week.

The greatest health benefit from exercise seems to come when people change from a sedentary lifestyle to exercising 30 minutes, three or four times weekly. There are additional health benefits when an individual exercises more than this (for example, 1 hour daily may be more effective for maintaining weight loss [36]), but these benefits are not as great as the benefit of moving from a sedentary lifestyle to exercising moderately. Most studies of the

TABLE 5.3
Leisure Activities

Activity	METS*
Biking	4–10
Walking	3.5–6
Running	8–13
Playing basketball	8
Shooting baskets	4.5
Playing baseball	5
Swimming	8
Playing tennis	8
Playing recreational football	5

*Ranges depend upon speed. Energy expenditure during exercise is expressed as metabolic equivalents (METS; multiples of resting energy expenditure). A 70-kg person would burn approximately 6 kcal/minute in a 5-MET activity.

effects of exercise on cardiovascular disease and diabetes have involved dynamic or aerobic exercise, such as brisk walking, jogging, swimming, dance, cycling, treadmill, hiking, rowing, tennis, racquetball, soccer, and basketball. This kind of activity is clearly of benefit for these medical problems. (See Table 5.3.)

Resistance or strength training is often recommended as an adjunct to dynamic exercise. Strength training builds muscle and changes body composition by increasing muscle and decreasing fat. However, these changes are gradual. Strength training is recommended two or three times per week as an adjunct to aerobic exercise.

Leisure Time Physical Activity vs Lifestyle Activity

Levels of leisure time physical activity are correlated with socioeconomic status (SES) (37). It may not be realistic for patients of lower SES to make time to exercise. People who cannot find the time to exercise should be advised to build more activity into their daily routine. Strategies include parking farther away than necessary, getting off the bus one stop earlier, and taking the stairs rather than the elevator. Small bouts of exercise, even if not continuous, may add up during the course of a day (38). Other people engage in pleasurable activities that may involve work or leisure, such as walking, gardening, yard work, housework, and dancing. The energy expended in these activities will contribute to weight loss but may not improve cardiovascular fitness (28).

Motivating Patients to Exercise

The techniques described in this chapter to help patients change dietary behaviors can be applied to exercise as well. People who exercise regularly report improvements in their overall health, feelings of well being and self-worth, sleep, and ability to stick with a diet. Thus, if clients stay with an exercise regimen long enough, they may discover that it becomes self-reinforcing (a positive addiction). Until that time, it is important to start gradually, with perhaps 5 minutes of exercise per day, emphasizing fun activities, injury avoidance, and achieving realistic goals. Using the principles of motivational interviewing, counselors can interview patients about the relationship between a sedentary lifestyle and their illness or health risks. Because all cultures have forms of acceptable physical activity, the challenge to the counselor is finding some form of exercise that can fit into the client's lifestyle. If it is not enjoyable, the activity may not be continued, so enjoyment must be the primary focus. Patients who are using exercise alone in their efforts to lose weight need to be cautioned that frequent, vigorous exercise is required for significant weight loss. Patients should be encouraged by intermediate endpoints (rather than weight loss), such as reduced blood pressure, lipid levels, improved feelings of well being, or how their clothes fit. They should also be reminded that exercise is the biggest predictor of weight maintenance after weight loss.

Measuring Exercise

Exercise can be classified by how much oxygen it requires. At rest the body uses 3 to 5 mL of oxygen per kilogram of body weight each minute. This equals 1 metabolic equivalent (MET). A 5-MET level of exercise uses five times the oxygen used at rest. There are two problems with the MET classification of exercise. Environmental factors such as wind, humidity, cold, hills, and heat can cause the cardiovascular system to work harder or easier at the same MET level. In addition, as a person's cardiovascular conditioning improves, a higher MET level is required to challenge the system.

Target heart rate is an alternative means of measuring exercise. Using the formula 220 minus age to calculate maximum heart rate, an individual can work at anywhere from 55% to 90% of maximum heart rate to challenge the cardiovascular system, burn energy, and improve conditioning. The difficulty with target heart rate is that the calculation of 220 minus age is an estimate; as conditioning improves, maximum heart rate may increase. The only way to really establish maximum heart rate is with an exercise stress test. Exercisers can measure their progress using a heart rate monitor. These monitors have electrodes that strap around the chest and transmit to a wristwatch display. The least expensive ones cost about $65; more expensive models have more features, but it is unclear whether anyone needs any features beyond simple heart rate and perhaps elapsed time. Heart rate monitors may be a convenient way of measuring exercise intensity.

Another means of measuring exercise is rating perceived exertion. This is done in gradations, such as very, very hard; very hard; hard; medium; light; very light. This method accounts for conditioning level and environmental variations, but it is very subjective.

Pedometers are becoming a popular way of keeping track of walking, jogging, or running so that one can improve fitness level. Pedometers were formerly built around a pendulum, but newer electronic models are more accurate and less expensive. All pedometers measure steps, and some models also calculate miles, kilometers, energy burned, speed in miles per hour, and exercise time. More expensive models may store some of these factors in memory. Pedometers cost between $11 and $40. Feedback about the number of steps taken each day can provide powerful motivation for increasing activity levels and achieving targets (eg, 10,000 steps per day is the equivalent of walking 3 miles a day).

Setting Physical Activity Goals and Monitoring Progress

Sedentary individuals should set a goal of 5 minutes of exercise per day. They should understand that there is a clear benefit of moderate dynamic exercise at 30 minutes per day, three or four times per week. Less exercise has some benefit, but the 30-minute/3- or 4-times-per-week threshold should be a long-term goal to achieve. Depending on body weight and physical condition, give the clients feedback if their goals are unrealistic. Gradual progress should be monitored weekly, in terms of total minutes per week and intensity of exercise. A 20% increase in intensity or duration every 6 weeks will lead to gradual performance improvements.

Example: Promoting Physical Activity Using the Five A Model

The five A model is a useful tool for helping clients increase physical activity (39).

- *Assess* your client's current and past physical activity level, abilities, beliefs, and knowledge.
- *Advise* your client about the health risks associated with his or her current level of physical activity and the potential benefits of regular exercise. Describe an appropriate amount, intensity, and type of physical activity.
- *Agree* on a mutually devised program that acknowledges the patient's interests and confidence. The program should get the patient from where he or she is now to where he or she would like to be in an appropriate time frame to avoid injury or other risks.
- *Assist* the client in identifying potential barriers to the successful implementation of this plan and strategies to address these barriers. Identify resources that can help the client reach goals. Encourage the client to enlist the help of social supports (family and friends).
- *Arrange* follow-up after an appropriate interval to monitor progress and troubleshoot problems.

CONCLUSION

Helping patients achieve long-term changes in eating behavior and physical activity generally requires intensive and consistent interventions for many months and even years. Using a combination of several models of behavior change allows health professionals the opportunity to maximize their attempts to help specific patients make multiple lifestyle changes. Dietitians should seek to become skilled at assessing the patient's readiness to change based on the transtheoretical model and then use motivational interviewing to help the patient move to the action stage. Clinicians must become familiar with the theories behind behavior change and then practice implementation of the various approaches to determine which works best for them. Additional methods, such as the five A and choices and changes approaches, may help specific patients strengthen their behavior change efforts.

The references cited in this chapter contain much more detail on some of the specific techniques, and further reading is highly recommended. In addition, Botelho has developed a self-learning module that can be accessed on-line to help train health professionals in behavior change strategies (7).

CASE STUDY: PRACTICAL APPLICATION FOR BEHAVIOR CHANGE*

SL is a 38-year-old woman referred by her primary care physician for nutrition therapy, diagnosis code 272.2 (hyperlipidemia, mixed). Table 5.4 shows her lipid levels. The physician's plan was a 3-month trial of diet and exercise at which point lipids would be rechecked and medication started as needed.

*Reprinted with permission from Latson B. Case study: using stages of change for counseling to reduce potential for metabolic syndrome. *On the Cutting Edge*. 2002;23:28-30.

TABLE 5.4
Initial Lipid Levels

Lipid Laboratory Tests	Patient's Lab Results (mg/dL) in June 2000	ATP III Reference Values (mg/dL)
LDL cholesterol	120	Optimal <100
Total cholesterol	230	Desirable <200
HDL cholesterol	27	>40
Triglycerides	474	Normal <150

All other laboratory values were normal. Her past medical history was unremarkable except for depression; Zoloft was her only medication. Her family history was positive for type 2 diabetes and hyperlipidemia in her father. With a weight of 220 pounds and height of 5 feet, 6 inches, her body mass index (BMI) was 36, indicating obesity II. She declined waist measurement. The social/lifestyle assessment included no alcohol or tobacco use, single, business executive. She reported no deliberate exercise although said she liked to walk.

Assessing Stages of Change

The stages of change from the transtheoretical model were used to assess SL's readiness for dietary change and to select the best counseling strategies focusing on her goals and preferences. Her adamant response to the question on what she wanted to accomplish included: "I don't want any kind of a weight-loss diet, my therapist has recommended that I not even talk about trying to lose weight because it's what makes me feel like the biggest failure." She also said that for more than a year she had tried to eat a very low-fat diet, not for weight loss, but because of her high cholesterol and she would be interested in a calculation of how much fat she was actually eating and might want to work on that.

SL was assessed to be in precontemplation for behavior change targeted to weight loss and in a maintenance stage of change for a low-fat diet—the latter based on patient-perceived intake. She was thanked for being direct and her self-efficacy was supported with praise for her attention to her mental health, validating the importance of both mental and physical health.

Stage-Matched Counseling Strategies

The stage-matched counseling strategies employed were to acknowledge SL's feelings about previous weight-loss efforts, support her decision to defer weight-loss goals while reinforcing her willingness to make diet changes targeted to lipid control. Her constellation of risk factors for metabolic syndrome (low HDL, high triglycerides [TGs], probable waist measurement greater than 35 inches) were explained along with the recommended interventions while stressing that selecting any one intervention was worthwhile. (See Table 7.1 in Chapter 7 for clinical criteria of the third Adult Treatment Panel [ATP III] for risk of metabolic syndrome [diagnosis code 277.7], which includes at least three of the following: hypertension, low HDL, elevated TGs, elevated fasting blood glucose, and abdominal obesity.)

Physical Activity

Increased physical activity is recommended by ATP III in the treatment of metabolic syndrome. The benefit of exercise to help raise HDL was explained to SL but she viewed exercise as targeted to weight loss and chose to defer this option.

Dietary Assessment

Preliminary assessment of SL's diet revealed a high calorie intake consistent with her weight, low total and saturated fat and cholesterol and high carbohydrate partly due to avoiding most meat, eggs, dairy, and all visible fat.

It was explained that this somewhat "skewed" diet could be worsening her TGs and HDL, and by making some equal-calorie food substitutions of monounsaturated fats and protein for carbohydrates, she should not feel hungry or deprived and her lipid profile might improve. SL was cautioned about the potential for unwanted weight gain with the higher-calorie fat foods.

Developing a Plan of Action

The specific changes the patient agreed to make included: (a) one bagel with 2 tablespoons of natural peanut butter at breakfast instead of her usual two bagels with jelly, (b) instead of 12 ounces of fruit juice twice a day, drink 4 ounce servings diluted with water or seltzer and could add 1 to 2 ounces of peanuts for snacks, (c) substitute 3 to 4 ounces of fish or lean meat for one bread serving at lunch and, (d) reduce usual pasta servings by half and enjoy an olive-oil based pesto dressing on this smaller portion. SL scheduled another appointment in 1 month and agreed to keep food records and fax them after 1 week.

A computerized nutrient analysis of SL's original diet showed intake of 2,861 kcal, 71% carbohydrate, 10% protein, and 19% fat. Analysis of the revised diet was 2,855 kcal, 60% carbohydrate, 15% protein and 25% fat.

Stages and Strategies Vary for Different Behaviors

At her next appointment the stage-matched strategy employed was skill building on food composition using nutrient analyses of the "before" and "after" diets. SL was asked what she thought about the breakdown of each diet, and she responded "I can see that I'm on my way to a more balanced diet with these changes."

Teaching skills and helping patients access resources needed for change are counseling strategies specific to the preparation stage of change. SL was assessed as being in the preparation stage for the more balanced style of eating, and she selected other food substitutions with her stated goal of "getting more balance in my diet." She verbalized surprise that beverages contribute so much carbohydrate and said she would think about that. Her weight was stable, and she said she felt good about being able to make diet changes without feeling hungry or guilty. In fact she reported her new diet was more palatable and varied.

The plan for the next month was (a) keep food records 4 days/week, (b) consider acceptable substitutions for her usual two fruit juice drinks per day, and (c) try the new recipes for avocado oil–based dressings and marinades.

At the second month follow-up, the patient presented with her own computerized diet records and analyses showing an average intake of 2,563 kcal, 50% carbohydrate, 20% protein, 30% fat with 15% from monounsaturated fats. The two juice drinks had been replaced by fruit-flavored, sugar-free tea with concomitant reduction of 300 kcal. SL was congratulated on her hard work both in computerized nutrient analysis and dietary behavior changes, thus supporting her decision to make this change. This reinforcement is stage-matched for the action stage of change into which SL now appeared to have moved. She commented that even if her labs did not improve next month, she would have learned a new computer program and added several new Mediterranean dishes to her culinary repertoire! Based on her reported lower calorie intake, her weight might be expected to be stable or lower but it was up 1.5 pounds. She said she was thinking about getting back to walking, and we discussed how this would fit in her daily schedule. Discussing barriers is an appropriate counseling strategy for the contemplation stage of change in which she was assessed to be for exercise.

Outcome

Immediately prior to the third month follow-up, the patient faxed in her new lab results (Table 5.5) where she had scrawled "We did it!"

SL's self-efficacy was almost visibly boosted, which in turn motivated her to continue making changes to improve her health. She began a daily walking program, and we discussed the benefits of using a step-counter for self-monitoring. Six months later SL, who had moved from the area, emailed that she was continuing to eat a more balanced diet, her weight was gradually decreasing, and she now felt ready to focus on specific weight-loss goals. She had moved from precontemplation to the preparation stage for behaviors targeted to weight loss (Table 5.6).

Case Study Summary

Advertisers say "results may vary," but elevated serum triglycerides is the component of the metabolic syndrome most readily responsive to dietary intervention. Changes in cholesterol take longer to achieve and are likely to be more limited. Working with clients with hypertriglyceridemia is particularly rewarding in that the ready response increases the client's self-efficacy, which becomes the foundation for further health-enhancing changes.

TABLE 5.5
Pretreatment and Posttreatment Lipid Levels

Lipid Laboratory Tests	Patient's Lab Results (mg/dL)		ATP III Reference Values (mg/dL)
	June	September	
LDL cholesterol	120	128	Optimal <100
Total cholesterol	230	191	Desirable <200
HDL cholesterol	27	45	>40
Triglycerides	474	69	Normal <150

TABLE 5.6
SLs Progress through Stages of Change

Stage	Targeted Behavior	Counseling Strategy
Precontemplation to preparation	Weight loss	Encourage expression of feelings.
Maintenance	Low-fat diet	
Contemplation to preparation to action to maintenance	Balanced diet	Identify/discuss barriers to change. Develop plan of action. Teach skills and provide resources. Reinforce action. Offer ideas to maintain change.
Precontemplation to contemplation to action	Exercise	Raise awareness of health concern.

REFERENCES

1. Prochaska JO, DiClemente CC, Norcross JC. In search of how people change: applications to addictive behaviors. *Am Psychol.* 1992;47:1102-1114.
2. Sutton K, Logue E, Jarhoura D, Baughman K, Smucker W, Capers C. Assessing dietary and exercise stage of change to optimize weight loss interventions. *Obes Res.* 2003;22:641-652.
3. Vallis M, Ruggiero L, Greene G, Jones H, Zinman B, Rossi S, Edwards L, Rossi JS, Prochaska JO. Stages of change for healthy eating in diabetes: relation to demographic, eating-related, health care utilization, and psychosocial factors. *Diabetes Care.* 2003;26:1468-1474.
4. Molaison EF. Stages of change in clinical nutrition. *Nutr Clin Care.* 2002;5:251-257.
5. Finckenor MA, Byrd-Bredbenner C. Nutrition intervention group program based on preaction stage–oriented change processes of the transtheoretical model promotes long-term reduction in dietary fat intake. *J Am Diet Assoc.* 2000;100:335-342.
6. Miller WR, Rollnick S. *Motivational Interviewing: Preparing People for Change.* 2nd ed. New York, NY: Guilford Publishing; 2002.
7. Take Back Your Health. Available at: http://www.motivatehealthyhabits.com. Accessed January 31, 2004.
8. Rollick SN, Miller WR. Motivational Interviewing. Available at: http://www.motivationalinterview.org/clinical/whatismi.html. Accessed December 23, 2003.
9. Miller WR. Motivation for treatment: a review with special emphasis on alcoholism. *Psych Bull.* 1985;98:84-107.
10. Coulehan JL, Block MR. *The Medical Interview: Mastering Skills for Clinical Practice.* 4th ed. Philadelphia, Pa: FA Davis; 2001.
11. Rogers CR. A theory of therapy, personality, and interpersonal relationships, as developed in the client-centered framework. *Psychology.* 1959;3:184-256.
12. Egan G. *The Skilled Helper: A Problem-Management Approach to Helping.* 7th ed. Pacific Grove, Calif: Brooks-Cole Publishing Co; 2001.
13. Miller WR, Rollnick S. *Motivational Interviewing: Preparing People to Change Addictive Behavior.* New York, NY: Guilford Press; 1991:55-62.
14. Bandura A. Self-efficacy: toward a unifying theory of behavioral change. *Psych Rev.* 1977;84:191-215.
15. Rimal RN. Closing the knowledge-behavior gap in health promotion: the mediating role of self-efficacy. *Health Commun.* 2000;12:219-237.
16. Becker MH. *The Health Beliefs Model and Personal Health Behavior.* Thorofare, NJ: CB Slack, Inc; 1974.
17. Zimmerman GL, Olsen CG, Bosworth MF. A "stages of change" approach to helping patients change behavior. *Am Fam Physician.* 2000;61:1409-1416.
18. Prochaska JO, Norcross JC, DiClemente CC. *Changing for Good.* New York, NY: William Morrow; 1994.
19. Greene GW, Rossi SR, Reed GR, Willey C, Prochaska JO. Stages of change for reducing dietary fat to 30% of energy or less. *J Am Diet Assoc.* 1994;94:1105-1110.
20. Gregg EW, Gerzoff RB, Thompson TJ, Williamson DF. Intentional weight loss and death in overweight and obese US adults 35 years of age and older. *Ann Intern Med.* 2003;138:383-389.
21. Botelho R. *Beyond Advice: Book 1, Becoming a Motivational Practitioner; Book 2, Developing Motivational Skills.* Rochester, NY: Motivate Healthy Habits; 2003.
22. Keller VF, White MK. Choices and changes: a new model for influencing patient health behavior. *J Clin Outcomes Manage.* 1997;4:33-36.
23. Glynn TJ, Manley MW. *How to Help Your Patients Stop Smoking: A National Cancer Institute Manual for Physicians.* Bethesda, Md: National Cancer Institute; 1989. NIH publication 89-3064.
24. Fletcher GF, Blair SN, Blumenthal J, Caspersen C, Chaitman B, Epstein S, Falls H, Froelicher ESS, Froelicher VF, Pina IL. Statement on exercise: benefits and recommendations for physical activity programs for all Americans. A statement for health professionals by the Committee on Exercise and Cardiac Rehabilitation of the Council on Clinical Cardiology, American Heart Association. *Circulation.* 1992;86:340-344.
25. Powell KE, Thompson PD, Caspersen CJ, Kendrick JS. Physical activity and the incidence of coronary heart disease. *Annu Rev Public Health.* 1987;8:253-287.
26. Ekelund L, Haskell WL, Johnson JL, Whaley FS, Criqui MH, Sheps DS. Physical fitness as a predictor of cardiovascular mortality in asymptomatic North American men: the Lipid Research Clinics Mortality Follow-up Study. *N Engl J Med.* 1988;319:1379-1384.
27. Sandvik L, Erikssen J, Thaulow E, Erikssen G, Mundal R, Rodahl K. Physical fitness as a predictor of mortality among healthy, middle-aged Norwegian men. *N Engl J Med.* 1993;328:533-537.
28. Blair SN, Jackson AS. Physical fitness and activity as separate heart disease risk factors: a meta-analysis. *Med Sci Sports Exerc.* 2001;33:762-764.
29. Paffenbarger RS, Hyde RT, Wing AL, Lee I, Jung DL, Kampert JB. The association of changes in physical activity level and other lifestyle characteristics with mortality among men. *N Engl J Med.* 1993;328:538-545.
30. Leon AS, Connett J. Physical activity and 10.5 year mortality in the Multiple Risk Factor Intervention Trial. *Int J Epidemiol.* 1991;20:690-697.
31. Jennings GL, Deakin G, Korner P, Meredith I, Kingwell B, Nelson L. What is the dose-response relationship between exercise training and blood pressure? *Ann Med.* 1991;23:313-318.

32. Paffenbarger RS, Wing AL, Hyde RT. Physical activity as an index of heart attack risk in college alumni. *Am J Epidemiol.* 1978;108:161-175.

33. Kraus WE, Houmard JA, Duscha BD, Knetzger KJ, Wharton MB, McCartney JS, Bales CW, Henes S, Samsa GP, Otvos JD, Kulkarni KR, Slentz CA. Effects of the amount and intensity of exercise on plasma lipoproteins. *N Engl J Med.* 2002;347:1483-1492.

34. Pollock ML, Gaesser GA, Butcher JD, Despres JP, Dishman RK, Franklin BA, Garber CE. American College of Sports Medicine Position Stand: the recommended quantity and quality of exercise for developing and maintaining cardiorespiratory and muscular fitness, and flexibility in healthy adults. *Med Sci Sports Exerc.* 1998;31:975-991.

35. Institute of Medicine. *Dietary Reference Intakes: Energy, Carbohydrate, Fiber, Fat, Fatty Acids, Cholesterol, Protein, and Amino Acids.* Washington, DC: National Academies Press; 2002:12-1.

36. National Heart, Lung, and Blood Institute, Obesity Education Initiative Expert Panel. *Clinical Guidelines on the Identification, Evaluation, and Treatment of Overweight and Obesity in Adults, the Evidence Report.* Bethesda, Md: National Institutes of Health; 1998. NIH publication 98-4038.

37. Parks SE, Houseman RA, Brownson RC. Differential correlates of physical activity in urban and rural adults of various socioeconomic backgrounds in the United States. *J Epidemiol Community Health.* 2003;57: 29-35.

38. DeBusk RF, Stenestrand U, Sheehan M, Haskell WL. Training effects of long versus short bouts of exercise in healthy subjects. *Am J Cardiol.* 1990;15;65:1010-1013.

39. Estabrooks PA, Glasgow RE, Dzewaltowski DA. Physical activity promotion through primary care. *JAMA.* 2003;289:2913-2916.

PART III

Medical Nutrition Therapy and Physical Activity

MEDICAL NUTRITION THERAPY IN THE PREVENTION AND MANAGEMENT OF CORONARY HEART DISEASE

Jo Ann S. Carson, PhD, RD, Scott M. Grundy, MD, PhD, Linda Van Horn, PhD, RD, and Neil Stone, MD; Dietary Recommendations for Total Fat section by Amy E. Binkoski, RD, and Penny M. Kris-Etherton, PhD, RD; case study by Jo Ann S. Carson, PhD, RD

Nutrition is important in the prevention and treatment of coronary heart disease (CHD). This chapter addresses the evidence and strategies underlying the role of nutrition in the prevention of CHD with a focus on the use of medical nutrition therapy (MNT) for patients with abnormal lipid profiles that place them at increased risk of CHD. Two documents provide the underpinnings of MNT for CHD in this chapter: the National Cholesterol Education Program's Third Adult Treatment Panel Report (ATP III) (1) and the American Dietetic Association's MNT Evidence-Based Guide for Practice for Hyperlipidemia (2). ATP III (1) provides the basic rationale for intervention, including nutrition advice, fostering physical activity, and drug therapy when needed to improve lipid profiles. The lifestyle interventions recommended in ATP III are the framework for the MNT Guide (2), which incorporates ATP III recommendations, as well as reviewing research on the impact of nutrition on serum lipids published since ATP III. After covering the rationale and principles of MNT for CHD, this chapter describes practical approaches for delivering MNT through individualized counseling, group classes, and Web sites. Diets appropriate for patients with congestive heart failure (CHF) or the dyslipidemia associated with renal disease are also addressed.

PREVENTION EFFORTS: AN OVERVIEW

Primary prevention of CHD centers on healthy lifestyle habits to reduce the risk factors discussed in Chapter 3. Maintaining a healthy weight, participating in regular physical activity, consuming fruits and vegetables daily, and eating a diet low in saturated fat should be habits established early in life to keep low-density lipoprotein (LDL) cholesterol at optimum levels. The Dietary

Guidelines for Americans (3) and the American Heart Association (AHA) guidelines (4) provide guidance for the general public on healthy eating that can reduce risk of heart disease.

During various stages of life, maintaining healthy lifestyle habits may require targeted interventions. For instance, as a young adult enters college or begins an office job, intentionally incorporating regular physical activity into his or her routine could reduce cardiovascular disease (CVD) risk and unhealthy weight gain (5). Pregnancy may be an opportune time to prompt smoking cessation. Later in life, specific attention to energy balance may be needed when activity decreases because of physiological changes or retirement from an active job. Encouraging physical activity and resistance exercise can avert the decline in muscle mass and increases in body fat that typically accompany aging.

Consistent messages about smoking cessation, weight control, and adherence to diet and medication regimens should be provided by multiple health care providers, including physicians, nurses, physician assistants, physical therapists, and registered dietitians. Recognition of national guidelines should provide the rationale for this approach and support consistency. Multidisciplinary communication via chart notes, electronic messages, and personal conversations can further enhance patient care.

In the presence of other risk factors, elevated LDL cholesterol and other lipoprotein abnormalities require more intensive intervention to forestall development of CHD. If CHD is present, aggressive dietary intervention and physical activity are indicated. Patients with atherosclerotic heart disease usually have multiple problems. In addition to elevated cholesterol, patients with CHD likely have metabolic syndrome, hypertension, or diabetes. (Chapters 7, 8, and 9 focus on these diagnoses.) The clinician must weave together principles of care for the multiple diagnoses associated with CVD as care for patients is individualized.

ATP III GUIDELINES

Practice guidelines for addressing diet, physical activity, and medication in the control of high blood cholesterol and management of CHD risk were outlined in 2001 by ATP III (1). The American Dietetic Association's MNT Evidence-Based Guide for Hyperlipidemia incorporates the ATP III guidelines as they relate to nutrition therapy (2). These and other national guidelines related to heart disease are listed in Box 6.1 (1,2,4,6-9). Chapter 3 discusses risk factors for CHD delineated by ATP III, as well as the steps for assessing a patient's risk factors and developing overall treatment plans.

After determining a patient's risk category, decisions can be made regarding initiation of MNT and physical activity (termed Therapeutic Lifestyle Changes [TLC] by ATP III) and, if needed, initiation of drug therapy. (See Table 3.4 in Chapter 3.)

Elements of TLC include the following recommendations:

- Nutrients that raise LDL cholesterol should be minimized.
  - Reduce dietary saturated fat to less than 7% of total energy.
  - Reduce dietary cholesterol to less than 200 mg/day.
  - Total dietary fat should be in the range of 25% to 35% of total energy.
- Therapeutic options may be added for further lowering of LDL cholesterol.
  - Plant stanols and sterols can be added (2 g/day).
  - Viscous fiber may be increased to 10 to 25 g/day.

Box 6.1 **National Guidelines Related to Prevention and Treatment of Coronary Heart Disease**

American Dietetic Association's Medical Nutrition Therapy Protocol for Hyperlipidemia (2)
  Available at: http://guidelines.gov
National Cholesterol Education Program's Third Adult Treatment Panel (1)
  Available at: http://www.nhlbi.nih.gov/guidelines/cholesterol/atp3_rpt.htm
American Heart Association (4)
  Available at: http://www.americanheart.org/dietaryguidelines
American Diabetes Association (6)
  Available at: http://care.diabetesjournals.org/cgi/contentfull/26/suppl_1/s51
Heart Failure (7)
  Available at: http://www.acc.org/clinical/guidelines/failure/hf_index.htm
US Preventive Services Task Force (8)
  Available at: http://www.ahrcpr.gov/clinic/3rduspstf/diet/dietrr.htm
National Kidney Foundation's Kidney Disease Outcome Quality Indicators (9)
  Available at: http://www.kidney.org/professionals/kdoqi/index.cfm

---

- Total energy intake should be adjusted to maintain desirable body weight and prevent weight gain.
- Physical activity should include moderate exercise to expend 200 or more kcal/day (1).

The macronutrient distribution for TLC is approximately 15% of energy from protein, 50% to 60% of energy from carbohydrate, and 25% to 35% of energy from fat. Further delineation is shown in Table 6.1 (1,10,11). From a macronutrient perspective, nutrition recommendations to reduce the risk of CHD include the following:

- Limit intake of cholesterol-raising saturated fat and *trans* fat. Replace with monounsaturated fat and, to some extent, polyunsaturated fat.
- Emphasize carbohydrate intake from whole grains, fruits, and vegetables to provide complex carbohydrate, dietary fiber, vitamins, and other antioxidants.

TABLE 6.1
ATP III Nutrient Recommendations Compared with the American Diet

Group	% Energy from Fat as				Cholesterol (mg)	Dietary Fiber (g)
	Total	SFA	MUFA	PUFA		
ATP III*	25–35	<7	≤20	≤10	<200	20–30
Men[†]	33.3	11.2	12.9	6.6	331	18.6
Women[†]	32.4	10.7	12.2	6.8	213	13.9
All individuals[†] (includes children)	32.8	11.3	12.5	6.4	256	15.1

Abbreviations: ATP III, Adult Treatment Panel III; MUFA, monounsaturated fat; PUFA, polyunsaturated fat; SFA, saturated fat.

*NCEP ATP III Requirements (1).

[†]American diet data are from Continuing Survey of Food Intakes by Individuals, 1994–1996 (10); 1989–1991 data indicate 2.6% of energy is from *trans* fatty acids (11).

- Choose protein from sources that limit saturated fat and can provide n-3 fatty acids, isoflavones, and monounsaturated fats (ie, fish, soy, and nuts) (12).

The AHA (4), ATP III (1), and the American Dietetic Association's MNT Evidence-Based Guide (2) provide guidelines for nutrition and heart disease. AHA provides food-based guidance for the public to prevent CHD. The other two sets of guidelines are more specific, nutrient-based guidelines designed for the primary and secondary prevention of CHD events in patients with risk factors for CHD. The current research base for each of the TLC components is reviewed in the next section.

EVIDENCE BASE FOR COMPONENTS OF THERAPEUTIC LIFESTYLE CHANGE

Diet for prevention and treatment of CHD has traditionally focused on lowering serum cholesterol, more specifically serum LDL cholesterol levels. Lowering dietary saturated fat and cholesterol in the general population can lower incidence of CHD by lowering serum cholesterol. If Americans limited intake of saturated fat to less than 10% of total energy intake and consumed less than 300 mg of cholesterol daily, as outlined in *Healthy People 2010* objectives (13), then total serum cholesterol in the population could be reduced by approximately 5% to 7%. A further reduction of saturated fat to less than 7% of energy intake and dietary cholesterol to less than 200 mg, as outlined in TLC, could lower serum cholesterol by an additional 3% to 7% (14,15). The key dietary strategies for lowering LDL cholesterol are summarized in Table 6.2.

The well-established scientific evidence for the relationship of nutrition to multiple factors influencing CHD is discussed in this and following chapters. Dietary saturated fat and cholesterol are known atherogenic factors that increase total and LDL cholesterol. This concept underlies dietary prevention and treatment of CHD. Nutrition also influences other major risk factors, including low high-density lipoprotein (HDL) cholesterol, high triglycerides, and elevated blood pressure. In addition to reporting the effects of nutritional manipulations on LDL cholesterol, considering the impact of diet on the total cholesterol–to–HDL cholesterol ratio heightens the importance of MNT for treating hyperlipidemia. Recently, the enumeration of other CHD risk factors has prompted questions as to how diet may influence

TABLE 6.2
Dietary Changes to Lower LDL Cholesterol Levels

Nutritional Strategy	Food-Based Advice
Decrease intake of saturated fat.	Limit portion size of meats; use lean meats and fat-free dairy products.
Replace saturated fat with MUFA or PUFA.	Use canola or olive oil for MUFA; can use safflower or corn oil for PUFA.
Limit intake of *trans* fatty acids.	Use tub or liquid margarine. Limit baked goods with partially hydrogenated oils. When eating out, select fresh and grilled foods rather than fried, especially at fast food restaurants.
Limit intake of cholesterol.	Limit egg yolks, organ meats, butterfat, and high-fat meats.

Abbreviations: LDL, low-density lipoprotein; MUFA, monounsaturated fat; PUFA, polyunsaturated fat.

TABLE 6.3
Dietary Sources of Saturated Fatty Acid

Saturated Fatty Acid	Source
Stearic acid (18:0)	Beef
	Chocolate
Palmitic (16:0)	Meats, dairy fat, and palm oil
Myristic (14:0)	Meat and dairy fat
Lauric acid (12:0)	Tropical oils—coconut, palm kernel

Source: Data are from references 20–23.

thrombotic tendency, hyperhomocysteinemia, systemic inflammation, endothelial dysfunction, and insulin sensitivity (12).

Saturated Fatty Acids

Reducing and maintaining low dietary saturated fat is a major step toward optimizing the serum lipids to prevent CHD and reduce risk. Dietary saturated fatty acids, as contrasted with unsaturated fatty acids, decrease synthesis and activation of receptors, raising serum LDL cholesterol and providing an environment conducive to atherogenesis (16). A 1% increase in energy from saturated fat raises serum LDL cholesterol approximately 2% (1).

The degree to which LDL cholesterol can be lowered can vary depending upon initial lipid levels and concomitant dietary changes, such as further restriction of dietary cholesterol or addition of soluble fiber. Yu Poth's meta-analysis (15) concluded that a diet with 30% energy from total fat, less than 10% energy from saturated fat, and less than 300 mg cholesterol/day lowered LDL cholesterol by 12%, and by 16% with further reduction of saturated fat and cholesterol. A recent clinical trial restricting energy from saturated fat to 7% and cholesterol to less than 200 mg lowered LDL cholesterol by 11% (17). Large, randomized clinical trials of a similar diet reported LDL cholesterol was lowered by 11% (18) and 8% (19).

How does the goal of lowering saturated fat to less than 7% of energy compare with the typical American diet? Based on the Continuing Survey of Food Intakes by Individuals (CSFII), Americans' saturated fat intake has decreased from 12.6% of energy in 1989–1991 to 11.3% in 1994–1996 (10). Further data from the 1994–1996 survey on fat in the American diet are shown in Table 6.1. National data are not yet available to adequately assess whether the popularity of low-carbohydrate diets has altered the trend in lowering saturated fat intake.

Saturated fat in the American diet is primarily from four specific fatty acids (lauric, myristic, palmitic, and stearic) (see Table 6.3) (20-23). A recent meta-analysis concluded lauric acid has the greatest LDL-raising effect, followed by myristic and then palmitic acids. Stearic acid lowers LDL cholesterol; however, both lauric and stearic acids lower the total cholesterol–to–HDL ratio, pointing to myristic and palmitic acids as the major dietary villains among fatty acids (24). Figure 6.1 provides a graphic representation of the saturated, monounsaturated, and polyunsaturated fat in common dietary fats (23).

The amount of meat and type of meat in the diet influence the saturated fat content of the diet. To study the impact of type of meat within a heart-healthy diet high in fiber, 18 men with hypercholesterolemia were provided with three different diets, each for 26 days. The fish, lean beef, and poultry diets each lowered LDL cholesterol with no significant difference based on the type of meat. The fish-based diet did raise HDL_2 cholesterol when compared with the lean beef diet (25).

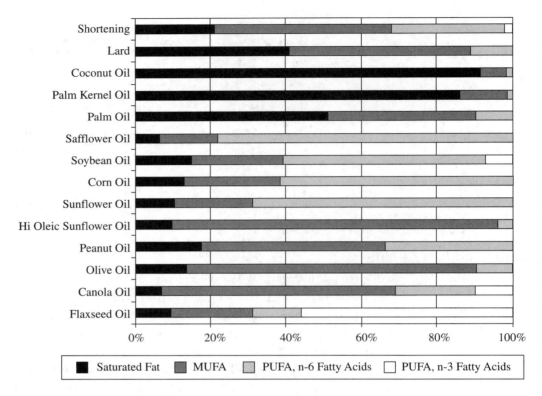

FIGURE 6.1
Distribution of types of fat in common sources of dietary fat. MUFA, monounsaturated fatty acids; PUFA, polyunsaturated fatty acids. Data are from reference 23.

Trans Fatty Acids

Trans-unsaturated fatty acids result when polyunsaturated fats, such as those in corn oil and soybean oil, are partially hydrogenated to produce stick margarine and shortening. In addition to use in frying fast foods, partially hydrogenated fats enhance shelf-life of bakery goods and snack foods. When substituted for energy from carbohydrates, *trans* fatty acids raise LDL cholesterol and the total cholesterol–to–HDL ratio, as well as possibly producing a smaller, more atherogenic LDL particle (24,26). Although these effects are detrimental for CHD at the population level, *trans* fatty acids are less significant in heart disease than saturated fatty acids, because they are less prevalent in the diet of most Americans.

Based on the 1989–1991 CSFII, Americans consume approximately 2.6% of energy from *trans* fatty acids, as contrasted with 12.3% from saturated fat (11). The Minnesota Heart Study found a decline in *trans* fatty acid intake from 8.3 g/day (3% of energy) in 1980–1982 to 6.2 g/day (2.2% of energy) in 1995–1997 (27). *Trans* fatty acids intake in Canadian pregnant women was estimated to be 3.5% of energy (28).

Several types of evidence indicate the detrimental effects of *trans* fatty acids. A meta-analysis of eight controlled clinical trials has allowed prediction of the effect of particular fats on total cholesterol–to–HDL cholesterol ratio as shown in Figure 6.2 (24). Although the prediction indicates coconut and palm kernel as slightly beneficial using the total cholesterol–to–HDL cholesterol ratio, these saturated fats are not encouraged based on their effect on LDL cholesterol. Of more significance in this figure is the depiction of how *trans* fatty acid sources such as stick margarine and shortening raise the total cholesterol–to–HDL

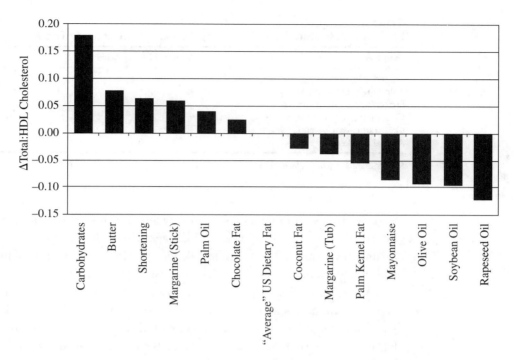

FIGURE 6.2

Predicted effects of various dietary fat sources on total cholesterol–to–HDL cholesterol ratio. Reprinted from Mensink RP, Zock PL, Kester ADM, Katan MB. Effects of dietary fatty acids and carbohydrates on the ratio of serum total to HDL cholesterol and on serum lipids and apolipoproteins: a meta-analysis of 60 controlled trials. *Am J Clin Nutr.* 2003;77:1146-1155. Reproduced with permission by the *American Journal of Clinical Nutrition.* © Am J Clin Nutr. American Society for Clinical Nutrition.

cholesterol ratio (24). One recent clinical trial provided six variations of diets to 50 normocholesterolemic men in a crossover design. When *trans* fatty acids replaced 8% of energy from carbohydrates, LDL cholesterol was raised 10% (29). In another study, metabolic diets using a spectrum of fat sources (butter, soybean oil, semiliquid margarine, shortening, or stick margarine) were provided to mildly hypercholesterolemic men and women older than 50 years. LDL cholesterol levels were highest when subjects were on the diet using butter and were reduced proportionately in diets using products with fewer or no *trans* fatty acids. LDL cholesterol levels were 5% lower when subjects used stick margarine, 9% lower when subjects used tub margarine, and 12% lower when subjects used soybean oil (30). Lichtenstein and associates (31) did not find that *trans* fatty acids altered other risk factors such as blood pressure and C-reactive protein. When Denke (32) fed 46 families baked goods made with either butter or tub margarine in a crossover study, LDL cholesterol levels were 11% lower during the 5-week margarine period.

Epidemiologic studies have correlated *trans* fatty acid intake with increased risk for CHD in both men and women (12,33,34). Although conjugated linoleic acid found in animal foods may perform differently from the *trans* fatty acids resulting from partial hydrogenation of vegetable oils (35), inadequate data preclude conclusions regarding individual *trans* fatty acids.

Exactly where are the *trans* fatty acids in our diet? About one fourth of the *trans* fatty acids originates naturally in foods such as milk and meat, whereas the majority of *trans* fatty acids are introduced into the diet through hydrogenated vegetable oils. The major sources of *trans* fatty

TABLE 6.4
Examples of Saturated and *Trans* Fatty Acid Contents of Snack Foods

Food Item	Saturated Fatty Acids (g)	*Trans* Fatty Acids (g)
Glazed doughnut, 1	2.5	4
Thin wheat crackers, 16	1	2
Frozen apple pie, ⅛ pie	3	4
Chocolate chip cookies, 3	2	1.5
Oat bran cereal, ¾ cup	2	1.5
Animal crackers, 8	0.5	1

Source: Data are from reference 36.

acids in the diets of pregnant Canadian women were baked goods (33% of *trans* fatty acid intake), fast foods (12%), breads (10%), snacks (10%), and margarine or shortening (8%) (28). An analysis performed for *Consumer Reports* provides a comparison of the saturated and *trans* fatty acid content of common snack foods (see Table 6.4) (36).

A Food and Drug Administration (FDA) regulation requires that manufacturers specify grams of *trans* fatty acids per serving on the Nutrition Facts label on packaged foods beginning January 1, 2006 (37). This requirement will likely prompt the food industry to use healthier fats in food preparation, as already observed when a major snack food producer switched to liquid oils and now lists 0 g *trans* fatty acids on food labels. Based on the amount of products sold across the United States, this change is expected to lower the *trans* fat intake of Americans by an average of 0.2 g/day (Robert Brown, personal communication).

As evidence pointing to the detrimental effects of *trans* fatty acids mounts, however, one should not lose sight of dietary sources of saturated fat. Occurring in at least a threefold greater proportion in the American diet, saturated fat is the major dietary factor contributing to LDL cholesterol.

Monounsaturated Fatty Acids

When saturated and *trans* fatty acids are limited in the diet, carbohydrate or unsaturated fat can replace the unhealthy fat, providing an equivalent amount of energy. Monounsaturated fatty acids occur naturally in the *cis* form in olive oil, canola oil, avocado, olives, pecans, peanuts, and other nuts. Several guidelines allow for individualization of macronutrient proportions to increase energy from monounsaturated fat (1,38). Work by Grundy (39) and Mattson (40) point to the benefit of replacing saturated fat with monounsaturated fat because the latter lowered LDL cholesterol levels without lowering HDL cholesterol levels. When substituted for carbohydrate, monounsaturated fat also reduces serum triglyceride levels (41).

A number of studies suggest the benefits of monounsaturated fat in optimizing serum lipid profiles. While maintaining saturated fat below 7% of energy, Kris-Etherton compared a diet consisting of 25% of energy from fat with three diets high in monounsaturated fats (34% total fat) from olive oil, peanut oil, or peanuts and peanut butter. The three test diets high in monounsaturated fat lowered LDL cholesterol levels comparably to the lower fat diet. However, they did not lower HDL cholesterol levels or increase triglyceride levels whereas the lower fat diet did (42).

When Gill decreased the proportion of saturated to monounsaturated fat in the diet from 2:1 to 1:2, LDL cholesterol levels decreased by almost 20% without a significant change in

HDL or triglyceride levels (41). In Kris-Etherton's study, diets were slightly higher in total fat (34% of energy) than in Gill et al's study in which 30% of energy came from total fat (42,43). With a 1:3 ratio of saturated to monounsaturated fat in a 34% fat diet, LDL cholesterol levels were lowered 14% (43). Although such trials suggest a benefit of liberal intake of monounsaturated fats, there are no large intervention trials testing the benefit of a higher monounsaturated fat intake on CHD events as endpoints.

The monounsaturated fat content of many nuts is one of the reasons for increasing attention to the benefit of nuts. In addition, they are a natural source of vitamin E and dietary fiber. A study of pecan intake by normolipidemic individuals reported significantly lower cholesterol in the small group randomized to include 2 ounces of pecans in the daily diet (44). Nuts are discussed further in Chapter 10.

Polyunsaturated Fatty Acids: N-3 and N-6

Polyunsaturated fatty acids, those containing more than one double bond, can be subdivided into n-3 and n-6 fatty acids. In n-3 fatty acids, the first double bond occurs after the third carbon from the methyl end of the compound; in n-6 the first double bond occurs after the sixth carbon. Of the two essential fatty acids, linoleic and linolenic, linoleic is the n-6 polyunsaturated fatty acid found in vegetable oils, such as corn, safflower, and sunflower oils. Alpha-linolenic is the n-3 polyunsaturated fatty acid, found primarily in flaxseed oil, but also present in canola, soybean, and mustard seed oil. Substitution of saturated fat with polyunsaturated fat lowers LDL cholesterol levels (1). N-3 fatty acids serve as precursors for eicosanoids, producing an environment that reduces platelet aggregation as well as possibly reducing inflammation. This benefit can arise from directly consuming the long-chain fish oils or ingesting the 18-carbon-alpha-linolenic acid that is elongated and desaturated within the body. N-3 fatty acids are discussed further in Chapter 10.

Hu and Willett (12) have summarized the clinical trials in several countries from the 1960s and 1970s that reduced saturated fat and increased polyunsaturated fat in the diet. Three of five trials found significant reduction in CHD or CHD events when polyunsaturated fat was increased along with reducing dietary saturated fat.

Views of the benefits of monounsaturated vs polyunsaturated fats have fluctuated during recent years. However, the current interpretation of research findings is that dietary saturated and *trans* fatty acids should be limited, and naturally occurring *cis*-monounsaturated and polyunsaturated fats are similarly heart healthy (45,46).

Dietary Cholesterol

Metabolic diet studies indicate that dietary cholesterol increases total serum cholesterol approximately 10 mg/dL for every 100 mg of dietary cholesterol consumed per 1,000 kcal (1). By controlling saturated fat intake, dietary cholesterol intake usually decreases. Egg yolks, the most common source of dietary cholesterol, should be limited. Weggemans and associates conducted meta-analysis of clinical trials that varied cholesterol intake by changes in egg consumption but controlled other aspects of the diet. The authors concluded that the dietary cholesterol in one egg yolk per day significantly worsened the total cholesterol–to–HDL cholesterol ratio (47). Knopp and colleagues (48) reported a nonsignificant increase in LDL cholesterol when two eggs per day were added to the diets of patients with hypercholesterolemia; however, the increase was significant among subjects with both elevated cholesterol and triglyceride levels.

Analysis of older epidemiologic results from the Zutphen, Western Electric, Irish Brothers, and Honolulu Heart studies found an independent additional increase in CVD risk associated with a higher dietary cholesterol intake. Risk was increased above the greater risk induced by the resultant increase in serum cholesterol (49). Recent prospective cohort studies that specifically addressed egg intake and risk of heart disease had varying results. A study in which half the subjects were vegetarians reported a relative risk of 2.68 for those consuming six eggs per week as contrasted with those who ate less than one egg per week (50). After controlling for confounding factors, the Nurses' Health Study and the Male Health Professionals Study reported no significant relationship between egg intake and risk of heart disease. However, analyses of the subgroup with diabetes found a twofold increase in risk of heart disease for individuals consuming one or more eggs per day compared with subjects who consumed less than one egg per week (51).

In promoting heart health, the AHA recommends inclusion of egg yolks within the overall daily cholesterol limit (52). ATP III suggests only two per week to keep dietary cholesterol less than 200 mg/day (1).

Additional Therapeutic Options

TLC includes use of sterol and stanol esters and soluble fiber for additional lowering of LDL cholesterol levels. These and several other specific strategies for reducing CHD risk are discussed in later chapters. Sterol and stanol esters in margarines and n-3 fatty acids are described in Chapter 10. The benefits of increased consumption of soluble fiber are reviewed in Chapters 9 and 10.

Weight Control

Weight control is an important factor for optimizing the lipid profile. Weight loss can lower LDL cholesterol levels somewhat but has its more dramatic benefit in lowering serum triglyceride levels. A recent Canadian study reported a 7.6% reduction in LDL cholesterol when body weight was reduced by 10% (53). Chapter 7 discusses the importance of weight loss and physical activity for patients with metabolic syndrome. Chapters 9, 12, and 14 provide additional information on approaches to weight control.

Physical Activity

Physical activity, whether it is a part of everyday activities or intentional, regular sessions designed to improve fitness, improves cardiovascular health. Epidemiologic data clearly indicate that regular physical activity reduces the likelihood of developing CHD, most likely by reducing CHD risk factors (54). For example, the HERITAGE family study enrolled 675 normolipidemic individuals who followed exercise prescriptions for 5 months. Triglyceride levels declined and HDL cholesterol increased significantly (55). A recent pilot study of 41 subjects found significant improvement in lipid profile when a supervised aerobic exercise program was added to dietary intervention (53). The TLC recommendation to expend at least 200 kcal/day in moderate activity translates into a brisk 2-mile walk. This is similar to the Centers for Disease Control and Prevention's and AHA's recommendations of 30 minutes or more of moderate intensity physical activity on most, if not all, days of the week (56). With an emphasis on preventing and reducing obesity, the Institute of Medicine Dietary Reference Intake (DRI) report on macronutrients recommends 60 minutes of daily moderate physical activity (57).

TABLE 6.5
Total Fat and Saturated Fatty Acid (SFA) Goals Based on Caloric Recommendations

Total Energy (kcal)	Total Fat (g)				SFA (g); <7% of Energy from Saturated Fat
	20% Energy from Fat	25% Energy from Fat	30% Energy from Fat	35% Energy from Fat	
1200	27	33	40	47	9
1400	31	39	47	54	11
1600	36	44	53	62	12
1800	40	50	60	70	14
2000	44	56	67	78	16
2200	49	61	73	86	17
2400	53	67	80	93	19
2600	58	72	87	101	20
2800	62	78	93	109	22
3000	67	83	100	117	23

DIETARY RECOMMENDATIONS FOR TOTAL FAT

In addition to ensuring a good fat quality by the inclusion of unsaturated rather than saturated fat, one needs to address the optimum proportion of total fat in the diet. Until recently, the long-standing dietary recommendation for total fat was that it be no more than 30% of total energy (58). Because no lower limit was set, questions were raised in clinical practice about what the specific level of total fat should be. Routinely, 30% became the target value; however, this goal was translated broadly and some health professionals advocated very-low-fat (< 15% to 20% of energy) diets.

Recently, new dietary recommendations include ranges for total fat intake. ATP III recommends 25% to 35% of energy from fat (1), and the DRI report on macronutrients recommends 20% to 35% of energy from fat (57). The lower limit is justified to achieve adherence because a diet even lower in total fat is difficult for most individuals living in developed countries to follow (57). The higher limit takes into consideration the potential for adverse effects on risk factors for CHD (1). Higher fat diets are moderately hypercaloric compared with lower fat diets in ad libitum conditions (57), and higher fat intake may be appropriate for the treatment of metabolic syndrome (1). The new ranges in total fat intake still raise questions about the ideal level of dietary fat for individuals. Clinical judgment must be applied. Table 6.5 shows the grams of fat for diets that provide 20%, 25%, 30%, and 35% of energy from fat over a range of different energy levels (from 1,200 to 3,000 kcal). Irrespective of level of total fat recommended, saturated fat should be kept low (< 7% of energy) to achieve and maintain desirable total and LDL cholesterol levels. Guidance is needed regarding the appropriate level of dietary fat to prescribe for practitioners who deal with many different patient profiles. Total fat affects important lipid risk factors beyond LDL cholesterol, notably, triglycerides, HDL cholesterol, non-HDL cholesterol, the ratios of total cholesterol–to–HDL cholesterol and LDL cholesterol–to–HDL cholesterol, and small, dense LDL particles. Total fat also affects postprandial plasma glucose and insulin levels, especially in individuals with type 2 diabetes (41,59). Elevated levels of postprandial plasma glucose and insulin over time may increase risk of diabetes and CHD (60). The preferred total fat intake is based on these parameters to reduce CHD risk. Control of energy intake must also be achieved to promote a healthy body weight and avoid overweight and obesity.

How Total Fat Affects CHD Risk

ATP III considers a low HDL cholesterol level (< 40 mg/dL) to be a major risk factor for CHD. Conversely, a high HDL cholesterol level (> 60 mg/dL) is considered to be a negative risk factor for CHD; that is, it removes one risk factor from the total count of risk factors present. Elevated triglycerides, defined as 150 mg/dL or higher, are associated with an increased risk for CHD; ATP III recommends that elevated serum triglycerides be targeted for reduction initially using a lifestyle approach. Non-HDL cholesterol (the sum of very-low-density lipoprotein [VLDL] and LDL cholesterol) is highly predictive of CHD risk, especially in persons with high triglyceride levels (≥ 200 mg/dL) (1).

The ratios of total cholesterol–to–HDL cholesterol and LDL cholesterol–to–HDL cholesterol are used frequently to assess CHD risk. Changes in these ratios reflect corresponding alterations in the component lipoproteins that comprise the ratio. Small, dense LDL particles are an emerging risk factor for CHD (1). As compared with the larger, more buoyant particles, these smaller, dense LDL particles have been associated with a greater risk of myocardial infarction (61), ischemic heart disease (62,63), and various types of CHD (64). Frequently, patients with elevated triglycerides or low HDL cholesterol or both have an accompanying elevation in small LDL particles. This combination of lipid risk factors is termed "atherogenic dyslipidemia." This profile frequently accompanies metabolic syndrome, which increases CHD risk. Metabolic syndrome consists of the following components: atherogenic dyslipidemia, elevated blood pressure, glucose intolerance, a prothrombotic state, and a proinflammatory state. The ATP III report (1) proposes a simple clinical scheme to allow for a clinical diagnosis. According to this scheme, if a person has three of the following five characteristics, this person can be said to have metabolic syndrome:

- Abdominal obesity (waist circumference > 40 inches in men; > 35 inches in women)
- Triglyceride levels of 150 mg/dL or more
- HDL cholesterol levels lower than 40 mg/dL in men, lower than 50 mg/dL in women
- Blood pressure of 130/85 mm Hg or higher
- Fasting glucose levels of 110 mg/dL or more (redefined as ≥ 100 mg/dL by the American Diabetes Association in 2003) (65). (See Chapter 7.)

A high postprandial glucose response might lead to the accumulation of glycated products or advanced glycation end products that promote atherogenesis (66). As discussed later in this chapter, there is evidence that total fat can affect these CHD risk factors. As a result, using these risk factors can help establish what the fat level should be to reduce CHD risk beyond that attained by lowering LDL cholesterol.

Effects on Triglycerides

Serum triglycerides rise when the percentage of energy from dietary fat is decreased as the percentage of energy from carbohydrate is increased (57). Increasing total fat at the expense of carbohydrate is associated with small decreases in triglycerides (57). Based on regression analysis, every 5% decrease in total fat is predicted to increase triglycerides by 6% (57). Emerging evidence further indicates that dietary fiber, particularly soluble fiber, may play a role in preventing the hypertriglyceridemic response that occurs when dietary fat is reduced (67).

Using data from the Dietary Approaches to Stop Hypertension (DASH) Study, Obarzanek (68) reported that a diet providing 27% total fat and 7% saturated fat, as well as high dietary fiber (30 g/day), significantly lowered total and LDL cholesterol levels without altering triglycerides compared with a control diet (37% total fat, 14% saturated fat, 11 g/day fiber). Triglycerides also were unchanged in a study comparing a typical Western diet (39% total fat, 15% saturated fat, 10 g fiber/1,000 kcal) to a TLC diet (28% total fat, 7% saturated fat, 16 g fiber/1,000 kcal) in subjects with moderate hypercholesterolemia (17). Chandalia et al (69) found that a high-fiber diet (50 g/day) significantly reduced triglycerides by 10.2% below that of a diet containing 24 g/day of dietary fiber in subjects with type 2 diabetes mellitus. Both diets contained 30% of energy from total fat and 7% from saturated fat. Inclusion of high-fiber foods may prevent an increase and possibly decrease triglycerides in individuals consuming diets reduced in total fat (ie, high in carbohydrate) compared with a reduced fat diet that is low in dietary fiber. In most patients, increasing fiber-rich foods while reducing total fat can optimize the lipid profile. Higher total fat may be appropriate for some patients to decrease triglyceride levels, but this should be recommended only with careful consideration of energy balance.

Effects on HDL Cholesterol

With weight held constant, decreasing total dietary fat and increasing carbohydrate are associated with reductions in HDL cholesterol levels. Regression analysis predicts a 2.2% reduction in HDL cholesterol for every 5% decrease in total fat in the diet (57), but individual results vary widely. Often low-fat diets result in greater LDL cholesterol lowering, yielding a significant improvement in the LDL cholesterol–to–HDL cholesterol ratio. According to some investigators the effects of reducing fat intake on HDL cholesterol level may be relatively small. For example, Asztalos (70) reported that, compared with an average American diet (37% of energy from fat), a reduced-fat diet was not detrimental for individuals with a low HDL cholesterol level (≤ 35 mg/dL). In these subjects, the HDL cholesterol level did not decrease on the cholesterol-lowering diet that provided 28% of energy from total fat and decreased only slightly (4%) on the 24% total fat diet. LDL cholesterol decreased substantially (8% and 15% on the 28% and 24% total fat diets, respectively), resulting in an 11% reduction in the LDL cholesterol–to–HDL cholesterol ratio following the 24% total fat diet. In subjects with a higher HDL cholesterol level (> 35 mg/dL), consumption of 28% and 24% total fat diets resulted in a significant decrease in the HDL cholesterol level (8% and 11.5%, respectively), as well as a decrease in the LDL cholesterol level (7.4% and 11.9%, respectively), resulting in an unchanged LDL cholesterol–to–HDL cholesterol ratio.

Similar results were reported by Ginsberg (18) in a heterogeneous group of subjects that varied in age, gender, and ethnicity in the Dietary Effects on Lipoproteins and Thrombogenic Activity study. Both LDL and HDL cholesterol levels were decreased in response to reductions in total and saturated fat, resulting in no significant changes in the total–to–HDL cholesterol ratio. The relationship between HDL cholesterol level and dietary fat must be considered when dietary fat prescriptions are made. For some individuals, a cholesterol-lowering diet that is lower in fat (within the recommended range) may be preferable, whereas for others a diet that is higher in fat (within the recommended range) is more appropriate to beneficially affect the HDL cholesterol level, and, in turn, the ratios of LDL cholesterol–to–HDL cholesterol and total cholesterol–to–LDL cholesterol.

LDL Subclass Patterns

Small, dense LDL (pattern B) increases risk for CHD when contrasted with large, buoyant LDL (pattern A) (62-64,71). Approximately one third of individuals who presented with large, buoyant LDL (pattern A) shifted to a pattern B LDL profile (smaller, denser LDL) in response to a diet much lower in total fat and saturated fat. In metabolic ward–type conditions, subjects with pattern A and subjects with pattern B both decreased LDL cholesterol levels when total fat was reduced from 46% to 24% and saturated fat reduced from 18.3% to 5.4%. The blood lipid lowering was approximately twofold greater for individuals with pattern B compared with pattern A individuals (72). Reduction in total fat and saturated fat may be especially beneficial for individuals with a stable B LDL profile because of LDL lowering potential. A moderate fat level may be more appropriate for individuals with pattern A to avoid a possible shift to pattern B that could occur with dramatic reductions in dietary fat. Weight loss has further been shown to induce a shift from pattern B to pattern A profile (73). Thus, for some overweight patients with a pattern B profile, a weight-loss diet that is reduced in total fat to achieve an energy deficit may be appropriate if weight loss is achieved and maintained. Alternatively, a moderate diet is more appropriate for weight loss for pattern A individuals to avoid a shift to pattern B, as well as for those subjects with pattern B profile who experienced difficulty with adherence to a weight-loss diet reduced in total fat. Physical activity is encouraged for all cases.

How does the practitioner consider the issue of LDL particle size in the clinical setting? Current methods used in research studies to determine pattern A or B, such as ultracentrifugation, gel electrophoresis, and magnetic resonance imaging, are not routinely run in a clinical laboratory, although development of methods suitable for clinical laboratories is under way (74). If a patient is very interested, there are specialty laboratories that can determine whether the patient has pattern A or B LDL. In general, pattern B is seen in patients with high triglycerides (> 150 mg/dL) and is uncommon when triglycerides are below 100 mg/dL. Consideration of a patient's subclass of LDL particles could guide the dietitian's final decision on the amount of total dietary fat; however, regardless of particle size, LDL cholesterol is atherogenic (75). Within the fat allowance, saturated fat should be limited to less than 7% of total energy.

Atherogenic Dyslipidemia

Atherogenic dyslipidemia is characterized by elevated apolipoprotein B and triglycerides, small dense LDL particles, and a low HDL cholesterol level. Often, individuals with atherogenic dyslipidemia are overweight or obese (especially abdominal obesity) and have insulin resistance. ATP III views this atherogenic dyslipidemia as a risk factor because each component (low HDL cholesterol level, small dense LDL particles, and elevated triglyceride-rich lipoprotein and apolipoprotein B) is individually atherogenic. Beyond LDL cholesterol–lowering strategies, lifestyle changes that promote weight reduction and physical activity favorably modify the components of atherogenic dyslipidemia; such changes are therefore key for treating overweight individuals. An overweight patient with atherogenic dyslipidemia may benefit from a weight-loss diet reduced in total fat to facilitate energy reduction and favorably affect the triglyceride and HDL cholesterol levels. Total fat should be individualized to promote adherence and achieve the maximum weight loss possible. Some overweight patients adhere better to a moderate-fat weight-loss diet. Increasing dietary carbohydrate above 60% of energy can reduce HDL cholesterol and increase triglycerides without additional LDL lowering (1,76). For normal-weight individuals with atherogenic dyslipidemia, total fat also must be individualized. As previously noted, a diet low in total fat has been shown to benefit persons with a low HDL cholesterol level (71), as well as persons with a stable pattern B LDL profile (72). However, because reductions in dietary fat can result in elevated triglycerides, high-fiber foods should be especially encouraged. A moderate-fat diet may be preferable in some patients to potentially raise HDL cholesterol levels, but the emphasis is on lowering triglyceride levels in patients with atherogenic dyslipidemia.

Body Weight

Because dietary fat is calorically dense, decreasing total fat intake can facilitate weight loss. Both the AHA Dietary Guidelines (4) and the National Heart, Lung, and Blood Institute (NHLBI) *Evidence Report on the Clinical Guidelines for the Identification, Evaluation, and Treatment of Overweight and Obesity in Adults* (77) recommend a total fat intake of no more than 30% as a means of decreasing total energy and facilitating weight loss. The DRI report on macronutrients (57) reviews 10 long-term ($\geq$ 1 year) weight-loss intervention studies that had a reduced fat intervention. The weight-loss diets provided 12% to 31% energy from fat and resulted in a + 1 to – 6 kg weight change. The National Weight Control Registry (NWCR) reports greater weight loss in individuals who followed self-selected weight-loss programs including a reduction in total fat (eg, 24% of energy) (78). There is also evidence that weight-loss diets moderate in total fat (approximately 35% of energy) achieve long-term weight loss (79,80). Obviously, an energy deficit is needed regardless of total fat intake. Collectively, studies conducted to date demonstrate the importance of individualizing total fat recommendations to best achieve weight loss.

NWCR, the largest database of individuals who have been successful in maintaining a substantial weight loss long term (a weight loss of $\geq$ 13.6 kg [30 lb] that has been maintained for $\geq$ 1 year), has shown that a modest reduction in total dietary fat is a successful approach to promote weight loss (78). Of the various dietary strategies used to achieve weight loss, 33.1% of participants limited their percentage of daily energy from fat. Dietary intakes of fat, protein, and carbohydrate as assessed by food-frequency questionnaire were 24%, 19%, and 56% of energy, respectively. In addition, individuals maintaining weight loss reported using more behavioral strategies to control their weight, including ongoing adherence to a low-fat diet and exercise regimen and continual monitoring of body weight (81).

McManus et al (79) reported that a moderate amount of dietary fat was associated with successful weight loss and maintenance of reduced body weight. Weight loss was evaluated in subjects consuming a 20% total fat diet compared with a moderate-fat, Mediterranean-style diet consisting of 35% energy from total fat. The participation rate was only 20% for the low-fat diet group, whereas participation in the moderate-fat diet group was 54% at the completion of the 18-month study. In addition to greater adherence to the diet, the moderate-fat diet group had a greater weight loss at the end of the study (– 4.1 kg), whereas the low-fat group had actually gained weight (+ 2.9 kg). Recently, Wien (80) evaluated the effects of a formula-based, almond-enriched (39% total fat), reduced-calorie diet compared with a self-selected, reduced-calorie, complex carbohydrate diet (18% total fat) on weight loss. During this 24-week intervention, subjects following the reduced-calorie, complex carbohydrate diet experienced a plateau at 16 weeks of the weight-loss intervention, whereas those following the almond-enriched diet continued to lose weight for the duration of the trial. These results support other findings documenting difficulties with adherence to a low-fat diet. A moderate-fat diet may offer the most effective approach for weight loss and long-term maintenance of reduced body weight through greater adherence compared with a much lower fat diet (18% to 20% of energy).

A key question for individual patients is "What is the appropriate level of total fat, within the fat recommendation range of 20% to 35%, to promote long-term weight loss and maintenance?" The available evidence suggests that a range of fat-intake levels can be used for successful weight-loss diets. The level of total fat selected is dependent on personal diet-adherence issues and what level facilitates long-term adherence to a calorie-controlled diet. Moderation is the key; dietary fat should not be too low or too high because dietary adherence is challenging with the former, and an adequate energy deficit can be difficult to achieve with the latter.

Glucose and Insulin Levels

It is well established that insulin resistance is a risk factor for the development of hyperglycemia. A high-carbohydrate (ie, low-fat) diet leads to a greater postprandial glucose and insulin response. The long-term consequences of repeated stimulation of insulin secretion are unknown. Some investigators postulate that it could accelerate beta-cell exhaustion (82,83). Moreover, a prolonged elevation in plasma glucose in response to a low-fat, high-carbohydrate diet theoretically could enhance production of glycated products or advanced glycated end products, both of which could be atherogenic. Thus, among individuals who have insulin resistance or type 2 diabetes, it may be prudent for some to follow a higher fat diet within the range recommended by ATP III (1), as well as the DRI (57).

Summary of the Effect of Total Fat on CHD Parameters

Given the range of total fat levels that are recommended, the following considerations should be addressed in treating individual patients:

- Assess the baseline laboratory values, body weight, and metabolic profile of the patient.
- Carefully monitor how CHD risk factors change in response to alterations in dietary fat level.
- Change the dietary fat level as needed to facilitate the most favorable CHD risk factor profile.

There is now an impressive armamentarium of approaches for treating risk factors that include individualizing dietary fat levels. Monitoring this array of risk factors is important for maximally reducing CHD risk. Dietary fat level is the starting point for optimizing the diet to reduce CHD risk to the greatest extent possible. Other nuances in prescribing the ideal diet require the unique skills of a registered dietitian. Examples of clinically relevant patient profiles with appropriate dietary fat recommendations follow. They are intended to guide selection of diets that vary in dietary fat levels for patients with different clinical profiles and dietary adherence issues.

Individualizing Total Fat Prescriptions in Clinical Practice for Treatment of Multiple CHD Risk Factors

Total fat recommendations allow great flexibility in planning and prescribing diets that are reduced in saturated fat and cholesterol to decrease LDL cholesterol and favorably affect other risk factors. The unique clinical skills of a registered dietitian must be used to prioritize and deal with individual risk factors, as well as clusters of risk factors in an individual. Consider the following patient examples:

Example 1

The patient is overweight with a normal LDL cholesterol level, increased fasting glucose, increased blood pressure, and increased waist circumference. This patient is diagnosed with metabolic syndrome because of the following: abdominal obesity (waist circumference > 40 inches in men; > 35 inches in women), blood pressure of 130/85 mm Hg or higher, and an elevated fasting glucose level (≥ 100 mg/dL) (1,65). The first priority for this patient is weight loss to decrease abdominal obesity, blood pressure, and the fasting glucose level. A diet reduced in total fat would be appropriate to reduce energy intake. However, a moderate-fat diet may be more appropriate to ensure adherence. The starting level of fat should be based on the patient's current intake and should not be too extreme. The diet prescription can then be changed as the patient's adherence and weight loss are monitored. For this patient, instruction in reducing energy intake is the primary goal to facilitate weight loss, regardless of the total fat content of the diet. Nonetheless, total fat is important from the perspective of adherence.

Example 2

The patient has normal weight, a normal LDL cholesterol level, elevated fasting triglycerides, a low HDL cholesterol level, and elevated blood pressure. Also diagnosed with metabolic syndrome, this patient's primary target is the lipid profile and not body weight. For this patient, a moderate-fat diet is appropriate to reduce triglycerides and possibly increase HDL cholesterol.

Example 3

The patient has elevated LDL cholesterol and triglyceride levels. The primary goal for this patient is to reduce saturated fat to reduce LDL cholesterol. A moderate-fat diet emphasizing unsaturated fatty acids, whole grains, and fiber-rich foods may be indicated. Alternatively, a diet at the lower end of the recommended range for total fat may be appropriate for this patient if fiber is increased to prevent an elevation in triglycerides.

Special Conditions

Certain conditions require reduction in dietary fat intake below recommended guidelines. When triglyceride levels exceed 500 mg/dL, patients are at an increased risk for acute pancreatitis. A very-low-fat diet (< 15% of total energy as fat) is recommended in addition to drug therapy to lessen the chylomicronemia, which contributes to very high triglycerides (1).

Highly motivated patients may be interested in intensive lifestyle change programs that recommend a very-low-fat diet. The Pritikin Program includes a diet high in complex carbohydrates and low in fat (< 10%) and cholesterol (< 25 mg/day) and includes daily exercise. Participants in a 26-day residential program experienced a 21% reduction in total cholesterol levels (84). Similar results (a 19% reduction) were reported in a group of individuals 70 years of age and older (85). Ornish and colleagues recommend a low-fat, whole foods diet with stress-management techniques, such as yoga and meditation, to promote relaxation and increase energy, moderate exercise, and social support. Patients with moderate to severe CHD who participated for 5 years in the Lifestyle Heart Trial (86) experienced regression of coronary atherosclerosis (a 7.9% relative improvement) at 5 years' follow-up. Participants consumed a 10% fat vegetarian diet that was rich in fruits, vegetables, grains, legumes, and soybean products. Such intensive programs illustrate cardiovascular benefits of not only a diet markedly reduced in total and saturated fat but also other accompanying lifestyle modifications. These programs offer options for very committed individuals who wish to make major lifestyle changes to decrease their risk of coronary disease.

Prescribing the appropriate level of dietary fat can maximally decrease CHD risk by affecting multiple CHD risk factors. Individualizing the dietary fat prescription can optimize the lipid profile and dietary adherence. Regardless of the specific level of dietary fat, saturated fat should be less than 7% of energy for desirable LDL cholesterol levels. Registered dietitians can identify and implement the most appropriate dietary fat prescription for an individual, monitor its effects, and modify it as needed.

OTHER ASPECTS OF DIET RELATED TO CHD

Fruits and Vegetables

Fruits and vegetables contain a number of components that may further reduce the development of CHD, including soluble fiber, antioxidant vitamins, folate, and minerals, such as calcium, potassium, and magnesium. However, published data on fruits and vegetables in relation to CHD are limited. Several cohort studies have not confirmed a benefit (87). The National Health and Nutrition Examination Survey Epidemiologic Follow-up Study did report that CVD mortality for subjects consuming three or more fruits and vegetables per day was 27% lower than for subjects consuming less than one serving per day. Deaths included those due to strokes and ischemic heart disease (88). Fruit and vegetable intake has also been associated with lower incidence of ischemic strokes in a Danish cohort (89).

Although the DASH Study has shown benefits from fruits and vegetables in control of hypertension, trials have not focused on ischemic heart disease. A Finnish 6-week trial provided either a higher polyunsaturated fat diet (using sunflower oil) or a higher monounsaturated fat diet (using high-oleic sunflower and olive oils), with or without the addition of vegetables, berries, and apples. Significant differences in parameters were not observed in serum lipids, homocysteine, and LDL oxidation (90).

B Vitamins and Homocysteine Levels

Hyperhomocysteinemia (greater than 12 μmol/dL) has been identified as an independent risk factor for CHD. Vitamins involved in homocysteine metabolism (folate, vitamin B-6, and vitamin B-12) are being prescribed by some lipid specialists to normalize homocysteine levels. Polymorphisms in the gene for the enzyme methyl tetrahydrofolate reductase (MTHFR), which converts the dimethyl form of tetrahydrofolate to the methyl form (N^5, N^{10} methylene tetrahydrofolate to N^5 methyl tetrahydrofolate), suggest that some individuals may need higher amounts of folate to maintain normal homocysteine levels (91).

TABLE 6.6
Theoretical Effect of Multiple Dietary Components Estimated by ATP III

Dietary Component	Dietary Change	Approximate LDL Cholesterol Reduction, %
Saturated fatty acids	<7% kcal	8–10
Cholesterol	<200 mg/d	3–5
Weight reduction	Lose 10 lb	5–8
Soluble fiber	5–10 g/d	3–5
Plant stanols	2 g/d	6–15
Cumulative Potential Effect		**20–30**

Abbreviations: ATP III, Adult Treatment Panel III; LDL, low-density lipoprotein.
Source: Adapted from Table V.5-2 in reference 1, based on data from reference 99.

In an effort to reduce neural tube defects, the US government in 1998 mandated that white, refined flour be fortified with 1.4 mg folate for each kg of flour. An additional benefit may be reduction of CHD by lowering serum homocysteine levels. Plasma homocysteine levels were significantly lower in the Framingham population after the initiation of folate fortification of flour (92). Failure to document significantly different homocysteine levels in a group of Mexican-American women with polymorphisms of MTHFR led to speculation that the now higher intake of folate due to flour fortification may compensate for genetic variations in MTHFR (93).

Although a number of studies report an association of elevated homocysteine levels with risk for CHD (94), results from published clinical trials are very limited. Two years of supplementation with 5 mg folic acid and 250 mg vitamin B-6 decreased subclinical atherosclerosis in siblings of patients with CVD (95). In the Swiss Heart Study, in patients receiving 6 months of supplementation with 1 mg folic acid, 400 μg vitamin B-12, and 10 mg vitamin B-6 after coronary angioplasty, the need for further revascularation was reduced by almost half (20% in those supplemented compared with 38% in the control patients) (96). On the other hand, even though serum homocysteine levels were reduced 18% among CHD patients given 0.5 mg folic acid daily, after 2 years mortality and vascular events were not significantly changed (97).

How much to supplement? A Danish dose-response study determined 400 μg/day of folate as the minimum dose for adequate homocysteine reduction in 50- to 75-year-old individuals (98). This is the amount contained in a multivitamin supplement. The Danish population did not have the benefit of folate fortification of flour, as in the United States. The use of B vitamin supplements is discussed further in Chapter 11.

Combining Nutrition Approaches

Having considered the effect of individual dietary factors on risk of CHD, questions arise regarding the potential synergistic benefits from combining these approaches. ATP III estimated the combined impact of its major dietary principles could lower LDL cholesterol levels by 20% to 30% (refer to Table 6.6) (1,99). Studies investigating these overall dietary approaches rather than specific nutrition components are increasingly popular.

In the Lyon Diet Heart Study, provision of a Mediterranean-style diet low in saturated fat, high in monounsaturated and n-3 polyunsaturated fatty acids, and rich in vegetables was associated with a significant reduction in recurrent heart disease (100). Intervention with a similar diet in India among patients at risk for heart disease found significantly fewer cardiovascular endpoints after 2 years in subjects consuming a diet high in fruits, vegetables, nuts, whole grains, legumes, and n-3 alpha-linolenic acid from mustard seed or soybean oil (101).

A cross-sectional study of Danish adults classified their diets into three patterns: cosmopolitan pattern (high in fried vegetables, salad, rice, chicken, fish, and wine), a traditional pattern (high in red meat and potatoes, limited in low-fat dairy products and fruit), and a "refined foods" pattern (including french fries, high-sugar beverages, and white bread). The cosmopolitan pattern was associated with higher HDL cholesterol levels and the refined foods with higher total cholesterol levels (102). A similar comparison of a prudent vs Western diet among men enrolled in the Health Professionals Follow-up Study found lower C-reactive protein and serum homocysteine levels among those consuming the prudent diet composed of fruits, vegetables, whole grains, and poultry, as contrasted with the Western diet higher in red meats, high-fat dairy products, and refined grains (103).

Recently, Jenkins and colleagues (104) provided a portfolio diet that not only met TLC recommendations for saturated fat, stanol esters, and soluble fiber but also provided protein through soy and nuts. Patients with moderate hypercholesterolemia stabilized on a diet with less than 7% saturated fat and less than 200 mg cholesterol per day were then randomized to a control diet, to the experimental portfolio diet, or to use of statin medication. Subjects consuming the dietary portfolio of stanol esters, soluble fiber, soy, and nuts lowered their LDL cholesterol to levels comparable to the levels of subjects receiving the statin medication (28.6% vs 30.9%). In addition, C-reactive protein levels were significantly lower in both the dietary portfolio and statin groups than in the control group.

Although nutritional parameters underlie overall dietary approaches to optimize heart health, communication to the public and patients is more meaningful when it focuses on foods. Kris-Etherton et al (105) carefully reviewed the effects of foods on lipid parameters. As the benefits of including nuts, fish, plant stanol margarines, and many other foods are communicated, attention to substitution rather than addition of foods is important for maintaining energy balance.

PRACTICAL ISSUES IN MNT

On the basis of this research evidence, when the patient's lipid profile and risk factors indicate the need for intervention (as shown in Chapter 3, Table 3.4), MNT is required. Individualized MNT in the clinical setting is currently the most common, but group-based nutrition intervention may also be appropriate and cost-effective in cardiac rehabilitation programs.

Table 6.7 summarizes food-based advice for complying with ATP III guidelines (1). In advising patients to adopt these dietary practices, counselors should recognize that some are more easily adopted than others. Using CSFII data and the fat-related questions of the Diet and Health Knowledge Survey, Capps et al (106) reported that almost half of Americans trim fat from meat, remove skin from chicken, and eat chips infrequently. Although one third of those surveyed used nonfat or low-fat milk, another third never do so. Less-frequent behaviors include use of low-fat cheese and having fruit for dessert.

Individualized MNT Sessions

Provision of MNT through individualized sessions is the most common mode for assisting patients in achieving long-term behavior change. The American Dietetic Association (ADA) offers the Medical Nutrition Therapy Protocol for Hyperlipidemia to standardize the process for dietitians' provision of MNT; this protocol is particularly beneficial for reimbursement for

TABLE 6.7
Food-Based Advice for Therapeutic Lifestyle Changes (TLC)

Food	Recommended Amount	These More Often	These Less Often
Breads and cereals	≥6 servings per day (adjust servings to balance energy needs)	Breads and cereals, especially whole grain; pasta; rice; potatoes; dry beans and peas; low fat crackers, pretzels, and cookies	High-fat bakery products, such as doughnuts, biscuits, croissants, Danish pastries, pies, cookies
Many grain-based snacks, including chips, cheese puffs, snack mix, regular crackers, buttered popcorn
Vegetables and fruits	3–5 servings vegetables per day
2–4 servings fruits per day	Fresh, frozen, or canned vegetables without added fat, sauce, or salt
Fresh, frozen, canned, or dried fruit	Vegetables fried or prepared with butter, cheese, or cream sauce
Fruits fried or served with butter or cream
Dairy products	2–3 servings per day	Nonfat, one-half percent, and low-fat milk, buttermilk, yogurt, and cottage cheese; fat-free and low-fat cheese	Whole milk, reduced-fat milk, whole-milk yogurt, ice cream, cream, half & half, cream cheese, sour cream, and cheese
Eggs	≤2 egg yolks per week	Egg whites or egg substitute	Whole eggs, egg yolk
Meat, fish, and poultry	≤5 ounces per day	Lean cuts, loin, leg, round; extra lean hamburger; cold cuts made with lean meat or soy protein; skinless poultry; fish; peanut butter; meat alternatives made with soy or textured vegetable protein	Higher fat meat cuts, ribs, t-bone steak, regular hamburger, bacon, sausage; cold cuts, salami, bologna, corned beef, hot dogs; organ meats, liver, brains, sweetbreads; poultry with skin; fried meat, poultry, and fish
Fats and oils	Amount adjusted to caloric level	Unsaturated oils; soft or liquid margarines and vegetable oil spreads, salad dressings, seeds, and nuts	Butter, shortening, stick margarine, chocolate, tropical oils, coconut, palm, and palm kernel

Source: Adapted from Table V.2-6 in reference 1.

MNT (2). The protocol can be accessed at the National Guideline Clearinghouse Web site (http://guidelines.gov). An analysis of the evidence base for nutrition interventions in hyperlipidemia provides the foundation for the detailed outline of assessment and counseling steps. Additional practice tools on CD-ROM can be purchased from the ADA (http://www.eatright.org).

Sikand et al (107) studied evidence of the effectiveness of individualized MNT by the dietitian in patients participating in lipid-lowering drug trials. The investigators reviewed LDL cholesterol levels in patients receiving multiple counseling sessions for stabilization on a cholesterol-lowering diet before initiation of medications. LDL cholesterol values were significantly lower after two, three, or four appointments with a dietitian. The trend of declining LDL levels continued beyond the second visit through the third and fourth visits. Approximately half of the patients no longer qualified for lipid-lowering medication according to the earlier ATP II guidelines in effect at the time. This group also reviewed charts of 75 patients with combined hyperlipidemia who participated in an 8-week dietitian intervention program. LDL cholesterol was lowered by 9% and triglycerides by 22%. Cost-benefit data further indicated a saving of $3 in medication cost for every dollar invested in MNT (108).

In Denmark, a comparison of individuals receiving one brief 10-minute counseling session with individuals receiving two 50-minute sessions found that 1 year later saturated fat intake had decreased significantly (from 11.9% to 9.6% of energy) among subjects receiving the two individualized sessions, but not among those who received only one brief session (10.9% to 10.1%) (109). According to the Cochrane database on evidence-based medicine, the few studies available suggest that nutrition counseling by the dietitian lowers LDL levels more than nutrition intervention by the physician alone (110). The US Preventive Services Task Force recommends intensive behavioral dietary counseling for adults with hyperlipidemia and other risk factors for heart disease. The task force concluded that there is "good evidence that medium- to high-intensity counseling" can produce medium-to-large changes in the average daily intake of saturated fat, fiber, fruit, and vegetables among adult patients at risk for diet-related chronic disease (8).

Guidelines for MNT Sessions

As outlined by ADA's MNT Evidence-Based Guide for Hyperlipidemia (2), an initial MNT session should include assessment, intervention, provision of self-management materials, and plans for measuring outcomes. Thorough assessment of clinical data should address risk factors (including smoking history), lipid profile, and medications. Nutrition assessment includes the following:

- Anthropometric measures, including body mass index (BMI) and waist circumference
- Biochemical laboratory values, including the lipid profile and serum proteins
- Change readiness and knowledge for lifestyle changes
- Dietary assessment, noting
  - Percentage of energy from fat in the diet and types of fat
  - Fiber and viscous fiber intake and sources of fiber
  - Fruit and vegetable intake
  - Use of specific items, such as fish, nuts, soy, and use of stanol- or sterol-fortified products
  - Use of dietary supplements
  - Physical activity levels

The intervention portion of the MNT session should facilitate self-management for identified goals. During this segment, the dietitian does the following:

- Discuss risk factors
- Explain role of diet and physical activity in lipid management
- Provide nutrition prescription based on TLC
- Explain value of different types of fat
- Provide information about special food products
- Discuss self-monitoring techniques, such as food records and pedometers
- Mutually establish goals, such as those related to serum lipids, BMI, waist circumference, eating behaviors, food intake, and physical activity

Written or Web-based materials should be customized to the client's needs. Patients typically need advice on how to purchase foods and plan and prepare meals, as well as guidance in how to apply principles when eating out, traveling, and celebrating special occasions.

Outcome measures can be derived from assessment data and individualized goals. Follow-up MNT sessions focus on assessment of response to nutrition therapy and the extent to which the patient has been able to adopt recommended lifestyle changes.

Behavioral Issues: Lifestyle Change

Assessment of the patient's stage of change allows for guiding the patient to long-term behavior change (see Chapter 5). It is helpful to recognize that a patient can be at different stages of change for different heart-healthy behaviors. For instance, a patient may be at the maintenance stage for using nonfat milk, but only at the contemplation stage for eating appropriate portion sizes of meat. Offering patients multiple strategies for dealing with a specific problem food, such as ice cream or bacon, can be helpful. Common strategies include the following:

- Reducing the portion size
- Preparing the food more healthfully
- Reducing the frequency it is eaten
- Substituting a more healthful food for the problem food

Self-monitoring, such as counting fat grams and recording food intake and physical activity, is essential.

Numerous sample programs, educational materials, and patient resources are available for helping patients achieve a heart-healthy diet. The ADA MNT Evidence-Based Guide for Hyperlipidemia (2) provides materials for use in MNT. Protocols used in clinical trials for reducing heart disease risk (111) and cancer (112) provide excellent ideas. Although developed a number of years ago, the interdisciplinary approach of the Multiple Risk Factor Intervention Trial (111) with individual and group sessions continues to provide a model for helping patients to achieve long-term dietary changes with flexible eating patterns. The Polyp Prevention Trial (112), which was designed to reduce recurrence of colon polyps, included campaigns to reduce total fat, increase fruit and vegetable intake, and focus on goal achievement. Frequent contact and an action orientation were teamed with novelty, fun, and rewards to enhance achievement of behavior change goals. A variety of resource materials available on the Internet are outlined in Table 6.8 (1,52,77,113-122).

Group Classes

Group sessions modeled after clinical trial protocols can be an efficient means of providing nutrition education and counseling to prevent and manage CHD. Target audiences include the general public, individuals with modifiable risk factors for CHD, and cardiac rehabilitation patients (post–myocardial infarction, coronary artery bypass graft, or angioplasty).

Single classes can increase the public's awareness of modifying lifestyle habits for reducing CHD risk and steer them to additional resources, such as Web sites, individual MNT, or a series of group classes. A short series for clients interested in lowering LDL cholesterol levels with dietary strategies could include three to four sessions, as outlined in Table 6.9. When resources permit, a supermarket tour, a cooking demonstration, and tastings can help clients and their families learn to purchase and prepare heart-healthy foods. Food preparation tips and a list of substitutions to lower total and saturated fat in recipes are provided in Box 6.2 (123) and are available at the AHA's Delicious Decisions Web site (114). A dinner session at a restaurant allows application of newly gained knowledge when selecting from the menu. The National Restaurant Association (116) and the AHA (52,114) provide tips at Web sites listed in Table 6.8.

TABLE 6.8
Web-Based Patient Education Resources

Organization and URL	Materials Available
American Diabetes Association (113) http://vgs.diabetes.org/grocery_tour.jsp	Virtual grocery store tour allows users to go to sections of the store to read information about wise selections and click to view nutrition label information on both packaged foods and fresh produce and meat; requires users to register (no cost).
American Heart Association (52,114) http://www.americanheart.org and http://www.deliciousdecisions.org	Many resources, fact sheets, and "Delicious Decisions" (an online tabbed book format with AHA Food Pyramid and label reading, supermarket shopping, eating out, fitness-weight control).
Bell Institute (115) http://www.bellinstitute.com/hearthealth/index.asp	"Destination Heart-Healthy Eating" provides patient booklet and instructor Power Point using behavior change principles for achieving ATP III guidelines.
National Cholesterol Education Program Adult Treatment Panel III (1) http://www.nhlbi.nih.gov/guidelines/cholesterol/index.htm	ATP III Web site includes interactive consumer section titled "Live Healthier, Live Longer," which provides information and activities divided for users who want to prevent CHD or who have CHD. In "Create-A-Diet," users select food items to see how nutrient contents stack up against ATP III guidelines.
National Restaurant Association (116) http://www.restaurant.org/dineout/nutrition.cfm	"Tips for Eating Smart in Restaurants" and an ask the nutritionist section to e-mail questions to a registered dietitian.
Centers for Disease Control and Prevention (117) http://www.cdc.gov	Information and links to other sites on nutrition, physical activity, and weight control.
Food and Drug Administration (118) http://www.cfsan.fda.gov/dms/foodlab.html	The booklet "Guidance on How to Understand and Use the Nutrition Facts Panel on Food Labels" explains each component of Nutrition Facts panel with sample labels.
National Heart, Lung, and Blood Institute: recipe Web pages (119–121) http://www.nhlbi.nih.gov/health/public/heart/other/syah/index.htm http://www.nhlbi.nih.gov/health/public/heart/other/chdblack/cooking.pdf http://www.nhlbi.nih.gov/health/public/heart/other/sp_recip.pdf	"Stay Young at Heart, The Heart Healthy Cooking Way" recipes for low-fat cooking "Heart Healthy Home Cooking, African-American Style:" 32-page cookbook filled with heart healthy recipes. "Latino Heart Healthy Recipes," 56-page Spanish/English translation recipe book.
National Heart, Lung, and Blood Institute: Obesity Education Initiative (77) http://www.nhlbi.nih.gov/about/oei/index.htm	Weight control information for consumers and health professionals.
Weight-Control Information Network (122) http://www.niddk.nih.gov/health/nutrit/nutrit.htm	"Healthy Eating and Physical Activity across Your Lifespan," provides a four-part series, including "Better Health for You" (for adults) and "Young at Heart" (older adults)

Additional Approaches to Behavior Change

Food Label Education

Educating patients on the use of food labels is a valuable step in helping them to make heart-healthy selections, especially in the supermarket. Such education usually includes helping patients define terms on the label, such as saturated fat, cholesterol, and fiber, as well as claims on the label, such as "low-fat," "lite," or "cholesterol free." Patients should also understand how the % Daily Value is derived and their daily goals for total fat, saturated fat, and fiber. The FDA's Web site has valuable education on use of the Nutrition Facts panel of the food label (see Table 6.8).

TABLE 6.9
Sample Outline of Group Classes

Topic	Learner Objectives
Overview of heart-healthy eating	Learners will be able to 1. Distinguish types of dietary fat and their effect on serum lipids. 2. Use the nutrition label to select heart-healthy oils and margarines. 3. Describe the benefit of generous inclusion of fruits, vegetables, and whole grains in a heart-healthy diet. 4. Discuss the potential benefit of including • Soluble fiber • Stanol-sterol ester fortified margarines • Soy products • Fish and other sources of n-3 fatty acids
Meal planning and food preparation	Learners will be able to 1. Identify ways to incorporate generous amounts of fruits, vegetables, and whole grains in a heart-healthy diet. 2. Explain how to stock their pantry and refrigerator for heart-healthy cooking.
Supermarket tour and use of nutrition label	Learners will be able to 1. Use the nutrition label to select heart-healthy • Dairy products • Cooking oils and salad dressings • Cereals • Preprepared entrees • Snack foods and desserts 2. Select heart-healthy • Meat and fish • Produce 3. Prepare new fruits and vegetables.
Special issues: eating out, traveling, and celebrations	Learners will be able to 1. Make heart-healthy menu selections using restaurant and fast food menus. 2. Describe strategies for maintaining a heart-healthy diet while traveling. 3. Describe ways to promote heart-healthy eating on special occasions, such as holidays.

Source: Adapted from Heart Challenge classes taught by Jo Ann S. Carson, PhD, RD.

The FDA has approved specific health claims that are allowed on food products (124,125). Those related to heart disease are listed in Table 6.10. The FDA has ascertained that scientific evidence is substantive enough to allow claims related to saturated fat, soluble fiber, soy protein, and stanol esters. More recently, qualified claims have been introduced that allow mention of the possible benefits of nuts, n-3 fatty acids, and the B complex vitamins—folate, B-6, and B-12—in relation to CHD.

Supermarket Nutrition Tours

Supermarket nutrition tours are a fun, interactive means of helping clients learn to select heart-healthy foods using the nutrition label. The store environment provides immediate access to new products and sometimes allows food tasting. Clients can apply new information in the context in which they will use it, such as making informed shopping decisions. In addition to comparing the types of fats in cooking oils, cheese, or margarine or the amount of fiber in breads and cereals, tour participants can receive tips on selecting and preparing items from the perimeter of the store—meats and produce. Resources available include *Supermarket Savvy Newsletter* and the companion tour training guide (126). The American Diabetes Association provides a virtual supermarket tour (see Table 6.8).

Box 6.2 Tips for Reducing Saturated Fatty Acids in Food Preparation

Food Preparation

- Prepare beef, pork, chicken, and fish by baking, broiling, roasting, stewing, or stir-frying.
- Trim all visible fat from beef and pork before cooking; select lean cuts, such as those with loin or round in the name.
- Defat ground meat by cooking meat and then draining off fat.
- Brown meats in pan lightly brushed or sprayed with oil.
- When preparing stews or soup, refrigerate the broth and skim off fat with a spoon before reheating and serving.
- Remove skin from chicken before serving.
- Instead of frying fish, try broiling, grilling, microwaving, baking with bread crumbs, or poaching in milk, tomato juice, or water flavored with a little lemon juice.
- When cooking foods such as eggs, French toast, and pancakes, brush the pan with oil just to coat it, or use a nonstick spray made from vegetable oil or a nonstick pan that requires no greasing.
- Flavor vegetables with lemon juice or herbs like dill, rosemary, or basil instead of adding fat.

Recipe Substitutions

In place of	Try
Whole egg	2 egg whites, or 1 egg white + 2 tsp nonfat milk powder + 2 tsp oil, or 1/4 cup egg substitute
Whole milk (1 cup)	1 cup nonfat milk, or 1 cup nonfat milk + 2 tsp oil, or 1/2 cup nonfat milk + 1/2 cup evaporated nonfat milk
Sour cream	Fat free sour cream, or nonfat or low-fat plain yogurt, or 1 cup low-fat cottage cheese blended with 2 tsp lemon juice
Butter, shortening, or lard	Regular tub margarine (not light)
Cream cheese	1 cup low-fat cottage cheese, rinsed under water and then blended with 1/4 c margarine
Baking chocolate (1 oz)	3 Tbsp unsweetened cocoa + 1 Tbsp margarine
Cream	Equal measure of canned evaporated nonfat milk
Bacon	Soy bacon-like bits (texturized vegetable protein)
Cheese	Fat-free and low-fat cheese and processed cheese

Source: Adapted from reference 123.

Computerized Nutrient Analysis

Given the number of recommendations stated in terms of percentage of energy, the patient attempting to follow a heart-healthy diet can often benefit from computerized nutrient analysis of a 3- to 4-day food record. Some patients find monitoring their diet with software on their home computer valuable. The Create-A-Diet Activity, available from the NHLBI (http://www.nhlbi support.com/chd1/create.htm), provides one means of assessing diet by computer (1).

Home-Delivered Diets

An innovative approach in helping patients adhere to dietary recommendations and control body weight is the use of a home-delivered diet. Gleason (127) demonstrated that providing meals with only 4% of energy from saturated fat for 8 weeks significantly lowered LDL

TABLE 6.10

Food and Drug Administration–Approved Health Claims Related to Cardiovascular Disease

Nutrient/Food	Approved Health Claim
Unqualified Health Claims	
Saturated fat and cholesterol	While many factors affect heart disease, diets low in saturated fat and cholesterol may reduce the risk of this disease.
Soluble fiber	Diets low in saturated fat and cholesterol and rich in fruits, vegetables, and grain products that contain some types of dietary fiber, particularly soluble fiber, may reduce the risk of heart disease, a disease associated with many factors. OR
	Soluble fiber from foods such as [name of soluble fiber source, and, if desired, name of food product], as part of a diet low in saturated fat and cholesterol, may reduce the risk of heart disease. A serving of [name of food product] supplies _____ grams of the [necessary daily dietary intake for the benefit] soluble fiber from [name of soluble fiber source] necessary per day to have this effect.
Soy protein	Twenty-five grams of soy protein a day, as part of a diet low in saturated fat and cholesterol, may reduce the risk of heart disease. A serving of [name of food] supplies _____ grams of soy protein. OR
	Diets low in saturated fat and cholesterol that include 25 grams of soy protein a day may reduce the risk of heart disease. One serving of [name of food] provides _____ grams of soy protein.
Stanol esters	Foods containing at least 0.65 gram per serving of vegetable oil sterol esters, eaten twice a day with meals for a daily total intake of at least 1.3 grams, as part of a diet low in saturated fat and cholesterol, may reduce the risk of heart disease. A serving of [name of food] supplies _____ grams of vegetable oil sterol esters. OR
	Diets low in saturated fat and cholesterol that include two servings of foods that provide a daily total of at least 3.4 grams of plant stanol esters in two meals may reduce the risk of heart disease. A serving of [name of food] supplies _____ grams of plant stanol esters.
Qualified Health Claims	
Nuts	Scientific evidence suggests but does not prove that eating 1.5 ounces per day of most nuts [such as name of specific nut] as part of a diet low in saturated fat and cholesterol may reduce the risk of heart disease. OR
	Supportive but not conclusive research shows that eating 1.5 ounces per day of walnuts as part of a diet low in saturated fat and cholesterol may reduce the risk of heart disease. See nutrition information for fat content. OR
	Scientific evidence suggests but does not prove that eating 1.5 ounces per day of most nuts, such as walnuts, as part of a diet low in saturated fat and cholesterol may reduce the risk of heart disease. See nutrition information for fat content.
n-3 fatty acids	Consumption of n-3 fatty acids may reduce the risk of coronary heart disease. FDA evaluated the data and determined that, although there is scientific evidence supporting the claim, the evidence is not conclusive.
Folate, B-6, B-12	As part of a well-balanced diet that is low in saturated fat and cholesterol, folic acid, vitamin B-6, and vitamin B-12 may reduce the risk of vascular disease. FDA evaluated the above claim and found that, while it is known that diets low in saturated fat and cholesterol reduce the risk of heart disease and other vascular diseases, the evidence in support of the above claim is inconclusive.

Source: Reprinted from references 123 and 124.

cholesterol by 7.5 mg/dL in the 35 men and women in the study. Participants received educational information from the dietitian by telephone.

Adapting for Cultural Differences

Behavior change is more likely when nutrition counseling to lower saturated fat and cholesterol is adapted to the cultural food patterns of the patient. Chapter 15 illustrates principles important in cultural adaptations. Sample TLC menus are provided in Diet Appendix B of ATP III for men and women using traditional American, lacto-ovo vegetarian, Southern, Asian, and Mexican-American foods (1 [pp B1-B10]).

Cardiac Rehabilitation Programs

Patients who have experienced CHD events, such as a myocardial infarction, or had coronary artery bypass grafts or angioplasty due to occluded coronary arteries are generally provided with a team-oriented cardiac rehabilitation program. This generally consists of 6 to 12 weeks of supervised exercise and a series of educational sessions on improving heart health. A comprehensive cardiac rehabilitation program includes exploration of risk factors, involvement of the patient and cardiac rehabilitation team in establishing patient goals, and development of a plan to achieve the goals.

Given the nature of events that place a patient in cardiac rehabilitation, these patients may have moved to the action stage of change. It is a prime time for helping patients initiate long-term lifestyle changes. Whether considering healthier eating, increasing physical activity, or smoking cessation, patients need to see the value of long-term change in place of aggressive short-term change with no lasting lifestyle changes.

Results from a series of 12 weekly nutrition classes for cardiac rehabilitation patients showed that almost half of the patients were already in the maintenance stage for reducing fat. This increased to 87% of the patients 2 years after the program was initiated. On the other hand, for the behavior of modifying fruit and vegetable intake, the most patients were at a stage before action at the start of the program and had moved beyond that stage 2 years later (128).

Ideally, a cardiac rehabilitation program includes several team members from various disciplines, such as medicine, exercise physiology, nursing, and nutrition (129). The dietetics professional's sessions are often similar to those enumerated in Table 6.9 for group classes. Although dietitians are often involved in cardiac rehabilitation programs, strained health care budgets sometimes limit such participation. In one program, the impact of including nutrition through two classes and one individual session was assessed. With or without specific nutrition sessions, patients improved in their ability to make dietary changes. The patients participating in the sessions with the dietitian completed the program with greater self-efficacy regarding eating healthfully, particularly in terms of eating out or when eating alone (130).

ADDITION OF MEDICATIONS TO OPTIMIZE LIPID PROFILE

Medications to Lower LDL Cholesterol Levels

In Chapter 3, Table 3.4 provides the recommendations from ATP III for when medication should be prescribed to lower serum lipids. Diet and medication are begun simultaneously in a patient with CHD and an LDL cholesterol level above 100 mg/dL or a patient with no risk factors but an LDL cholesterol level greater than 190 mg/dL.

Both patients and practitioners should recognize that lifestyle changes should be initiated or maintained when medications are initiated. Although patients may regularly be referred to the dietitian for weight loss and nutrition therapy for diabetes, some physicians may routinely prescribe a statin without addressing MNT. Eighty percent of primary care physicians who responded to a survey in the Midwestern United States agreed that diet can be effective in controlling cholesterol levels; 70% indicated they initiate diet therapy for CHD patients with LDL cholesterol levels greater than 130 mg/dL (131). Baseline data reported for *Healthy People 2010* indicated 65% of physician office visits for hyperlipidemia include nutrition counseling (132). Chart prompts can be an effective means of supporting primary care providers in following practice guidelines (133). Given that the trials documenting the effectiveness of statin drugs included stabilization on cholesterol-lowering diets, diet should be included in treatment plans that incorporate cholesterol-lowering medications (107).

When medications are indicated, they are prescribed based on the lipid abnormalities. Standard doses of 3-hydroxy-3-methylglutaryl coenzyme A (HMG-CoA) reductase inhibitors (statins) lower LDL cholesterol levels approximately 30% to 40%. Higher doses can reduce levels up to 50%. Bile acid sequestrants and ezetimibe are alternative means of lowering LDL cholesterol, particularly when a statin is contraindicated or not tolerated well. These agents also can be used in combination with statins to lower LDL levels more (see Table 6.11) (1).

Medications to Lower Serum Triglycerides

Nicotinic acid is used to lower triglycerides, as well as LDL cholesterol levels. Fibrates are used similarly without the bothersome side effect of flushing of nicotinic acid. Table 6.11 summarizes medications available.

MNT FOR SPECIAL MEDICAL ISSUES

Genetic Hypertriglyceridemia

The patient with elevated triglycerides likely has either metabolic syndrome (addressed in Chapter 7) or a genetic hyperlipidemia. When triglycerides are above 150 mg/dL, ATP III indicates use of a non-HDL cholesterol goal rather than an LDL cholesterol goal. The non-HDL goal is determined by adding 30 mg/dL to the LDL cholesterol goal established based on risk category (see Chapter 3, Table 3.4). When triglycerides are between 150 and 200 mg/dL, treatment focuses on achieving the LDL cholesterol goal and weight management, including physical activity. For triglycerides between 200 and 500 mg/dL, fibrate or nicotinic acid can be considered. They are particularly useful in combination with a statin. If the combination of fibrate and statin is used, the fibrate should be fenofibrate, and not gemfibrozil. The combination of gemfibrozil and statin carries too high a risk for severe myopathy. Triglycerides greater than 500 mg/dL are treated to prevent pancreatitis by the following (1):

- Use of nicotinic acid or fibrate
- A very-low-fat diet (≤ 15% of energy)
- Weight management and physical activity
- Avoidance of alcohol

Hyperlipidemia in Renal Disease

Increased levels of blood urea nitrogen (BUN) resulting from kidney failure can produce hyperlipidemia, partly due to inhibition of both lipoprotein lipase and hepatic lipase. With reduced lipase activity for releasing fatty acids from lipoproteins, VLDL and chylomicrons tend to increase in the blood. The LDL particles tend to be smaller and denser in nature because they are more atherogenic. Similar to ATP III guidelines, the National Kidney Foundation has established guidelines for addressing serum lipids in patients with kidney disease (9). Patients with stage 5 chronic kidney disease (CKD) should have a lipid profile completed on presentation and annually thereafter, as well as within 2 to 3 months of a change in treatment. For patients on hemodialysis, the blood sample should be taken before hemodialysis or on an alternate day. Treatment in these patients is indicated with the following lipid levels: an LDL cholesterol level greater than 100 mg/dL, a non-HDL cholesterol level greater than 130 mg/dL, or triglycerides greater than 500 mg/dL. Although clinical trials testing low-fat, low-cholesterol diets have not been conducted in patients with CKD, elevated lipids are treated similarly using TLC within any additional restraints of the patient's renal diet, such as limitations on sodium, phosphorus, and potassium. The ADA MNT Evidence-Based Guide for Practice: Chronic Kidney Disease provides guidelines on nutrition therapy for various stages of CKD (134). Fish oil supplementation may have multiple benefits for the patient with kidney failure, including reducing risk of CVD (135).

Congestive Heart Failure

Extensive CHD places extra demands upon the heart and can precipitate CHF. As the heart pumps harder to meet the increased demands, it enlarges, causing cardiomegaly. When it can no longer meet the increasing challenges, CHF results. The body is then overloaded with fluid and sodium. Fatigue, shortness of breath, and edema are common symptoms. Heart failure is divided into four stages (7):

- Stage A—High Risk. Patient has no signs or symptoms of heart failure but has conditions strongly associated with development of heart failure.
- Stage B—Asymptomatic. The patient has a structural disorder, such as an enlarged ventricle, but no signs or symptoms are present.
- Stage C—Symptomatic. The patient has a structural disorder and currently has signs or symptoms, or the patient has a structural disorder and had signs or symptoms in the past.
- Stage D—Advanced Disease. The patient has advanced structural disease and symptoms present even when at rest.

MNT for CHF includes the following:

- Limit sodium to less than 2 to 3 g/day (7)
- Limit fluid intake to 1.5 to 2 liters/day, especially when hyponatremia is present (7).
- Energy intake appropriate for maintaining adequate nutritional status, but promoting weight loss in obese patients.

Close adherence to sodium and fluid restrictions can be promoted by including a registered dietitian in a multidisciplinary team for treating CHF and investing time and resources

TABLE 6.11
Medications Used to Treat Dyslipidemias

Medication Type	Generic (Brand Name)	Mechanism	Lipid Effects	Safety	Major Side Effects	Contraindications
Statins	• Lovastatin (Mevacor) • Pravastatin (Pravachol) • Simvastatin (Zocor) • Fluvastatin (Lescol) • Atorvastatin (Lipitor) • Rosuvastatin (Crestor)	Reduce endogenous cholesterol synthesis by inhibiting HMG-CoA reductase	Lower LDL 18%–55% Raise HDL 5%–15% Lower TG 7%–30%	Side effects were minimal in clinical trials	Myopathy, increased liver transaminases	Absolute: active or chronic liver disease Relative: use of cyclosporine, macrolide antibiotics, various antifungal agents, and cytochrome P-450 inhibitors
Bile acid sequestrants	• Cholestyramine (Questran) • Colestipol (Colestid) • Colesevelam (WelChol)	Binds bile acids in gastrointestinal tract, prompting fecal excretion of bile acids resulting in increased use of cholesterol for bile salts	Lower LDL 15%–30% Raise HDL 3%–5% No effect or raises TG	Lack of systemic effect in clinical trials; GI side effects are common	Upper and lower GI complaints Decreased absorption of other drugs	Absolute: familial dysbetalipoproteinemia; TG > 400 mg/dL Relative: TG > 200 mg/dL
Other inhibitors of cholesterol absorption	• Ezetimibe (Zetia)	Block absorption of cholesterol	Adding Zetia to statin treatment lowered LDL an additional 25% and TG an additional 9% beyond the statin effect	Similar minimal side effects as with statins, when used in combination with statin	Myopathy and increased liver transaminases when used with statin; none when used alone	Because of unknown effects, not recommended for those with moderate or severe hepatic insufficiency
Nicotinic acid	• Immediate release (crystalline): sold over the counter • Extended release: sold over the counter and by prescription (Advicor [niacin and lovastatin]) • Sustained-release: sold by prescription (Niaspan)	Appears to inhibit lipoprotein synthesis and decrease VLDL production in the liver	Lower LDL 5%–25% Raise HDL 15%–35% Lower TG 20%–50%	Serious long-term effects rare for crystalline form; hepatoxicity may occur with sustained-release form	Flushing, hyperglycemia, hyperuricemia or gout, upper GI distress, hepatoxicity	Absolute: chronic liver disease, gout Relative: hyperuricemia; high doses in type 2 diabetes
Fibric acid derivatives	• Gemfibrozil (Lopid) • Fenofibrate (Tricor) • Clofibrate	Complex mechanism of action involving action as an agonist with nuclear transcription factor PPAR-alpha	Lower LDL 5%–20%, may increase in hypertriglyceridemia Raise HDL 10%–35% Lower TG 20%–50%	Long-term effects do not seem to occur; early trials with clofibrate showed an increase in non-CHD deaths, but recent clinical trials have shown no adverse effects of fibrate therapy	Dyspepsia, gallstones, myopathy	Absolute: severe hepatic or renal insufficiency

Abbreviations: CHD, coronary heart disease; GI, gastrointestinal; HDL, high-density lipoprotein; HMG-CoA, 3-hydroxy-3-methylglutaryl coenzyme A; LDL, low-density lipoprotein; PPAR alpha, peroxisome proliferator-activated receptor alpha; TG, triglyceride; VLDL, very-low-density lipoprotein.

Source: Data from Tables VI.2-1 through VI.2-4 in reference 1.

in patient counseling. These steps can prevent exacerbations and reduce hospitalizations. A program described by Kuehneman and associates (136) included sessions in the ambulatory care setting for patients at their initial visit to the Heart Failure Team, at 2 to 3 months, and again at 6 to 9 months. Patients' sodium and fluid intake was reduced significantly during participation in the program. In another CHF clinic, Neily et al (137) delineated topics to cover with patients and family members: recommended level of dietary sodium, use of the nutrition label, and ways to distinguish between high and low sources of sodium. In addition, patients should learn to manage sodium intake in nonroutine situations, such as travel, holidays, and times when a spouse is ill or hospitalized. Kuehneman's program included assistance with reducing sodium in family recipes and providing samples of spices, salt substitutes, and low-sodium products.

Initial nutrition assessment of the patient should include attention to weight status, medications, quality of life, and stage of CHF. Subsequent patient visits should address weight fluctuations, paying attention to fluid changes as well as the possibility of loss of body mass due to inadequate intake of protein and energy. Early satiety resulting from lower functional gastric volume can reduce intake, as can fatigue and reduced palatability of lower sodium diets. Patients needing to increase energy intake can try small, frequent meals and liquid supplements. Body weight and serum albumin levels are not good indicators of nutritional status, given the potential for excessive fluids inflating weight or diluting serum proteins.

Although physical activity is limited for patients with CHF, randomized controlled trials of increased physical activity document improvement in maximum oxygen consumption (VO_{2max}). The National Institutes of Health are currently supporting a large, prospective randomized trial titled "Heart Failure—a Controlled Trial Investigating Outcomes of Exercise Training." The trial's goal is to measure the impact of formal exercise training vs usual care on mortality and hospitalization rates in patients with CHF (138).

SUMMARY

The ATP III guidelines provide a basic framework, cut points, and rationale for assessing risk and implementing lifestyle changes to achieve serum lipid goals for prevention of CHD and related events. The ATP III guidelines also specify MNT as the treatment of choice in initiating therapy. ADA's MNT Evidence-Based Guide for Practice for Hyperlipidemia further specify the four parameters of TLC: lowering LDL-raising saturated and *trans* fatty acids, adding use of stanol or sterol esters and soluble fiber, promoting a healthy weight, and being physically active daily. The previous ATP II guideline advocating less than 30% of energy from fat has been broadened to a range of 25% to 35% of energy to accommodate individuals with elevated serum triglyceride levels or low HDL cholesterol levels who might benefit from slightly higher unsaturated fat levels. Attention to quality of fat is important, encouraging the use of unsaturated fat, as monounsaturated or polyunsaturated fat, including n-3 polyunsaturated fat.

Both MNT by the dietitian and numerous Web-based materials can assist patients in achieving long-term lifestyle changes to manage serum lipids and reduce risk for CHD. When necessary, medications can be included in the treatment regimen. Patients with specific medical problems, such as CHF and CKD, require intensive nutrition management integrated within their medical care.

TABLE 6.12
Laboratory Values

Laboratory Test Results	Patient's Results	Reference Values
LDL cholesterol (mg/dL)	140	Optimal <100
Total cholesterol (mg/dL)	209	Desirable <200
HDL cholesterol (mg/dL)	42	>40
Triglycerides (mg/dL)	125	Normal <150
Glucose (mg/dL)	105	65–110
Creatinine (mg/dL)	1.0	0.6–1.2
Blood urea nitrogen (mg/dL)	10	7–21
TSH (µU/L)	28.0	0.2–4.5
Free T4 (ng/mL)	0.4	0.8–1.8

Abbreviations: HDL, high-density lipoprotein; LDL, low-density lipoprotein; TSH, thyroid-stimulating hormone (thryotropin); T4, thyroxine.

CASE STUDY: HYPERLIPIDEMIA

Past Medical History, Family, and Social History

JM is a 58-year-old postmenopausal white woman who presents to the General Internal Medicine Clinic for establishment of a primary care physician after moving from another state. Her hypertension diagnosed 4 years ago is well controlled on Maxzide (hydrochlorothiazide and triamterene); last menses was 2 years ago. A nonsmoker, she usually drinks a glass of wine with dinner. She walks 2 miles three to four times per week. Her 82-year-old mother is alive and well; her father had a fatal myocardial infarction at age 77.

Dietary Intake

JM tries to eat a heart-healthy diet. She eats meat approximately four times per week and uses nonfat milk. She enjoys salads, fresh vegetables, and whole-grain breads and cereal. Her saturated fat intake comes primarily from 4 to 6 ounces of regular cheese per week, an occasional hamburger, one or two servings of ice cream per week, afternoon candy snacks, and sometimes a slice of pie with her husband in the evening. She has been careful to limit her sodium intake by not adding salt and avoiding high-sodium, processed foods. A computerized nutrient analysis of her 3-day food record indicated that she eats approximately 1,980 kcal per day with 31% of energy from fat, 11% of energy from saturated fat, and 180 mg of dietary cholesterol.

Physical Examination and Laboratory Data

On physical examination JM had a heart rate of 68 beats per minute and blood pressure of 130/83 mm Hg. She is 5 feet, 6 inches in height (168 cm) and weighs 148 lb (67 kg). After a stable weight of 135 lb for many years, she has gained 10 lb in the last 2 years. Her BMI is 24 and waist circumference is 31 inches. Her physical exam was otherwise unremarkable. Laboratory values are shown in Table 6.12.

Medical Treatment Goals

ATP III (Table 3.4 in Chapter 3) provides a means for assessing JM's lipid profile and establishing an LDL cholesterol goal for her. JM has two CVD risk factors: age (being a woman older than 55 years) and hypertension. Although her father died of a myocardial infarction, there is no evidence of family history of premature heart disease, such as her father having CHD before the age of 55. With two risk factors, her 10-year risk for CHD is estimated as 5% (see Table 3.5 in Chapter 3). According to ATP III guidelines, her LDL goal is therefore less than 130 mg/dL. New AHA recommendations (see Chapter 14) suggest an LDL goal of less than 100 mg/dL for high-risk women.

In considering treatment for JM, one should not overlook her hypothyroidism. As a secondary cause for hyperlipidemia, her thyroid status should be normalized before assessing whether a cholesterol-lowering medication should be added. The hypothyroidism may have contributed to her recent weight gain.

Treatment goals for JM include achieving euthyroid status and lowering LDL cholesterol. In addition, energy balance should be achieved to halt her recent weight gain trend. The physician prescribed Synthroid as supplemental thyroid hormone and referred her to a registered dietitian for MNT to lower LDL cholesterol.

Reduction of Risk Factors Using National Guidelines

Given JM's hypertension and hyperlipidemia, the DASH diet (see Chapter 7) can provide for optimizing serum lipids, as well as managing her blood pressure. However, after review of the problem areas in JM's diet and her stable blood pressure, her first session with the dietitian focused on lowering saturated fat in her diet. From her computerized nutrient analysis she identified cheese, ice cream, candy, and pie as contributors of saturated fat. In addition, crackers and pie were circled as sources of *trans* fatty acids. Given options, she was able to select substitutions lower in saturated fat, including fat-free cheese for sandwiches and cooking, mini carrots or dried fruit for afternoon snacks, and fat-free frozen yogurt in place of ice cream. Eliminating evening desserts would reduce saturated fat and energy intake.

Follow-Up

A follow-up appointment with the physician is scheduled for 6 weeks to reassess thyroid status and serum lipids. An appointment on the same day is scheduled with the dietitian. If her LDL cholesterol goal has not been reached, a focus on inclusion of soluble fiber can reduce the energy density of her diet while providing additional LDL-lowering benefits. Increasing her 2-mile walks to most days of the week is another strategy that can be added to her regimen to support weight control and HDL cholesterol levels.

REFERENCES

1. Expert Panel on Detection, Evaluation, and Treatment of High Blood Cholesterol in Adults. Executive summary of the third report of the national cholesterol education program (NCEP) expert panel on detection, evaluation, and treatment of high blood cholesterol in adults (Adult Treatment Panel III). *JAMA.* 2001;285:2486-2497. Full report: National Institutes of Health. *Third Report of the National Cholesterol Education Program Expert Panel on Detection, Evaluation, and Treatment of High Blood Cholesterol in Adults (Adult Treatment Panel III).* Bethesda, Md: National Institutes of Health; 2001. NIH Publication 01-3670. Available at: http://www.nhlbi.nih.gov/guidelines/cholesterol/atp3_rpt.htm. Accessed March 29, 2004.
2. American Dietetic Association. *Medical Nutrition Therapy Evidence-Based Guides for Practice: Hyperlipidemia—Medical Nutrition Therapy Protocol.* Chicago, Ill: American Dietetic Association; 2004 (in press).
3. US Departments of Agriculture and Health and Human Services. *Nutrition and Your Health: Dietary Guidelines for Americans.* 5th ed. Washington, DC: US Departments of Agriculture and Health and Human Services; 2000. Home and Garden Bulletin No. 232.

4. Krauss RM, Eckel RH, Howard B, Appel LJ, Daniels SR, Deckelbaum RJ, Erdman JW, Kris-Etherton P, Goldberg IJ, Kotchen TA, Lichtenstein AH, Mitch WE, Mullis R, Robinson K, Wylie-Rosett J, St Jeor S, Suttie J, Tribble DL, Bazzarre TL. AHA dietary guidelines. Revision 2000: a statement for healthcare professionals from the nutrition committee of the American Heart Association. *Circulation.* 2000;102:2284-2299.

5. Carnethon MR, Gidding SS, Nehgme R, Sidney S, Jacobs DR Jr, Lui K. Cardiorespiratory fitness in young adulthood and the development of cardiovascular disease risk. *JAMA.* 2003;290:3092-3100.

6. American Diabetes Association. Evidence-based nutrition principles and recommendations for the treatment and prevention of diabetes and related complications. *Diabetes Care.* 2003;26(suppl 1):S51-S61.

7. Hunt SA, Baker DW, Chin MH, Cinquegrani MP, Feldman AM, Francis GS, Ganiats TG, Goldstein S, Gregoratos G, Jessup ML, Noble RJ, Packer M, Silver MA, Stevenson LW. ACC/AHA guidelines for the evaluation and management of chronic heart failure in the adult: executive summary of a report of the American College of Cardiology/American Heart Association Task Force on Practice Guidelines (committee to revise the 1995 guidelines for the evaluation and management of heart failure). *Circulation.* 2001;104:2996-3007.

8. US Preventive Services Task Force. Healthy diet—counseling. Available at: http://www.ahrq.gov/clinic/uspstf/uspsdiet.htm. Accessed April 3, 2004.

9. National Kidney Foundation. K/DOQI clinical practice guidelines for managing dyslipidemias in chronic kidney disease. *Am J Kidney Dis.* 2003;41(suppl 3):S1-S92.

10. Agriculture Research Service. Continuing Survey of Food Intake by Individuals (1994–1996). Available at http://www.barc.usda.gov/bhnrc/foodsurvey/pdf/Csfii3yr.pdf. Accessed December 13, 2003.

11. Allison DB, Egan SK, Barraj LM, Caughman C, Infante M, Heimbach JT. Estimated intakes of *trans* fatty and other fatty acids in the US population. *J Am Diet Assoc.* 1999;99:166-169.

12. Hu FB, Willett WC. Optimal diets for prevention of coronary heart disease. *JAMA.* 2002;288:2569-2578.

13. US Health and Human Services. *Healthy People 2010.* 2nd ed. Washington, DC: US Department of Health and Human Services; 2000.

14. Van Horn L, McDonald A, Peters E, Gernhofer N. Dietary management of cardiovascular disease: a year 2002 perspective. *Nutr Clin Care.* 2001;4:314-331.

15. Yu-Poth S, Zhao G, Etherton T, Naglak M, Jonnalagadda S, Kris-Etherton PM. Effects of the National Cholesterol Education Program's Step I and II dietary intervention programs on cardiovascular disease risk factors: a meta-analysis. *Am J Clin Nutr.* 1999;69:632-646.

16. Grundy SM. Nutrition and diet in the management of hyperlipidemia and atherosclerosis. In: Shils ME, Olson JA, Shike M, Ross AC, eds. *Modern Nutrition in Health and Disease.* 9th ed. Baltimore, Md: Williams & Wilkins; 1999:1199-1216.

17. Lichtenstein AH, Ausman LM, Jalbert SM, Vilella-Bach M, Jauhiainen M, McGladdery S, Erkkila AT, Ehnholm C, Frohlich J, Schaefer EJ. Efficacy of a Therapeutic Lifestyle Change/Step 2 diet in moderately hypercholesterolemic middle-aged and elderly female and male subjects. *J Lipid Res.* 2002;43:264-273.

18. Ginsberg HN, Kris-Etherton P, Dennis B, Elmer PJ, Ershow A, Lefevre M, Pearson T, Roheim P, Ramarkrishnan R, Reed R, Stewart K, Stewart P, Phillips K, Anderson N, for the Delta Research Group. Effects of reducing dietary saturated fatty acids on plasma lipids and lipoproteins in healthy subjects. The Delta Study, Protocol 1. *Arterioscler Thromb Vasc Biol.* 1998;18:441-449.

19. Walden CE, Retzlaff BM, Buck BL, McCann BS, Knopp RH. Lipoprotein lipid response to the National Cholesterol Education Program Step II diet by hypercholesterolemic and combined hyperlipidemic women and men. *Arterioscler Thromb Vasc Biol.* 1997;17:375-382.

20. Denke MA, Role of beef and beef tallow, an enriched source of stearic acid, in a cholesterol-lowering diet. *Am J Clin Nutr.* 1994;60(suppl):1044S-1049S.

21. Kris-Etherton PM, Mustad VA. Chocolate feeding studies: a novel approach for evaluating the plasma lipid effects of stearic acid. *Am J Clin Nutr.* 1994;60(suppl):1029S-1036S.

22. Sacks FM, Katan M. Randomized clinical trials on the effects of dietary fat and carbohydrate on plasma lipoproteins and cardiovascular disease. *Am J Med.* 2002;113(suppl 9B):13S-24S.

23. US Department of Agriculture. National Nutrient Database for Standard Reference. Available at: www.ars.usda.gov/fnic/foodcomp/search/index.html. Accessed March 27, 2004.

24. Mensink RP, Zock PL, Kester ADM, Katan MB. Effects of dietary fatty acids and carbohydrates on the ratio of serum total to HDL cholesterol and on serum lipids and apolipoproteins: a meta-analysis of 60 controlled trials. *Am J Clin Nutr.* 2003;77:1146-1155.

25. Beauchesne-Rondeau E, Gascon A, Bergeron J, Jacqeus H. Plasma lipids and lipoproteins in hypercholesterolemic men fed a lipid-lowering diet containing beef, lean fish or poultry. *Am J Clin Nutr.* 2003;77:587-593.

26. Mauger J-F, Lichenstein AH, Ausman LM, Jalbert SM, Jauhiainen M, Ehnholm C, Lamarche B. Effect of different forms of dietary hydrogenated fats on LDL particle size. *Am J Clin Nutr.* 2003;78:370-375.

27. Harnack L, Lee S, Schakel SF, Duval S, Luepker RV, Arnett DK. Trends in the *trans*-fatty acid composition of the diet in a metropolitan area: The Minnesota Heart Survey. *J Am Diet Assoc.* 2003;103:1160-1166.

28. Elias SL, Innis SM. Bakery foods are the major dietary source of *trans*-fatty acids among pregnant women with diets providing 30 percent energy from fat. *J Am Diet Assoc*. 2002;102:46-51.

29. Judd J, Baer D, Clevidence B, Kris-Etherton P, Muesing R. Dietary *cis* and *trans* monounsaturated and saturated fatty acids. *Lipids*. 2002;37:123-131.

30. Lichtenstein AH, Ausman LM, Jalbert SM, Schaefer EJ. Effects of different forms of dietary hydrogenated fats on serum lipoprotein cholesterol levels. *N Engl J Med*. 1999;340:1933-1940.

31. Lichtenstein AH, Erkkila AT, Lamarche B, Schwab US, Jalbert SM, Ausman LM. Influence of hydrogenated fat and butter on CVD risk factors: remnant like particles, glucose and insulin, blood pressure and C-reactive protein. *Atherosclerosis*. 2003;171:97-107.

32. Denke MA, Adams-Huet B, Nguyen AT. Individual cholesterol variation in response to a margarine- or butter-based diet: a study in families. *JAMA*. 2000;284:2740-2747.

33. Baylin A, Kabagambe EK, Ascherio A, Spiegelman D, Campos H. High 18:2 *trans* fatty acids in adipose tissue are associated with increased risk of nonfatal acute myocardial infarction in Costa Rican adults. *J Nutr*. 2003;133:1186-1191.

34. Oomen CM, Ocke MC, Feskens EJM, van Erp-Baart MAJ, Kok FJ, Kromhout D. Association between *trans* fatty acid intake and 10-year risk of coronary heart disease in the Zutphen Elderly Study: a prospective population-based study. *Lancet*. 2001;357:746-751.

35. Belury M. Not all *trans*-fatty acids are alike: what consumers may lose when we oversimplify nutrition facts. *J Am Diet Assoc*. 2002;102:1606-1607.

36. Bad fats in common foods. *Consumer Reports*. 2003(March). Available at: http://www.consumerreports.org/main/detailv2.jsp?CONTENT%3C%3Ecnt_id=300683&FOLDER%3C%3Efolder_id=162689&bmUID=1062861309750. Accessed September 5, 2003.

37. USHHS Food and Drug Administration. Food labeling: *trans* fatty acids in nutrition labeling, nutrient content claims and health claims. *Fed Regist*. 2003;68:41433-41506.

38. Kris-Etherton PM. Monounsaturated fatty acids and risk of cardiovascular disease. *Circulation*. 1999;100:1253-1258.

39. Grundy SM. Comparison of monounsaturated fatty acids and carbohydrates for lowering plasma cholesterol. *N Engl J Med*. 1986;314:745-748.

40. Mattson FH, Grundy SM. Comparison of effects of dietary saturated, monounsaturated, and polyunsaturated fatty acids on plasma lipids and lipoproteins in man. *J Lipid Res*. 1985;26:115-126.

41. Garg A. High-monounsaturated-fat diets for patients with diabetes mellitus: a meta-analysis. *Am J Clin Nutr*. 1998;67(suppl):577S-582S.

42. Kris-Etherton PM, Pearson TA, Wan Y, Hargrove RL, Moriarty K, Fishell V, Etherton TD. High-monounsaturated fatty acid diets lower both plasma cholesterol and triacylglycerol concentrations. *Am J Clin Nutr*. 1999;70:1009-1015.

43. Gill JMR, Brown JC, Caslake MJ, Wright DM, Cooney J, Bedford D, Hughes DA, Stanely JC, Packard CJ. Effects of dietary monounsaturated fatty acids on lipoprotein concentrations, compositions, and subfraction distributions and on VLDL apolipoprotein B kinetics: dose-dependent effects on LDL. *Am J Clin Nutr*. 2003;78:47-56.

44. Morgan WA, Clayshulte BJ. Pecans lower low-density lipoprotein cholesterol in people with normal lipid levels. *J Am Diet Assoc*. 2000;100:312-318.

45. Lada AT, Rudel LL. Dietary monounsaturated versus polyunsaturated fatty acids: which is really better for protection from coronary heart disease? *Curr Opin Lipidol*. 2003;14:41-46.

46. Grundy SM. What is the desirable ratio of saturated, polyunsaturated, and monounsaturated fatty acids in the diet? *Am J Clin Nutr*. 1997;66(suppl):988S-990S.

47. Weggemans RM, Zock PL, Katan MB. Dietary cholesterol from eggs increases the ratio of total cholesterol to high-density lipoprotein cholesterol in humans: a meta-analysis. *Am J Clin Nutr*. 2001;73:885-891.

48. Knopp RH, Retzlaff RB, Walden CE, Dowdy AA, Tsunehara CH, Austin MA, Nguyen T. A double-blind, randomized, controlled trial of the effects of two eggs per day in moderately hypercholesterolemic and combined hyperlipidemic subjects taught the NCEP Step I Diet. *J Am Coll Nutr*. 1997;16:551-561.

49. Stamler J, Shekelle R. Dietary cholesterol and human coronary heart disease: the epidemiologic evidence. *Arch Pathol Lab Med*. 1988;112:1032-1040.

50. Mann JI, Appleby PN, Key TJA, Thorogood M. Dietary determinants of ischaemic heart disease in health-conscious individuals. *Heart*. 1997;78:450-455.

51. Hu FB, Stampfer JM, Rimm EB, Manson JE, Ascherio A, Colditz GA, Rosner BA, Speigelman D, Speizer FE, Sacks FM, Hennekens CH, Willett WC. A prospective study of egg consumption and risk of cardiovascular disease in men and women. *JAMA*. 1999;281:1387-1394.

52. American Heart Association Web site. Available at: http://www.americanheart.org. Accessed March 23, 2004.

53. Lalonde L, Gray-Donald K, Lowensteyn I, Marchand S, Dorais M, Michaels G, Llewellyn-Thomas HA, O'Connor A, Grover SA, for the Canadian Collaborative Cardiac Assessment Group. Comparing the benefits of diet and exercise in the treatment of dyslipidemia. *Prev Med*. 2002;35:16-24.

54. Blair SN, Jackson AS. Physical fitness and activity as separate heart disease risk factors: a meta-analysis. *Med Sci Sports Exerc*. 2001;33:762-764.

55. Leon AS, Rice T, Mandel S, Despres JP, Bergeron J, Gagnon J, Rao DC, Skinner JS, Wilmore JH, Bouchard

C. Blood lipid response to 20 weeks of supervised exercise in a large biracial population: the HERITAGE Family Study. *Metabolism.* 2000;49:513-520.

56. Thompson PD, Buchner D, Pina IL, Balady GJ, Wiliams MA, Marcus BH, Berra K, Blair SN, Costa F, Franklin B, Fletcher GF, Gordon NF, Pate RR, Rodriguez B, Yancey AK, Wenger NK. Exercise and physical activity in the prevention and treatment of atherosclerotic cardiovascular disease: a statement from the Council on Clinical Cardiology (Subcommittee on Exercise, Rehabilitation, and Prevention) and the Council on Nutrition, Physical Activity, and Metabolism (Subcommittee on Physical Activity). *Circulation.* 2003;107:3109-3116.

57. Institute of Medicine. *Dietary Reference Intakes: Energy, Carbohydrate, Fiber, Fat, Fatty Acids, Cholesterol, Protein, and Amino Acids.* Washington, DC: National Academies Press; 2002.

58. US Department of Agriculture. *Report of the Dietary Guidelines Advisory Committee on the Dietary Guidelines for Americans to the Secretary of Agriculture and the Secretary of Health and Human Services.* Washington, DC: US Department of Agriculture; 1980, 1985, 1990, 1995.

59. Garg A, Bantle JP, Henry RR, Coulston AM, Griver KA, Raatz SK, Brinkley L, Chen YD, Grundy SM, Huet BA. Effects of varying carbohydrate content of diet in patients with non-insulin dependent diabetes mellitus. *JAMA.* 1994;271:1421-1428.

60. Ginsberg HN. New perspectives on atherogenesis. Role of abnormal triglyceride-rich lipoprotein metabolism. *Circulation.* 2002;106:2137-2142.

61. Gardner CD, Fortmann SP, Krauss RM. Association of small, dense lipoprotein particles with incidence of coronary artery disease in men and women. *JAMA.* 1996;276:875-881.

62. Lamarche B, St-Perre AC, Ruel IL, Cantin B, Dagenais GR, Despres JP. A prospective, population-based study of low-density lipoprotein particle size as a risk factor for ischemic heart disease in men. *Can J Cardiol.* 2001;17:859-865.

63. St-Pierre AC, Ruel IL, Cantin B, Dagenais GR, Bernard PM, Despres JP, Larmarche B. Comparison of various electrophoretic characteristics of LDL particles and their relationship to the risk of ischemic heart disease. *Circulation.* 2001;104:2295-2299.

64. Koba S, Hirano T, Kondo T, Shibata M, Suzuki H, Murakami M, Geshi E, Katagiri T. Significance of small dense low-density lipoproteins and other risk factors in patients with various types of coronary heart disease. *Am Heart J.* 2002;144:1026-2035.

65. The Expert Committee on the Diagnosis and Classification of Diabetes Mellitus. Follow-up report on the diagnosis of diabetes mellitus. *Diabetes Care.* 2003;26:3160-3176.

66. Lopes-Virella MF, Virella G. Modified lipoproteins, cytokines and macrovascular disease in non-insulin dependent diabetes mellitus. *Ann Med.* 1996;28:347-354.

67. Anderson J. Dietary fiber prevents carbohydrate-induced hypertriglyceridemia. *Curr Athero Rep.* 2000;2:536-541.

68. Obarzanek E, Sacks F, Vollmer W, Bray G, Miller E, Lin PH, Karanja N, Most-Windhauser M, Moore T, Swain J, Bales C, Proschan M, for the DASH Research Group. Effects on blood lipids of a blood pressure-lowering diet: the Dietary Approaches to Stop Hypertension (DASH) Trial. *Am J Clin Nutr.* 2001;74:80-89.

69. Chandalia M, Garg A, Lutjohann D, von Bergmann K, Grundy SM, Brinkley LJ. Beneficial effects of high dietary fiber intake in patients with type 2 diabetes mellitus. *N Engl J Med.* 2000;342:1392-1398.

70. Asztalos B, Lefevre M, Wong L, Foster TA, Tulley R, Windhauser M, Zhang W, Roheim PS. Differential response to low-fat diet between low and normal HDL-cholesterol subjects. *J Lipid Res.* 2000;41:321-328.

71. Austin MA, Rodriguez BL, McKnight B, McNeely MJ, Edwards KL, Curb JD, Sharp DS. Low-density lipoprotein particle size, triglycerides, and high-density lipoprotein cholesterol as risk factors for coronary heart disease in older Japanese-American men. *Am J Cardiol.* 2000;86:412-416.

72. Krauss RM, Dreon DM. Low-density-lipoprotein subclasses and response to a low-fat diet in healthy men. *Am J Clin Nutr.* 1995;62(suppl):478S-487S.

73. Williams PT, Krauss RM, Vranian KM, Wood PD. Changes in lipoprotein subfractions during diet-induced and exercise-induced weight loss in moderately overweight men. *Circulation.* 1990;81:1293-1304.

74. Hoefner DM, Hodel SD, O'Brien JF, Branum EL, Sun D, Meissner I, McConnell JP. Development of a rapid, quantitative method for LDL subfractionation with use of the Quantimetrix Lipoprint LDL System. *Clin Chem.* 2001;47:266-274.

75. Sacks FM, Campos H. Low-density lipoprotein size and cardiovascular disease: a reappraisal. *J Clin Endocrinol Metab.* 2003;88:4525-4532.

76. Knopp RH, Retzlaff B, Walden C, Fish B, Buck B, McCann B. One-year effects of increasingly fat-restricted, carbohydrate-enriched diets on lipoprotein levels in free-living subjects. *Proc Soc Exp Biol Med.* 2000;225:191-199.

77. National Institutes of Health/National Heart, Lung, and Blood Institute/Obesity Education Initiative Expert Panel. *Clinical Guidelines on the Identification, Evaluation, and Treatment of Overweight and Obesity in Adults.* The Evidence Report. NIH; 1998. Available at: http://www.nhlbi.nih.gov/about/oei/index.htm. Accessed December 10, 2003.

78. Klem ML, Wing RR, McGuire MT, Seagle HM, Hill JO. A descriptive study of individuals successful at long-term maintenance of substantial weight loss. *Am J Clin Nutr.* 1997;66:239-246.

79. McManus K, Antinoro L, Sacks F. A randomized controlled trial of a moderate-fat, low-energy diet compared with a low-fat, low-energy diet for weight loss in overweight adults. *Int J Obes.* 2001;25:1503-1511.

80. Wien MA, Sabate JM, Idle DN, Cole SE, Kandeel FR. Almonds vs complex carbohydrates in a weight reduction program. *Int J Obes Relat Metab Disord.* 2003;27:1365-1372.

81. McGuire MT, Wing RR, Klem ML, Hill JO. Behavioral strategies of individuals who have maintained long-term weight losses. *Obes Res.* 1999;7:334-341.

82. Reaven GM. Pathophysiology of insulin resistance in human disease. *Physiol Rev.* 1995;75:473-486.

83. Gerich JE. Is reduced first-phase insulin release the earliest detectable abnormality in individuals destined to develop type 2 diabetes? *Diabetes.* 2002;51(suppl 1):S117-S121.

84. Rosenthal MB, Barnard RJ, Rose DP, Inkeles S, Hall J, Pritikin N. Effects of a high-complex-carbohydrate, low-fat, low-cholesterol diet on serum levels of serum lipids and estradiol. *Am J Med.* 1985;78:23-27.

85. Weber F, Barnard RJ, Roy D. Effects of a high-complex-carbohydrate, low-fat diet and daily exercise on individuals 70 years of age and older. *J Gerontol.* 1983;38:155-161.

86. Ornish D, Scherwitz LW, Billings JH, Brown SE, Gould KL, Merritt TA, Sparler S, Armstrong WT, Ports TA, Kirkeeide RL, Hogeboom C, Brand RJ. Intensive lifestyle changes for reversal of coronary heart disease. *JAMA.* 1998;280:2001-2007.

87. Ness AR, Powles JW. Fruits and vegetables and cardiovascular disease: a review. *Int J Epidemiol.* 1997;26:1-13.

88. Bazzano LA, He J, Ogden LG, Loria CM, Vupputuri S, Myers L, Whelton PK. Fruit and vegetable intake and risk of cardiovascular disease in US adults: the first National Health and Nutrition Examination Survey Epidemiologic Follow-up Study. *Am J Clin Nutr.* 2002;76:93-99.

89. Johnsen SP, Overvad K, Stripp C, Tjonneland A, Husted SE, Sorensen HT. Intake of fruit and vegetables and the risk of ischemic stroke in a cohort of Danish men and women. *Am J Clin Nutr.* 2003;78:57-64.

90. Freese R, Alfthan G, Jauhiainen M, Basu S, Erlund I, Salminen I, Aro A, Mutanen M. High intakes of vegetables, berries, and apples combined with a high intake of linoleic or oleic acid only slightly affect markers of lipid peroxidation and lipoprotein metabolism in healthy subjects. *Am J Clin Nutr.* 2002;76:950-960.

91. Jacques PF, Bostom AG, Williams RR, Ellison RC, Eckfeldt JH, Rosenberg IH, Selhub J, Rozen R. Relation between folate status, a common mutation in methylenetetrahydrofolate reductase, and plasma homocysteine concentrations. *Circulation.* 1996;93:7-9.

92. Jacques PF, Selhub J, Bostom AG, Wilson PWF, Rosenberg IH. The effect of folic acid fortification on plasma folate and total homocysteine concentrations. *N Engl J Med.* 1999; 340:1449-1454.

93. Esfahani ST, Cogger EA, Caudill MA. Heterogeneity in the prevalence of MTHFR gene polymorphisms in women of different ethnic groups. *J Am Diet Assoc.* 2003;103:200-207.

94. Bazzano LA, He J, Ogden LG, Loria CM, Vupputuri S, Myers L, Whelton PK. Dietary intake of folate and risk of stroke in US men and women: NHANES I Epidemiologic Follow-up Study. National Health and Nutrition Examination Survey. *Stroke.* 2002;33:1188-1189.

95. Vermeulen EG, Stehouwer CD, Valk J, Van Der Knaap M, Van Den Berg M, Twisk JW, Prevoo W, Rauwerda JA. Effect of homocysteine-lowering treatment with folic acid plus vitamin B6 on progression of subclinical atherosclerosis: a randomized, placebo-controlled trial. *Lancet.* 2000;355:517-522.

96. Schnyder G, Roffi M, Pin R, Flammer Y, Lange H, Eberli FR, Meier B, Turi ZG, Hess OM. Decreased rate of coronary restenosis after lowering of plasma homocysteine levels. *New Engl J Med.* 2001;345:1593-1600.

97. Liem A, Reynierse-Buitenwerf GH, Zwinderman AH, Jukeme JW, van Veldhuisen DJ. Secondary prevention with folic acid: effects on clinical outcomes. *J Am Coll Cardiol.* 2003;41:2105-2113.

98. Van Oort FV, Melse-Boonstra A, Brouwer IA, Clarke R, West CE, Katan MB, Verhoef P. Folic acid and reduction in plasma homocysteine concentrations in older adults: a dose-response study. *Am J Clin Nutr.* 2003;77:1318-1323.

99. Jenkins DJ, Kendall CW, Axelsen M, Augustin LS, Vuksan V. Viscous and nonviscous fibres, nonabsorbable and low glycaemic index carbohydrates, blood lipids and coronary heart disease. *Curr Opin Lipidol.* 2000;11:49-56.

100. de Lorgeril M, Salen P, Martin JL, Monjaud I, Delaye J, Mamelle N. Mediterranean diet, traditional risk factors, and the rate of cardiovascular complications after myocardial infarction: final report of the Lyon Diet Heart Study. *Circulation.* 1999;99:779-785.

101. Singh RB, Dubnov G, Niaz MA, Ghosh S, Singh R, Rastogi SS, Manor O, Pella D, Berry EM. Effect of an Indo-Mediterranean diet on progression of coronary artery disease in high-risk patients (Indo-Mediterranean Diet Heart Study): a randomized single-blind trial. *Lancet.* 2002;260:1455-1461.

102. Van Dam RM, Giervink L, Ocke MC, Feskens EJ. Patterns of food consumption and risk factors for cardiovascular disease in the general Dutch population. *Am J Clin Nutr.* 2003;77:1156-1163.

103. Fung TT, Rimm EB, Spiegelman D, Rifai N, Tofler GH, Willett WC, Hu FB. Association between dietary patterns and plasma biomarkers of obesity and cardiovascular disease risk. *Am J Clin Nutr.* 2001;73:61-67.

104. Jenkins DJ, Kendall CW, Marchie A, Faulkner DA, Wong JM, de Souza R, Emam A, Parker TL, Vidgen E, Lapsley KG, Taurtwein EA, Josse RG, Leiter LA, Connelly PW. Effects of a dietary portfolio of cholesterol-lowering foods vs lovastatin on serum lipids and C-reactive protein. *JAMA.* 2003;290:502-510.

105. Kris-Etherton PM, Etherton TD, Carlson J, Gardner C. Recent discoveries in inclusive food-based approaches and dietary patterns for reduction in risk for cardiovascular disease. *Curr Opin Lipidol.* 2002;13:397-407.

106. Capps O, Cleveland L, Park J. Dietary behaviors associated with total fat and saturated fat intake. *J Am Diet Assoc.* 2002;102:490-496,501-502.

107. Sikand G, Kashyap ML, Yang I. Medical nutrition therapy lowers serum cholesterol and saves medication costs in men with hypercholesterolemia. *J Am Diet Assoc.* 1998;98:889-894.

108. Sikand G, Kashyap ML, Wong ND, Hsu JC. Dietitian intervention improves lipid values and saves medication costs in men with combined hyperlipidemia and a history of niacin noncompliance. *J Am Diet Assoc.* 2000;200:218-224.

109. Dalgard C, Thuroe A, Haastrup B, Haghfelt T, Stender S. Saturated fat intake is reduced in patients with ischemic heart disease 1 year after comprehensive counseling but not after brief counseling. *J Am Diet Assoc.* 2001;101:1420-1424,1429.

110. Thompson RL, Summerbell CD, Hooper L, Higgins JPT, Little PS, Talbot D, Ebrahim S. Dietary advice given by a dietitian versus other health professional or self-help resources to reduce blood cholesterol. *Cochrane Database Syst Rev.* 2003;3.

111. Dolecek TA, Stamler J, Caggiula A, Tillotson JL, Buzzard IM. Methods of dietary and nutritional assessment and intervention and other methods in the Multiple Risk Factor Intervention Trial. *Am J Clin Nutr.* 1997;65(suppl):196S-210S.

112. Lanza E, Schatzkin LE, Daston C, Corle D, Freedman L, Ballard-Barbash R, Caan B, Lance P, Marshall J, Iber F, Shike M, Weissfeld J, Slattery M, Paskett E, Matreski D, Albert P. Implementation of a 4-y, high-fiber, high-fruit-and-vegetable, low-fat dietary intervention: results of dietary changes in the Polyp Prevention Trial. *Am J Clin Nutr.* 2001;74:387-401.

113. American Diabetes Association. Virtual grocery store. Available at: http://vgs.diabetes.org/grocery_tour.jsp. Accessed April 13, 2004.

114. American Heart Association. Delicious decisions. Available at: http://www.deliciousdecisions.org. Accessed December 14, 2003.

115. Bell Institute. Healthy destinations. Available at: http://www.bellinstitute.com/hearthealth/index.asp. Accessed on January 12, 2004.

116. Cohn S. Want to watch calories when dining out? Available at: http://www.restaurant.org/dineout/nutrition.cfm. Accessed April 13, 2004.

117. Centers for Disease Control and Prevention Web site. Available at: http://www.cdc.gov. Accessed November 14, 2003.

118. US Food and Drug Administration. Guidance on how to understand and use the nutrition facts panel on food labels. Available at: http://www.cfsan.fda.gov/~dms/foodlab.html. Accessed April 13, 2004.

119. National Heart, Lung and Blood Institute. Stay young at heart—cooking the heart healthy way. Available at: http://www.nhlbi.nih.gov/health/public/heart/other/syah/index.htm. Accessed April 13, 2004.

120. National Heart, Lung and Blood Institute. *Heart-healthy cooking at home: African-American style.* Available at: http://www.nhlbi.nih.gov/health/public/heart/other/chdblack/cooking.pdf. Accessed November 14, 2003.

121. National Heart, Lung and Blood Institute. *Platillos Latinos—sabrosos y saludables: delicious heart-healthy Latino recipes.* Available at: http://www.nhlbi.nih.gov/health/public/heart/other/sp_recip.pdf. Accessed November 14, 2003.

122. Weight-control Information Network. Weight loss and control. Available at: http://www.niddk.nih.gov/health/nutrit/nutrit.htm. Accessed November 14, 2003.

123. National Institutes of Health. National Cholesterol Education Program. *Report of the Expert Panel on Blood Cholesterol Levels in Children and Adolescents.* Bethesda, Md: National Institutes of Health; 1992. NIH publication 2732.

124. US Food and Drug Administration. Qualified health claims. Available at: http://www.cfsan.fda.gov/~dms/lab-qhc.html. Accessed April 13, 2004.

125. US Food and Drug Administration. Food labeling guide. Available at: http://www.cfsan.fda.gov/~dms/flg-toc.html. Accessed April 13, 2004.

126. McDonald L. Supermarket savvy. Available at: http://www.supermarketsavvy.com. Accessed April 13, 2004.

127. Gleason JA, Bourdet KL, Koehn K, Holay S, Schaefer EJ. Cardiovascular risk reduction and dietary compliance with a home-delivered diet and lifestyle modification program. *J Am Diet Assoc.* 2002;102:1445-1451.

128. Frame CJ, Green CG, Herr DG, Taylor ML. A 2-year stage of change evaluation of dietary fat and fruit and vegetable intake behaviors of cardiac rehabilitation patients. *Am J Health Promot.* 2003;17:361-368.

129. Cavallaro V, Dwyer J, House RF, Shores K, Canez I, Hong A, Altman K, Helmic E, Murphy JN. Influence of dietitian presence on outpatient cardiac rehabilitation nutrition services. *J Am Diet Assoc.* 2004;104:611-614.

130. Timlin MT, Shores KV, Reicks M. Behavior change outcomes in an outpatient cardiac rehabilitation program. *J Am Diet Assoc.* 2002;102:664-671.

131. McBride PM, Schrott HC, Plane MB, Underbakke G, Brownh RL. Primary care practice adherence to National Cholesterol Education Program Guidelines for patients with coronary heart disease. *Arch Intern Med.* 1998;185:1238-1244.

132. Winstead B. Missed opportunities in preventive counseling for cardiovascular disease—United States, 1995. *MMWR Morb Mortal Wkly Rep.* 1998;47:91-95.

133. Evans AT, Rogers LQ, Peden JG, Seelig CB, Lane RD, Levine MA, Levin ML, Grossman RS, Darden PM, Jackson SM, Ammerman AS, Settle MB, Stritter FT, Fletcher SW, for the CADRE Study Group. Teaching dietary counseling skills to residents: patient and physician outcomes. *Am J Prev Med*. 1996;12:259-265.

134. American Dietetic Association. *Medical Nutrition Therapy Evidence-Based Guides for Practice: Chronic Kidney Disease—Medical Nutrition Therapy Protocol*. Chicago, Ill: American Dietetic Association; 2002.

135. Vergili-Nelson JM. Benefits of fish oil supplementation for hemodialysis patients. *J Am Diet Assoc*. 2003;103:1174-1177.

136. Kuehneman T, Saulsbury D, Splett P, Chapman DB. Demonstrating the impact of nutrition intervention in a heart failure program. *J Am Diet Assoc*. 2002;102:1790-1794.

137. Neily JB, Toto KH, Gardner EB, Rame JE, Yancy CW, Sheffield MA, Dries DL, Drazner MH. Potential contributing factors to noncompliance with dietary sodium restriction in patients with heart failure. *Am Heart J*. 2002;143:29-33.

138. Pina IL, Apstein CS, Balady GJ, Belardinelli R, Chaitman BR, Duscha BD, Fletcher BJ, Fleg JL, Myhers JN, Sullivan MJ. Exercise and heart failure: ADA scientific statement. *Circulation*. 2003;107:1210-1225.

CHAPTER 7

METABOLIC SYNDROME: TIME FOR ACTION

Lisa A. Hark, PhD, RD, Rex Parker, BS, Darwin D. Deen, MD, MS, and
F. Xavier Pi-Sunyer, MD, MPH; case study by Frances M. Burke, MS, RD

"To lengthen thy life, lessen thy meals"
Benjamin Franklin

INTRODUCTION

Metabolic syndrome (MES) has been given a variety of names: syndrome X, insulin resistance syndrome, the deadly quartet, and the multiple metabolic syndrome. It consists of a cluster of risk factors responsible for much of the cardiovascular disease (CVD) morbidity among overweight and obese patients and those with type 2 diabetes mellitus (1). The National Cholesterol Education Program (NCEP) Adult Treatment Panel III report (ATP III) (2) has identified MES as an independent risk factor for CVD and considers it an indication for intensive lifestyle modification. This conclusion is based on a review of numerous nonintervention trials.

DEFINITION OF MES

Although definitions have varied, the major characteristics of MES include insulin resistance (IR), abdominal obesity, elevated blood pressure, and lipid abnormalities: elevated triglycerides and low high-density lipoprotein (HDL) cholesterol levels. Table 7.1 compares the definitions of MES from ATP III (2) and the World Health Organization (3). MES is also associated with a proinflammatory, prothrombotic state that may include elevated C-reactive protein, endothelial dysfunction, increased platelet aggregation, elevated uric acid levels, microalbuminuria, and a shift toward small dense low-density lipoprotein (LDL) particles (4). IR has been implicated in the polycystic ovarian syndrome and nonalcoholic steatohepatitis (NASH).

TABLE 7.1
ATP III and WHO Diagnostic Criteria for Metabolic Syndrome

Component	WHO Diagnostic Criteria (High fasting glucose criteria plus two of the following)	ATP III Diagnostic Criteria (Three of the following)
Abdominal-central obesity	Waist-to-hip ratio >0.90 in men Waist-to-hip ratio >0.85 in women *or* BMI >30	Waist circumference >102 cm (40 in) in men Waist circumference >88 cm (35 in) in women
Hypertriglyceridemia	TG ≥ 150 mg/dL (>1.695 mmol/L)	TG ≥ 150 mg/dL (≥1.695 mmol/L)
Low HDL cholesterol	HDL <35 mg/dL (<0.9 mmol/L) in men HDL <39 mg/dL (<1.0 mmol/L) in women	HDL <40 mg/dL (<1.036 mmol/L) in men HDL <50 mg/dL (<1.295 mmol/L) in women
High blood pressure	BP ≥ 160/90 mm Hg or documented use of antihypertensive therapy	BP ≥ 130/85 mm Hg or documented use of antihypertensive therapy
High fasting glucose	Impaired glucose tolerance, impaired fasting glucose, insulin resistance, or diabetes	Glucose ≥ 100 mg/dL (≥6.1 mmol/L)
Microalbuminuria	Urinary albumin-to-creatinine ratio = 20 mg/g *or* Albumin excretion rate = 20 µg/min	

Abbreviations: ATP III, Adult Treatment Panel III; BMI, body mass index; BP, blood pressure; HDL, high-density lipo-protein; TG, triglycerides; WHO, World Health Organization.
Source: Data are from references 2 and 3.

BACKGROUND AND SIGNIFICANCE

Differences in body fat distribution (gynecoid vs android) associated with an altered metabolic profile were reported in the medical literature as early as 50 years ago (5,6). In 1988 Reaven named this altered metabolic profile "syndrome X" (7). Each component of the syndrome has been associated with increased CVD risk (8). In patients with diabetes mellitus, MES predicts proteinuria, CVD, and other complications (9). Nevertheless, some clinicians have been slow to recognize the importance of aggressive intervention for patients with MES.

EPIDEMIOLOGY AND PREVALENCE

The prevalence of MES varies by definition used and population studied (10). Recent calcu-lations, based on data from the Third National Health and Nutrition Examination Survey, estimate that 22% to 24% of the adult US population has MES (11). Among comparable age groups, prevalence of MES in the United States is highest in Mexican Americans and lowest in blacks (12). (Refer to Figure 7.1.) The prevalence of MES increases with age and with increasing body weight. Given the aging American population and the current epidemic of overweight and obesity, MES is likely to soon overtake cigarette smoking as the primary con-tributor to risk of CVD (13).

ETIOLOGY

Although the etiology of MES has not been definitively established, two theories have been proposed. Abdominal obesity, independent of body mass index (BMI), plays a role in both

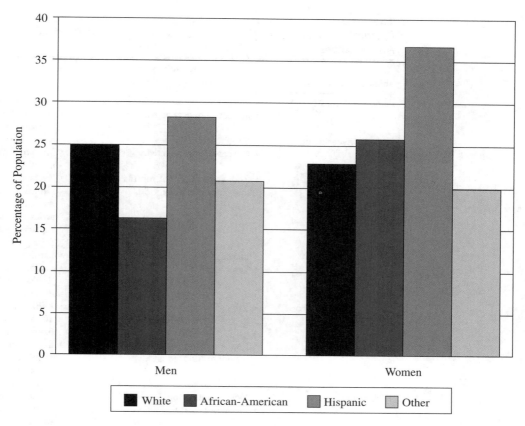

FIGURE 7.1

Prevalence of metabolic syndrome among US adults. Data are from reference 11.

theories. One hypothesis assumes that the primary lesion is IR, which correlates with abdominal fat measured by waist circumference or waist-to-hip ratio. Supporting this theory, data from the Nurses' Health Study showed a threefold increased risk of CVD in women with a waist circumference above 38 inches (after adjusting for age and other known risk factors) (14). The link between IR and CVD is probably mediated by oxidative stress, which produces endothelial cell dysfunction, promoting vascular damage and atheroma formation (15). A second hypothesis places importance on hormonal changes, principally elevated serum cortisol levels (caused by chronic stress) (16).

Regardless of which theory proves to be correct (if either), skeletal muscle has been shown to play an important role in determining IR. Despres (17) demonstrated that the accumulation of visceral adipose tissue is associated with increased hepatic lipase and decreased muscle lipoprotein lipase (LPL). These changes in the proportion of lipase in liver and muscle may explain the accumulation of fat in the liver because less fat is burned in the muscle. This mechanism provides a clue to possible effective therapies for IR and MES.

CLINICAL EVALUATION

A routine medical and family history helps to identify patients at risk for MES. Questions in the review of systems about recent or past weight changes and efforts to gain or lose weight

TABLE 7.2

Practical Advice for Lifestyle Interventions to Target Specific Metabolic Syndrome Abnormalities

Abnormality	Diet and Physical Activity Interventions	Practical Advice
Abdominal obesity	• Weight reduction • Increase physical activity	• Reduce portion sizes to cut calories • 30 min of moderate intensity exercise daily
Hypertriglyceridemia	• Weight reduction • Increase physical activity	• Reduce portion sizes to cut calories • 30 min of moderate intensity exercise daily
	• Reduce total carbohydrates; increase low-glycemic index foods	• Replace refined carbohydrates (white bread, potatoes, pasta) with monounsaturated fats (nuts, avocado, canola oil, or olive oil); replace soda and juices with water, seltzer, and diet beverages
	• Increase n-3 fatty acids • Limit alcohol	• Eat fish at least once a week • Limit alcohol to no more than two drinks per day for men and one drink per day for women
Low HDL cholesterol	• Weight reduction • Increase physical activity	• Reduce portion sizes to cut calories • 30 min of moderate intensity exercise daily
	• Replace carbohydrates with monounsaturated fat	• Eat fish, nuts, avocado; use olive or canola oils in salad dressing and for cooking
	• Quit smoking	• Join a smoking cessation program
High blood pressure	• Weight reduction • Increase physical activity	• Reduce portion sizes to cut calories • 30 min of moderate intensity exercise daily
	• Reduce sodium intake	• Reduce salt intake to no more than 2.4 g/d or 6 g/d NaCl by using more herbs in cooking; read labels for sodium content; skip the salt shaker
	• Reduce saturated fat intake; increase fruits and vegetables • Increase low-fat dairy products	• Consume at least five servings of fruits and vegetables every day • Drink or eat three servings of low-fat dairy daily
	• Moderate alcohol consumption	• Limit alcohol to no more than two drinks per day for men and one drink per day for women
High fasting glucose	• Weight reduction • Increase physical activity	• Reduce portion sizes to cut calories • 30 min of moderate intensity exercise daily
	• Reduce total carbohydrates; replace carbohydrates with monounsaturated fat; increase low-glycemic index foods	• Replace refined grains with whole grains, such as oatmeal, brown rice, corn, and whole wheat and monounsaturated fats (nuts, avocado, canola oil, or olive oil)
	• Increase dietary fiber (>30 g/d)	• Add legumes for soluble fiber

Source: Developed by Darwin Deen, MD, Albert Einstein College of Medicine, and Lisa Hark, PhD, RD, University of Pennsylvania School of Medicine. 2004. Used by permission of the authors.

may provide important information. A diet and physical activity history, including both occupational and leisure-time physical activity, should be part of the routine patient evaluation (18,19). Have patients estimate how many hours a day they are sedentary (watching TV or sitting at a desk). Questions about typical food intake and efforts to reduce dietary fat or other specific dietary changes help to provide a clue to patients' awareness of CVD risk and help to estimate their readiness to change lifestyle habits (see Table 7.2).

PHYSICAL EXAMINATION

Height and weight, as well as blood pressure and waist circumference, should be measured as part of the physical examination. Waist circumference is measured just above the iliac crest. (See Chapter 4 for specific measurement instructions for waist circumference.) Waist circumference appears to be a better predictor of CVD risk than waist-to-hip ratio (20). BMI, defined as weight (kg) divided by height squared (m²), should be assessed to classify patients as underweight, normal weight, overweight, or obese (see Table 4.3 in Chapter 4).

LABORATORY EVALUATION

Clinicians should obtain a fasting glucose level and a fasting lipid profile on patients suspected of having MES. Fasting insulin levels or glucose levels after a glucose challenge can be measured to establish a diagnosis of IR. However, these levels are not as accurate as a euglycemic clamp, which is used in research studies but is impractical in the clinical setting. Fasting blood glucose or fasting insulin levels are both good indicators of IR, but measuring insulin levels is probably not necessary in most situations. It is not necessary to measure apolipoprotein B levels if LDL is normal because low HDL cholesterol and high triglyceride (TG) levels are predictive of small dense LDL particles, which raise apo B levels. Although there is no consensus on how to treat elevated C-reactive protein (CRP) levels, the American Heart Association (AHA) recommends measuring CRP in high-risk patients (21). Baseline uric acid levels and routine liver function tests, such as alanine aminotransferase (ALT), aspartate aminotransferase (AST), and gamma-glutamyltranspeptidase (γ GTP) levels, screen for NASH, but fatty liver can be present even in the absence of elevated liver function tests.

A word of caution in interpreting the results of laboratory studies: the lack of any individual component of the syndrome does not mean a patient is free of risk. Many patients who do not meet the full criteria of MES have an increased risk of CVD from the components of the syndrome they do have.

TREATMENT STRATEGIES

To date, no randomized controlled trials aimed specifically at treating MES have been published. By aggressively managing the individual components of the syndrome, the goal is to prevent or delay the onset of diabetes, hypertension, and CVD. All patients diagnosed with MES should be encouraged to attempt to change their diet and exercise habits as primary therapy (2). Weight loss improves all aspects of MES and reduces all-cause morbidity and CVD mortality (22). Goals for treatment of each facet of MES are summarized in Table 7.3. Although many patients find weight loss difficult to achieve, dietary changes can lower blood pressure and improve lipid levels. Increasing exercise can improve insulin sensitivity even in the absence of weight loss (23).

Exercise and Physical Activity

As an insulin-sensitive tissue, skeletal muscle is a primary target for affecting IR. Physical training has been shown to reduce skeletal muscle lipid levels and IR for individuals across the BMI range (24). Exercise training increases the muscle's ability to take up and oxidize free fatty acids and increases muscle LPL activity. Exercise has been shown to lower systolic blood

TABLE 7.3

Adult Treatment Panel III Guidelines for Treatment of Metabolic Syndrome

Targeted Area	Goal
Treat LDL Cholesterol First	
CHD and CHD risk equivalent (10-y risk for CHD >20%)	<100 mg/dL
Multiple (≥2) risk factors and 10-y risk ≤20%	<130 mg/dL
Institute weight control	Decrease by 10% from baseline
Institute physical activity	30 to 40 min/d for 3 to 5 d/wk
Monitor treatment of hypertension	<130/85 mm Hg
Treat Elevated Triglycerides and Low HDL Cholesterol	
Goal of non-HDL cholesterol for patients with triglyceride ≥ 200 mg/dL and ≤ 499 mg/dL	High CHD risk: <130 mg/dL Intermediate CHD risk: <160 mg/dL Low CHD risk: <190 mg/dL

Abbreviations: CHD, coronary heart disease; HDL, high-density lipoprotein; LDL, low-density lipoprotein.

Source: Data are from reference 1.

pressure by an average of 4 to 9 mm Hg in patients with elevated blood pressure. Regular exercise reverses the age-related decline in insulin sensitivity independent of weight loss or increases in maximum oxygen consumption (VO_{2max}) (23). The impact of exercise on insulin sensitivity is evident for 24 to 48 hours and disappears within 3 to 5 days. Thus, regular physical activity should be a part of any effort to reverse the effects of IR (25).

Exercise alone has not been shown to reduce body weight; thus, the importance of exercise for weight loss is unclear (26). Exercise, however, is the best predictor of weight-loss maintenance (27) and has been shown to improve hemoglobin A1c in patients who have not lost weight. In a meta-analysis of studies published on the impact of exercise in patients with type 2 diabetes, Boule and colleagues concluded that exercise should be considered a desirable end point and not just a means to achieve weight loss (26).

Exercise Prescription

The Institute of Medicine's *Dietary Reference Intakes for Energy, Carbohydrates, Fiber, Fat, Protein, and Amino Acids (Macronutrients)* (2002) recommends 1 hour of physical activity daily for health maintenance (28). This recommendation has been made to prevent continued weight gain in the population. The greatest health benefits from an increase in physical activity occur when sedentary individuals incorporate moderate-intensity exercise as part of their lifestyle. Despres (17) has coined the term "metabolic fitness" to distinguish the level of exercise needed to prevent cardiovascular risk from the more commonly accepted cardiorespiratory fitness defined by VO_{2max}.

Low-intensity exercise can have a significant impact on cardiorespiratory fitness. It is easier to get patients to comply with less-intensive and less-frequent exercise regimens. Compliance (and efficacy) decline as frequency increases (29). This finding highlights the importance of encouraging patients to find their own comfort level for physical activity rather than assigning them a specific task. The goal is to help patients find a level of activity that they can accomplish over the long term (30,31). A combination of resistance and aerobic exercise is advised, but any activity is better than none, and patients who have been sedentary need to start slowly and increase duration and intensity gradually (31). Patients should be encouraged to do some type of aerobic and resistance exercise on alternating days. Low-weight dumbbells, stretchy bands, or even 16-ounce food cans provide the needed resistance.

Circuit-type resistance training machines, if available, maximize the impact of muscle strengthening. The ultimate goal may be 1 hour of daily physical activity (walking or any combination of lifestyle activities), but in working up to that goal, patients should start with 1 to 2 days per week for 5 to 10 minutes at 50% of maximal heart rate and increase gradually.

Medical Nutrition Therapy

Medical nutrition therapy (MNT) for patients with MES should focus on the patients' specific metabolic alterations. The most important aspect of any dietary change is to limit energy intake enough to produce an energy deficit as an attempt to reduce weight. As previously stated, all aspects of MES improve with modest weight reduction (32). However, remind patients that their efforts to alter their lifestyle may be rewarded with improved health and reduced CVD risk even in the absence of weight loss.

Macronutrients

The first step in developing a diet prescription is the evaluation of the patient's current diet. This is most easily done during the course of the history with a few pertinent questions. The primary emphasis of the diet for MES should focus on reducing CVD risk. If the patient has elevated LDL cholesterol, recommend a low-fat, moderate-carbohydrate diet (total fat 25% to 35% of energy, saturated fat less than 7%, with carbohydrate as 45% to 60% of energy). Both epidemiologic data and clinical trial results have shown this diet to be effective in reducing LDL cholesterol and lowering CVD risk (33,34).

Although the NCEP recommends that carbohydrates comprise the major source of energy (50% to 60% of total energy), patients need to be aware of both the quantity and quality of their carbohydrate intake because excessive consumption of carbohydrates may increase TG levels while depressing HDL cholesterol levels (35). (See Chapter 6 for further discussion of the impact on serum lipids of the fat-to-carbohydrate ratio in the diet.)

According to the AHA and ATP III, the intake of added sugars should be minimized, while the intake of whole grains that are higher in fiber should be increased (2,36). The glycemic index (GI) categorizes or ranks carbohydrate-containing foods according to the extent to which they raise blood glucose levels after eating. Initial studies analyzed the blood glucose response using 50 g of pure glucose compared with 50 g of a carbohydrate-containing food. However, the standard to which carbohydrate foods are now compared has been changed to white bread (37). Diets tailored to lower the GI have been shown in small studies to reduce TG levels and raise HDL cholesterol levels (38). A recent observational study further supports a high-fiber, low-GI diet for patients at risk for MES (39). Because many variables affect the blood glucose response of a particular carbohydrate-containing food, some controversy exists concerning the usefulness of GI as a tool in the nutrition management of MES, diabetes, or hyperlipidemia. Whether GI-tailored diets are effective, acceptable, and understandable to patients over the long term is under investigation (37,39). Table 7.4 shows how to improve patients' carbohydrate choices. (See Chapter 9 on GI.)

Fiber

ATP III recommends the inclusion of 20 to 30 g/day of dietary fiber, 10 to 25 g/day of which should come from soluble or viscous fiber (2). In the United States the average fiber intake is only 15 g/day (40). Oatmeal, beans, citrus fruits, split peas, and broccoli are some of the best sources of soluble fiber, with approximately 2 to 4 g per serving. (See Table 9.4 in Chapter 9 for a list of soluble-fiber foods.) In addition, foods that contain dietary fiber often take longer

TABLE 7.4
Improving Carbohydrate Choices

Poor Carbohydrate Choice*	Better Carbohydrate Source[†]
Apple juice (presweetened)	Apple (whole, with skin)
Potato (russet, baked)	Sweet potato, yam (baked)
Rice (white, long grain)	Brown rice (steamed)
Corn, sweet (cooked)	Lentils (boiled)
Bran muffin	Oatmeal (rolled oats)
White bread or bagel	Seven-grain or whole wheat bread
Croissant	English muffin
Doughnut	Whole-wheat waffles
Fried tortilla or corn chips	Baked tortilla or corn chips
Corn flakes cereal	Raisin bran cereal
Chocolate chip cookies	Oatmeal cookies
Carrot cake	Angel food cake with fresh fruit

*Low in fiber, some high in sugar and fat, and high glycemic index.

[†]High in fiber, low in sugar and fat, and low glycemic index.

Source: Developed by Darwin Deen, MD, Albert Einstein College of Medicine, and Lisa Hark, PhD, RD, University of Pennsylvania School of Medicine. Copyright 2004. Used by permission of the authors.

to eat and may increase satiety by delaying gastric emptying, which may assist in glucose handling and weight management. Observational studies have also reported that diets high in fiber can even delay the onset of diabetes (41). The quality and quantity of carbohydrate intake can easily be assessed by asking patients four simple questions, discussed below. Box 7.1 lists other useful questions to ask patients.

Asking Key Nutrition History Questions

What Do You Like to Drink During the Day? How Many Glasses?

Regular soda, sugar-sweetened iced tea, soft drinks, sports drinks, and fruit juices contribute a significant amount of energy and sugar, both of which can affect body weight and TG levels. Quantifying patients' beverage intake and guiding them to substitute plain or seltzer water or other calorie-free beverages with meals and snacks can save hundreds of kilocalories per day. If they are able to make only one dietary change, this may be the most realistic and effective one.

In addition, alcohol intake should always be quantified. Although alcohol has been shown to be cardioprotective in certain patients, it contributes a significant amount of energy and can raise TG levels (42). For example, 6 ounces of red wine has approximately 120 kcal and 12 ounces of regular beer has 150 kcal, equivalent to a 12-ounce can of regular soda. In addition, excessive alcohol consumption may cause hypertension, atrial arrhythmias, stroke, cirrhosis, pancreatitis, breast cancer, and accidents. Finally, alcohol can weaken an individual's resolve to control calorie intake.

What Type of Snacks and Desserts Do You Eat?

Snacks and desserts such as cookies, crackers, pretzels, candy bars, cakes, pies, and ice cream contain large amounts of sugar as well as fat and calories, which could contribute to weight gain and increased TG levels in patients with MES. Remind patients to check the labels of snack foods for hidden sugars in the guise of ingredients such as brown sugar, molasses, honey, high-fructose corn syrup, sorbitol, and juice concentrate. Substituting fresh fruit for desserts

Box 7.1   Key Diet History Questions for Patients with Metabolic Syndrome

Questions for All Patients

- How many meals and snacks do you eat every day?
- How often do you eat out? What kinds of restaurants?
- What do you like to drink during the day, including alcohol? How many glasses?
- How often do you eat fruits and vegetables?
- How often do you eat dairy products? Low fat or regular type?
- Do you usually finish what is on your plate or leave food?
- How often do you exercise, including walking?
- How many hours of television do you watch every day?

In addition to the questions above

Questions for Patients with Dyslipidemia

- How often do you eat fatty meats? (hot dogs, bacon, sausage, salami, pastrami, corned beef)
- How often do you eat fish? How is it prepared?
- What do you spread on your bread?
- What types of fats do you use in cooking?
- What type of snacks and desserts do you eat?

Questions for Patients with High Blood Pressure

- Do you use a salt shaker at the table or in cooking?
- Do you read food labels for sodium content? (< 400 mg per serving permitted)
- How often do you eat canned, smoked, frozen, and processed foods?

Questions for Patients with Elevated Fasting Glucose Levels

- What time do you take your diabetes medication (including insulin)?
- What time do you eat your meals and snacks?
- Do you ever skip meals during the day?
- How many servings of starchy foods such as breads, cereals, pastas, corn, peas, or beans do you eat during a typical day?

Source: Reprinted from Hark LA, Bowman M, and Bellini L. Overview of nutrition in clinical practice. In: Hark LA, Morrison G, eds. *Medical Nutrition and Disease: A Case-Based Approach.* 3rd ed. Malden, Mass: Blackwell Pulishing; 2003. Used by permission of the author, Lisa Hark, PhD, RD.

helps reduce total fat and energy intake, but patients should also be advised to skip the snack and share the dessert. If a patient needs a snack, suggest a piece of fruit or 1 tablespoon of unsalted dry roasted peanuts, almonds, pecans, or walnuts. These small servings of nuts help increase monounsaturated-fat intake, which can improve the dyslipidemia associated with MES.

How Much Bread, Pasta, and Potatoes Do You Generally Eat?

In American culture, people tend to eat far too much of these foods, leading to excessive carbohydrate and energy intake. Ask specifically about white bread, dinner rolls, bagels, white pasta, white rice, and mashed or fried potatoes. Unless fortified, these foods tend to be low in nutrient value and high in energy. Suggest that patients eat whole grains such as wheat, rye, or pumpernickel breads, wheat pasta, brown rice, or baked potatoes with skin. Advise them to try one substitution every 2 weeks as a way of introducing new foods. (See Table 7.4.)

How Often Do You Eat Fruits and Vegetables?

Fruits and vegetables are ideal carbohydrate-rich foods. They are high in fiber and contain important polynutrients such as antioxidant vitamins and flavonoids. The epidemiologic evidence strongly supports the inverse association between the intake of fruits and vegetables and CVD (43). Unfortunately, fewer than 25% of Americans eat five or more daily servings of these two food groups combined. Thus, following the recommendations of both the AHA and American Cancer Society, patients with MES should be encouraged to eat at least five servings of fruits and vegetables every day.

Investigators for the Dietary Approaches to Stop Hypertension (DASH) trial found that diets low in saturated fat and sodium that included eight to ten servings of fruits and vegetables (at least four of each) and three to four servings of low-fat dairy per day were effective in lowering systolic blood pressure by 3 to 6 mm Hg (44). Thus, increasing fruit and vegetable intake addresses both the glucose and blood pressure abnormalities in patients with MES. Helpful suggestions to reach the goal of five servings a day include snacking on fresh fruit, celery, or carrot sticks or drinking a glass of a low-sodium vegetable juice.

Assessing Fat Intake: Substituting Good Fats for Bad Fats

Saturated fat and *trans* unsaturated fats, the so-called bad fats, are associated with an increased risk of CVD, primarily through negative effects on LDL cholesterol concentration. The average saturated-fat intake in the American diet has declined during the last several decades from about 20% to 11% of total energy (40). The current AHA and ATP III guidelines, however, recommend that saturated-fat intake be limited to less than 7% of total energy intake (2,36).

Saturated fat is often solid at room temperature and is found predominantly in animal products, as well as palm and coconut oils, which are often used in baked goods. Foods containing saturated fat include red meats (beef and lamb), full-fat dairy products (such as butter, cheese, and ice cream), hot dogs, bacon, sausage, and many baked desserts. The use of partially hydrogenated fats to lengthen the shelf life of products has increased dietary *trans* fatty acids, found primarily in stick margarines, fried foods (such as french fries and fried chicken), and processed baked goods (doughnuts and cakes).

Counsel patients with MES to substitute monounsaturated fatty acids (MUFAs) and n-3 polyunsaturated fatty acids (n-3 PUFAs) for saturated and *trans* fats. For patients with MES, MUFAs are the preferred dietary fats because they have desirable effects on lipid levels, insulin sensitivity, platelet function, and blood pressure and may thus reduce CVD risk (45-47). The most common MUFA, oleic acid, is the predominant fatty acid in olives and olive oil. Other dietary sources of MUFAs include tree nuts, peanuts, tahini paste, canola oil, and avocados. Epidemiologic and clinical trial data suggest that diets rich in nuts and olive oil can reduce cardiovascular risk (48). Thus, substituting some energy from MUFAs that might otherwise come from saturated fat or carbohydrates can reduce the LDL cholesterol concentration without lowering HDL cholesterol or raising TG levels. This has been recognized by the NCEP

Therapeutic Lifestyle Change (TLC) diet, which has increased the recommended intake of MUFAs to 20% of total energy (2). The caveat in increasing dietary MUFAs is that these foods are energy dense and may cause weight gain if not substituted for saturated fats and carbohydrates. Advising patients on appropriate portion sizes of food sources of MUFAs helps patients control their body weight.

PUFAs have also been associated with improved lipid profiles. More specifically, n-3 PUFAs have been shown to consistently lower fasting TG levels, reduce platelet adhesion, and improve hemostatic function, blood pressure, and endothelial function (45). More importantly, diets rich in n-3 PUFAs have been shown to reduce the risk of death from CVD and all-cause mortality in both observational and intervention studies (49). Although most n-3 PUFAs are derived from fish, alpha-linolenic acid (ALA), which comes from certain plants, has also been associated with lower cardiovascular risk (50). To assess a patient's dietary balance between good and bad fats, ask the following three simple questions and use the answers as a platform for specific dietary recommendations.

How Often Do You Eat Fatty Meats and Luncheon Meats?

Processed meats, such as bacon, sausage, luncheon meats (bologna, pastrami, corned beef, salami), and hot dogs, are high in saturated fat, sodium, and energy and should be limited. Although LDL cholesterol levels are most affected by saturated-fat intake, these types of meats can also contribute a significant amount of sodium, which may raise blood pressure. Encourage patients to increase their intake of lower fat meats, such as white-meat chicken and turkey, fish, pork loin, and filet mignon.

In place of high-saturated-fat foods, patients with MES can substitute MUFA-rich sources of fat, such as walnuts, peanuts, peanut butter, almonds, avocado, and olives, although portion control is crucial. One serving (50 kcal or 3 g) of MUFA is found in 1 teaspoon of virgin olive oil, one eighth of a medium avocado, 8 black olives, 6 almonds, 6 cashews, or 1.5 teaspoons of peanut butter. Suggest that patients substitute peanut butter for luncheon meats, add unsalted almonds to a salad, or snack on a few cashews instead of pretzels.

How Often Do You Eat Fish?

Fish is an excellent alternative to meat and poultry because it is low in energy and higher in n-3 fatty acids. N-3 fatty acids include the very-long-chain eicosapentanoic acid (EPA) and docosahexanoic acid (DHA) found in fish, and the 18-carbon ALA found in plants (flaxseeds and flaxseed oil and, to some extent, canola and soybean oils). EPA and DHA are found in cold-water fish, including salmon, mackerel, sardines, herring, and, to a lesser extent, tuna and trout.

Encourage patients to increase their intake of fish. The AHA recommends eating fish two times per week. Patients can order it when dining out, requesting that it be grilled or broiled with lemon and herbs rather than fried. For vegetarian patients and those who do not like fish, ALA-rich foods such as flaxseeds, walnuts, soy, and leeks are good sources of n-3 PUFAs. Flaxseeds can be ground into powder and sprinkled onto salads or mixed into cereals and low-fat, low-sugar yogurts.

Patients with MES who cannot consume 1 to 3 g/day of n-3 PUFAs from conventional foods can consider concentrated fish-oil supplements (two to four capsules daily) (51) (see Tables 10.4 and 10.5 in Chapter 10). Higher dosages of fish-oil supplements (six to nine capsules daily) are reserved as adjunctive therapy in treating patients with severe hypertriglyceridemia (TG levels greater than 1,000 mg/dL).

Which Fats and Oils Do You Use in Cooking?

Epidemiologic data suggest that Mediterranean diets, rich in MUFAs and n-3 PUFAs, are associated with a lower incidence of CVD and a 25% total reduction in mortality (52). Moreover, evidence suggests that a diet containing up to 35% of total energy from fat is not only cardioprotective, but also preferable to the high-carbohydrate diets prescribed in the past (53). Diets in which the majority of energy is derived from carbohydrates can lead to increases in plasma TG concentrations while concomitantly lowering levels of HDL cholesterol (35). In contrast, diets high in MUFAs have been shown to decrease plasma TG levels relative to both high–saturated-fat and high-carbohydrate diets (54). Based on these compelling data, encourage patients to use only olive or canola oils for sauteing and cooking, substituting them for animal fats (lard, bacon fat), butter, margarine, and other vegetable oils (corn, sunflower).

Assessing Sodium and Calcium Intake

According to the Joint National Committee on Prevention, Detection, Evaluation, and Treatment of High Blood Pressure (JNC 7), diet and lifestyle changes should be first line therapy for hypertension (55). Aside from the benefits of sodium restriction, investigators from the original DASH study found that incorporating two servings of low-fat dairy products into a low-fat, high-fiber diet was optimal for lowering blood pressure (56). In the follow-up DASH-Sodium trial, investigators found that different levels of sodium restriction (3,300 mg/day, 2,400 mg/day, and 1,500 mg/day) in addition to the combined DASH diet further reduced blood pressure (57). The following two questions address sodium and calcium intake:

Do You Use the Salt Shaker at the Dinner Table or in Cooking?

Foods that contribute the most sodium to the diet are canned, smoked, and processed foods, including frozen and prepared dinners, deli meats, and fast food. Condiments and snack foods also contain significant amounts of sodium. Recommend that patients with MES and prehypertension (blood pressure 130/85 mm Hg) limit their sodium intake to 2,000 to 3,000 mg/day of sodium, which is equivalent to about 5 to 7.5 g/day of salt (1 to 1.5 teaspoons per day). In practice, this means not adding table salt to foods during preparation and not using it at meals. Encourage patients to substitute fresh herbs, pepper, or salt substitutes made from potassium chloride (such as Mrs. Dash and NuSalt) for table salt. The salt substitutes provide the salt flavoring as well as contributing small amounts of potassium, which has been shown to reduce blood pressure.

How Often Do You Consume Dairy Products?

Patients should be asked about their intake of dairy foods and advised to select low-fat and fat-free sources. Low-fat and nonfat mozzarella, ricotta, cottage, and farmer cheese are available. Low-fat or nonfat yogurt or nonfat sour cream alternatives can be used to make dips and salad dressings. Lactose-intolerant patients should be encouraged to use lower-fat and nonfat varieties of lactose-free dairy foods. Lactase supplements, in the form of caplets, tablets, and chewable tablets, may be helpful and can be ingested along with dairy products for lactose-intolerant individuals.

Encourage patients to eat at least two to three servings of low-fat or nonfat dairy products every day. If it is not possible for certain patients to achieve a satisfactory calcium intake in this way, daily supplements should be recommended. Greater compliance has been found with flavored calcium supplements.

Finally, because individuals respond differently to dietary changes, laboratory tests should be monitored. If patients develop hypertriglyceridemia or fail to show improvements in serum lipid levels, then fiber intake can be increased (with a goal of 25 to 35 g/day) or carbohydrate intake can be reduced and replaced with MUFA (54,58). This diet should still emphasize high-fiber, lower GI foods (39,59) (see Chapter 9, Table 9.4). The long-term effects of low-carbohydrate diets have not been adequately studied, but short term, these diets have been shown to lower TGs, raise HDL cholesterol, and reduce body weight (59). If patients choose a low-carbohydrate diet plan, advise them to select lean meats and MUFAs and to limit saturated fats.

Pharmacotherapy

Diet and exercise prescriptions for patients with MES are outlined above. After lifestyle adjustment has been addressed, the treatment of MES focuses on treating any cardiovascular or diabetes risk factors the patient may have.

ATP III guidelines classify MES as a secondary therapeutic target after the initial treatment of any LDL cholesterol abnormalities (2). Treatment of LDL cholesterol with statins has proven to be effective in reducing cardiovascular events in patients with diabetes, a population with a high proportion of patients with MES (60). The Heart Protection Study, a placebo-controlled, randomized trial, included a subpopulation of nearly 6,000 patients with diabetes. This study showed that in a high-risk population including those with diabetes, simvastatin not only lowered LDL cholesterol levels but significantly reduced vascular events (61).

For patients with hypertriglyceridemia, fibrates such as gemfibrozil or fenofibrate are peroxisome proliferator-activated receptor (PPAR)-alpha agonists, which act primarily by increasing fatty-acid oxidation and thus lead to reductions in TG synthesis and very-low-density lipoprotein (VLDL) secretion. Moreover, fibrates increase the expression of apo A-I, consequently leading to a beneficial increase in HDL cholesterol level. In the Veteran Affairs High-Density Lipoprotein Intervention Study (VA-HIT), gemfibrozil treatment was associated with a 35% decrease in relative risk for a combined cardiovascular end point among patients with diabetes (62).

Although the use of niacin was previously contraindicated in patients with IR because it may increase levels of blood glucose and aggravate IR, recent trials indicate a potential role for niacin therapy in patients with MES. A report on the Arterial Disease Multiple Intervention Trial showed an association between niacin therapy and decreased TG levels, as well as increased HDL cholesterol, in patients with diabetes (63). And although this study did confirm that niacin raises blood glucose in people both with and without diabetes, the levels of glycated hemoglobin did not change in the patients with diabetes. Thus, the study indicates that niacin therapy may be a useful adjunct in the treatment of individuals with diabetes or IR, although care must be taken to monitor glucose levels.

Antihypertensive agents should be included when blood pressure needs to be lowered. Beta-blocker therapy has been withheld from patients with either diabetes or IR because of its ability to mask hypoglycemic symptoms. However, beta-blockers can significantly reduce cardiovascular mortality among patients with diabetes and hypertension and should consequently receive consideration (64). Also, there is compelling evidence not only that treatment of hypertension with angiotensin-converting enzyme inhibitors (ACE inhibitors) is beneficial for its effect on lowering blood pressure, but that it may also prove to reduce the risk of other complications of diabetes such as nephropathy and CVD (65,66).

Finally, IR can be treated with the use of thiazolidinediones. These drugs are PPAR-gamma agonists, which, in addition to promoting fatty-acid oxidation, also increase insulin sensitivity (67). Thiazolidinediones have also been shown to be effective in delaying the onset of diabetes in those with IR. Overall, the combination of smoking cessation, blood pressure control, blood sugar control in diabetics, aggressive LDL-lowering therapy, weight reduction, regular exercise, and daily aspirin use can lower CVD risk by up to 50% in 5 years (16).

PREVENTION

The US Preventive Services Task Force recommends intensive behavior and dietary counseling for adult patients with known risk factors for CVD. The task force's literature review supports the notion that intensive counseling delivered by primary care clinicians or dietitians rates a category B recommendation (68). The Diabetes Prevention Program (69) demonstrated that vigorous lifestyle intervention could prevent the onset of diabetes by more than 50% (from 11% to 4.8%). Patients randomized to the control, metformin, or lifestyle interventions all ate fewer total calories. The control and metformin groups reduced their daily energy intake by 250 and 300 kcal, respectively, whereas the lifestyle group reduced their intake by 400 kcal. Patients initially consumed 34% of their energy from fat; with dietary instruction, they reduced their fat intake by 6.6%. Although the many individual counseling sessions provided to each patient during 2 to 3 years is clearly beyond what physician practices can offer as part of routine care, efforts are being made to educate family physicians on how to conduct brief counseling sessions for patients with MES (70). It is heartening that these dramatic results were obtained with only half of patients meeting their rather modest weight-loss goal (7% of body weight). The authors calculated that only seven patients needed to be treated for 3 years to prevent one case of diabetes.

So what should clinicians do if MES is suspected?

- Recognize the problem, make the diagnosis, inform patient and physician.
- Provide a clear and consistent message to patients about what needs to be done.
- Initiate lifestyle behavior change.
- Help the patients to identify specific changes to be made.
- Arrange follow-up to do the following
  - monitor progress
  - reinforce success
  - identify barriers
  - keep the process of change going

CASE STUDY: METABOLIC SYNDROME*

Past Medical History, Family and Social History

CS is a 55-year-old male who presents to the clinic for cardiovascular risk assessment. His past medical history is significant for hypercholesterolemia for the past 5 years. He has no history

---

*Updated and reprinted from Burke F. Case report: clinical application of the NCEP ATP III Guidelines. *On the Cutting Edge.* 2002;23.

of hypertension, diabetes, or thyroid abnormalities. His family history is notable for premature CVD and type 2 diabetes mellitus. CS is an ex-cigarette smoker of 15 years and drinks one glass of wine one to two times per week. He exercises routinely on a treadmill, 30 minutes, three times per week. He is currently not taking any medications or dietary supplements and he has no known food allergies.

Dietary Intake

CS eats a vegetarian diet at home. His usual breakfast consists of 10 ounces of orange juice, 2 cups raisin bran cereal with 4 ounces of reduced-fat (2%) milk, one banana, coffee with cream and 2 teaspoons sugar. Lunch usually includes french onion or creamed soup, a caesar salad, and a diet beverage. Dinner consists of a large plate of semolina pasta and Italian bread. CS orders red meat on occasion, more typically pasta and fish entrees, or Chinese food while eating out at least three nights a week. Throughout the day, CS snacks on dried fruit, pretzels, and hard candy and drinks fruit juice.

Physical Examination and Laboratory Data

On physical examination CS had a heart rate of 59 beats per minute and blood pressure of 115/79 mm Hg. He is 5 feet 9 inches in height (175 cm) and weighs 196 pounds (89 kg). His BMI is 29 and his waist circumference is 39 inches. His physical exam was otherwise unremarkable. His lipid laboratory values are shown in Table 7.5. His homocysteine is 15.4 μmol/L (< 12 μmol/L), glucose 112 mg/dL (70 to 100 mg/dL), and hemoglobin A1c is 5.4 (4%-6%).

In summary, CS, a 55-year-old white male, is at moderately high CVD risk due to (*a*) his positive family history of CVD, (*b*) his age, and (*c*) his lipid profile, suggestive of familial combined hyperlipidemia. Based on the Framingham scoring system, his 10-year CHD risk is 20% (2). CS also presents with MES, as suggested by a low HDL cholesterol and elevated triglyceride and glucose levels (2,71). In addition, he has an elevated homocysteine level and a BMI of 29, which classifies him as overweight. Secondary causes of hyperlipidemia, such as hypothyroidism or steroid medication therapy, were ruled out. CS has never taken lipid-lowering medication and prefers to avoid medication to treat his dyslipidemia, if possible.

Medical Treatment Goals

The initial recommendation for CS is lifestyle modification for the next 3 months. Given his family history of premature heart disease and desire to avoid lipid-lowering medication, CS is very motivated to make lifestyle and behavioral changes, which include incorporating various dietary strategies into his current eating pattern.

His goals are to lower LDL cholesterol and triglycerides, raise HDL cholesterol, and reduce his body weight. In addition CS should be prescribed a folic acid supplement to lower his homocysteine to normal levels (36,72) and 81 mg aspirin to lower his CVD risk (73).

TABLE 7.5
Lipid Levels

Laboratory Test	Patient's Results (mg/dL)	ATP III Reference Values (mg/dL)
LDL cholesterol	167	Optimal <100
Total cholesterol	288	Desirable <200
HDL cholesterol	36	>40
Triglycerides	302	Normal <150

Abbreviations: ATP III, Adult Treatment Panel III; HDL, high-density lipoprotein; LDL, low-density lipoprotein.

Reduction of Risk Factors Using National Guidelines

Using ATP III guidelines, LDL cholesterol reduction is the primary focus to reduce his CVD risk. CS's target LDL cholesterol goal is less than 130 mg/dL because he presents with more than two risk factors (2). CS's current LDL cholesterol is 167 mg/dL. By adhering to the TLC diet, which limits saturated fat to less than 7% of total energy, CS may reduce his LDL cholesterol by an average of 10% (2). Although CS eats a predominantly vegetarian diet, his choices include Chinese shrimp fried rice, spring rolls, cheese pizza, eggplant parmigiana, caesar salad, lobster bisque, and baked desserts. Thus, his dietary intake is high in energy, saturated fat, and low-fiber carbohydrates. Major sources of saturated fat in CS's diet include cheese, cream, fried foods, and baked desserts. Reducing *trans* fatty acids in CS's diet may also have some cardioprotective benefits. CS should be encouraged to limit his intake of fried foods, crackers, desserts, and foods containing hydrogenated fat (36).

ATP III recommends treatment beyond LDL cholesterol reduction in patients with triglyceride levels greater than 200 mg/dL (2). CS's triglyceride level is 302 mg/dL. Often a very-low-fat, high-carbohydrate diet (> 60% of energy) can lead to an elevation in triglycerides or, in this case, aggravate the existing metabolic abnormality (36). The liver synthesizes triglyceride-rich VLDL particles following consumption of a high-carbohydrate meal. For patients with low HDL cholesterol and high triglyceride levels, increasing total fat up to 35% of energy while limiting both carbohydrate and energy intake to allow for weight reduction can have a beneficial effect. Monounsaturated fat should be favored in place of both saturated fat and *trans* fat (74).

Dietary recommendations to help CS reduce his saturated-fat and sugar intake include substituting 1 cup cooked oatmeal, ½ cup low-fat (1%) milk, and a small navel orange for breakfast. If used, fruit juice should be limited to 4 to 6 ounces per day, and low-sugar, high-fiber cereals should be chosen more often. The focus should be to reduce sugar and increase soluble fiber. The TLC diet includes the option to increase soluble fiber to 10 to 25 g/day (2). Soluble fiber has a modest effect on lowering LDL cholesterol. The viscous fibers are thought to bind bile acids in the gut and interfere with the dietary absorption of both cholesterol and fat (see Chapter 10). Other ways to incorporate soluble fiber in CS's diet would be to increase his fresh fruit, vegetable, bean, and legume intake to a minimum of three to five servings per day. Because nuts are a major source of monounsaturated fat and contain fiber, they could be recommended as a snack choice in 1-ounce portions, replacing dried fruits, hard candy, and baked goods. Emphasis on portion control is necessary as a means to manage weight. Other menu suggestions can include whole grain pasta, veggie burgers containing soy protein, as well as the consumption of grilled or broiled fish containing n-3 fatty acids, such as salmon, at least twice weekly. Based on evidence from clinical trials, the AHA recommends the consumption of soy protein especially for individuals with elevated total and LDL cholesterol levels (36,75). Additional sources of soy protein include soy milk, tofu, tempeh, soy energy bars, soy cheese, and soy nuts.

Weight reduction and increased physical activity are recommended for the management of MES (2). CS is likely eating approximately 2,600 to 2,800 kcal/day (89 kg × 30 kcal/kg) to maintain his weight. Counseling CS to reduce his intake by 500 kcal/day and increase his physical activity to 4 days/week could result in a weight loss of 1 lb per week. Sustained weight loss of as little as 5% to 10% of body weight (10 to 20 lb in this patient) may enhance LDL cholesterol and triglyceride lowering and increase HDL cholesterol, as well as improve nonlipid risk factors such as blood glucose elevation (76).

Follow-Up

The patient should be reevaluated at 6 weeks with a follow-up fasting lipid profile. If CS's LDL cholesterol level remains greater than 130 mg/dL, counseling on the use of margarines containing plant stanol or sterol esters would be appropriate (2). The recommended intake of 2 to 3 g/day (which is contained in approximately 2 tablespoons) has the potential to lower LDL cholesterol up to 14% (77). Stanol and sterol esters have no effect on HDL cholesterol or triglycerides (36). If CS does not reach his LDL cholesterol target after 3 months of lifestyle modifications, lipid-lowering medication should be initiated. In addition, if CS fails to achieve an adequate response to folate supplementation for his hyperhomocysteinemia, vitamins B-12 and B-6 may also be considered. CS should be followed every 4 to 6 months thereafter to monitor laboratory values, drug efficacy, and the possible development of type 2 diabetes.

REFERENCES

1. Vega GL. Obesity, metabolic syndrome, and cardiovascular disease. *Am Heart J.* 2001;142:1108-1116.
2. National Heart, Lung, and Blood Institute *Third Report of the National Cholesterol Education Program Expert Panel on Detection, Evaluation, and Treatment of High Blood Cholesterol in Adults (Adult Treatment Panel III). Executive Summary.* Bethesda, Md: National Institutes of Health; 2001. NIH publication 01-3670.
3. Alberti KG, Zimmet PZ. Definition, diagnosis and classification of diabetes mellitus and its complications. Part 1. Diagnosis and classification of diabetes mellitus, provisional report of a WHO consultation. *Diabetes Med.* 1998;15:539-553.
4. Bray GA, Champagne CM. Obesity and the metabolic syndrome: implications for dietetics practitioners. *J Am Diet Assoc.* 2004;104:86-89.
5. Vague J. La differenciation sexuelle, facture determinant des formes de l'obesite. *Presse Med.* 1947;30:339-340.
6. Vague J. The degree of masculine differentiation of obesities: a factor determining the predisposition to diabetes, atherosclerosis, gout, and uric calculous disease. *Am J Clin Nutr.* 1956;4:20-28.
7. Reaven GM. Role of insulin resistance in human disease. *Diabetes.* 1988;37:1595-1607.
8. Lamarche B, Tchernof A, Mauriege P, Cantin B, Dagenais GR, Lupien PJ, Despres JP. Fasting insulin and apolipoprotein B levels and low-density lipoprotein particle size as risk factors for ischemic heart disease. *JAMA.* 1998;279:1955-1961.
9. Isomaa B, Henricsson M, Almgren P, Tuomi T, Taskinen MR, Groop L. The metabolic syndrome influences the risk of chronic complications in patients with type II diabetes. *Diabetologia.* 2001;44:1148-1154.
10. Ford ES, Giles WH. A comparison of the prevalence of the metabolic syndrome using two proposed definitions. *Diabetes Care.* 2003;26:575-581.
11. Ford E, Giles W, Dietz W. Prevalence of the metabolic syndrome among US adults. *JAMA.* 2002;287:356-359.
12. Park Y, Zhu S, Palaniappan L, Heshka S, Carnethon MR, Heymsfield SB. The metabolic syndrome: prevalence and associated risk factor findings in the US populations from the Third National Health and Nutrition Examination Survey, 1988–1994. *Arch Intern Med.* 2003;163:427-436.
13. Zimmet P, Alberti KG, Shaw J. Global and societal implications of the diabetic epidemic. *Nature.* 2001;414:782-787.
14. Rexrode KM, Carey VJ, Hennekens CH, Walters EE, Colditz GA, Stampfer MJ, Willett WC, Manson JE. Abdominal adiposity and coronary heart disease in women. *JAMA.* 1998;280:1843-1848.
15. Lopez-Candales A. Metabolic syndrome X: a comprehensive review of the pathophysiology and recommended therapy. *J Med.* 2001;32:283-300.
16. Björntorp P. Heart and soul: stress and the metabolic syndrome. *Scand Cardiovasc J.* 2001;35:172-177.
17. Despres JP. Visceral obesity, insulin resistance, and dyslipidemia: contribution of endurance exercise training to the treatment of the plurimetabolic syndrome. *Exerc Sport Sci Rev.* 1997;25:271-300.
18. Hark LA, Deen D. Taking a nutrition history: a practical approach for family physicians. *Am Fam Physician.* 1999;59:1521-1528.
19. Hark LA, Bowman M, Bellini L. Overview of nutrition in clinical care. In: Hark LA, Morrison G, eds. *Medical Nutrition and Disease.* 3rd ed. Malden, Mass: Blackwell Publishing; 2003:3-38.
20. Pouliot MC, Despres JP, Lemieux S, Moorjani S, Bouchard C, Tremblay A, Nadeau A, Lupien PJ. Waist circumference and abdominal sagittal diameter: best simple anthropometric indexes of abdominal visceral adipose tissue accumulation and related cardiovascular risk in men and women. *Am J Cardiol.* 1994;73:460-468.

21. Pearson TA, Mensah GA, Alexander RW, Anderson JL, Cannon RO III, Criqui M, Fadl YY, Fortmann SP, Hong Y, Myers GL, Rifai N, Smith SC Jr, Taubert K, Tracy RP, Vinicor F. Centers for Disease Control and Prevention. American Heart Association. Markers of inflammation and cardiovascular disease: application to clinical and public health practice: a statement for healthcare professionals from the Centers for Disease Control and Prevention and the American Heart Association. *Circulation.* 2003;107:499-511.

22. Williamson DF, Pamuk E, Thun M, Flanders D, Byers T, Heath C. Prospective study of intentional weight loss and mortality in never-smoking overweight US white women aged 40-64. *Am J Epidemiol.* 1995;141:1128-1141.

23. Duncan GE, Perri MG, Theriaque DW, Hutson AD, Eckel RH, Stacpoole PW. Exercise training, without weight loss, increases insulin sensitivity and post heparin plasma lipase activity in previously sedentary adults. *Diabetes Care.* 2003;26:557-562.

24. Goodpaster BH, He J, Watkins S, Kelly DE. Skeletal muscle lipid content and insulin resistance: evidence for a paradox in endurance-trained athletes. *J Clin Endocrinol Metab.* 2001;86:5755-5761.

25. Pratt M. Benefits of lifestyle activity vs structured exercise. *JAMA.* 2001;281:375-376.

26. Boule NG, Haddad E, Kenny GP, Wells GA, Sigal RJ. Effects of exercise on glycemic control and body mass in type 2 diabetes mellitus: a meta-analysis of controlled clinical trials. *JAMA.* 2001;286:1218-1227.

27. Wing RR, Hill JO. Successful weight loss maintenance. *Annu Rev Nutr.* 2001;21:323-341.

28. Institute of Medicine. *Dietary Reference Intakes for Energy, Carbohydrates, Fiber, Fat, Protein, and Amino Acids (Macronutrients).* Washington, DC: National Academy Press; 2002.

29. Keller C, Trevino RP. Effects of two frequencies of walking on cardiovascular risk factor reduction in Mexican American women. *Res Nurs Health.* 2001;24:390-401.

30. Shangold MM. Beyond the exercise prescription: making exercise a way of life. *Sports Phys Med.* 1998;26:35-36.

31. Jones TF, Eaton CB. Exercise prescription. *Am Fam Physician.* 1995;52:543-549.

32. Busetto L. Visceral obesity and the metabolic syndrome: effects of weight loss. *Nutr Metab Cardiovasc Dis.* 2001;11:195-204.

33. Lui S, Manson JE. Dietary carbohydrates, physical inactivity, obesity, and the "metabolic syndrome" as predictors of coronary heart disease. *Curr Opin Lipidol.* 2001;12:395-404.

34. Storlien LH, Tapsell LC, Fraser A, Leslie E, Ball K, Higgins JA, Helge JW, Owen N. Insulin resistance: influence of diet and physical activity. *World Rev Nutr Diet.* 2001;90:26-43.

35. Howard BV, Wylie-Rosset J. Sugar and cardiovascular disease: a statement for healthcare professions from the Committee on Nutrition of the Council on Nutrition, Physical Activity, and Metabolism of the American Heart Association. *Circulation.* 2002;106:523-527.

36. Krauss RM, Eckel RH, Howard B, Appel LJ, Daniels SR, Deckelbaum RJ, Erdman JW, Kris-Etherton P, Goldberg IJ, Kotchen TA, Lichtenstein AH, Mitch WE, Mullis R, Robinson K, Wylie-Rosett J, St Jeor S, Suttie J, Tribble DL, Bazzarre TL. AHA Dietary Guidelines: revision 2000: a statement for healthcare professionals from the Nutrition Committee of the American Heart Association. *Circulation.* 2000;102:2284-2299.

37. Pi-Sunyer FX . Glycemic index and disease. *Am J Clin Nutr.* 2002;6(suppl):290S-298S.

38. Ludwig DS. The glycemic index: physiological mechanisms relating to obesity, diabetes, and cardiovascular disease. *JAMA.* 2002;287:2414-2423.

39. McKeown NM, Meigs JB, Liu S, Saltzman E, Wilson PW, Jacques PF. Carbohydrate nutrition, insulin resistance, and the prevalence of the metabolic syndrome in the Framingham Offspring cohort. *Diabetes Care.* 2004;27:538-546.

40. USDA Human Nutrition Research Center. What we eat in America (CSF II data tables). Available at: http://www.barc.usda.gov/bhnrc/foodsurvey/home.htm. Accessed September 4, 2003.

41. Liu S. Whole-grain foods, dietary fiber, and type 2 diabetes: searching for a kernel of truth. *Am J Clin Nutr.* 2003;77:527-529.

42. Pownall HJ. Alcohol: lipid metabolism and cardioprotection. *Curr Atheroscler Rep.* 2002;4:107-112.

43. Bazzano LA, He J, Ogden LG, Loria CM, Vupputuri S, Myers L, Whelton PK. Fruit and vegetable intake and risk of cardiovascular disease in US adults: the first National Health and Nutrition Examination Survey Epidemiologic Follow-up Study. *Am J Clin Nutr.* 2002;76:93-99.

44. Lopes HF, Martin KL, Nashar K, Morrow JD, Goodfriend TL, Egan BM. DASH diet lowers blood pressure and lipid-induced oxidative stress in obesity. *Hypertension.* 2003;41:422-430.

45. Kris-Etherton P, Daniels SR, Eckel RH, Engler M, Howard BV, Krauss RM, Lichtenstein AH, Sacks F, St Jeor S, Stampfer M, Eckel RH, Grundy SM, Appel LJ, Byers T, Campos H, Cooney G, Denke MA, Kennedy E, Marckmann P, Pearson TA, Riccardi G, Rudel LL, Rudrum M, Sacks F, Stein DT, Tracy RP, Ursin V, Vogel RA, Zock PL, Bazzarre TL, Clark J. Summary of the scientific conference on dietary fatty acids and cardiovascular health: conference summary from the nutrition committee of the American Heart Association. *Circulation.* 2001;103:1034-1039.

46. Rivellese AA, Maffettone A, Vessby B, Uusitupa M, Hermansen K, Berglund L, Louheranta A, Meyer BJ, Riccardi G. Effects of dietary saturated, monounsaturated and n-3 fatty acids on fasting lipoproteins, LDL size and post-prandial lipid metabolism in healthy subjects. *Atherosclerosis.* 2003;167:149-158.

47. Kris-Etherton PM. AHA Science Advisory. Monounsaturated fatty acids and risk of cardiovascular disease: American Heart Association, Nutrition Committee. *Circulation.* 1999;100:1253-1258.

48. Kris-Etherton P, Eckel RH, Howard BV, St Jeor S, Bazzarre TL. Nutrition Committee Population Science Committee and Clinical Science Committee of the American Heart Association. AHA Science Advisory: Lyon Diet Heart Study: benefits of a Mediterranean-style, National Cholesterol Education Program/American Heart Association Step 1 dietary pattern on cardiovascular disease. *Circulation*. 2001;103:1823-1825.

49. Hu FB, Cho E, Rexrode KM, Albert CM, Manson JE. Fish and long-chain omega-3 fatty acid intake and risk of coronary heart disease and total mortality in diabetic women. *Circulation*. 2003;107:1852-1857.

50. Bemelmans WJ, Broer J, Feskens EJ, Smit AJ, Muskiet FA, Lefrandt JD, Bom VJ, May JF, Meyboom-de Jong B. Effect of an increased intake of alpha-linolenic acid and group nutritional education on cardiovascular risk factors: the Mediterranean Alpha-linolenic Enriched Groningen Dietary Intervention (MARGARIN) study. *Am J Clin Nutr*. 2002;75:221-227.

51. Lewis CJ. US Food and Drug Administration, Center for Food Safety and Applied Nutrition. Letter regarding dietary supplement health claim for omega-3 fatty acids and coronary heart disease. Available at: http://www.cfsan.fda.gov/~dms/ds-ltr11.html. Accessed March 30, 2004.

52. Trichopoulou A, Costacou T, Bamia C, Trichopoulos D. Adherence to a Mediterranean diet and survival in a Greek population. *New Engl J Med*. 2003;348:2599-2608.

53. Grundy SM, Abate N, Chandalia M. Diet composition and the metabolic syndrome: what is the optimal fat intake?. *Am J Med*. 2002;113(suppl 9B):25S-29S.

54. Grundy SM. Comparison of monounsaturated fatty acids and carbohydrates for lowering plasma cholesterol. *N Engl J Med*. 1986;314:745-748.

55. The Seventh Report of the Joint National Committee on Prevention, Detection, Evaluation, and Treatment of High Blood Pressure JNC VII. *JAMA*. 2003;289:2560-2572.

56. Appel LJ, Moore TJ, Obarzanek E, Vollmer WM, Svetkey LP, Sacks FM, Bray GA, Vogt TM, Cutler JA, Windhauser MM, Pao-Hwa L, Karnja N. A clinical trial of the effects of dietary patterns on blood pressure: DASH Collaborative Research Group. *New Engl J Med*. 1997;336:1117-1124.

57. Sacks FM, Svetkey LP, Vollmer WM, Appel LJ, Bray GA, Harsha D, Obarzanek E, Conlin PR, Miller ER III, Simons-Morton DG, Karanja N, Lin PH. Effects on blood pressure of reduced dietary sodium and the Dietary Approaches to Stop Hypertension (DASH) diet. DASH-Sodium Collaborative Research Group. *New Engl J Med*. 2001;344:3-10.

58. Szapary PO, Hark LA, Burke FM. The metabolic syndrome: a new focus for lifestyle modification. *Patient Care*. 2002;36:75- 88.

59. Foster GD, Wyatt HR, Hill JO, McGuckin BG, Brill C, Mohammed BS, Szapary PO, Rader DJ, Edman JS, Klein S. A randomized trial of a low-carbohydrate diet for obesity. *N Engl J Med*. 2003;348:2082-2090.

60. Koshiyama H. The impact of statin treatment on diabetic patients. *Curr Opin Investig Drugs*. 2003;4:395-400.

61. MRC/BHF Heart Protection Study of cholesterol lowering with simvastatin in 20,536 high-risk individuals: a randomized placebo-controlled trial. *Lancet*. 2002;360:7-22.

62. Rubins HB, Robins SJ. Conclusions from the VA-HIT study. *Am J Cardiol*. 2000;86:543-544.

63. Elam MB, Hunninghake DB, Davis KB, Garg R, Johnson C, Egan D, Kostis JB, Sheps DS, Brinton EA. Effect of niacin on lipid and lipoprotein levels and glycemic control in patients with diabetes and peripheral arterial disease: the ADMIT study: a randomized trial. *JAMA*. 2000;284:1263-1270.

64. Landray MJ, Toescu V, Kendall MJ. The cardioprotective role of beta-blockers in patients with diabetes mellitus. *J Clin Pharm Ther*. 2002;27:233-242.

65. Lewis EJ, Hunsicker LG, Clarke WR, Berl T, Pohl MA, Lewis JB, Ritz E, Atkins RC, Rohde R, Raz I; Collaborative Study Group. Renoprotective effect of the angiotensin-receptor antagonist irbesartan in patients with nephropathy due to type 2 diabetes. *N Engl J Med*. 2001;345:861-869.

66. Heart Outcomes Prevention Evaluation Study Investigators. Effects of ramipril on cardiovascular and microvascular outcomes in people with diabetes mellitus: results of the HOPE study and MICRO-HOPE substudy. *Lancet*. 2000;355:253-259.

67. Bell DS. Beneficial effects resulting from thiazolidinediones for treatment of type 2 diabetes mellitus. *Postgrad Med*. 2003;May(spec no):35-44.

68. US Preventive Services Task Force. Healthy diet—counseling. Available at: http://www.ahrq.gov/clinic/uspstf/uspsdiet.htm. Accessed December 16, 2003.

69. Diabetes Prevention Program Research Group. Reduction in the incidence of type 2 diabetes with lifestyle intervention or metformin. *New Engl J Med*. 2002;346:393-403.

70. Deen D. Metabolic syndrome: a practical guide for clinicians. *Am Fam Physician*. 2004;69:2875-2882.

71. Wilson PW, Kannel WB, Silbershatz H, D'Agostino RB. Clustering of metabolic factors and coronary heart disease. *Arch Intern Med*. 1999;159:1104-1109.

72. Bunout D, Garrido A, Suazo M, Kauffman R, Venegas P, de la Maza P, Petermann M, Hirsch S. Effects of supplementation with folic acid and antioxidant vitamins on homocysteine levels and LDL oxidation in coronary patients. *Nutrition*. 2000;16:107-110.

73. Hayden M, Pignone M, Phillips C, Mulrow C. Aspirin for the primary prevention of cardiovascular events: a summary of the evidence for the US Preventive Services Task Force. *Arch Intern Med*. 2002;136:161-172.

74. Kris-Etherton PM, Zhao G, Pelkman CL, Fishell VK, Coval SM. Beneficial effects of a diet high in monounsaturated fatty acids on risk factors for cardiovascular disease. *Nutr Clin Care*. 2000;3:153-162.

75. Anderson JW, Johnstone BM, Cook-Newell M. Meta-analysis of the effects of soy protein intake on serum lipids. *N Engl J Med.* 1995;333:276-282.

76. Pasanisi F, Contaldo F, de Simone G, Mancini M. Benefits of sustained moderate weight loss in obesity. *Nutr Metab Cardiovasc Dis.* 2001;11:401-406.

77. Miettinen TA, Puska P, Gylling H, Vanhanen H, Vartiainen E. Reduction of serum cholesterol with sitonstanol-ester margarine in a mildly hypercholesterolemic population. *N Engl J Med.* 1995;333:1308-1312.

CHAPTER 8

LIFESTYLE MODIFICATION IN THE PREVENTION AND TREATMENT OF HYPERTENSION

Frances M. Burke, MS, RD, and Emma A. Meagher, MD

Hypertension is an independent risk factor for both coronary heart disease (CHD) and stroke. This relationship is both continuous and consistent (1,2). Hypertension is defined as having a systolic blood pressure (SBP) of 140 mm Hg or greater, having a diastolic blood pressure (DBP) of 90 mm Hg or greater, or taking antihypertensive medication. Macrovascular disease resulting from hypertension includes heart failure, stroke, and renal insufficiency. High blood pressure has recently been associated with endothelial dysfunction. Hypertension frequently coexists with other cardiovascular disease (CVD) risk factors, including obesity, lipid abnormalities, insulin resistance, and glucose intolerance (3). Antihypertensive therapy has been associated with mean reductions of 35% to 40% in stroke incidence; 20% to 25% in myocardial infarction; and more than 50% in heart failure in clinical trials (2). Therefore, hypertension management is a critical component of preventive therapies for reducing morbidity and mortality from CVD.

This chapter reviews the proven nonpharmacologic strategies for the management of high blood pressure as recommended by the Seventh Report of the Joint National Committee on Prevention, Detection, Evaluation, and Treatment of High Blood Pressure (JNC 7) issued by the National High Blood Pressure Education Program (NHBPEP) in May 2003 (2). JNC 7 provides an evidence-based approach to the prevention and treatment of hypertension in adults. Key messages contained in JNC 7 include the following (2):

- For persons older than 50 years of age, SBP greater than 140 mm Hg is more important than DBP as a CVD risk factor.
- Individuals who are normotensive at age 55 years have a 90% lifetime risk for developing hypertension.
- The risk of CVD doubles with each increment elevation in blood pressure of 20/10 mm Hg starting at 115/75 mm Hg.

TABLE 8.1
Classification and Management of Blood Pressure for Adults Aged 18 Years or Older

| | | | | | Management* | |
| | | | | | Initial Drug Therapy | |
BP Classification	Systolic BP, mm Hg*		Diastolic BP, mm Hg*	Lifestyle Modification	Without Compelling Indication	With Compelling Indications‡
Normal	<120	and	<80	Encourage		
Prehypertension	120–139	or	80–89	Yes	No antihypertensive drug indicated	Drug(s) for the compelling indications‡
Stage 1 hypertension	140–159	or	90–99	Yes	Thiazide-type diuretics for most; may consider ACE inhibitor, ARB, β-blocker, CCB, or combination	Drug(s) for the compelling indications Other hypertensive drugs (diuretics, ACE inhibitor, ARB, β-blocker, CCB) as needed
Stage 2 hypertension	≥160	or	≥100	Yes	2-Drug combination for most (usually thiazide-type diuretic and ACE inhibitor or ARB or β-blocker or CCB)§	Drug(s) for the compelling indications Other hypertensive drugs (diuretics, ACE inhibitor, ARB, β-blocker, CCB) as needed

Abbreviations: ACE, angiotensin-converting enzyme; ARB, angiotensin-receptor blocker; BP, blood pressure; CCB, calcium channel blocker.

*Treatment determined by highest BP category.

†Compelling indications for antihypertensive drugs include heart failure, postmyocardial infarction, high coronary disease risk, diabetes, chronic kidney disease, and recurrent stroke prevention.

‡Treat patients with chronic kidney disease or diabetes to BP goal of less than 130/80 mm Hg.

§Initial combined therapy should be used cautiously in those at risk for orthostatic hypertension.

Source: Reprinted from reference 2.

- Individuals with an SBP of 120 to 139 mm Hg or a DBP of 80 to 89 mm Hg should be considered as prehypertensive and counseled on lifestyle interventions to prevent CVD (see Table 8.1) (2).
- To treat most patients with uncomplicated hypertension, thiazide-type diuretics should be used either alone or in combination with antihypertensive drugs from other classes.
- Most hypertensive patients require two or more medications to achieve their blood pressure goal (< 140/90 mm Hg, or < 130/80 mm Hg for patients with diabetes or chronic kidney disease).
- Patient motivation is an essential component in blood pressure control.

CLASSIFICATION

JNC 7 has simplified the classification of blood pressure for adults 18 years of age and older by creating fewer categories than the previous JNC 6 report (refer to Table 8.1) (2). Blood pressure is classified according to severity and is based on the average of at least two blood pressure readings properly measured on at least two different occasions with the patient in a seated position. Data from the Framingham Heart Study (4) have shown that for adults with blood pressure levels between 130/85 and 139/89 mm Hg, those younger than 65 years of age have a 37.3% chance of developing sustained hypertension within 4 years compared with a 49.5% chance for adults 65 years old and older. In contrast, the rate of developing hypertension for adults with blood pressure levels below 120/80 mm Hg is much less: 5.3% for adults younger than 65 years of age and 16% for adults 65 years old and older. Therefore, for those considered prehypertensive (defined by an SBP of 120 to 139 mm Hg or a DBP of 80 to 89 mm Hg), developing healthy lifestyle habits may delay or prevent the onset of hypertension (2). Individuals diagnosed with stage 1 or 2 hypertension should also be informed that lifestyle interventions can lower blood pressure, enhance the efficacy of antihypertensive medications, and lower cardiovascular risk (2).

PREVALENCE

The prevalence of hypertension is related to age, gender, and ethnicity. Contrary to earlier reports of a declining trend in the prevalence of hypertension in the United States from 1960 to 1991, the most recent National Health and Nutrition Examination Survey (NHANES) shows an overall increase in the prevalence of hypertension. According to the 1999 to 2000 NHANES age-adjusted data, collected by the National Center for Health Statistics, 28.7% of the participants had hypertension. This represents an estimated 58.4 million individuals and an increase in the prevalence of hypertension by 3.7% compared with 1988 to 1991. Non-Hispanic blacks have the highest prevalence of hypertension, and Mexican Americans have the lowest (refer to Figure 8.1) (5).

Hypertension prevalence increases with age (65.4% among those aged 60 years or older), and tends to be higher in women (30.1%) (5). The greater prevalence among older women is presumably linked to the onset of menopause. Different prevalence rates between certain population and age groups have been attributed in part to the degree of societal industrialization.

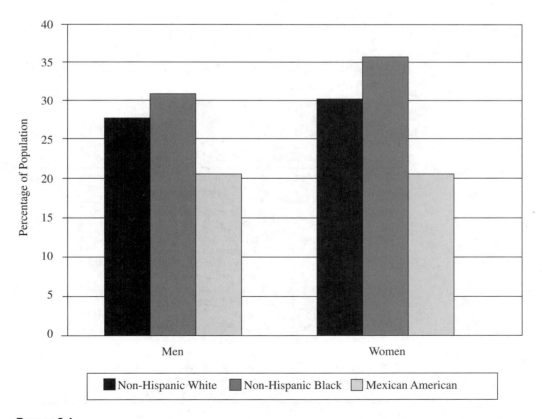

FIGURE 8.1
Age-adjusted prevalence of hypertension by sex, race, and ethnicity in the US population, 1999-2000. Data are from reference 5.

However, it has been suggested that certain modifiable factors, including dietary patterns and intake of certain nutrients, could account for these differences as well (5).

In 1999 to 2000, almost 30% of all hypertensive individuals were unaware of their illness, 59% were being treated, and at the time their blood pressure was measured, only 34% had their hypertension controlled (2). The goal of the US Department of Health and Human Services is that 50% of Americans with hypertension will have their blood pressure controlled by the year 2010 (6). Since 1988, however, little progress has been made in the treatment and control of hypertension, and it remains an important public health problem.

NONPHARMACOLOGIC TREATMENT OF HYPERTENSION

As is the case for the treatment of hyperlipidemia, medical nutrition therapy (MNT) is considered to be the cornerstone of treatment for patients with hypertension. Dietary modification and lifestyle changes have typically produced only modest reductions in blood pressure. Poor compliance is thought to largely account for these modest reductions. Patients should be strongly encouraged to adopt and adhere to lifestyle interventions, particularly if they have additional risk factors for CVD. Lifestyle modification may not completely obviate the need for antihypertensive medications, but it can dramatically reduce the amount of antihypertensive medication required to reach target blood pressure goals. The recent guidelines of the National High Blood Pressure Education Program estimate that a reduction in SBP of as little as 2 mm Hg could save more than 70,000 lives in the United States each year (1).

The specific nonpharmacologic dietary and lifestyle interventions recommended by JNC 7 include the following:

- Weight reduction
- Dietary Approaches to Stop Hypertension (DASH) eating plan
- Dietary sodium reduction

TABLE 8.2
Effects of Lifestyle Interventions to Manage Hypertension

Modification	Recommendations	Approximate Systolic Blood Pressure Reduction
Weight reduction	Maintain normal body weight (BMI 18.5–24.9)	5–20 mm Hg/10 kg weight loss
Adapt DASH eating plan	Consume diet rich in fruits, vegetables, and low-fat dairy products with a reduced content of saturated and total fat	8–14 mm Hg
Dietary sodium reduction	Reduce sodium intake to no more than 2.4 g/day sodium or 6 g/day NaCl	2–8 mm Hg
Increase physical activity	Engage in regular aerobic exercise such as brisk walking (30 min/day on most days of the week)	4–9 mm Hg
Moderate alcohol consumption	Limit alcohol to no more than two drinks per day for men and one drink per day for women	2–4 mm Hg

Abbreviations: BMI, body mass index; DASH, Dietary Approaches to Stop Hypertension.
Source: Data are from reference 2.

- Aerobic physical activity
- Moderation of alcohol consumption

Table 8.2 (2) summarizes the approximate reductions in SBP that can be achieved with dietary and lifestyle interventions based on the evidence discussed below.

Weight Reduction

Body weight is one of the strongest determinants of blood pressure. Obesity, as defined by a body mass index (BMI) equal to or greater than 30, is significantly associated with elevated blood pressure. An estimated 64% of the US adult population is either overweight or obese (7). NHANES III data shows that the age-adjusted prevalence of high blood pressure increases as BMI increases for both men and women (see Figure 8.2) (8). The prevalence of high blood pressure among individuals with BMIs equal to or greater than 30 is 41.9% for men and 37.8% for women, compared with 14.9% for men and 15.2% for women with BMIs less than or equal to 25 (8).

Although the exact mechanism of obesity-induced hypertension is unknown, several hypotheses have been proposed. Excess body weight is associated with an increased circulating blood volume. This is believed to impose a hemodynamic burden on the cardiovascular system that may elevate blood pressure (9-11). In addition, obesity is commonly associated with increases in both sympathetic nervous system activity and insulin resistance. Increased

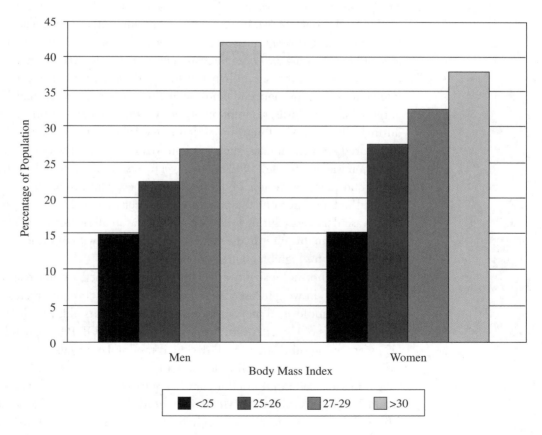

FIGURE 8.2
NHANES III age-adjusted prevalence of hypertension according to BMI. Data are from reference 8.

sympathetic activity increases catecholamine production, which may adversely affect blood pressure through vascular effects. Furthermore, weight loss has been shown to lower blood pressure by decreasing plasma renin activity (12). Finally, leptin, a hormone secreted by adipocytes, acts on the central nervous system to suppress appetite and increase sympathetic nervous system activity. Several studies have linked hypertension with high leptin levels, which are commonly elevated in obesity. High circulating leptin concentrations suggest that leptin resistance may contribute to obesity and possibly obesity-related hypertension (11,13).

In both hypertensive and normotensive individuals, there is strong support for the efficacy of weight loss in reducing blood pressure or the need for antihypertensive medication. The National Heart, Lung, and Blood Institute (NHLBI) *Clinical Guidelines on the Identification, Evaluation, and Treatment of Overweight and Obesity in Adults* provide a comprehensive review of the effects of weight reduction on blood pressure (12). Results from a number of randomized controlled trials of individuals with hypertension have demonstrated that a weight loss of 10 kg (22 lb) is associated with an average reduction of 7 mm Hg SBP and 3 mm Hg DBP (12). A recent meta-analysis performed by Neter et al (14) included 4,874 participants from different ethnic populations and showed reductions in SPB and DBP of approximately 1 mm Hg for each 1-kg reduction in body weight.

The Trial of Nonpharmacologic Interventions in the Elderly (TONE) was designed to determine whether weight loss or reduced sodium intake is effective in the treatment of hypertensive adults 60 to 80 years of age (15). TONE involved 975 participants with an SBP less than 145 mm Hg and a DBP less than 85 mm Hg on single-drug therapy for hypertension. The participants were assigned to six groups. Of the total, 585 subjects were obese and were randomized to one of the following: reduced-sodium intake alone, weight loss alone, reduced-sodium intake and weight loss combined, or usual care (no active intervention by investigators). The remaining 390 nonobese subjects were randomized to reduced-sodium intake or usual care. Withdrawal of antihypertensive medication was accomplished after 3 months of intervention. The primary end point was a blood pressure greater than 150/90 mm Hg at one or more follow-up visits, resumption of antihypertensive medication, or a cardiovascular event during follow-up. The follow-up period lasted from 15 to 36 months (median 29 months). Compared with usual care, mean weight loss was about 4.5 kg (10 lb) and mean sodium reduction was 40 mmol/day (920 mg/day). The results of this trial demonstrated that the combined end points were less frequent among obese and nonobese subjects assigned to the reduced-sodium intervention and in obese subjects assigned to weight loss. The frequency of cardiovascular events during follow-up was similar in all six treatment groups. Thus, it can be concluded from this study that a reduced-sodium intake with or without weight loss is an effective treatment for high blood pressure in older adults.

Trials in normotensive overweight adults produced similar results in blood pressure reductions when weight loss was achieved through dietary interventions. Involving 2,382 overweight middle-aged men and women, 30 to 54 years old, with high normal blood pressure, the Trials of Hypertension Prevention Phase I (TOHP I) (16) and Phase II (TOHP II) (17) were among the larger, well-designed randomized trials. Participants were randomly assigned to receive counseling for weight loss, sodium restriction, or a combination of weight loss and sodium restriction, or to a control group, and followed for 18 months (phase I) and 3 to 4 years (phase II). Mean reductions in weight of 4.4 kg (9.7 lb) at 6 months and 2.0 kg (4.4 lb) at 36 months were achieved in subjects assigned to the weight-loss and combined weight-loss and sodium-restricted groups. Throughout the 36-month follow-up period, SBP and DBP decreased more in all of the active treatment groups compared with the control group. The authors noted that blood pressure was reduced 3.7/2.7 mm Hg in the weight-loss group, 2.9/1.6 mm Hg in the sodium-restricted group, and 4.0/2.8 mm Hg in the combined group at 6 months. In addition, participants who were able to lose 4.4 kg (9.7 lb) and maintain the weight loss through the 36-month period of follow-up experienced average reductions in SBP and DBP of 5.0 and 7.0 mm Hg, respectively. Weight loss reduced hypertension incidence by 20% to 50% after 18 months and by 19% at 3 years. A positive correlation was demonstrated between the degree of weight loss and degree of blood pressure reduction.

DASH Eating Plan

The DASH and the later DASH-Sodium trials have demonstrated the benefit of a comprehensive dietary approach for the prevention and treatment of hypertension (18). The original multicenter study funded by the NHLBI enrolled 459 healthy adults with SBP levels less than 160 mm Hg and DBP levels between 80 to 95 mm Hg. Participants were randomized to three groups: (a) the control diet, which resembled the typical dietary intake in the United States (low in fruits, vegetables, and dairy), (b) a diet high in fruits and vegetables (8 to 10 servings per day), and (c) a "combination" diet that was high in fruits, vegetables, and low-fat dairy products and low in both total and saturated fat. Dietary sodium intake (3 g/day compared with 3 to 4 g/day currently consumed in the United States) remained constant for all three diets, and body weight was maintained throughout the study. The mean SBP and DBP levels at baseline were 131.3 ± 10.8 mm Hg and 84.7 ± 4.7 mm Hg, respectively. After 8 weeks, the combination or DASH diet reduced SBP and DBP levels by 5.5 and 3.0 mm Hg more, respectively, than the control diet. Among the 133 mildly hypertensive subjects, the mean SBP and DBP reduction was 11.4 mm Hg and 5.5 mm Hg, respectively, in response to the DASH diet. African Americans represented 60% of the study participants, and their blood pressure reduction on the DASH diet was greater than the reduction seen in whites. Among hypertensive African Americans, the DASH diet lowered blood pressure levels by 13.2/6.1 mm Hg compared with 6.3/4.4 mm Hg in hypertensive white participants (19). The fruit and vegetable diet lowered blood pressure half as much as the DASH diet. The effects of the DASH diet were attributed to relatively high intakes of dietary potassium (4.4 g/day), magnesium (480 mg/day), and calcium (1,265 mg/day) and low total and saturated fat intakes. (Refer to Tables 8.3 [20] and 8.4 [18].) The NHLBI has published a practical guide to the DASH diet, which can be accessed on-line (20).

The results of the PREMIER trial reaffirmed the conclusions of the DASH trial. PREMIER was the first multicenter trial to evaluate the effectiveness of the combination of proven lifestyle therapies on blood pressure levels among free living subjects (21). The PREMIER study investigated multiple lifestyle interventions in 810 mostly overweight and sedentary individuals with SBPs of 120 to 159 mm Hg and DBPs of 80 to 85 mm Hg. At the start of the trial, 38% of the subjects were hypertensive. Subjects were randomly assigned to one of three groups: Advice-Only, Established, and Established-plus-DASH. The Advice-Only group received one counseling session with a nutritionist; the Established group received both individual and group counseling sessions and was encouraged to keep a diet and activity log; and the Established-plus-DASH group received the same intervention schedule as the Established group but was taught to follow the DASH diet plan as well. All three groups received printed materials containing information and recommendations on blood pressure and lifestyle modification. A reduction in blood pressure was demonstrated in all

TABLE 8.3
Following the DASH Eating Plan*

Food Group	Daily Servings (except as noted)	Serving Sizes	Examples and Notes	Significance of Each Food Group to the DASH Eating Plan
Grains and grain products	7–8	1 slice bread 1 oz dry cereal[†] ½ cup cooked rice, pasta, or cereal	Whole-wheat bread, English muffin, pita bread, bagel, cereals, grits, oatmeal, crackers, unsalted pretzels, and popcorn	Major sources of energy and fiber
Vegetables	4–5	1 cup raw leafy vegetable ½ cup cooked vegetable 6 oz vegetable juice	Tomatoes, potatoes, carrots, green peas, squash, broccoli, turnip greens, collards, kale, spinach, artichokes, green beans, lima beans, sweet potatoes	Rich sources of potassium, magnesium, and fiber
Fruits	4–5	6 oz fruit juice 1 medium fruit ½ cup dried fruit ½ cup fresh, frozen, or canned fruit	Apricots, bananas, dates, grapes, oranges, orange juice, grapefruit, grapefruit juice, mangoes, melons, peaches, pineapples, prunes, raisins, strawberries, tangerines	Important sources of potassium, magnesium, and fiber
Low-fat or fat-free dairy foods	2–3	8 oz milk 1 cup yogurt 1½ oz cheese	Fat-free (skim) or low-fat (1%) milk, fat-free or low-fat buttermilk, fat-free or low-fat regular or frozen yogurt, low-fat and fat-free cheese	Major sources of calcium and protein
Meats, poultry, and fish	2 or less	3 oz cooked meats, poultry, or fish	Select only lean; trim away visible fats; broil, roast, or boil instead of frying; remove skin from poultry	Rich sources of protein and magnesium
Nuts, seeds, and dry beans	4–5 per week	⅓ cup or 1½ oz nuts 2 Tbsp or ½ oz seeds ½ cup cooked dry beans	Almonds, filberts, mixed nuts, peanuts, walnuts, sunflower seeds, kidney beans, lentils, peas	Rich sources of energy, magnesium, potassium, protein, and fiber
Fats and oils[‡]	2–3	1 tsp soft margarine 1 Tbsp low-fat mayonnaise 2 Tbsp light salad dressing 1 tsp vegetable oil	Soft margarine, low-fat mayonnaise, light salad dressing, vegetable oil (such as olive, corn, canola, or safflower)	DASH has 27% of calories as fat, including fat in or added to foods
Sweets	5 per week	1 Tbsp sugar 1 Tbsp jelly or jam ½ oz jelly beans 8 oz lemonade	Maple syrup, sugar, jelly, jam, fruit-flavored gelatin, jelly beans, hard candy, fruit punch, sorbet, ices	Sweets should be low in fat

*The Dietary Approaches to Stop Hypertension (DASH) eating plan shown here is based on 2,000 kcal per day. The number of daily servings in a food group may vary from those listed, depending on an individual's caloric needs. This chart can be used to help plan menus, or individual's can take it with them when they go to the store.

[†]Equals ½–1¼ cups, depending on cereal type. Check the product's Nutrition Facts Label.

[‡]Fat content changes serving counts for fats and oils: For example, 1 Tbsp of regular salad dressing equals 1 serving; 1 Tbsp of a low-fat dressing equals ½ serving; 1 Tbsp of a fat-free dressing equals 0 servings.

Source: Adapted from reference 20.

three groups after 6 months, but the reduction was greatest in the Established-plus-DASH group. On average, SBP and DBP decreased by 11.1 mm Hg and 6.4 mm Hg, respectively, in the Established-plus-DASH group. In addition, the percentage of those subjects with hypertension in the Established-plus-DASH group decreased 25% compared with 12% in the Advice-Only group. Another key result of this trial was that significant weight loss occurred in all three groups. The authors concluded that not only was it feasible and realis-

TABLE 8.4
Nutrient Comparison of Dietary Approaches to Stop Hypertension (DASH) "Combination Diet" and Control Diet

Nutrient	DASH Diet	Control Diet
Total fat (% of total kcal)	26	36
Saturated fat	7	14
Monounsaturated fat	10	12
Polyunsaturated fat	7	6
Carbohydrate (% of total kcal)	57	51
Protein (% of total kcal)	18	14
Cholesterol (mg/d)	151	233
Potassium (mg/d)	4415	1752
Magnesium (mg/d)	480	176
Calcium (mg/d)	1265	443
Sodium (mg/d)	2859	3028

Source: Data are from reference 18.

tic for Americans to follow the DASH diet, but they could lose weight and reduce their risk of developing high blood pressure while doing so.

Sodium

Sodium is the nutrient most often linked to high blood pressure, and it is the nutrient that has received the most attention from investigators. It is widely accepted that sodium restriction is associated with lower blood pressure, particularly among older, hypertensive, or African-American individuals. It is debatable whether younger individuals derive a blood pressure benefit from a sodium restriction as well.

A plethora of scientific evidence has linked a high sodium intake with high blood pressure (22), and several clinical trials, including TONE, TOPH Phase II, and the DASH Sodium trial (23), have demonstrated that hypertensive and normotensive individuals can achieve a reduction in blood pressure with moderate reductions in daily sodium intake (40 to 50 mEq [920 to 1,150 mg]).

Increased sodium intake does not elevate blood pressure in all individuals. Studies that have looked at individual differences in blood pressure response to sodium intake have used a very-low-sodium diet (10 to 20 mEq/day [230 to 460 mg/day]) for several days followed by a very high sodium intake, provided as a saline intravenous infusion or a diet supplemented with sodium chloride tablets. Individuals who experience a blood pressure rise in response to a high-sodium diet or a fall in blood pressure with sodium restriction are referred to as "salt sensitive." Several factors are thought to influence salt sensitivity, including obesity, age, race, plasma renin level, sympathetic nervous system activity, and presence of other diseases such as diabetes or renal failure (24). Approximately 50% of hypertensive and approximately 25% of normotensive individuals are salt sensitive. The prevalence of salt-sensitive hypertensive African Americans is thought to approach 75% (24).

Salt-sensitive individuals may benefit most from sodium restriction (24). It is difficult to accurately predict who will respond favorably to sodium restriction. It is reasonable to expect that most hypertensive individuals would benefit by moderately restricting sodium intake to no more than 100 mEq/day (approximately 2,300 mg) (2). Extreme sodium restriction is discouraged because it may result in deleterious effects on cardiovascular morbidity and mortality (25).

The DASH-Sodium trial (23), like DASH, was a randomized controlled-feeding study of 412 persons with an average SBP of 120 to 159 mm Hg and an average DBP of 80 to 95 mm Hg. It compared the effects of three different dietary sodium intake levels, as measured by 24-hour urine collections, on blood pressure in patients assigned to either the DASH diet or a typical American diet. A reduction in daily sodium intake from a high level of 142 mEq (approximately 3,300 mg) to an intermediate level of 107 mEq (approximately 2,400 mg) reduced SBP by 2.1 mm Hg with the usual American control diet and by 1.3 mm Hg with the DASH diet. The lower sodium diet of 65 mEq/day (1,500 mg/day) resulted in an additional reduction in SBP of 4.6 mm Hg with the control diet and 1.7 mm Hg with the DASH diet. These findings are consistent with the current US Department of Agriculture Dietary Guidelines for Americans, which recommend a moderate daily intake of dietary sodium of 2,000 to 3,000 mg (approximately 6 g of sodium chloride). Compared with the higher-sodium control diet, the DASH diet with lower sodium reduced SBP by 7.1 mm Hg in normotensive individuals and by 11.5 mm Hg in hypertensive individuals. Thus, the DASH-Sodium trial demonstrated that the combined effect on blood pressure of a lower sodium intake and a diet rich in fruits, vegetables, and low-fat dairy and low in saturated fat is greater than the effect of either the DASH diet or reduced sodium intake alone. This combined dietary effect on blood pressure was similar to that of single-drug therapy for hypertensive participants. In addition, reducing sodium intake with either the control diet or the DASH diet resulted in a lower SBP in both normotensive and hypertensive participants, providing a scientific basis for the current dietary sodium recommendations.

Evidence from clinical trials has demonstrated that a moderate reduction in sodium intake is associated with a reduction in blood pressure levels in both hypertensive and normotensive individuals. Thus, a recommendation to limit dietary sodium intake directed at all Americans is essential for the primary prevention of hypertension in the US population. Data from NHANES between 1974 and 1994 suggest an increasing trend in sodium intake, which is not surprising considering the increasing consumption of commercially prepared foods and foods eaten outside the home (26). Current daily consumption of sodium in the United States is estimated to be between 140 and 150 mEq (approximately 3.5 grams sodium or 8 to 9 grams salt) (27).

National Recommendations for Dietary Sodium Intake

The American Heart Association (28) and JNC 7 (2) guidelines recommend a dietary sodium intake of no more than 2.4 g (2,400 mg) or approximately 100 mEq sodium per day (1 mEq sodium = 1 mmol sodium = 23 mg sodium). This translates to 6 g sodium chloride (table salt) per day (2). Citing the adverse effects of high sodium intakes on blood pressure levels as its scientific rationale, the Institute of Medicine has set a tolerable upper intake level (UL) of 2.3 g (2,300 mg or 100 mEq) of sodium per day. An adequate intake level (AI) of 1.5 g (1,500 mg or 65 mEq) of sodium per day is recommended for young adults 50 years of age and younger (29). To achieve a diet in the range of 2,000 to 3,000 mg/day of sodium, the use of salt should be limited. It can be replaced with herbs, spices, natural flavorings, or lower sodium seasonings and condiments. Minimally processed foods should be encouraged because many processed foods (including low-fat choices) can be significant sources of sodium (see Table 8.5) (30). Because foods prepared outside of the home often contain added salt, more home preparation of food and care in food selection when dining in restaurants are advised.

Since the Nutrition Labeling and Education Act of 1990 (NLEA), most processed foods display the Nutrition Facts panel, which provides sodium content to help monitor intake. During

TABLE 8.5
Sodium Content of Foods

Food	Sodium Content (mg)
Condiments and Miscellaneous Food	
Bacon bits (0.25 oz)	220
Barbeque sauce (1 Tbsp)	150–200
Bouillon (1 cube)	1200
Salad dressing (1 Tbsp)	125–280
Garlic and onion salt (1 tsp)	1480
Catsup (1 Tbsp)	150–200
Mustard, prepared (1 tsp)	65–80
Olives (1 medium)	35–100
Pickle relish (1 Tbsp)	120–165
Pickles, sweet or dill (1 large)	330–830
Regular soy sauce (1 Tbsp)	800–900
Steak sauce (1 Tbsp)	250–300
Teriyaki sauce (1 Tbsp)	650–700
Worcestershire sauce (1 Tbsp)	200–250
Baking powder, regular (1 tsp)	400–550
Baking soda, regular (1 tsp)	1370
Canned Foods	
Deviled ham (1.5 oz)	380
Soup (⅓ cup)	490–860
Tuna/salmon (⅓ cup)	250–325
Sauerkraut (½ cup)	780
Tomato sauce (½ cup)	150–370
Snack Foods	
Brownie (2 inch square)	50–150
Cake (1/12 cake)	115–430
Pretzels (1 oz)	500–700
Potato or corn chips (1 oz)	150–300
Dairy	
Cheese, American (1 oz)	400
Cheese, cheddar (1 oz)	180
Meat and Meat Products	
Sausage, smoked 1 link	400–500
Bologna (1 slice)	300
Frankfurter, beef (2 oz)	600
Ham, cured boiled (1 oz)	275
Fast Foods	
Cheeseburger, 1 sandwich	790
Double cheeseburger	1220
Chicken tenders, 6 pieces	670
French fries, (medium)	290

Source: Data are from reference 30.

the last several decades, many lower sodium products have become available, offering greater variety to individuals who wish to maintain a low-sodium diet. The NLEA regulates nutrient-content claims used on food packages to describe the amount of nutrients per serving. Labeling claims for the sodium content of foods and beverages include the following:

- Low: less than or equal to 140 mg sodium per serving; products labeled "no added salt" are usually low in sodium but are not sodium-free because they contain naturally occurring sodium.

- Reduced or less: at least 25% less sodium per reference amount.
- Light or lite: at least 50% less sodium per reference amount. A "lightly salted" product has 50% less added sodium than is normally added to the food; the label must declare "not a low sodium food" if the product contains 140 mg sodium or more.

In some products, potassium chloride may be substituted for sodium chloride. Patients should check with their physician before using potassium chloride supplements or "salt sub-stitutes" because the additional potassium may be contraindicated in certain conditions, such as renal insufficiency and CVD. Potassium supplements should also be avoided when taking certain medications, such as angiotensin-converting enzyme (ACE) inhibitors and potassium-sparing diuretics, because of the possibility of drug-nutrient interactions.

Potassium

Observational studies have shown that a high potassium intake is beneficial in reducing blood pressure in both the general population and individuals with high blood pressure. This effect appears to be greater among African Americans, the elderly, and individuals consuming a high-sodium diet (31). Several small intervention studies have shown that potassium supple-mentation results in a modest hypotensive effect. A meta-analysis performed by Whelton et al (31) identified 33 randomized, controlled trials in both hypertensive ($n = 2,565$) and nor-motensive ($n = 1,005$) individuals, in which the effect of dietary potassium on blood pressure was assessed. With median potassium supplementation of 75 mEq per day (approximately 3,000 mg), significant but modest reductions of 3 mm Hg SBP and 2 mm Hg DSP were demonstrated. Interestingly, there was a greater reduction in blood pressure among subjects with higher levels of urinary sodium excretion.

Several mechanisms have been proposed to explain the blood pressure–lowering effects of potassium supplementation. These include naturesis, inhibition of renin release, and direct arterial vasodilatation via decreased thromboxane production. Foods high in potassium include oranges, orange juice, potatoes (especially with the skins), and bananas (refer to Table 8.6) (30). In the United States, the combination of increased consumption of processed foods, which are low in potassium, and a reduction in fruit and vegetable intake has resulted in low-potassium diets. The average potassium intake in the United States varies between 30 and 100 mEq per day (1,200 to 4,000 mg) (32). The DASH diet, which includes 8 to 10 servings of fruits and vegetables per day, helps to ensure a higher potassium intake. This may have con-tributed to the efficacy of the DASH diet in lowering blood pressure in the DASH trials.

The kidney closely regulates potassium balance so that excretion matches intake. How-ever, urinary excretion of potassium is influenced by many factors, including sodium con-centration. Potassium supplementation has a more pronounced effect on lowering blood pres-sure when sodium intake is high than when sodium intake is low (33). The urinary ratio of sodium to potassium also appears to be more closely associated with blood pressure response than is intake or excretion of either mineral alone. A high concentration of sodium in the dis-tal tubules of the kidney enhances urinary potassium excretion. Diuretic therapy, a first line modality for treating hypertension, frequently induces potassium wasting. Increasing dietary potassium intake in these patients may obviate the need for synthetic potassium supplements, which require close monitoring.

In addition to its hypotensive effect, potassium supplementation may have an effect on reducing the risk of stroke. Bazzano et al (34), using the participants (9,805 US adults) in the

TABLE 8.6
Potassium Content of Foods

Food	Potassium Content (mg)
Vegetables (½ cup serving unless otherwise noted)	
Asparagus (6 spears)	144
Beans, kidney, boiled	357
Beans, lentils, boiled	365
Beans, black, boiled	306
Lima beans, boiled	370
Broccoli, boiled, chopped	166
Broccoli, raw, chopped	143
Brussels sprouts, boiled	247
Carrot, raw, 1 medium	233
Carrots, boiled	177
Cauliflower, raw	152
Cauliflower, boiled	125
Celery, raw, 1 stalk	115
Corn, canned	160
Green beans, boiled	185
Peas, canned	147
Potato, baked with skin	844
Potato, boiled without skin	512
Sweet potato, baked with skin	397
Spinach, boiled	419
Tomato, raw, 1 medium	273
Tomato juice, 6 fl oz	400
Zucchini, raw	161
Fruits and Fruit Juices	
Apple, with skin, 1 medium	159
Apricots, fresh, 3 medium	314
Avocado, 1 medium	1097
Banana, 1 medium	451
Fig, 1 medium	116
Fruit cocktail, canned, juice pack, ½ cup	118
Cherries, sweet, 10 raw	152
Cantaloupe, 1 cup cubed	494
Mango, 1 medium	323
Peach, 1 medium	171
Grapefruit, raw, ½ medium	175
Oranges, navel, 1 medium	233
Watermelon, 1 cup cubed	186
Papaya, 1 medium	781
Pineapple, canned, juice pack, 1 cup	305
Prunes, dried, cooked, ½ cup	354
Strawberries, fresh, 1 cup	247
Apricot nectar, 8 fl oz, canned	286
Orange juice, 8 fl oz from frozen concentrate	473
Prune juice, 8 fl oz, canned	707
Miscellaneous	
Milk, low-fat, 8 fl oz	381
All-Bran cereal, Kellogg's, ½ cup	310
Raisin Bran cereal, Post, 1 cup	380
Almonds, dry roasted, 1 oz	218
Peanuts, dry roasted, 1 oz	187
Salt Substitutes (containing potassium chloride)	
Morton lite salt, ⅛ tsp	350
Morton salt substitute, ⅛ tsp	600
Morton seasoned salt substitute, ⅛ tsp	480

Manufacturers: Kellogg's, Battle Creek, MI 49016; Post Cereal (division of Kraft Foods), Northfield, IL 60093; Morton Salt, Chicago, IL 60606.

Source: Data are from reference 30.

first National Health and Nutrition Examination Survey (NHANES I) Epidemiologic Follow-up Study, examined the relationship between a low-potassium diet and the risk of stroke and CHD. Study participants who were followed for an average of 19 years had 927 stroke and 1,847 CHD events. After adjusting for several CVD risk factors, those who had consumed the lowest quartile of potassium experienced a 28% higher risk of stroke than the remainder of the cohort. Similarly, in two much larger cohorts, the US Health Professional Follow-up Study and the Nurses' Health Study (35), a high potassium intake was associated with a lower risk of stroke. Epidemiologic studies identify association but do not confirm causality. Therefore, randomized clinical trials of potassium supplementation and risk of stroke are needed to demonstrate the exact nature of this association.

Calcium and Magnesium

An interesting aspect of the association between blood pressure and intakes of calcium and magnesium is that the metabolism of each of these minerals is interrelated with sodium metabolism. Urinary calcium excretion is more closely associated with dietary levels of sodium than dietary levels of calcium. In fact, the association between sodium intake and blood pressure is strongest when calcium intake is low (36). In general, studies have shown a small and inconsistent effect on blood pressure lowering with calcium supplementation (37). However, an adequate calcium intake is essential for a healthy diet. The inclusion of two to three servings of low-fat dairy products per day as part of the DASH diet did reduce blood pressure more than the fruit and vegetable diet. The dietary reference intake (DRI) for calcium is 1,000 mg/day for adults ages 19 to 50 and 1,200 mg/day for adults older than 50 (38).

Magnesium's interaction with sodium is the least understood of the minerals examined. Current evidence suggests only a weak and inconsistent hypotensive effect of magnesium on blood pressure (39). A meta-analysis performed by Jee et al noted a dose-dependent reduction in blood pressure from magnesium supplementation; however, more clinical trials are needed to confirm this relationship (40). Therefore, magnesium supplementation is not recommended at this time, but it is still important to eat a varied diet containing foods high in magnesium. Dietary sources of magnesium include dark-green leafy vegetables, legumes, beans, nuts, and whole grains, all of which are also high in fiber. With the increased consumption of processed foods, dietary intake of magnesium has decreased. The DRI for magnesium is 310 mg/day for women ages 19 to 30, 320 mg/day for women older than 30 years, 400 mg/day for men ages 19 to 30, and 420 mg/day for men older than 30 years (38).

Dietary modifications for the management of hypertension should include an emphasis on foods rich in calcium, potassium, and magnesium in the diet plan and a reduction in high-sodium foods. Increased intakes of calcium, potassium, and magnesium should augment the effectiveness of sodium restriction on blood pressure response. For individuals who are at reasonable body weights and are not responsive to sodium restriction, increased intakes of these other minerals may provide an additional means for improving blood pressure response with or without medications.

Physical Activity

Individuals who participate in moderate physical activity have a lower mortality rate than individuals who are sedentary. The amount of physical activity is much more important than achieving a high level of cardiorespiratory fitness (41). Therefore, sedentary individuals can favorably affect their risk profile by walking for as little as 10 minutes three times daily. Individuals should be encouraged, however, to strive for an activity level that increases fitness in addition to decreasing their risk of disease.

Physical activity influences blood pressure and overall CVD risk. Numerous epidemiologic studies have suggested an inverse association between physical activity and blood pressure levels. An extensive body of evidence now strongly supports the assertion that physical activity, in the context of a healthy lifestyle, may delay or prevent the development of hypertension. (42). The risk for high blood pressure is thought to increase by as much as 30% to 50% in sedentary individuals (43). Other reported benefits to regular physical activity besides reduction in blood pressure levels are discussed in Chapter 5.

In both normotensive and hypertensive adults, significant reductions in blood pressure have been achieved with moderate aerobic physical activity, such as walking, jogging, cycling, or swimming, performed routinely three to five times per week (44). In a recent meta-analysis of 54 randomized, controlled clinical trials, Whelton et al (43) found significant postexercise reductions for both SBP and DBP levels of 3.8 and 2.6 mm Hg, respectively. Aerobic exercise had a slightly greater effect on blood pressure in hypertensive compared with normotensive participants.

A number of interventional studies support the effectiveness of regular aerobic exercise in reducing blood pressure in people with mild to moderate hypertension (45,46). The magnitude of reduction is approximately 8 to 11 mm Hg for SBP and 7 to 8 mm Hg for DBP. In these studies, no gender, race, or age-related differences were seen in blood pressure response to exercise, and the effects appeared to be independent of weight changes (12,46).

Resistance or strength training exercise (weight lifting) has not consistently demonstrated a reduction in blood pressure levels (47). Therefore, the American College of Sports Medicine (ACSM) does not recommend strength training as the only form of exercise for individuals with elevated blood pressure (48). Aerobic exercise more effectively modifies CVD risk factors. In the past, patients with heart disease were advised to avoid resistance exercises because of the risk of dysrhythmia and the fear of an exaggerated blood pressure response. However, when appropriately prescribed, resistance exercises are critical for maintaining flexibility, bone health, and strength, especially in older people, and should therefore be an adjunct to a general health and fitness program. Contraindications to resistance training include unstable angina, uncontrolled hypertension (SBP ≥ 160 Hg or DBP ≥ 100 mm Hg), uncontrolled dysrhythmias, and recent onset of congestive heart failure (49).

The mechanisms by which physical activity mediates a reduction in blood pressure are complex and poorly understood. A single bout of physical activity can have an immediate and temporary dilating effect on peripheral blood vessels. However, exercise training can attenuate the sympathetic nervous system, which may cause a hypotensive effect by reducing the activity of the renin-angiotensin system, thereby promoting vasodilatation. The concomitant improvement in insulin sensitivity reduces circulating insulin levels, which may in turn contribute to blood pressure reduction by decreasing insulin-mediated sodium reabsorption by the kidney (41). Improved endothelial function has also been suggested as another possible mechanism (46).

The JNC 7 guidelines recommend 30 minutes of regular aerobic physical activity, such as brisk walking, on most days of the week (2). This recommendation is consistent with recommendations from the ACSM (50), as well as from the Centers for Disease Control and Prevention and the Surgeon General's Report on Physical Activity and Health (41). A moderate-intensity physical activity is considered to be 60% to 79% of predicted maximum heart rate

(PMHR; 220 minus the subject's age) (46). Walking at a brisk pace of 3 to 4 miles per hour qualifies as a moderate-intensity activity. Some authors have concluded that moderate exercise has a blood pressure–lowering effect similar to or possibly even greater than vigorous exercise, although few studies have directly compared the effects of different exercise intensities on blood pressure reduction (42). Although more studies addressing this issue are needed, getting individuals to participate in a moderate activity, such as walking, is probably more realistic and achievable than expecting them to engage in high-intensity activities. Patients need to know the level of exercise intensity that is safe for them. Additional recommendations to assist patients in their efforts to exercise are discussed in Chapter 5.

Alcohol

A large number of epidemiologic studies have established a relationship between alcohol consumption and blood pressure (51). Chronic excess consumption of alcohol can adversely affect blood pressure and blood pressure responsiveness to antihypertensive medications (52). Sustained elevation in blood pressure resulting from heavy alcohol consumption has been estimated to account for about 3% to 12% of diagnosed cases of hypertension (53). In the Atherosclerosis Risk in Communities Study, one in five cases of hypertension were estimated to be attributed to a daily intake of alcohol equal to or greater than 30 g (54).

Numerous epidemiologic studies support the J-shaped relationship of alcohol consumption and CVD (55). Nondrinkers and heavy drinkers have higher rates of CVD mortality than do moderate drinkers (see Figure 8.3) (56). Moderate alcohol consumption is shown to be associated with a lower incidence of atherosclerotic CVD. The cardioprotective effects associated with alcohol intake may be related to increases in high-density lipoprotein and

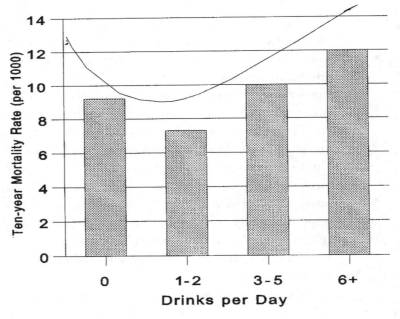

FIGURE 8.3
Total mortality rate compared with alcohol consumption. The J-shaped curve shows that moderate drinkers appear to live longer than either heavy drinkers or abstainers. Adapted with permission from Klatsky AL, Friedman GD, Siegelaub AB. Alcohol and mortality. A ten-year Kaiser-Permanente experience. Ann Intern Med. 1981;95:139-145.

apolipoproteins A-I and A-II, antioxidant polyphenols (quercetin, resveratrol, catechin), and reduced platelet aggregation (52,57,58).

Randomized clinical trials support the association between chronic alcohol consumption and elevated blood pressure. Results from a meta-analysis of 15 clinical trials demonstrate that alcohol reduction was associated with a significant reduction in mean SBP and DBP of 3.3 mm Hg and 2.0 mm Hg, respectively. Those with higher blood pressure levels at baseline demonstrated a greater reduction in blood pressure following the intervention (51). In addition, the greater the reduction in alcohol intake, the greater was the observed response in blood pressure reduction. A rule of thumb derived from these studies is that for each reduction in alcoholic drink per day both SBP and DBP is lowered by approximately 1 mm Hg (52).

It appears that the relationship between alcohol and blood pressure is dependent on the amount and not the type of alcohol ingested. The relationship is independent of the effects of obesity, smoking, and a high sodium intake (55). A standard drink in the United States is defined as 14 g of alcohol. This amount of alcohol is in 12 ounces of beer, 5 ounces of table wine, and 1.5 ounces of 80 proof (40% alcohol) liquor. Both the epidemiologic and randomized controlled trials provide strong evidence that in persons who drink three or more alcoholic drinks per day, a reduction in alcohol consumption can effectively lower blood pressure (52,54).

Several potential mechanisms have been identified for the relationship between alcohol and elevated blood pressure, including hormonal and catecholaminergic effects, increased vascular tone, and abdominal obesity. Although an immediate effect of alcohol intake is vasodilation, sustained chronic alcohol intake is associated with increased formation of the vasoconstrictor, thromboxane (52).

In addition to its effects on blood pressure, increased alcohol consumption is associated with an increased risk of cardiomyopathy, hemorrhagic and ischemic strokes, certain cancers, cirrhosis, pancreatitis, gastritis, suicides, and accidents (52,57). Therefore, the current public health recommendation is moderation in alcohol consumption, which is defined as two drinks per day for men and one drink per day for women (28). With 7 kcal/g, alcohol also contributes empty (nutrient-poor) energy to the diet and can displace nutrient-dense foods. In patients where weight reduction is a consideration, abstaining from alcohol can aid in weight management. During clinical encounters, all hypertensive patients should be questioned about their current drinking habits, including quantity and frequency.

SUMMARY

Extensive research documenting the specific mechanisms and all aspects of blood pressure homeostasis support the efficacy of dietary and lifestyle factors on the prevention and treatment of high blood pressure. Blood pressure may be either favorably or adversely affected by dietary factors through effects on plasma volume and cardiac output; sympathetic nervous system activity and peripheral vascular resistance; concentrations of vasoactive prostacyclins, thromboxanes, and cytokines; and membrane ion transport activity.

The control of blood pressure by dietary means offers an approach to the management of all patients with hypertension. Dietary and lifestyle changes often reduce and sometimes eliminate the need for medications and the development of adverse drug side effects that may accompany high dosages. In clinical practice, a nonpharmacologic approach to the treatment of hypertension should emphasize weight control; moderate sodium restriction; moderation of alcohol intake; a diet rich in food sources of calcium, potassium, and magnesium; and physical activity. These nonpharmacologic approaches, although small, can have an enormous impact when applied to whole population groups.

REFERENCES

1. National High Blood Pressure Education Program Coordinating Committee. Primary prevention of hypertension: clinical and public health advisory from the National High Blood Pressure Education Program. *JAMA*. 2002;288:1882-1888.
2. National High Blood Pressure Education Program Coordinating Committee. The seventh report of the Joint National Committee on Prevention, Detection, Evaluation, and Treatment of High Blood Pressure. The JNC 7 Report. *JAMA*. 2003;289:2560-2572.
3. Reaven GM, Lithell H, Landsburg L. Hypertension and associated metabolic abnormalities: the role of insulin resistance and the sympathoadrenal system. *N Engl J Med*. 1996;334:374-381.
4. Vasan RS, Larson MG, Leip EP, Kannel WB, Levy D. Assessment of frequency of progression to hypertension in nonhypertensive participants in the Framingham Heart Study: a cohort study. *Lancet*. 2001;358:1682-1686.
5. Hajjar I, Kotchen T. Trends in the prevalence, awareness, treatment, and control of hypertension in the United States, 1988–2000. *JAMA*. 2003;290:199-206.
6. US Department of Health and Human Services; *Healthy People 2010*. 2nd ed. Washington, DC: US Department of Health and Human Services; 2000.
7. Flegal KM, Carroll MD, Ogden CL, Johnson CL. Prevalence and trends in obesity among US adults, 1999–2000. *JAMA*. 2002;288:1723-1727.
8. Brown CD, Higgins M, Donato KA, Rohde FC, Garrison R, Obarzanek E, Ernst ND, Horan M. Body mass index and the prevalence of hypertension and dyslipidemia. *Obes Res*. 2000;8:605-619.
9. Reisin E. Weight reduction in the management of hypertension: epidemiologic and mechanistic evidence. *Can J Physiol Pharmacol*. 1986;64:818-824.
10. Landsberg L, Krieger DR. Obesity, metabolism and the sympathetic nervous system. *Am J Hypertension*. 1989;2:125S-132S.
11. Thakur V, Zhang R, Morse S, Reisin E. Obesity Hypertension: the effects on cardiovascular and renal systems. *Cardiovasc Rev Rep*. 2002;23:213-219.
12. National Heart, Lung, and Blood Institute, *Clinical Guidelines on the Identification, Evaluation, and Treatment of Overweight and Obesity in Adults: The Evidence Report*. Bethesda, Md: National Institutes of Health; 1998. NIH publication 98-4083. Available at: http://www.nhlbi.nih.gov/guidelines/obesity/ob_gdlns.pdf. Accessed April 22, 2004.
13. Mark AL, Correia ML, Rahmouni K, Haynes WG. Selective leptin resistance: a new concept in leptin physiology with cardiovascular implications. *J Hypertens*. 2002;20:1245-1250.
14. Neter JE, Stam BE, Kok FJ, Grobbee DE, Geleijnse JM. Influence of weight reduction on blood pressure. A meta-analysis of randomized controlled trials. *Hypertension*. 2003;42:878-884.
15. TONE Collaborative Research Group. Sodium reduction and weight loss in the treatment of hypertension in older persons: a randomized controlled trial of nonpharmacologic interventions in the elderly (TONE). *JAMA*. 1998;279:839-846.
16. The Trials of Hypertension Prevention Collaborative Research Group. The effects of non-pharmacologic interventions on blood pressure of persons with high normal levels: results of the Trials of Hypertension Prevention, Phase I. *JAMA*. 1992;267:1213-1220.
17. The Trials of Hypertension Prevention Collaborative Research Group. Effects of weight loss and sodium reduction intervention on blood pressure and hypertension incidence in overweight people with high-normal blood pressure: the Trials of Hypertension Prevention, Phase II. *Arch Intern Med*. 1997;157:657-667.
18. Appel LJ, Moore TJ, Obarzanek E, Vollmer WM, Svetkey LP, Sacks FM, Bray GA, Vogt TM, Cutler JA, Windhauser MM, Lin PH, Karanja N. A clinical trial of the effects of dietary patterns on blood pressure. *N Engl J Med*. 1997;336:1117-1124.
19. Svetkey LP, Simons-Morton D, Vollmer WM, Appel LJ, Conlin PR, Ryan DH, Ard J, Kennedy BM. Effects of dietary patterns on blood pressure. Subgroup analysis of the dietary approaches to stop hypertension (DASH) randomized clinical trial. *Arch Intern Med*. 1999;159:285-293.
20. National Heart, Lung, and Blood Institute. *Facts about the DASH Eating Plan*. Bethesda, Md: National Institutes of Health; 2003. NIH publication 03-4082. Available at: http://www.nhlbi.nih.gov/health/public/heart/hbp/dash/new_dash.pdf. Accessed April 22, 2004.
21. Working Group of the PREMIER Collaborative Research Group. Effects of comprehensive lifestyle modification on blood pressure control. Main results of the PREMIER clinical trial. *JAMA*. 2003;289:2083-2093.
22. Chobanian AV, Hill M. National Heart, Lung, and Blood Institute Workshop on sodium and blood pressure. A critical review of current scientific evidence. *Hypertension*. 2000;35:858-863.
23. Sacks FM, Svetkey LP, Vollmer WM, Appel LJ, Bray GA, Harsha D, Obaranek E, Conlin PR, Miller ER III, Simons-Morton DG, Karanja N, Lin PH, for the DASH-Sodium Collaborative Research Group. Effects on

blood pressure of reduced dietary sodium and the Dietary Approaches to Stop Hypertension (DASH) diet. *N Engl J Med.* 2001;344:3-10.

24. Weinberger MH. Salt sensitivity of blood pressure in humans. *Hypertension.* 1996;27:481-490.

25. Alderman MH. Salt, blood pressure, and human health. *Hypertension.* 2000;36:890-893.

26. Loria, CM, Obarzanek E, Ernst ND. Choose and prepare foods with less salt: dietary advice for all Americans. *J Nutr.* 2001;131:536S-551S.

27. Elliott P. Salt and blood pressure. In: Izzo JL Jr, Black HR, eds. *Hypertension Primer: The Essentials of High Blood Pressure.* 3rd ed. Dallas, Tex: American Heart Association; 2003:277-279.

28. American Heart Association Scientific Statement, AHA Dietary Guidelines. Revision 2000: a statement for healthcare professionals from the Nutrition Committee of the American Heart Association. *Circulation.* 2000;102:2284-2299.

29. Institute of Medicine. *Dietary Reference Intakes for Water, Potassium, Sodium, Chloride, and Sulfate.* Washington, DC: National Academy Press; 2004. Available at: http://www.nap.edu/books. Accessed March 30, 2004.

30. Pennington J. *Food Values of Portions Commonly Used.* 17th ed. Philadelphia, Pa: Lippincott; 1998.

31. Whelton PK, He J, Cutler JA, Brancati FL, Appel LJ, Follmann D, Klag MJ. Effects of oral potassium on blood pressure: meta-analysis of randomized controlled clinical trials. *JAMA.* 1997;277:1624-1632.

32. Suter PM, Sierro C, Vetter W. Nutritional factors in the control of blood pressure and hypertension. *Nutr Clin Care.* 2002;5:9-19.

33. Skrabal F, Aubock J, Hortagl H. Low sodium/high potassium diet for prevention of hypertension: possible mechanisms of action. *Lancet.* 1985;2:895-900.

34. Bazzano LA, He J, Ogden LG, Loria C, Vupputuri S, Myers L. Whelton PK. Dietary potassium intake and risk of stroke in US men and women. National Health and Nutrition Examination Survey I Epidemiologic Follow-up Study. *Stroke.* 2001;32:1473-1480.

35. Joshipura KJ, Ascherio A, Manson JE, Stampfer MJ, Rimm EB, Speizer FE, Hennekens CH, Spiegelman D, Willett WC. Fruit and vegetable intake in relation to risk of ischemic stroke. *JAMA.* 1999;282:1233-1239.

36. Kotchen TA, McCarron DA. Dietary electrolytes and blood pressure. A statement for healthcare professionals from the American Heart Association Nutrition Committee. *Circulation.* 1998;98:613-617.

37. Allender PS, Cutler JA, Follman D, Cappuccio FP, Pryer J, Elliot P. Dietary calcium and blood pressure: a meta-analysis of randomized clinical trials. *Arch Intern Med.* 1996;124:825-831.

38. Institute of Medicine. *Dietary Reference Intakes for Calcium, Phosphorus, Magnesium, Vitamin D, and Fluoride.* Washington, DC: National Academy Press; 1997. Available at: http://www.nap.edu/books. Accessed March 30, 2004.

39. Appel LJ. Calcium, magnesium, heavy metals and blood pressure. In: Izzo JL Jr, Black HR, eds. *Hypertension Primer: The Essentials of High Blood Pressure.* 3rd ed. Dallas, Tex: American Heart Association; 2003:283-285.

40. Jee SH, Miller ER III, Guallar E, Singh VK, Appel LJ, Klag MJ. The effect of magnesium supplementation on blood pressure: a meta-analysis of randomized clinical trials. *Am J Hypertens.* 2002;15:691-696.

41. National Center for Chronic Disease Prevention and Health Promotion. *Physical Activity and Health: A Report of the Surgeon General.* Atlanta, Ga: US Department of Health and Human Services, Centers for Disease Control and Prevention; 1996:103-112.

42. Simons-Morton DG. Physical activity and blood pressure. In: Izzo JL Jr, Black HR, eds. *Hypertension Primer: The Essentials of High Blood Pressure.* 3rd ed. Dallas, Tex: American Heart Association; 2003:288-290.

43. Whelton SP, Chin A, Xin X, He J. Effect of aerobic exercise on blood pressure: a meta-analysis of randomized, controlled trials. *Ann Intern Med.* 2002;136:493-503.

44. Kelley GA, Kelley KS, Tran ZV. Aerobic exercise and resting blood pressure: a meta-analytic review of randomized, controlled trials. *Prev Cardiol.* 2001;4:73-80.

45. Hagberg JM, Park JJ, Brown MD. The role of exercise training in the treatment of hypertension: an update. *Sports Med.* 2000;30:193-206.

46. Kokkinos PF, Narayan P, Papedemetriou V. Exercise as hypertension therapy. *Cardiol Clin.* 2001;19:507-516.

47. Kelley GA, Kelley KS. Progressive resistance exercise and resting blood pressure: a meta-analysis of randomized controlled trials. *Hypertension.* 2000;35:838-843.

48. American College of Sports Medicine. Position stand: exercise and hypertension. *Med Sci Sports Exerc.* 2004;36:533-553.

49. Pollock ML, Franklin BA, Balady GJ, Chaitman BL, Fleg JL, Fletcher B, Limacher M, Pina IL, Stein RA, Williams M, Bazzarre T. AHA Science Advisory. Resistance exercise in individuals with and without cardiovascular disease. Benefits, rationale, safety, and prescription. An advisory from the Committee on Exercise, Rehabilitation, and Prevention, Council on Clinical Cardiology, American Heart Association. *Circulation.* 2000;101:828-836.

50. American College of Sports Medicine. Position stand: the recommended quantity and quality of exercise for developing and maintaining cardiorespiratory and muscular fitness and flexibility in healthy adults. *Med Sci Sports Exerc.* 1998;30:975-991.

51. Xin X, He J, Frontini MG, Ogden LG, Motsamai OI, Whelton PK. Effects of alcohol reduction on blood pressure: a meta-analysis of randomized controlled trials. *Hypertension.* 2001;38:1112-1117.

52. Cushman WC. Alcohol use and blood pressure. In: Izzo JL Jr, Black HR, eds. *Hypertension Primer: The Essentials of High Blood Pressure.* 3rd ed. Dallas, Tex: American Heart Association; 2003:290-294.

53. Larbi EB, Stamler J, Dyer A, Cooper R, Paul O, Shekelle RB, Lepper M. The population attributable risk of hypertension from heavy alcohol consumption. *Public Health Rep.* 1984;99:316-319.

54. Fuchs FD, Chambless LE, Whelton PK, Nieto FJ, Heiss G. Alcohol consumption and the incidence of hypertension. The Atherosclerosis Risk in Communities Study. *Hypertension.* 2001;37:1242-1250.

55. Klatsky AL. Alcohol and hypertension. *Clin Chim Acta.* 1996;246:91-105.

56. Klatsky AL, Friedman GD, Siegelaub AB. Alcohol and mortality. A ten year Kaiser-Permanente experience. *Ann Intern Med.* 1981;95:139-145.

57. Goldberg IJ, Mosca L, Piano MR, Fisher EA. AHA Science Advisory. Wine and your heart. *Stroke.* 2001;103:591-594.

58. De Oliveira e Silva ER, Foster D, McGee Harper M, Seidman CE, Smith JD, Breslow JL, Brinton EA. Alcohol consumption raises HDL cholesterol levels by increasing the transport rate of apolipoproteins A-I and A-II. *Circulation.* 2000;102:2347-2352.

CHAPTER 9

PREVENTING CARDIOVASCULAR COMPLICATIONS IN DIABETES

Joyce P. Barnett, MS, RD, and Abhimanyu Garg, MD

INTRODUCTION

The importance of medical nutrition therapy (MNT) and the role of the registered dietitian in diabetes management have come to the forefront with the recognition that dietary modifications are an effective means to improve a patient's glucose control and prevent long-term complications in this chronic disease. The benefit of intensive lifestyle interventions upon glucose levels was recently highlighted by the results of the Diabetes Prevention Program. Including moderate-intensity daily physical activity and a low-fat diet reduced development of type 2 diabetes by 58% during a 3-year period in obese men and women with impaired glucose tolerance (1).

Diabetes is a significant risk factor for cardiovascular disease (CVD), and therefore there are links between MNT protocols for both of these conditions. MNT is provided with the goal of reaching biochemical measures established by an evidence base for reducing morbidity for coronary heart disease (CHD) and diabetes. As discussed in Chapter 3, the Third Adult Treatment Panel of the National Cholesterol Education Program (ATP III) has defined diabetes as a CHD equivalent. Therefore, the low-density lipoprotein (LDL) cholesterol goal for patients with diabetes is less than 100 mg/dL (2). As a measure of glycemic control, elevations in glycosylated hemoglobin (HbA_{1c}) have been linked to increased risk for cardiac events (3-5).

An article assessing the quality of diabetes care in the United States in the 1990s found that whereas 85% of patients with diabetes had their cholesterol checked every 2 years, only 42% had LDL cholesterol levels less than 130 mg/dL. Hemoglobin A_{1c} levels greater than 9.5% were reported in 18% of patients, and only 38% monitored their blood glucose level at least once a day (6). From this article, it appears that there is much room for improving the cardiovascular risk of patients with diabetes.

In 2002 the American Diabetes Association issued evidence-based guidelines for MNT in diabetes mellitus (7,8). The 2002 nutrition principles and recommendations address the importance of energy balance, as well as the proportion of energy from carbohydrate, protein, and fat in the diet. The purpose of this chapter is to review the nutrition recommendations, as well as discuss practical aspects of implementing a diet that has a positive influence on the overall health of the person with diabetes mellitus.

WEIGHT MANAGEMENT

Adequate energy must be provided for normal growth and development throughout the various stages of the life cycle. Determining energy needs for weight management is a key step in MNT for patients with diabetes. At the time of diagnosis, individuals with type 1 diabetes often need additional energy beyond maintenance levels. Energy needs are also increased during times of infection, in a postoperative period, or when chronic hyperglycemia occurs. The energy requirement for the person with type 2 diabetes is especially noteworthy in relation to both CVD and diabetes management. Because obesity increases a person's risk for type 2 diabetes, weight management is a critical element in the prevention of diabetes in the predisposed individual. Figure 4.3 in Chapter 4 illustrates the increasing degree of disease risk with increasing body mass index (BMI) and waist circumference as defined by the National Heart, Lung, and Blood Institute's (NHLBI's) *Clinical Guidelines on the Identification, Evaluation, and Treatment of Overweight and Obesity in Adults* (9). Obesity is a recognized risk factor for diabetes, hypertension, and CVD. Diet, physical activity, and behavioral therapy are the treatment modalities recommended when the BMI is 25 or higher, especially when comorbid conditions exist. A recent meta-analysis of clinical studies on the effect of weight loss in obese individuals with diabetes also concludes that people with diabetes should achieve and maintain a BMI of less than or equal to 25 (10). In many patients, however, this may not be practical. In those cases, smaller amounts of weight loss (5% to 10% of body weight) or a reduction of BMI by 2 can be beneficial.

A negative energy balance is required for someone to lose weight. The factors that can contribute to an energy deficit are reducing energy intake and increasing energy expenditure. A combination of these two methods increases the likelihood of achieving and maintaining a reduced body weight. Research supports the premise that even a small amount of weight loss, 5% to 15%, can improve glycemic control and serum lipid levels, as well as decrease blood pressure (1,11-14). Factors associated with successful maintenance of reduced body weight include consumption of a low-calorie, low-fat diet and continued physical activity (15,16).

In addition to overall adiposity, distribution of body fat is an important factor in assessment of risk for CVD and diabetes. Insulin resistance and risk for development of diabetes are increased with even mild truncal obesity (17,18). The threshold for development of insulin resistance in response to increased body fat varies in different ethnic groups and among individuals in those groups (19). Increased intra-abdominal fat, even in individuals not considered overweight by BMI classification, may be detrimental. Therefore, these individuals could benefit from a reduction in body fat.

Dietary Management

Table 9.1 (9) outlines the components of the low-calorie diet (LCD) in the *Clinical Guidelines on the Identification, Evaluation, and Treatment of Overweight and Obesity in Adults* (9). The LCD is one approach to achieve reduced energy intake. An LCD consists of 800 to 1,500 kcal/day to achieve weight loss of approximately 0.5 to 1 kg per week. This approach represents a reduction of 500 to 1,000 kcal/day, as suggested in the American Diabetes Association's

TABLE 9.1
Low-Calorie Diet

Nutrient	Recommended Daily Intake	Comments
Energy	500 to 1,000 kcal less than usual intake	Promotes weight loss of 1 to 2 lb/wk.
Total fat	30% or less of total energy intake	Fat-modified foods may be helpful, but must also be low in calories with no compensation from other foods.
Saturated fatty acids	8% to 10% of total energy intake	Reduce to <7% if hypercholesterolemic.
Monounsaturated fatty acids	Up to 15% of total energy intake	
Polyunsaturated fatty acids	Up to 10% of total energy intake	
Cholesterol	<300 mg	Reduce to <200 mg if hypercholesterolemic.
Protein	Approximately 15% of total energy intake	Choose from plant sources and lean animal protein.
Carbohydrate	55% or more of total energy intake	Choose complex carbohydrates from fruits, vegetables, and whole grains.
Sodium chloride	Approximately 2.4 g of sodium or 6 g of sodium chloride	
Calcium	1,000 to 1,500 mg	Choose low-fat dairy products. Maintain adequate intake of vitamins and other minerals during weight loss efforts.
Fiber	20 to 30 g	Choose foods high in soluble fiber. Recommended upper limit for fiber is 35 g.

Source: Adapted from reference 9.

guidelines and the NHLBI obesity guidelines (7-9). From a practical standpoint, a 1,000-kcal reduction can be difficult to sustain for an extended period of time. A different approach to achieve reduced intake is to decrease current intake by 250 to 500 kcal/day for a weight loss of 0.25 to 0.5 kg per week. This method requires a realistic account of current dietary intake, highlighting the importance of a detailed dietary history or accurate food intake records. Targeting a specific food or beverage that contributes a significant proportion of the energy in an individual's daily energy intake is an alternate technique to achieve the desired energy intake reduction. Patients are often able to pinpoint with good accuracy one or more food items that contribute to excess energy intake.

Very-low-calorie diets (VLCDs) that provide less than 800 kcal/day have been effectively used to achieve rapid weight loss; however, long-term results for VLCDs are no better than for LCDs (9). A VLCD is not recommended for mildly overweight individuals (BMI < 30). A VLCD requires close medical supervision for safe implementation. Significant side effects include rapid loss of lean body mass, electrolyte imbalances, cardiac arrhythmias, gout, and gallstones.

Controversy exists about whether a high-carbohydrate or a high-fat diet is more effective in causing weight loss. Studies have revealed that total energy consumption is higher on a high-fat diet than a high-carbohydrate diet (20,21). Longer studies are needed to determine whether the excess energy consumption on the high-fat diet continues long term. It is also unclear whether those cultures habituated to a high-carbohydrate diet, such as Asian or African cultures, would consume excess energy if given a high-fat diet similar to the one consumed in the United States.

Studies show that reduction in total energy is more important than the source of the energy for achieving weight loss (22). Although the high-fat, low-carbohydrate diet has been promoted as an effective method for inducing weight loss for many years, there are limited clinical trials to support its efficacy compared with the high-carbohydrate, low-fat diet. A recent study with a small number of obese, nondiabetic subjects compared the low-carbohydrate, high-protein, high-fat diet with a conventional high-carbohydrate, low-fat, energy-deficit diet (23). The low-carbohydrate diet resulted in greater weight loss in the first 3 months, but at the end of 12 months there was no significant difference in amount of weight lost between the two different diet groups. After 3 months the serum total and LDL cholesterol levels were not significantly different between the two groups. Serum triglyceride levels were lower and high-density lipoprotein (HDL) cholesterol levels were higher on the low-carbohydrate, high-fat diet than on the conventional high-carbohydrate, low-fat diet. Promoters of the high-fat, low-carbohydrate diet propose that carbohydrate stimulates insulin secretion, thus contributing to insulin resistance. In this study comparing the two types of diet, insulin sensitivity improved on both diets. Attrition was high and adherence was low in both the high-carbohydrate and low-carbohydrate diet groups, emphasizing the difficulty in long-term maintenance of reduced body weight. Although some risk factors for CVD improved with the low-carbohydrate, high-fat diet, further research is needed to determine whether this type of diet is both safe and effective for long-term weight loss. Side effects of low-carbohydrate, high-fat, high-protein diets include induction of ketosis, increased risk of kidney stones, dehydration, and constipation. The restriction of carbohydrate intake and limited variety of foods consumed leads to a reduction in total energy resulting in weight loss. In addition, these dietary restrictions also reduce intake of fiber, vitamins, and minerals because of limited intake of grains, fruits, and vegetables. The emphasis in selecting a weight-control diet should be placed on the reduction of total energy intake rather than the source of energy.

Physical Activity Management

The degree of overweight can be a critical factor in whether an individual can use increased physical activity as a means to achieve the desired energy deficit. The recent movement to encourage use of a pedometer can provide a simple way for individuals to assess their current level of activity. This tool can motivate individuals to gradually increase their level of activity. In addition to number of steps, some pedometers record active time, which may be a more practical parameter than actual number of steps for the person with limited mobility. Walking is a good form of activity with which to start because distance and time can be gradually increased as fitness improves and no special equipment, other than good walking shoes, is required. Obese individuals often have significantly limited mobility because of the physical problems associated with the excess weight; therefore, alternate types of activity may need to be identified and encouraged. Chair exercises or water aerobics may be useful alternatives for people with mobility problems or impaired balance. Following appropriate guidelines for initiating an exercise program is especially important for individuals who already have established CVD or other chronic diseases. After obtaining physician approval for initiating an exercise plan, the following steps can be helpful:

- Assess current activity level using pedometer
- Set a realistic goal for increasing level of activity
- Find an enjoyable activity that requires movement
- Keep a log of activity

The National Institute on Aging has published an inexpensive guide to exercises designed to improve strength, balance, flexibility, and endurance for older people. The book, *Exercise:*

A Guide from the National Institute on Aging, also addresses safety issues, overcoming barriers to physical activity, and good basic nutrition (24).

Sweeteners and Fat Replacers in Weight Management

Are reduced-fat, fat-free, or sugar-free products useful adjuncts in weight control or diabetes management? If the patient is an informed consumer and does not overindulge to compensate for the reduced energy of the product, these products can be useful dietary adjuncts. The patient's use of these types of products and level of understanding about the product contents must be carefully assessed. Often these products are only slightly lower in total energy, requiring an astute shopper to detect the small difference between a regular and a modified product. The stated portion size may be much smaller than the amount normally consumed. Education on label reading is essential to ensure that the patient does not equate sugar-free or fat-free with calorie-free or energy-free.

Sweeteners

Nutritive and nonnutritive sweeteners can provide reduced-calorie options for beverages and desserts (25). The nutritive sweeteners need to be accounted for when evaluating total carbohydrate and energy intake. These include the sugar alcohols, or polyols, that provide 2 to 3 kcal/g compared with sucrose or fructose (26). Products containing sugar alcohols as sweetening agents may not be lower in energy content than the regular product they replace because fat content is often increased to enhance flavor or texture when the sugar alcohol replaces sucrose. Table 9.2 shows a guide for incorporating polyols into the diet developed by Warshaw and Powers (26). An unpleasant side effect of sugar alcohols is gastrointestinal discomfort in the form of cramping and diarrhea if consumed in large amounts (20 to 50 g). Small children may be particularly susceptible to diarrhea from ingestion of as little as 0.5 g/kg body weight (27). Because sugar alcohols do not raise blood glucose levels as much as glucose, they should not be used to treat hypoglycemia.

Nonnutritive sweeteners include saccharin, aspartame, acesulfame K, and sucralose. Saccharin and acesulfame K provide no energy because they are excreted from the body unchanged. Saccharin has been removed from the list of potential carcinogens, but some concerns still exist about its use in pregnancy because it is reported to cross the placenta and be cleared slowly by the fetus (25,28). The small amount of aspartame (4 kcal/g) needed for sweetening results in a negligible amount of energy. Aspartame is not recommended for use

TABLE 9.2
Fitting Foods with Polyols into a Meal Plan

Total Carbohydrate,* g	Count As
0–5	Do not count
6–10	½ carbohydrate serving or ½ starch, fruit, or milk serving
11–20	1 carbohydrate serving or 1 starch, fruit, or milk serving
21–25	1½ carbohydrate servings or 1½ starch, fruit, or milk servings
26–35	2 carbohydrate servings or 2 starch, fruit, or milk servings

*Use these guidelines when polyols are in the food: Guideline 1. If all the carbohydrate comes from polyols and is <10 g, consider it a free food. Guideline 2. If all the carbohydrate comes from polyols and the grams of polyols are >10, then subtract one half of the polyol grams from the total carbohydrate and count the remaining grams of carbohydrate into the meal plan. Guideline 3. If there are several sources of carbohydrate including polyols, then subtract one half of the polyol grams from the total carbohydrate and count the remaining grams of carbohydrate into the meal plan.

Source: Reprinted from Warshaw HS, Powers MA. A search for answers about foods with polyols (sugar alcohols). *Diabetes Educator.* 1999;25:319, with permission from *The Diabetes Educator,* American Association of Diabetes Educators, 1999.

in cooking because of heat instability. Aspartame is metabolized to phenylalanine and there-fore should not be used by people with phenylketonuria. Sucralose (trichlorogalactosucrose) provides many new options as a sweetening agent for people with diabetes. It is heat stable and can be used in desserts, confections, and beverages. No side effects have been reported from its use. Because sucralose is not absorbed by the intestines, it provides no energy; therefore, a substantial reduction in energy and carbohydrate content of a product occurs when sucralose is substituted for sucrose. The commercial version of sucralose is packaged with a small amount of dextrose that contributes a minimal amount of energy.

Fat Replacers

Some reduced-fat products provide a substantial savings in energy when compared with the regular full-fat product. Other reduced-fat products, however, have only slightly reduced energy content when compared with the full-fat versions. In cases where the energy saved is minimal, the reduced-fat product is of questionable benefit when weight management is important, as it is in type 2 diabetes. An additional problem is that the reduced-fat product may not have the satiety value of the regular item and could lead to consumption of a larger portion and excessive energy intake.

Fat replacers can be made from fat, protein, or carbohydrate. Fat-based substitutes are either synthetic or modified fat (29). Olestra, a sucrose polyester, is an example of a synthetic com-pound that tastes like fat but it is not digested or absorbed and therefore contributes no energy. If consumed in large quantities, olestra can cause gastrointestinal distress and may reduce the absorption of fat-soluble vitamins. Modified fats used as fat replacers include caprenin and salatrim, which have been altered to decrease absorption. Both of these products provide approx-imately 5 kcal/g. Salatrim is a modified triglyceride that consists of acetic, propionic, and stearic acids. Caprenin contains caprylic, capric, and behenic acids, which are known to raise serum cholesterol concentrations; therefore, it is not a good choice for a person at increased risk for CVD (30). Protein-based fat replacers are used in a number of products such as salad dressings and frozen dessert items. They are made of microparticulated egg white or milk protein and pro-vide 1 to 4 kcal/g (29). Because these fat replacers are made of protein, they are subject to coag-ulation at higher temperatures, which limits the types of products to which they can be added. Carbohydrate-based fat replacers raise special concerns for the person with diabetes. A consid-erable amount of carbohydrate can be consumed in a reduced-fat product containing a carbohydrate-based fat replacer. These products consist of gels, gums, and maltodextrins that contribute creaminess and texture to foods, such as salad dressings. Sugar or other nutritive sweet-eners may also be added to these products. Label-reading skills are very important for the per-son with diabetes to identify products that may not usually be considered a source of carbohy-drate. A typical fat-free salad dressing may contain 10 to 12 g carbohydrate per 2 tablespoon serving, compared with less than 5 g for a regular salad dressing. Reduced-fat peanut butter is an example of a product to which additional sugar is added when fat is removed, sometimes dou-bling the amount of carbohydrate when compared with regular peanut butter.

NUTRITION RECOMMENDATIONS: MACRONUTRIENTS

Dietary Carbohydrate

Carbohydrate is the macronutrient that most acutely influences blood glucose levels. Good glycemic control has been shown to decrease the incidence of complications in patients with type 1 and type 2 diabetes. The focus for carbohydrate in diabetes management has shifted from type to total amount of carbohydrate in the diet. For years, it was commonly believed that sugars were absorbed more rapidly than starches and thus would lead to a wider fluctuation in blood glucose levels. Research has shown, however, that similar increases in plasma glucose levels occur following ingestion of equal amounts of starch or sugar (31-34). Fructose ingestion causes a reduced glycemic excursion compared with sucrose (35-38). With CVD risk in mind, there are other concerns about the effects of some sugars, especially fructose. Research, although not consistent, has shown that both sucrose and fructose intake may increase serum triglyceride and cholesterol concentrations compared with starch intake (38,39). A recent randomized, crossover study in healthy adults compared a diet containing 17% of energy from fructose with a diet containing 3% of energy from fructose. After 6 weeks on the high-fructose diet, fasting and postprandial plasma triglyceride concentrations were increased in men, but not in women (40). Animal studies suggest that high fructose intake may increase de novo lipogenesis, the rate at which the body makes fatty acids from metabolism of sugars (41,42). Some researchers now hypothesize that because fructose does not stimulate insulin production, it may contribute to insulin resistance by adversely affecting leptin and adiponectin production, thus interfering with long-term energy regulatory mechanisms (43).

Intake of naturally occurring fructose is estimated to be approximately 15 to 16 g per day, or about 3% of total energy. Table 9.3 shows the amount of fructose in some commonly consumed foods (44). Naturally occurring fructose in fruit and vegetables is unlikely to cause metabolic problems. During the past 30 years, high-fructose corn syrup (HFCS) has replaced sucrose in many foods and beverages, and fructose consumption is estimated to have increased by 26% (43). Products containing added fructose should be limited (7,45,46). HFCS is a predominant sweetener used in soft drinks and fruit drinks and is estimated to contain approximately 55% fructose. Because sucrose consists of equal parts of glucose and fructose, the 55% HFCS represents only a 5% increase in fructose content compared with a product sweetened with sucrose (47). However, overall consumption of soft drinks and fruit drinks has increased significantly in recent years, thereby contributing to the increased intake of fructose. Soft drink consumption has doubled since the late 1970s in children and adolescents and consumption of noncitrus fruit drinks has increased by 300% in young children (48). Because food preferences are learned early in life, this pattern of increased consumption of HFCS-sweetened beverages is likely to continue as these children become adults. Fructose, in the form of HFCS, may contribute 10% of total energy when only two fructose-sweetened beverages are included as part of a 2,000-kcal diet (43).

Although naturally occurring sugars in fruits, vegetables, and low-fat dairy products are to be encouraged as part of a healthy diet, inclusion of added sugars present in processed foods has additional implications when considering cardiovascular risk. High-calorie foods containing added sugars may also include considerable amounts of total fat and cholesterol-raising saturated and *trans* fats. These dessert-type items can quickly sabotage weight-loss efforts if consumed on a daily basis.

The glycemic index (GI) of foods is a ranking of foods based on their immediate effect on blood glucose levels. The GI is widely used in Australia, Canada, and Europe as a guide to selection of carbohydrate-containing foods (49,50). A number of factors affect the GI of a food. Differences in processing and cooking methods, as well as the molecular and physical structure of the item, influence the response. In addition, there are variations in response from person to person. In a meta-analysis of 14 studies using low-GI diets, Brand-Miller and associates concluded that choosing low-GI rather than high-GI foods can result in a small improvement in medium-term glycemic control as measured by HbA_{1c} or fructosamine. A number of the

TABLE 9.3
Fructose Content of Commonly Eaten Foods

Food	Portion	Fructose, g	Total Carbohydrate, g
Soft drinks, sweetened with HFCS	12 oz	22*	40.0
Fruits			
Pear, fresh	1 medium	10.3	25.7
Apple, fresh with skin	1 medium	8.1	19.1
Pineapple, canned juice pack	½ cup	8.1	19.5
Grapes, red or green fresh	½ cup	6.3	13.9
Banana, fresh	1 medium	5.7	27.0
Strawberries, fresh sliced	1 cup	4.2	12.7
Orange juice, unsweetened from concentrate	½ cup	3.2	13.4
Cantaloupe	1 cup cubes	3.0	13.1
Peach, raw	1 medium	1.5	9.3
Vegetables			
Tomato, fresh	1 medium	1.7	4.8
Asparagus, cooked	½ cup	0.7	3.7
Sweet potato, cooked mashed	½ cup	0.7	29.1
Potato, baked	1 medium	0.6	36.6
Broccoli, cooked	½ cup	0.6	5.6
Pepper, green, cooked	¼ cup	0.5	2.3
Corn, yellow cooked	½ cup	0.4	20.6

*Estimated value, based on 55% fructose in high-fructose corn syrup.
Source: Data are from reference 44.

studies were of short duration with a small number of subjects. Brand-Miller et al noted that additional long-term randomized, controlled trials are needed to determine whether the GI is effective in decreasing the risk of complications of diabetes (51).

The GI of a food represents the carbohydrate quality of a food. More recently, a measure that includes carbohydrate quantity has been introduced. Glycemic load is the product of the GI and the amount of available carbohydrate in the food. Both GI and glycemic load values are provided in an extensive list of foods published in 2002 (50).

Experts express concern about some methodologies used to evaluate the glycemic response (52). Portion sizes used in the test are often different from the actual portion size likely to be eaten. The short 2-hour testing time may not be appropriate for people with type 2 diabetes because it may take longer than 2 hours for blood glucose to return to premeal values. Depending on the individual's premeal blood glucose level, foods may also have a different effect after breakfast than after lunch or dinner. Given these concerns, the American Diabetes Association does not recommend the GI as a primary tool in nutrition management of diabetes (53).

Another method for selecting carbohydrate-containing foods may be based upon total fiber, particularly soluble fiber content. Foods with a high amount of soluble fiber may improve blood glucose and lipid levels (54). Total fiber content of foods is listed on the Nutrition Facts panel of food labels, and soluble fiber content is provided in Table 9.4 (55).

Protein

Adequate protein intake is essential for maintenance of lean body mass in adults. Typical intake of protein ranges from 15% to 20% of total energy, which usually exceeds the recommended dietary allowance (RDA) amount of 0.8 g protein per kilogram (56). Meat, poultry, and dairy products tend to be the major sources of saturated fat and cholesterol in the diet in

TABLE 9.4
Soluble Fiber Content of Foods

Food*	Portion	Soluble Fiber, g
Vegetables		
Winter squash, cooked: acorn, hubbard, butternut	½ cup	0.7–3.1
Summer squash, cooked: spaghetti, chayote, zucchini	½ cup	0.5–0.6
Green vegetables, cooked:		
Brussels sprouts, collards, green peas, broccoli, turnip greens, okra	½ cup	1.0–1.9
Green cabbage, kale, green peppers, spinach	½ cup	0.6–0.8
Other Vegetables, Cooked (except as noted)		
Jicama (raw), sweet potato, carrots, onion,	½ cup	1.0–1.7
Baked potato, Chinese cabbage, cauliflower, eggplant	½ cup	0.3–0.7
Beans/Legumes, Cooked from Dried (except as noted)		
Lima beans, kidney beans, navy beans	½ cup	2.2–3.5
Pinto beans, soybeans (green), garbanzo beans, split peas	½ cup	1.1–1.9
Cowpeas, lentils	½ cup	0.6–0.7
Grains†		
Amaranth (dry), All Bran Buds (Kellogg's)	½ cup	3.8–4.7
Wheat germ, oat bran, Post 100% Bran (Kraft)	½ cup	1.2–1.8
Oatmeal (cooked), barley (cooked), All Bran (Kellogg's), spelt	½ cup	0.8–0.9
Fruits		
Pear, fresh	1 medium	
Prunes, apricots, peaches (cooked from dried)	½ cup	
Orange	1 medium	
Avocado (California type)	½ each	1.5–2.1
Figs, fresh	½ cup	
Mango, fresh	1 each	
Blackberries, fresh	1 cup	
Grapefruit	½ medium	
Dates	½ cup	1.0–1.4
Apricots, fresh	½ cup	
Apple, fresh	1 medium	
Raisins	½ cup	
Nectarine, peach	1 medium	
Cranberries (dried), plum (fresh), guava (fresh),	½ cup	
fruit cocktail (canned), star fruit (carambola)	½ cup	
Kiwi, fresh	1 medium	0.5–0.9
Grapes, fresh	1 cup	
Papaya, fresh	½ cup	
Cherries, fresh	½ cup	

*Foods within categories listed in descending order of soluble fiber content.
†Manufacturers: Kellogg's, Battle Creek, MI 49016; Kraft Foods, Glenview, IL 60025.
Source: Data are from reference 55.

the United States. If animal products are chosen as the source of protein in the diet, the best choices to reduce cardiovascular risk are lean meats and low-fat dairy products. When eaten in moderation, these foods can provide important nutrients such as calcium, iron, and zinc, yet still fit within guidelines for a healthy diet. Plant-based diets can also provide adequate amounts of protein with less saturated fat and cholesterol content. Lacto-ovo vegetarian diets provide approximately 12% to 14% of energy from protein, whereas vegan diets provide about 10% to 12% energy from protein. Plant-based diets may have other positive effects for people with diabetes or CVD because of the increased intake of associated components, such as soluble and insoluble fiber and beneficial phytochemicals (57). Soy protein has some cholesterol-lowering effects, attributed at least in part to the isoflavones, but the mechanisms are still unclear (58). The use of soy or other plant-based protein in the diet may be an appropriate adjunct for achieving modest cholesterol lowering (see Chapter 10).

Dietary Fat

Because they are at increased risk for CVD, individuals with diabetes need appropriate guidance on the amount and type of fat they should consume. In addition to elevated LDL cholesterol, patients with diabetes frequently have low HDL and elevated very-low-density lipoprotein (VLDL) levels, along with high serum triglyceride levels (59). Selecting types of fat that lower serum LDL and triglyceride levels while enhancing HDL levels is desirable.

As discussed in Chapter 6, dietary fats can be categorized depending upon the configuration of the molecules and are usually a mixture of saturated, monounsaturated, or polyunsaturated fatty acids. The recommended range of fat in the diet is 25% to 35% of total energy intake (2,56). Current recommendations are to limit saturated and *trans*-unsaturated fatty acids in the diet as much as possible to maximize reduction of serum LDL cholesterol. Two thirds of the saturated fat in the diet comes from animal products, with approximately 90% of total dietary fat coming from fats and oils, red meat, poultry, fish, and dairy products. People with diabetes need to be particularly attentive in their food selection; they should choose lower-fat options to limit the risk of the cholesterol-raising fatty acids. Invisible or hidden fats in foods are often overlooked as sources of cholesterol-raising fatty acids.

Saturated Fatty Acids

Consistent with the Therapeutic Lifestyle Changes (TLC) diet of ATP III, the American Diabetes Association recommends limiting saturated fatty acids to approximately 7% of total energy for patients with diabetes and elevated serum lipids (2,7). Lauric (C12:0; 12-carbon chain length, no double bond), myristic (C14:0) and palmitic (C16:0) acids are the most potent in terms of cholesterol-raising effect (60). The medium-chain fatty acids, caprylic (C8:0) and capric (C10:0) acids, and the long-chain fatty acid behenic acid (C22:0) have also been shown to raise serum LDL cholesterol levels (30,60).

Polyunsaturated Fatty Acids

Polyunsaturated fatty acids should be limited to 10% or less of total energy (2,7). Polyunsaturated fatty acids may be classified as n-3 or n-6, depending upon the location of the first double bond in relation to the methyl end of the carbon chain. Intake of approximately 2% to 3% of total energy from n-6 fatty acids provides sufficient essential fatty acids, linoleic (C18:2) and alpha-linolenic (C18:3) acids. Linoleic acid is a precursor for arachidonic and gamma-linolenic acids. When substituted for saturated fatty acids in the diet, linoleic acid lowers LDL cholesterol levels but not triglycerides. Large intakes of linoleic acid may lead to a decrease in HDL cholesterol.

N-3 fatty acids in the diet include alpha-linolenic acid, eicosapentaenoic acid (EPA) (C20:5), and docosahexaenoic acid (DHA) (C22:6). Dietary intake of n-3 fatty acids in the United States is primarily from alpha-linolenic acid, representing less than 1% of total energy intake. Less than 15% of the n-3 fatty acid intake is from EPA or DHA found in fish oils (61,62). Canola and soybean oils are the predominant dietary sources of alpha-linolenic in the United States. Flaxseed, flaxseed oil, and English walnuts are good sources of alpha-linolenic acid, but they are not widely consumed (63).

By competitively inhibiting hepatic triglyceride synthesis, long-chain n-3 fatty acids (EPA and DHA) reduce serum triglyceride levels. EPA and DHA are found in marine fish oils.

Intake of large amounts of fish oil (up to 5 to 10 g of n-3 polyunsaturated fatty acids per day) can cause hyperglycemia due to increased hepatic glucose output. Hyperglycemia has not been noted when energy intake is adequately controlled and small doses of fish oil (less than 6 g per day, which usually provide up to 3 g of n-3 fatty acids) are used (64). Patients with hypertriglyceridemia may experience a small increase in serum LDL cholesterol concentrations when fish oils are consumed (65,66). A potential cardiovascular benefit of fish oils for patients with diabetes is decreased platelet aggregation, which could reduce risk of acute myocardial infarction. To increase the consumption of n-3 fatty acids, people with diabetes should increase their intake of fish rather than take supplements because there is more epidemiologic data on fish intake than fish oil supplement intake. Some studies suggest that one serving of fish per week can lead to a reduction in sudden cardiac death (63,67). Patients with diabetes who have hypertriglyceridemia require moderate to large doses of fish oil to achieve reduction in serum triglycerides. For further discussion of n-3 supplementation, see Chapter 10.

cis-monounsaturated Fatty Acids

For centuries the Mediterranean diet has been rich in cis-monounsaturated fatty acids, and epidemiologic studies have demonstrated lower CHD mortality in the Mediterranean region. When oleic acid (C18:1) is substituted for saturated fatty acids, the serum LDL cholesterol level decreases in similar amount as when polyunsaturated fatty acids are substituted (68-70). In patients with type 2 diabetes, diets rich in monounsaturated fatty acids, compared with a diet high in carbohydrate, reduce plasma triglycerides and VLDL cholesterol levels and increase HDL cholesterol levels and apolipoprotein A-I concentrations. Plasma glucose and insulin concentrations are also reduced (71). A meta-analysis of nine randomized, crossover trials comparing high-carbohydrate with high-cis-monounsaturated-fat diets revealed that high-cis-monounsaturated-fat diets reduce fasting plasma triglycerides by 19% and VLDL cholesterol concentrations by 22%. No adverse effect on LDL cholesterol levels was noted, and there was a modest increase in HDL cholesterol levels (72). A study in subjects with type 1 diabetes also found the high-monounsaturated-fat diet to have a positive effect on serum lipids (73).

Overall energy intake must be controlled if weight loss is needed for management of type 2 diabetes. Use of monounsaturated oils, such as olive or canola oil, may improve the likelihood of compliance for the patient who has been consuming a high-fat diet. Other good sources of cis-monounsaturated fatty acids include mustard and peanut oils, avocados, olives, and some nuts. Genetically modified varieties of safflower and sunflower oils are also rich in cis-monounsaturated fatty acids. Cis-monounsaturated fatty acids, other than oleic acid, may have potential to lower cholesterol in patients with diabetes, but studies on these fatty acids are limited at this time.

Trans Fatty Acids

Dietary trans fatty acids have been shown to raise serum LDL cholesterol and apolipoprotein B levels and, with relatively high intake, may lower serum HDL cholesterol and apolipoprotein A-I levels (74,75). Because intake of dietary trans fatty acids has been associated with increased risk of CHD, this type of cholesterol-raising fatty acid should be limited as much as possible in the diets of individuals with diabetes (76,77). A study comparing relative risk reported that intake of trans fatty acids may increase the risk of type 2 diabetes in women more than total fat or saturated fat intake (78).

Dietary Cholesterol

High intake of dietary cholesterol raises both serum total cholesterol and LDL cholesterol levels. Current recommendations are to limit dietary cholesterol intake to 300 mg or less per day. For the patient with dyslipidemia, the recommendation is to further reduce dietary cholesterol intake to 200 mg or less per day to achieve maximum lowering of serum LDL cholesterol levels, consistent with TLC of ATP III (2,7). Because animal products are the sole source of cholesterol in the diet, their use should be limited in quantity and emphasis should be placed on choosing lower-fat items. Lean cuts of meat, poultry, and fish should be limited to 5 ounces or less per day, and egg yolks should be limited to two or fewer per week. Two to three servings daily of nonfat or low-fat dairy products are recommended.

Dietary Fiber

Actual dietary fiber intake is much lower than the current amount of 20 to 35 g per day recommended by the American Diabetes Association (7). Usual intake of dietary fiber in the United States is 16 to 17 g per day, and in other Western countries it is only slightly higher (approximately 22 g per day) (79,80). Dietary fiber can be classified as soluble or insoluble. Insoluble fibers, such as cellulose, lignin, and some hemicelluloses, increase stool volume and shorten intestinal transit time. Serum cholesterol levels are not affected by insoluble fiber. Addition of 5 to 10 g of soluble fiber to the diet, however, can reduce serum cholesterol levels by approximately 5% (2). Examples of soluble fiber include gums, pectin, mucilages, and some hemicelluloses. See Table 9.4 for fruits, grains, and vegetables that are the primary dietary sources of soluble fiber (55).

One study of subjects with type 2 diabetes used natural high-fiber foods to demonstrate the effectiveness of soluble fiber in lowering serum lipids and glucose. Without the use of a fiber supplement, a diet high in total dietary fiber (50 g) and soluble fiber (25 g) was compared with a moderate-fiber diet (24 g of total dietary fiber and 8 g of soluble fiber). A 10% reduction in 24-hour plasma glucose, a 12% reduction in plasma insulin, and decreased daily urinary glucose excretion were reported with the high-fiber diet. Plasma cholesterol level was reduced by 7%, triglyceride level by 10%, and VLDL cholesterol level by 12.5% (54). The National Health and Nutrition Examination Survey (NHANES) I Epidemiologic Follow-up Study, representing an average of 19 years of subject follow-up, found that higher intake of dietary fiber, especially soluble fiber, reduced risk of CHD (81).

An epidemiologic study of clinic patients with type 1 diabetes in 31 European countries reported that total dietary fiber intake was inversely related to HbA_{1c} levels and that risk of severe ketoacidosis decreased with higher dietary fiber intake. The average intake of natural dietary fiber for these patients with type 1 diabetes was approximately 17 g per day, with a range of 14 to 22 g. In this study, men with higher intakes of dietary fiber had lower LDL cholesterol levels. Both men and women with higher intakes of total dietary fiber had higher HDL cholesterol levels. A protective effect against CVD for total fiber intake was reported for women, but not for men (82).

Alcohol

Guidelines for alcohol consumption for patients with diabetes are the same as those for the general public. Certain individuals, including pregnant women and people with a history of alcohol abuse, gastritis, severe hypertriglyceridemia, or pancreatitis, should abstain from alcohol intake. Low to moderate intake of alcohol on a regular basis by individuals who do not have diabetes has been observed to increase serum HDL cholesterol and apolipoprotein A-I levels, which could lead to decreased cardiovascular risk. However, this potential benefit could be negated by an increase in blood pressure and a decrease in concentration of antithrombin III (83). Consumption of large amounts of alcohol causes peripheral insulin resistance and may lead to hyperglycemia, hypertriglyceridemia, and hypertension (84-86). Studies show that when alcohol is consumed along with fat, particularly saturated fat, hypertriglyceridemia is worse than when the alcohol is consumed alone (87). This is believed to result from inhibition of lipolysis of intestinally derived lipoproteins when alcohol is consumed. In a study comparing moderate drinkers with men who abstained or drank large amounts of alcohol, an increased risk for development of type 2 diabetes was observed in both the abstainers and the heavy drinkers (88).

Some of the metabolic effects of alcohol are especially problematic for people with diabetes. Alcohol ingestion may contribute to truncal obesity, leading to increased cardiovascular risk. Development of fatty liver is another potential negative effect of alcohol (89,90). If a person with diabetes binge drinks or fails to consume food along with alcohol, the risk for development of hypoglycemic events is greater because of enhanced glucose-stimulated insulin secretion and reduced gluconeogenesis following ingestion of alcohol. Risk of hypoglycemic unawareness also increases with alcohol ingestion (91). To decrease the risk of hypoglycemic events, food should never be omitted to compensate for alcohol when insulin injections are part of the treatment regimen for diabetes. Patients with type 2 diabetes on oral antidiabetes medications, particularly the elderly, are at risk for hypoglycemia when alcohol is consumed, but not as much as insulin-dependent patients with type 1 diabetes (92). Any patient taking insulin should always consume food when ingesting alcohol.

In the presence of good glycemic control, moderate ingestion of alcohol, defined as two drinks per day for men and one drink per day for women, has a limited acute effect on blood glucose levels. When weight management is a concern, as in type 2 diabetes, the extra energy intake from alcohol (7 kcal/g) needs to be considered. In patients with type 2 diabetes, alcohol can be substituted for fat servings in the diet to compensate for the additional energy intake.

NUTRITION RECOMMENDATIONS: VITAMINS AND MINERALS

People who eat a variety of foods and consume adequate energy for maintenance of normal body weight have little need for vitamin and mineral supplements (93). Individuals who follow energy-restricted diets for weight loss for an extended period of time are at greater risk for consuming less than recommended amounts of nutrients. A thorough assessment of dietary intake can identify patients who may be in need of supplemental vitamins and minerals. People who regularly eat meals and snacks away from home are more likely to consume higher amounts of energy and fat and lower amounts of vitamins and minerals than those who prepare and eat meals at home. During times of stress and illness, increased nutrient requirements should be assessed and provided as necessary.

Because of the increased risk of CVD with diabetes, antioxidant vitamins are of particular interest. Although vitamins C and E have been shown to protect LDL particles from oxidation (94), clinical trials supplementing with these vitamins have not reported a benefit (95). Likewise, clinical studies with beta carotene supplements have not substantiated a beneficial effect, and, in fact, a slightly increased risk for lung cancer has been reported in some subjects receiving the supplements. Therefore, consumption of naturally occurring beta carotene, vitamin A, and vitamin C from a variety of fruits and vegetables is preferable to supplementation (96).

Calcium

The NHLBI recommends a calcium intake for adults of 1,000 to 1,500 mg per day (9). This amount can be difficult to obtain from dietary sources if dairy products are not consumed on a regular basis. Individuals should be advised to choose low-fat dairy products to limit saturated fat and cholesterol intake. To reduce risk of osteoporosis, calcium supplementation may be needed if dietary intake does not meet recommended levels. Some recent intriguing research suggests that increased dietary calcium intake from dairy sources may play a role in energy metabolism by inhibiting adipocyte fatty acid synthase expression and activity and by stimulation of lipolysis. An inverse relationship between dietary calcium intake and body fat was found in NHANES III (97,98). This mechanism may offer another tool in the weight management arena if additional research supports the role of calcium in energy balance.

Chromium

As a potentiator of insulin activity, chromium affects glucose uptake by the cells. However, supplementation with chromium does not improve glucose tolerance unless an individual is deficient in chromium. Assessment of chromium status is limited by lack of specific tests to accurately measure it. A diet consistent with the guidelines discussed in this chapter is likely to provide higher chromium intake than a diet consisting of highly refined and processed foods. Food sources of chromium include meats, whole grains, cheese, nuts, and brewer's yeast.

Magnesium

Patients with uncontrolled diabetes and chronic glycosuria may experience low magnesium levels because of increased magnesium excretion. Repletion with oral magnesium chloride is recommended only when hypomagnesemia has been confirmed (99). Green leafy vegetables, legumes, and nuts are good food sources of magnesium. Patients with diabetes who maintain good glycemic control and eat a nutritionally balanced diet with adequate energy should be able to obtain adequate magnesium from their food.

Potassium

Hypokalemia can occur in diabetes, especially when the patient has hypertension and potassium-wasting diuretics are part of the treatment regimen. As with magnesium levels, potassium levels can be readily monitored with laboratory testing. Potassium is widespread in the diet, and many fruits and vegetables are good food sources of potassium. (See Chapter 8, Table 8.6.) Supplementation with potassium chloride may be needed to maintain normal levels if urinary potassium losses are substantial. Excessive intake of potassium from dietary sources alone rarely occurs with normal kidney function, but for those patients with renal insufficiency secondary to diabetes, use of a potassium-containing salt substitute may add sufficient potassium to cause hyperkalemia.

Sodium

Reduction of sodium intake is effective in lowering blood pressure in subjects with hypertension, and good blood pressure control is a very important element in preventing complications of diabetes (100-102). Salt sensitivity varies, but it seems to increase with age and may be more prevalent in individuals with diabetes (103). Sodium intake usually far exceeds the minimum needed for normal body function because of consumption of processed and convenience foods and frequent meals away from home. Moderate restriction of sodium (2,400 mg per day) is recommended for patients with hypertension (104). Sodium should be limited to 2,000 mg per day for individuals with diabetic nephropathy (7). Due to perceived decreased palatability, even a mild to moderate sodium restriction may limit total intake, especially in frail elderly patients, leading to undernutrition. Reduction of sodium intake can be difficult to achieve unless someone in the household is willing and able to make the time to prepare meals using fresh foods rather than processed and convenience products. Label reading is essential when working to control dietary sodium intake. Sodium is now added to a number of meat and poultry products that in the past would have been low in sodium. Use of herbs and spices to enhance flavors can help patients in the transition to a lower sodium intake.

MAXIMIZING DIABETES CONTROL WITH MEAL PLANNING

For patients using set doses of insulin or taking oral antidiabetes agents, day-to-day consistency and meal-to-meal consistency in carbohydrate intake are needed to maintain good glycemic control. Many experts recommend dietary carbohydrate–based calculation (carbohydrate-to-insulin ratio) of mealtime insulin dosage in patients with type 1 diabetes. Multiple daily injections of insulin or use of an insulin pump provide greater flexibility for patients in timing of meals, as well as in variation of amount of carbohydrate. The multiple injection and pump regimens require a high level of commitment from the patient and in-depth instruction from a registered dietitian or certified diabetes educator. The additional effort required for these intensive management regimens is usually rewarded with improved glucose control, thus reducing risk for CVD. Insulin injections should be matched to the peak glucose excursion following meals and snacks. If more than 5 hours of time elapse between meals, a snack is usually recommended to prevent a potential hypoglycemic event, especially for children or physically active adults.

Carbohydrate counting is a popular and effective method for maintaining consistency in carbohydrate intake. The rationale for carbohydrate counting as a meal-planning approach is that carbohydrate is the macronutrient that most acutely influences blood glucose levels and insulin requirements. The carbohydrate-containing food groups (starch, fruit, milk, and other carbohydrates) have approximately 15 g of carbohydrate for each serving, or "carbohydrate choice." The nonstarchy vegetables provide 5 g carbohydrate per serving. A carbohydrate-counting meal plan provides guidance by giving a range of either grams of carbohydrate or number of carbohydrate choices for each meal and snack. The carbohydrate-counting method works especially well for children because of the focus on one nutrient. As children grow and develop, overall sound nutrition principles can be incorporated into their meals plans to provide for long-term cardiovascular benefits. Overweight individuals with type 2 diabetes, who are at increased risk for CVD, need appropriate guidance on total energy and amount and type of fat intake when using carbohydrate counting as a meal-planning tool.

Multiple small meals may provide an advantage for the person with type 2 diabetes because this regimen has been shown to have a positive effect on serum lipids and lipoprotein, insulin, and postprandial glucose when compared with a pattern of less-frequent meals (105-107). Frequency of feeding does not appear to affect rate of weight loss, but a pattern of more frequent eating may limit a tendency to binge eat that arises from increased hunger when long periods of time elapse between feedings. When breakfast, a meal often skipped, is eaten, there is a tendency toward less-impulsive eating and a reduced fat intake (108). Analysis of NHANES III data on more than 16,000 subjects confirms that breakfast skippers (20% of subjects) tend to have higher BMIs than individuals who eat breakfast. One exception to this was that subjects who ate meat and eggs for breakfast (approximately 11% of subjects) had the highest energy intake and higher BMIs. Subjects who ate cooked or ready-to-eat cereals or quick breads had lower BMIs than individuals who skipped breakfast or ate meat and eggs. Almost 55% of the subject had BMIs equal to or greater than 25 (109). To prevent hypoglycemic events, patients taking oral antidiabetes agents or using insulin should always be advised not to skip meals.

Obstacles to Diabetes Management

Health issues requiring changes in behavior, such as diabetes and CVD, are challenging. There are many obstacles, or barriers, to overcome to achieve and sustain positive changes. The present-day hectic lifestyle and competing demands on a person's time are at the top of the list of identified obstacles to behavior change (110,111). For the patient with diabetes, factors contributing to this often overwhelming scenario include the following:

- Time constraints
- Financial constraints
- Portions and selections available when eating out
- Denial or unwillingness to make changes

The importance of the patient as an active participant in the care team is well known. Table 9.5 presents tips on how the dietitian and the patient can work together to overcome the obstacles to lifestyle changes and good nutrition practices. (See also Chapter 5 on Behavior Change.)

MNT has been shown to be effective in improving metabolic control in diabetes (112-116). Individualization and simplification of meal plans along with assistance with time-management skills are necessary to overcome the obstacles to behavior change. Long-term, constructive dietary changes are very difficult for most people to implement. Guidance from a registered dietitian providing MNT can facilitate the necessary changes. One study of patients with type 2 diabetes reported that lack of physician referral was the reason that approximately half of the patients did not see a dietitian (117). Infrequent referral has been found to be as ineffective in facilitating change as no referral at all (118). The Diabetes Control and Complications Trial demonstrated the importance of following a meal plan for improved glycemic control (119,120). Adherence to meal plans improves when follow-up counseling sessions take place (121). Often, however, MNT referrals are not made for patients with diabetes of long duration, even though they may face many obstacles to lifestyle change and may have poor metabolic control. These are the individuals who are most likely to benefit from intensive nutrition therapy (122). Emphasis is needed on increased self-glucose monitoring and the fact that complications of diabetes can be prevented with good glycemic control.

The patient and dietitian have a wide range of tools available to facilitate meal planning that fosters heart health and good glycemic control to prevent short- and long-term complications of diabetes. The choice of meal-planning tools can be as simple or as complex as

TABLE 9.5
Working Together to Overcome Obstacles: Intervention Plus Action Equals Success

Dietitian's Intervention	Patient's Action
Individualize and simplify meal plan as needed by adapting for cultural preferences, financial constraints, and educational level.	Ask your physician for a referral to a registered dietitian. Follow your meal plan. Read labels. Limit number of restaurant meals by preparing more meals at home. packing a lunch.
Promote healthy weight by teaching appropriate food choices.	Choose low saturated fat and low cholesterol foods. Increase intake of whole grains, vegetables, and fruits. Choose foods wisely when you do eat out. Practice portion control. Monitor weight at least once a week.
Encourage increased physical activity.	Check with your physician before starting an exercise regimen. Plan to decrease sedentary time. Find an enjoyable activity requiring movement. Use a pedometer to track current level of activity. Gradually increase number of steps per day.
Teach time-management skills.	Evaluate lifestyle. Set priorities. Make good diabetes control a high priority. Schedule times to eat and exercise.
Educate to prevent short- and long-term complications: (a) Assist in identifying obstacles to good diabetes control. (b) Explain target blood glucose range for good diabetes control. (c) Emphasize importance of glucose self-monitoring.	Discuss diabetes management problems with health care providers. Monitor blood glucose levels regularly. Identify situations that affect blood glucose levels. Identify foods that affect blood glucose levels.

needed to meet the patient's requirements. A few examples of the diabetes management tools available are provided in Table 9.6.

SUMMARY

The goals of MNT for diabetes and CVD are so interrelated that it is difficult to separate them. Adequate energy to achieve and maintain a healthy body weight is a primary concern for both conditions. Even modest weight loss (5% to 10%) for patients with type 2 diabetes promotes improved diabetes control. Physical activity consistent with a patient's physical abilities supports weight management efforts, decreases insulin resistance, and improves glycemic control and lipid profiles. As long as energy intake is controlled, a diet rich in carbohydrate with emphasis on foods high in soluble fiber or a diet rich in *cis*-monounsaturated fats can be used. A healthful lifestyle includes selection of a diet rich in whole grains, fresh fruits, and vegetables and low in cholesterol and cholesterol-raising saturated and *trans*-unsaturated fats. Establishing a realistic and individualized meal plan is essential to ensure adequate nutrition and to meet the metabolic goals set for glucose and lipids. Frequent follow-up and encouragement to maintain positive diet and lifestyle changes increases the likelihood of prevention of diabetes and cardiovascular complications.

TABLE 9.6
Examples of Diabetes Management Tools

Tools	Description	Source*
Basic Carbohydrate Counting	Beginning-level patient education brochure on carbohydrate counting	American Dietetic Association or American Diabetes Association
Advanced Carbohydrate Counting	Advanced-level patient education booklet for carbohydrate counting; includes how to determine insulin-to-carbohydrate ratios	American Dietetic Association or American Diabetes Association
Eating Healthy with Diabetes: Easy Reading Guide	Simple, easy-to-read booklet with pictures to illustrate foods for basic meal planning	American Dietetic Association or American Diabetes Association
The First Step in Diabetes Meal Planning [El Primer paso en planear sus comidas de diabetes]	Brochure based on the Food Guide Pyramid, useful for newly diagnosed patients. Available in English and Spanish	American Dietetic Association or American Diabetes Association
Healthy Food Choices	Simplified meal-planning guide based on exchange meal planning	American Dietetic Association or American Diabetes Association
Exchange Lists for Meal Planning [Listas de Intercambios para Planificacion de Comidas]	Advanced-level patient education booklet for meal planning using exchanges; contains extensive lists of foods and provides more information about types of fats and other nutrients than beginning level materials; a good choice for the detail-oriented patient. Available in English and Spanish	American Dietetic Association or American Diabetes Association
American Dietetic Association Guide to Eating Right When You Have Diabetes	Comprehensive, yet easy-to-read book for the patient with diabetes; includes sample menus for a variety of calorie levels, food exchange lists, fast food and ethnic food guides, other nutrition information, tips on preventing low blood glucose, and activity safety guidelines	American Dietetic Association
Small Steps, Big Rewards— Walking Your Way to Better Health	Easy-to-read Fast Fact Series pocket book with illustrations on who, what, when, where, why, and how of walking; can be purchased with or without a step-counting pedometer	American Diabetes Association
Carb Counting Made Easy for People with Diabetes	Easy-to-read Fast Fact Series pocket book with illustrations and tips for carbohydrate counting	
Idaho Plate Method Meal Planning Guide	Simple tool using a picture of a plate to illustrate meal planning, helpful for the newly diagnosed patient with diabetes, or for those with low literacy level. Two-sided, 11"-by-17" brochure, available in English and Spanish	Idaho DCE Plate Method

*American Dietetic Association, 800/877-1600, ext 5000, http://www.eatright.org/catalog. American Diabetes Association, 800/232-6733, http://store.diabetes.org. Idaho DCE Plate Method, LLC, PO Box 441, Rexburg, ID 83440-0441, http://www.platemethod.com.

REFERENCES

1. Knowler WC, Barrett-Connor E, Fowler SE, Hamman RF, Lachin JM, Walker EA, Nathan DM; Diabetes Prevention Program Research Group. Reduction in the incidence of type 2 diabetes with lifestyle intervention or metformin. N Engl J Med. 2002;346:393-403.

2. Expert Panel on Detection, Evaluation, and Treatment of High Blood Cholesterol in Adults. Executive summary of the Third Report of the National Cholesterol Education Program (NCEP) Expert Panel on Detection, Evaluation, and Treatment of High Blood Cholesterol in Adults (Adult Treatment Panel III). JAMA. 2001;285:2486-2497. Full report: National Institutes of Health. Third Report of the National Cholesterol Education Program Expert Panel on Detection, Evaluation, and Treatment of High Blood Cholesterol in Adults (Adult Treatment Panel III). Bethesda, Md: National Institutes of Health; 2001. NIH Publication 01-3670. Available at: http://www.nhlbi.nih.gov/guidelines/cholesterol/atp3_rpt.htm. Accessed March 29, 2004.

3. Kelin R. Hyperglycemia and microvascular and macrovascular disease in diabetes. Diabetes Care. 1995;18:258-268.

4. Turner RC, Millns H, Neil HA, Stratton IM, Manley SE, Matthews DR, Homan RR. Risk factors for coronary artery disease in non-insulin dependent diabetes mellitus: United Kingdom Prospective Diabetes Study (UKPDS 23). Br Med J. 1998;316:823-828.

5. Laakso M. Glycemic control and the risk for coronary heart disease in patients with non-insulin-dependent diabetes mellitus: the Finnish studies. *Ann Intern Med.* 1996;124:127-130.

6. Saaddine JB, Engelgau MM, Beckles GL, Gregg EW, Thompson TJ, Narayan KMV. A diabetes report card for the United States: quality of care in the 1990s. *Ann Intern Med.* 2002;136:565-574.

7. American Diabetes Association Position Statement. Evidence-based nutrition principles and recommendations for the treatment and prevention of diabetes and related complications. *Diabetes Care.* 2002;25:S50-S60.

8. Franz MJ, Bantle JP, Beebe CA, Brunzell JD, Chiasson JL, Holzmeister LA, Hoogwerf B, Mayer-Davis E, Mooradian AD, Purnell JQ, Wheeler M. Evidence-based nutrition principles and recommendations for the treatment and prevention of diabetes and related complications, Technical Review. *Diabetes Care.* 2002;25:148-198.

9. National Heart, Lung, and Blood Institute, Obesity Education Initiative Expert Panel. *Clinical Guidelines on the Identification, Evaluation, and Treatment of Overweight and Obesity in Adults: The Evidence Report.* Bethesda, Md: US Department of Health and Human Services; 1998. NIH publication 98-4038. Available at: http://www.nhlbi.nih.gov/guidelines/obesity/ob_gdlns.pdf. Accessed May 25, 2004.

10. Anderson JW, Kendall CWC, Jenkins DJA. Importance of weight management in type 2 diabetes: review with meta-analysis of clinical studies. *J Am Coll Nutr.* 2003;22:331-339.

11. Markovic TP, Jenkins AB, Campbell LV, Furler SM, Kraegen EW, Chisholm DJ. The determinants of glycemic responses to diet restriction and weight loss in obesity and NIDDM. *Diabetes Care.* 1998;21:687-694.

12. Bosello O, Armellini F, Zamboni M, Fitchet M. The benefits of modest weight loss in type II diabetes. *Int J Obesity.* 1997;21(suppl 1):S10-S13.

13. Van Gaal LF, Wauters MA, De Leeuw IH. The beneficial effects of modest weight loss on cardiovascular risk factors. *Int J Obes.* 1997;21(suppl 1):S5-S9.

14. Wing RR, Koeske R, Epstein LH, Nowalk MP, Gooding W, Becker D. Long-term effects of modest weight loss in type II diabetic patients. *Arch Intern Med.* 1987;147:1749-1753.

15. Shick SM, Wing RR, Klem ML, McGuire MT, Hill JO, Seagle H. Persons successful at long-term weight loss and maintenance continue to consume a low-energy, low-fat diet. *J Am Diet Assoc.* 1998;98:408-413.

16. Klem ML, Wing RR, McGuire MT, Seagle HM, Hill JO. A descriptive study of individuals successful at long-term maintenance of substantial weight loss. *Am J Clin Nutr.* 1997;66:239-246.

17. Abate N, Garg A. Heterogeneity in adipose tissue metabolism: causes, implications and management of regional adiposity. *Prog Lipid Res.* 1995;34:53-70.

18. Abate N, Garg A, Peshock RM, Stray-Gundersen J, Adams-Huet B, Grundy SM. Relationship of generalized and regional adiposity to insulin sensitivity in men with NIDDM. *Diabetes.* 1996;45:1684-1693.

19. Chandalia M, Abate N, Garg A, Stray-Gundersen J, Grundy SM. Regional adiposity and insulin resistance in Asian Indian migrant men to the United States. *J Invest Med.* 1995;43(suppl 2):303A.

20. Romieu I, Willett WC, Stampfer MJ, Colditz GA, Sampson L, Rosner B, Hennekens CH, Speizer FE. Energy intake and other determinants of relative weight. *Am J Clin Nutr.* 1988;47:406-412.

21. Gazzaniga JM, Burns TL. Relationship between diet composition and body fatness, with adjustment for resting energy expenditure and physical activity in preadolescent children. *Am J Clin Nutr.* 1993;58:21-28.

22. Shah M, Garg A. High-fat and high-carbohydrate diets and energy balance. *Diabetes Care.* 1996;19:1142-1152.

23. Foster GD, Wyatt HR, Hill JO, McGuckin BG, Brill C, Mohammed BS, Szapary PO, Rader DJ, Edman JS, Klein S. A randomized trial of a low-carbohydrate diet for obesity. *N Engl J Med.* 2003;348:2082-2090.

24. National Institute on Aging. Exercise: A Guide from the National Institute on Aging. Bethesda, Md: National Institutes of Health; 1999. NIH publication 99-4258.

25. American Dietetic Association. Position of the American Dietetic Association: use of nutritive and nonnutritive sweeteners. *J Am Diet Assoc.* 2004;104:255-275.

26. Warshaw HS, Powers MA. A search for answers about foods with polyols (sugar alcohols). *Diabetes Educator.* 1999;25:307-321.

27. Payne ML, Craig WJ, Williams AC. Sorbitol is a possible risk factor for diarrhea in young children. *J Am Diet Assoc.* 1997;97:532-534.

28. Pitkin R, Reynolds W, Filer LJ, Kling TG. Placental transmission and fetal distribution of saccharin. *Am J Obstet Gynecol.* 1971;111:280.

29. American Dietetic Association. Position paper on fat replacers. *J Am Diet Assoc.* 1998;98:463-468.

30. Cater NB, Denke MA. Comparison of effects of behenate oil, high oleic acid sunflower oil, and palm oil on lipids and lipoproteins in humans [Abstract]. *Circulation.* 1996;94:I-97.

31. Bantle JP, Swanson JE, Thomas W, Laine DC. Metabolic effects of dietary sucrose in type II diabetic subjects. *Diabetes Care.* 1993;16:1301-1305.

32. Peters AL, Davidson MB, Eisenberg K. Effect of isocaloric substitution of chocolate cake for potato in type I diabetic patients. *Diabetes Care.* 1990;13:888-892.

33. Hollenbeck CB, Coulston A, Donner CC, Williams RA, Reaven GM. The effects of variations in percent of naturally occurring complex and simple carbohydrates on plasma glucose and insulin response in individuals with non-insulin-dependent diabetes mellitus. *Diabetes.* 1985;34:151-155.

34. Coulston AM, Hollenbeck CB, Donner CC, Williams R, Chiou YA, Reaven GM. Metabolic effects of added dietary sucrose in individuals with non-insulin-dependent diabetes mellitus (NIDDM). *Metabolism.* 1985;34:962-966.

35. Bantle JP, Swanson JE, Thomas W, Laine DC. Metabolic effects of dietary fructose in diabetic subjects. *Diabetes Care.* 1992;15:1468-1476.

36. Bantle JP. Current recommendations regarding the dietary treatment of diabetes mellitus. *Endocrinologist.* 1994;4:189-195.

37. Crapo PA, Kolterman OG, Henry RR. Metabolic consequence of two-week fructose feeding in diabetic subjects. *Diabetes Care.* 1986;9:111-119.

38. Malerbi DA, Paiva ESA, Duarte AL, Wajchenberg BL. Metabolic effects of dietary sucrose and fructose in type II diabetic subjects. *Diabetes Care.* 1996;19:1249-1256.

39. Grant KI, Marais MP, Dhansay MA. Sucrose in a lipid-rich meal amplifies the postprandial excursion of serum and lipoprotein triglyceride and cholesterol concentrations by decreasing triglyceride clearance. *Am J Clin Nutr.* 1994;59:853-860.

40. Bantle JP, Raatz SK, Thomas W, Georgopoulos A. Effects of dietary fructose on plasma lipids in healthy subjects. *Am J Clin Nutr.* 2000;72:1128-1134.

41. Martinez FJ, Rizza RA, Romero JC. High-fructose feeding elicits insulin resistance, hyperinsulinism, and hypertension in normal mongrel dogs. *Hypertension.* 1994;23:456-463.

42. Thorburn AW, Storlien LH, Jenkins AB, Khouri S, Kraegen EW. Fructose-induced in vivo insulin resistance and elevated plasma triglycerides in rats. *Am J Clin Nutr.* 1989;49:1155-1163.

43. Elliott SS, Keim NL, Stern JS, Teff K, Havel PJ. Fructose, weight gain, and the insulin resistance syndrome. *Am J Clin Nutr.* 2002;76:911-922.

44. US Department of Agriculture, Agricultural Research Service. 2002. USDA National Nutrient Database for Standard Reference, Release 15. Nutrient Data Laboratory Home Page. Available at: http://www.nal.usda.gov/fnic/foodcomp. Accessed June 10, 2004.

45. Jeppesen J, Chen Y-DI, Zhou M-Y, Schaaf P, Coulston A, Reaven GM. Postprandial triglyceride and retinyl ester responses to oral fat: effects of fructose. *Am J Clin Nutr.* 1994;61:787-791.

46. Jeppesen J, Chen Y-DI, Zhou M-Y, Wang T, Reaven GM. Effect of variations in oral fat and carbohydrate load on postprandial lipemia. *Am J Clin Nutr.* 1995;62:1201-1205.

47. Coulston AM, Johnson RK. Sugar and sugars: myths and realities. *J Am Diet Assoc.* 2002;102:351-353.

48. Levine B. Role of liquid intake in childhood obesity and related diseases. *Curr Concepts Perspect Nutr.* 1996;8:1-8.

49. Wolever TM, Jenkins DJ, Jenkins AL, Josse RG. The glycemic index: methodology and clinical implications. *Am J Clin Nutr.* 1991;54:846-854.

50. Foster-Powell K, Holt SH, Brand-Miller JC. International table of glycemic index and glycemic load values: 2002. *Am J Clin Nutr.* 2002;76:5-56.

51. Brand-Miller J, Hayne S, Petocz P, Colagiuri S. Low-glycemic index diets in the management of diabetes. *Diabetes Care.* 2003;26:2261-2267.

52. Pi-Sunyer FX. Glycemic index and disease. *Am J Clin Nutr.* 2002;76(suppl):290S-298S.

53. Franz M. The glycemic index: not the most effective nutrition therapy intervention. *Diabetes Care.* 2003;26:2466-2468.

54. Chandalia M, Garg A, Lutjohann D, von Bergmann K, Grundy SM, Brinkley LJ. Beneficial effects of high dietary fiber intake in patients with type 2 diabetes mellitus. *N Engl J Med.* 2000;342:1392-1398.

55. Schakel SF, Pettit J, Himes JH. Dietary fiber values for common foods (Appendix Table A.1). In: Spiller GA, ed. *CRC Handbook of Dietary Fiber in Human Nutrition.* 3rd ed. Boca Raton, Fla: CRC Press; 2001:615.

56. Institute of Medicine. *Dietary Reference Intakes for Energy, Carbohydrate, Fiber, Fat, Fatty Acids, Cholesterol, Protein and Amino Acids.* Washington, DC: National Academy Press; 2002.

57. Jenkins DJA, Kendall CWC, Marchie A, Jenkins AL, Augustin LSA, Ludwig DS, Barnard ND, Anderson JW. Type 2 diabetes and the vegetarian diet. *Am J Clin Nutr.* 2003;78(suppl):610S-616S.

58. Jenkins DJA, Kendall CWC, Jackson CC, Connelly PW, Parker T, Faulkner D, Vidgen E, Cunnane SC, Leiter LA, Josse RG. Effects of high- and low-isoflavone soyfoods on blood lipids, oxidized LDL, homocysteine, and blood pressure in hyperlipidemic men and women. *Am J Clin Nutr.* 2002;76:365-372.

59. American Diabetes Association. Management of dyslipidemia in adults with diabetes. *Diabetes Care.* 2004;27(suppl):S68-S69.

60. Cater NB, Heller HJ, Denke MA. Comparison of the effects of medium-chain triacylglycerols, palm oil, and high oleic acid sunflower oil on plasma triacylglycerol fatty acids and lipid and lipoprotein concentrations in humans. *Am J Clin Nutr.* 1997;65:41-45.

61. Kris-Etherton PM, Taylor DS, Yu-Poth S, Huth P, Moriarty K, Fishell V, Hargrove RL, Zhao G, Etherton TD. Polyunsaturated fatty acids in the food chain in the United States. *Am J Clin Nutr.* 2000;71(suppl):179S-188S.

62. Kris-Etherton PM, Harris WS, Appel LJ. Fish consumption, fish oil omega-3 fatty acids, and cardiovascular disease. *Circulation.* 2002;106:2747-2757.

63. Harper CR, Jacobson TA. The fats of life. *Arch Intern Med.* 2002;161:2185-2192.

64. Prince MJ, Deeg MA. Do n-3 fatty acids improve glucose tolerance and lipemia in diabetics? *Curr Opin Lipidol.* 1997;8:7-11.

65. Connor WE, Prince MJ, Ullman D, Riddle M, Hatcher L, Smith FE, Wilson D. The hypotriglyceridemic effect of fish oil in adult-onset diabetes without adverse glucose control. *Ann N Y Acad Sci.* 1993;683:337-340.

66. Rivellese AA, Mafettone A, Iovine C, Di Marino L, Annuzzi G, Mancini M, Riccardi G. Long-term effects of fish oil on insulin resistance and plasma lipoproteins in NIDDM patients with hypertriglyceridemia. *Diabetes Care.* 1996;19:1207-1213.

67. Albert CM, Hennekens CH, O'Donnell CH, Christopher J, Ajani UA, Carey VJ, Willett WC, Ruskin JN, Manson JE. Fish consumption and risk of sudden cardiac death. *JAMA.* 1998;279:23-28.

68. Gill JMR, Brown JC, Caslake MJ, Wright DM, Cooney J, Bedford D, Hughes DA, Stanley JC, Packard CJ. Effects of dietary monounsaturated fatty acids on lipoprotein concentrations, compositions, and subfraction distributions and on VLDL apolipoprotein B kinetics: dose-dependent effects on LDL. *Am J Clin Nutr.* 2003;78:47-56.

69. Mensink RP, Katan MB. Effects of dietary fatty acids on serum lipids and lipoproteins: A meta-analysis of 27 trials. *Arterioscler Thromb.* 1992;12:911-919.

70. Dreon DM, Vranizan KM, Krauss RM, Austin MA, Wood PD. The effects of polyunsaturated fat vs monounsaturated fat on plasma lipoproteins. *JAMA.* 1990;263:2462-2466.

71. Garg A, Bonanome A, Grundy SM, Zhang ZJ, Unger RJ. Comparison of a high-carbohydrate diet with a high-monounsaturated-fat diet in patients with non-insulin-dependent diabetes mellitus. *N Engl J Med.* 1988;319:829-834.

72. Garg A. High-monounsaturated-fat diets for patients with diabetes mellitus: A meta-analysis. *Am J Clin Nutr.* 1998;67(suppl):577S-582S.

73. Strychar I, Ishac A, Rivard M, Lussier-Cacan S, Beauregard H, Aris-Jilwan N, Radwan F, Yale JF. Impact of a high-monounsaturated-fat diet on lipid profile in subjects with type 1 diabetes. *J Am Diet Assoc.* 2003;103:467-74.

74. Mensink RP, Katan MB. Effect of dietary trans fatty acids on high-density and low-density lipoprotein cholesterol levels in healthy subjects. *N Engl J Med.* 1990;323:439-445.

75. Lichtenstein A. *Trans* fatty acids and cardiovascular disease risk. *Curr Opin Lipidol.* 2000;11:37-42.

76. Hu FB, Stampfer MJ, Manson JE, Rimm E, Colditz GA, Rosner BA, Hennekens CH, Willett WC. Dietary fat intake and the risk of coronary heart disease in women. *N Engl J Med.* 1997;337:1491-1499.

77. Hu FB, Van Dam RM, Luis S. Diet and risk of type II diabetes: the role of types of fat and carbohydrate. *Diabetologia.* 2001;44:805-817.

78. Salmeron J, Hu FB, Manson JE, Stampfer MJ, Colditz GA, Rimm EB, Willett WC. Dietary fat intake and risk of type 2 diabetes in women. *Am J Clin Nutr.* 2002;73:1019-1026.

79. National Health and Nutrition Examination Survey III, 1988–1994. NCHS CD-ROM series 11. No. 2A. ASCII version. National Center for Health Statistics: April 1998.

80. Eeley EA, Stratton IM, Hadden DR, Turner RC, Holman, RR. UKPDS 18: estimated dietary intake in type 2 diabetic patients randomly allocated to diet, sulphonylurea, or insulin therapy. UK Prospective Diabetes Study Group. *Diabet Med.* 1996;13:656-662.

81. Bazzano LA, He J, Ogden LG, Loria CM, Whelton PK. Dietary fiber intake and reduced risk of coronary heart disease in US men and women. The National Health and Nutrition Examination Survey I Epidemiologic Follow-up Study. *Arch Intern Med.* 2003;163:1897-1904.

82. Toeller M. Fibre consumption, metabolic effects and prevention of complications in diabetic patients: epidemiologic evidence. *Dig Liver Dis.* 2002;34(suppl 2):S145-S149.

83. Kiechl S, Willeit J, Poewe W, Egger G, Oberhollenzer F, Muggeo M, Bonora E. Insulin sensitivity and regular alcohol consumption: large, prospective, cross sectional population study (Bruneck study). *BMJ.* 1996;313:1040-1044.

84. Ben G, Gnudi L, Maran A, Gigante A, Duner E, Iori E, Tiengo A, Avogaro A. Effects of chronic alcohol intake on carbohydrate and lipid metabolism in subjects with type II (non-insulin-dependent) diabetes. *Am J Med.* 1991;90:70-76.

85. Puhakainen I, Koivisto VA, Yki-Jarvinen H. No reduction in total hepatic glucose output by inhibition of gluconeogenesis with ethanol in NIDDM patients. *Diabetes.* 1991;40:1319-1327.

86. Yki-Jarvinen H, Koivisto VA, Ylikahri R, Taskinen MR. Acute effects of ethanol and acetate on glucose kinetics in normal subjects. *Am J Physiol.* 1988;254:E175-E180.

87. Pownell HJ, Ballantyne CM, Kimball KT, Simpson SL, Yeshurun D, Gotto AM Jr. Effect of moderate alcohol consumption on hypertriglyceridemia. *Arch Intern Med.* 1999;159:981-987.

88. Wei M, Gibbons LW, Mitchell TL, Kampert JB, Blair SN. Alcohol intake and incidence of type 2 diabetes in men. *Diabetes Care.* 2000;23:18-22.

89. Bjorntorp P, Rosmond R. Visceral obesity and diabetes. *Drugs.* 1999;58(suppl 1):S13-S18.

90. Naveau S, Giraud V, Borotto E, Aubert A, Capron F, Chaput JC. Excess weight risk factor for alcoholic liver disease. *Hepatology.* 1997;25:108-111.

91. Kerr D, Macdonald IA, Heller SR, Tattersall RB. Alcohol causes hypoglycaemic unawareness in healthy volunteers and patients with type 1 (insulin-dependent) diabetes. *Diabetologia.* 1990;33:216-221.

92. Burge MR, Zeise T-M, Sobhy TA, Rassam AG, Schade DS. Low-dose ethanol predisposes elderly fasted patients with type 2 diabetes to sulfonylurea-induced low blood glucose. *Diabetes Care.* 1999;22:2037-2043.

93. Mooradian AD, Failla M, Hoogwerf B, Maryniuk M, Wylie-Rosett J. Selected vitamins and minerals in diabetes. *Diabetes Care.* 1994;17:464-479.
94. Jialal I, Grundy SM. Effect of combined supplementation with alpha-tocopherol, ascorbate, and beta-carotene on low-density lipoprotein oxidation. *Circulation.* 1993;88:2780-2786.
95. Yusuf S, Dagenais G, Pogue J, Bosch J, Sleight P. Vitamin E supplementation and cardiovascular events in high-risk patients. The Heart Outcomes Prevention Evaluation Study Investigators. *N Engl J Med.* 2000;342:154-160.
96. Albanes D, Heinonen OP, Taylor PR, Virtamo J, Edwards BK, Rautalahti M, Hartman AM, Palmgren J, Freedman LS, Haapakoski J, Barrett MJ, Pietinen P, Malila N, Tala E, Liippo K, Salomaa ER, Tangrea JA, Teppo L, Askin FB, Taskinen E, Erozan Y, Greenwald P, Huttunen JK. Alpha-tocopherol and beta-carotene supplements and lung cancer incidence in the alpha-tocopherol, beta-carotene cancer prevention study: Effects of base-line characteristics and study compliance. *J Natl Cancer Inst.* 1996;88:1560-1570.
97. Zemel MB, Shi H, Greer B, Dirienzo D, Zemel PC. Regulation of adiposity by dietary calcium. *FASEB J.* 2000;14:1132-1138.
98. Lin Y, Lyle RM, McCabe LD, McCabe GP, Weaver CM, Teegarden D. Dairy calcium is related to changes in body composition during a two-year exercise intervention in young women. *J Am Coll Nutr.* 2000;19:754-760.
99. Lima JDL, Cruz T, Pousada JC, Rodrigues LE, Barbosa K, Cangucu V. The effect of magnesium supplementation in increasing doses on the control of type 2 diabetes. *Diabetes Care.* 1998;21:682-686.
100. UK Prospective Diabetes Study Group (UKPDS). Tight blood pressure control and risk of macrovascular and microvascular complications in type 2 diabetes (UKPDS 38) [erratum in *BMJ.* 1999;318:29]. *BMJ.* 1998;317:703-713.
101. UK Prospective Diabetes Study Group (UKPDS). Efficacy of atenolol and captopril in reducing risk of macrovascular and microvascular complications in type 2 diabetes (UKPDS 39). *BMJ.* 1998;317:713-720.
102. Midgley JP, Matthew AG, Greenwood CM, Logan AG. Effect of reduced dietary sodium on blood pressure: A meta-analysis of randomized controlled trials. *JAMA.* 1996;275:1590-1597.
103. Overlack A, Ruppert M, Kolloch R, Kraft K, Stumpe KO. Age is a major determinant of the divergent blood pressure responses to varying salt intake in essential hypertension. *Am J Hypertens.* 1995;8:829-836.
104. National Heart, Lung, and Blood Institute, National Institutes of Health, US Department of Health and Human Services. JNC 7 Express: The Seventh Report of the Joint National Committee on Prevention, Detection, Evaluation, and Treatment of High Blood Pressure. Available at: http://www.nhlbi.nih.gov/guidelines/hypertension/express.pdf. Accessed October 10, 2003.
105. Jenkins DJA, Ocana A, Jenkins AL, Wolever TMS, Vuksan V, Katzman L, Hollands M, Greenberg G, Corey P, Patten R, Wong G, Josse RG. Metabolic advantages of spreading the nutrient load: effects of increased meal frequency in non-insulin-dependent diabetes. *Am J Clin Nutr.* 1992;55:461-467.
106. Bertelsen J, Christiansen C, Thomsen C, Poulsen PL, Vestergaard S, Steinov A, Rasmussen LH, Rasmussen O, Hermansen K. Effect of meal frequency on blood glucose, insulin, and free fatty acids in NIDDM subjects. *Diabetes Care.* 1993;16:4-7.
107. Jenkins DJA, Wolever TMS, Vuksan V, Brighenti F, Cunnane SC, Venketeshwer R, Jenkins AL, Buckley G, Patten R, Singer W, Corey P, Josse RG. Nibbling versus gorging: Metabolic advantages of increased meal frequency. *N Engl J Med.* 1989;321:929-934.
108. Schlundt DG, Hill JO, Sbrocco T, Pope-Cordle J, Sharp T. The role of breakfast in the treatment of obesity: a randomized clinical trial. *Am J Clin Nutr.* 1992;55:645-651.
109. Cho S, Dietrich M, Brown CJP, Clark CA, Block G. The effect of breakfast type on total daily energy intake and body mass index: Results from the third National Health and Nutrition Examination Survey (NHANES III). *J Am Coll Nutr.* 2003;22:296-302.
110. Schlundt DG, Rea MR, Kline SS, Pichert JW. Situational obstacles to dietary adherence for adults with diabetes. *J Am Diet Assoc.* 1994;94:874-876, 879.
111. Williamson AR, Hunt AE, Pope JF, Tolman NM. Recommendations of dietitians for overcoming barriers to dietary adherence in individuals with diabetes. *Diabetes Educ.* 2000;26:272-279.
112. Johnson EQ, Valera S. Medical nutrition therapy in non-insulin-dependent diabetes mellitus improves clinical outcome. *J Am Diet Assoc.* 1995;95:700-701.
113. Franz MJ, Pastors JG, Warshaw H, Daly AE. Does "diet" fail? *Clin Diabetes.* 2000;18:162-168.
114. Franz MJ, Warshaw H, Daly AE, Green-Pastors J, Arnold MS, Bantle J. Evolution of diabetes medical nutrition therapy. *Postgrad Med J.* 2003;79:30-35.
115. Pastors JG, Warshaw H, Daly A, Franz M, Kulkarni K. The evidence for the effectiveness of medical nutrition therapy in diabetes management. *Diabetes Care.* 2002;25:608-613.
116. Pastors JG, Franz MJ, Warshaw H, Daly A, Arnold MS. How effective is medical nutrition therapy in diabetes care? *J Am Diet Assoc.* 2003;103:827-831.
117. Arnold MS, Stepien CJ, Hess GE, Hiss RG. Guidelines vs. practice in the delivery of diabetes nutrition care. *J Am Diet Assoc.* 1993;93:34-39.
118. Close EJ, Wiles PG, Lockton JA, Walmsley D, Oldham J, Wales JK. The degree of day-to-day variation in food intake in diabetic patients. *Diabet Med.* 1993;10:514-520.
119. The Diabetes Control and Complication Trial (DCCT) Research Group. Nutrition interventions for intensive therapy in The Diabetes Control and Complications Trial. *J Am Diet Assoc.* 1993;93:768-772.

120. Delahanty LM, Halford BN. The role of diet behaviors in achieving improved glycemic control in intensively treated patients in the diabetes control and complications trial. *Diabetes Care.* 1993;16:1453-1458.

121. Travis T. Patient perceptions of factors that affect adherence to dietary regimens for diabetes mellitus. *Diabetes Educ.* 1997;23:152-156.

122. Franz MJ, Monk A, Barry B, McClain K, Weaver T, Cooper N, Upham P, Bergenstal R, Mazze RS. Effectiveness of medical nutrition therapy provided by dietitians in the management of non-insulin-dependent diabetes mellitus: a randomized, controlled clinical trial. *J Am Diet Assoc.* 1995;95:1009-1017.

Complementary and Alternative Approaches

CHAPTER 10

FUNCTIONAL FOODS IN THE PREVENTION OF CARDIOVASCULAR DISEASE

Philippe O. Szapary, MD, FACP, and Maureen E. Conway, MBA, MA, RD

"Let your food be your medicine and your medicine be your food."
Hippocrates

INTRODUCTION

Coronary heart disease (CHD) remains the leading cause of morbidity and mortality in the Western world. The most recent statistics suggest that 2,600 Americans die of CHD each day, an average of one death every 33 seconds (1). Although great medical advances have been made in the last 40 years in treating CHD, especially in the acute setting, there is still ample opportunity for both primary and secondary prevention of CHD. Changes in lifestyle are perhaps one of the most cost-effective methods in preventing CHD morbidity (2). Specifically, adoption of more healthful diet patterns and an increase in physical activity are the two most important features of a comprehensive lifestyle change that has been shown to reduce the burden of CHD. These two factors were recognized by the National Cholesterol Education Program (NCEP) in its most recent guidelines (3). In the Adult Treatment Panel (ATP) III recommendations, the NCEP introduced the concept of Therapeutic Lifestyle Changes (TLC) as the first step in treating hypercholesterolemia and preventing CHD. In addition to dietary patterns, there has been an increasing interest in specific foods and their bioactive constituents as a therapeutic approach to CHD. These foods, often termed "functional foods" or "nutraceuticals," are defined by the American Dietetic Association (ADA) as "whole, fortified, enriched, or enhanced foods that have a potentially beneficial effect on health when consumed as part of a varied diet on a regular basis, at effective levels" (4). Although the definition of functional foods is a matter of debate, their therapeutic and economic importance is clear. For example, the NCEP has recently recognized two functional foods, plant sterols and stanols and soluble fiber, as approved therapies in managing hypercholesterolemia. This chapter summarizes the scientific basis for the efficacy, safety, and applicability of the most recognized functional foods used for cardiovascular risk reduction.

PLANT STEROLS AND STANOLS

Background and Mechanisms

Plant sterols and stanols, collectively known as phytosterols, are natural components of plants. The average daily consumption of plant sterols and stanols in typical American and Western European diets is about 300 mg, and vegetarian diets provide about 500 mg/day (5). Important sources of sterols and stanols include vegetable oils and nuts (6,7).

Plant sterols have chemical structures that are similar to cholesterol. Differences between phytosterols and cholesterol are seen only in their side chains, which presumably account for their differences in intestinal absorption (5,6). Whereas cholesterol is absorbed to a significant degree, plant sterols are absorbed to a much lower degree. The two most abundant plant sterols are campesterol and sitosterol (refer to Figure 10.1). Plant stanols can be produced by the hydrogenation of plant sterols and have no double bond in their sterol ring structure (refer to Figure 10.2). Presumably because of this minor difference from plant sterols and cholesterol, plant stanols are virtually not absorbed in the intestinal tract. Plant stanols are found in nature in smaller amounts, with sitostanol and campestanol being the major plant stanols (8).

The chemical structures of both plant sterols and stanols can be further modified by attaching fatty acid esters to the sterol rings. Esterification of plant sterols and stanols increases their solubility in food (3). Once in the small intestine, esters are readily cleaved by esterases to yield free sterol or stanol. Although their exact mechanism of action is unknown, the effect of plant sterols and stanols in reducing cholesterol absorption is well established (9,10). Both plant sterols and stanols compete with the absorption of dietary and biliary cholesterol in the

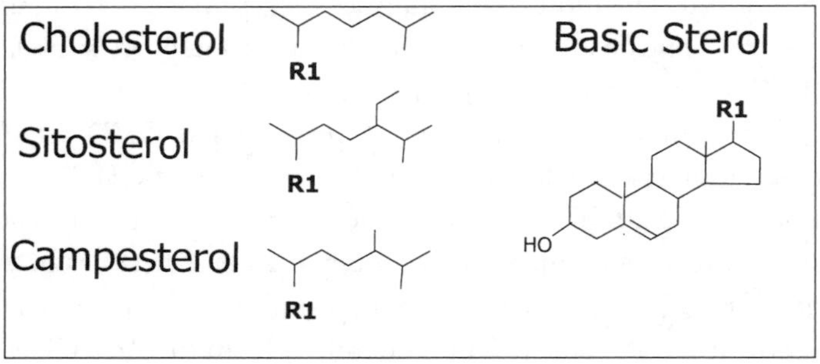

Figure 10.1
Structures of the most abundant sterols.

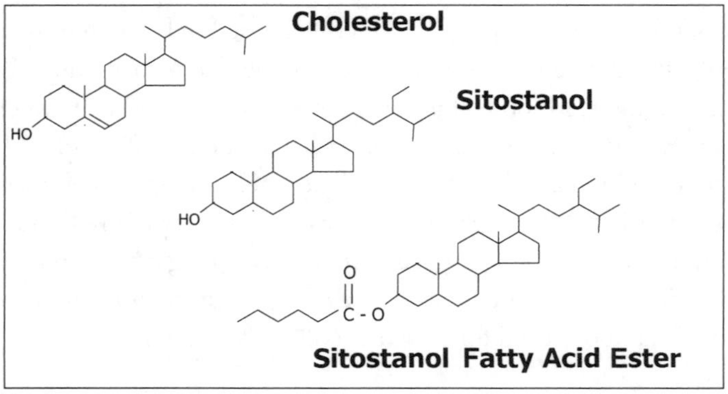

Figure 10.2
Structures of plant stanol esters.

intestinal lumen. By competing with cholesterol and replacing it in the mixed micelles, sterols and stanols reduce cholesterol absorption. Studies have shown that a minimum amount of 800 to 1,000 mg/day of esterified forms of plant stanols or sterols must be added to the diet to produce a significant reduction in cholesterol absorption and low-density lipoprotein (LDL) cholesterol levels (5).

It has recently been suggested that sterols and stanols also modulate the adenosine triphosphate-binding cassette (ABCA) transport proteins that promote transport of cholesterol from the enterocyte back into the intestinal lumen. (See Chapter 2 for explanation of ABCA1.) It is hypothesized that plant stanols—and possibly plant sterols—increase ABCA1-mediated cholesterol efflux back into the intestinal lumen and contribute to a decrease in cholesterol absorption (11). Delivering less cholesterol to the liver leads to increased cholesterol synthesis and increased LDL receptor activity, which results in a reduction of serum LDL cholesterol (5).

Efficacy Studies

More than any other functional food, phytosterols have a wealth of data supporting their role in cholesterol reduction. The hypocholesterolemic benefits of plant sterols were first recognized in the 1950s. Between then and the early 1990s, liquid suspensions, granules, and powders of non-esterified plant sterols were used in investigational studies. These formulations posed problems in terms of palatability, and reliable efficacy required doses that were quite large (between 10 and 50 g/day). In addition, there were concerns about excessive serum sterol levels being linked to atherosclerosis (5,7,12). It was then recognized that plant stanols might be more advantageous because they are virtually not absorbed (5). The esterification process was developed to facilitate incorporation of plant stanols into fat-based foods. These foods had been shown to be the best vehicles for delivering sterols and stanols to within proximity of mixed micelles and thus produce consistent reductions in cholesterol absorption and blood cholesterol levels. An esterification process for plant sterols was subsequently developed. Esterification allows for lower amounts of stanols and sterols (0.8 to 3.0 g/day) to be used (13). Although sterol esters are more readily absorbed than stanol esters, both sterol and stanol esters have been shown to have very good safety profiles (5).

In 1995, results of a landmark trial demonstrated that a plant stanol ester spread that provided 2.6 g/day of plant stanols reduced total cholesterol levels by 10% and LDL cholesterol levels by 14% in a mildly hypercholesterolemic Northern European population (14). These reductions were sustained during the rest of the year-long trial. In 2003 the results of a similarly designed year-long trial demonstrated that plant sterol ester spread, which provided 1.8 g/day of plant sterols, reduced total cholesterol levels by 4% and LDL cholesterol levels by 6% (15).

Numerous well-designed, shorter-term studies have consistently documented the efficacy of both plant sterol and stanol esters in reducing serum cholesterol both in monotherapy, with and without a low-fat diet, and in combination with prescription lipid-lowering drugs (16). For example, the effects of incorporating a reduced-fat, sterol-enriched margarine into a diet with less than 10% saturated fat were studied in people with mildly to moderately elevated cholesterol levels (17). In a randomized control trial, subjects consumed either a reduced-fat spread or a reduced-fat spread enriched with plant sterol esters to achieve intakes of 0, 1.1, or 2.2 g/day. LDL cholesterol levels were 7.6% and 8.1% lower in the low-sterol and high-sterol groups, respectively, than in the control group (17). Thus, the addition of a sterol-enriched spread resulted in an additional significant cholesterol reduction beyond that achieved with a lipid-lowering diet alone (17). These reductions in LDL cholesterol, although modest, are predicted to reduce the risk of heart disease by 25% (16).

Interest in non-esterified phytosterols has reemerged as investigators have sought ways to expand the range of potential foods in which these substances can be included. Non-esterified stanols and sterols have been incorporated into cereal, bread, and canola oil–based margarine (18), as well as butter (19) and beverages such as orange juice (20,21), at doses equivalent to those currently used in commercially available spreads. Results from clinical trials have demonstrated that these products produce a hypocholesterolemic effect comparable to sterol- and stanol-ester-enriched spreads when consumed with meals. It should be noted, however, that non-esterified forms have not been studied extensively for their cholesterol-lowering effects and that studies to date are lacking regarding their efficacy at amounts lower than 2 g/day. Moreover, food matrix and emulsification techniques may affect the efficacy of these products (8). In one study, plant sterol–fortified milk consumed with meals lowered LDL cholesterol levels more than plant sterol–fortified cereal or bread (22). Further evaluation is clearly warranted.

The minimum amount of sterols or stanols required to produce a clinically significant reduction of LDL cholesterol levels is in the range of 0.8 to 1 g/day (23,24). A dose-response relationship is apparent at doses up to 2 g/day. These findings have been supported in a single-blind, dose-range-finding study (23). Improvements in cholesterol at doses up to 3 g/day are not dramatically larger than improvements with 2 g/day, leading health and regulatory agencies to recommend intakes of 2 g/day (3,25,26).

Other studies have reported that the effects of plant stanol esters and sterol esters are additive to the effects of statins (27-30) and bile acid sequestrants (30). In one study, LDL cholesterol was reduced by an additional 17% (vs 7% for placebo) when 3 g/day of plant stanol in ester form was added to the diet of patients on a stable statin dose (28).

Safety Profile

The safety of stanol and sterols has been reviewed by regulatory agencies in the United States, Europe, and several other countries. The US Food and Drug Administration (FDA) has determined plant stanols and sterols to be generally recognized as safe (GRAS). The FDA has also issued a health claim that foods containing plant stanols and sterols may reduce the risk of heart disease (31). In April 2000 the Directorate-General of the European Commission on Health and Consumer Protection concluded that margarines with either plant stanols or sterols were safe for human use (32). Foods containing plant stanol esters have been available in Europe since 1995, and in the United States since 1999. Foods containing plant sterol esters were introduced in the United States and Europe in 1999. Although it has been determined that they do not pose a safety concern, the addition of sterols and stanols to dietary regimens has been found to have some effects on the absorption of some fat-soluble vitamins, specifically beta carotene (8,16). The reductions, however, were not found to be clinically significant and can be alleviated by the addition of one extra serving of a high-carotenoid fruit or vegetable to the daily diet (6,16,33).

Recommendations

Phytosterols have received approval as a cardiovascular nutraceutical by a wide body of non-profit and government agencies. In 2000 the FDA approved an interim final health claim that foods containing either plant stanol or sterol esters may reduce the risk of CHD by lowering total and LDL cholesterol (34) (see Chapter 6). The health claim was approved specifically for the following: (*a*) foods fortified with either stanol ester or sterol ester in margarine spreads, salad dressings, and snack bars and (*b*) dietary supplements in soft gel capsules containing plant stanol esters. In 2003 the FDA issued a letter of enforcement discretion that allowed for a more expanded use of the health claim, until a final ruling is issued, which was pending at press time. The discretionary letter allowed for non-esterified forms of stanols or sterols to also bear the health claim, provided they contain 400 mg per serving, with a recommendation of two servings per day (800 mg/day of sterols or stanols) consumed with meals (35). These products should be used as part of a diet low in saturated fat and cholesterol and must contain no more than 13 g of total fat per serving.

The clinical practice guidelines of the ATP III (3), the American Heart Association (AHA) (25), and the American Diabetes Association (26) recommend a level of intake of 2 g/day of sterols or stanols as adjuncts to LDL cholesterol–lowering strategies for cardiovascular disease (CVD) risk reduction. Thus, these guidelines recommend a higher level of daily intake than the minimum amount of 800 mg/day stated in the FDA health claim.

Phytosterols in Practice

In the United States, there are currently two cholesterol-lowering spreads on the market that contain either plant stanol or sterol esters. Both come in regular and light spreads, which can be used in place of margarine and butter in most applications. The regular versions of both products are formulated so they can be used in cooking, frying, and baking, in addition to using them as traditional spreads. Plant stanol esters are also available as a dietary supplement. All products begin to work after 2 weeks of consuming two to three servings per day with meals. More information on Benecol, the only product with plant stanol esters, can be obtained from the product Web site (http://www.benecol.com). For more on Take Control, the only product with plant sterol esters, see its Web site (http://www.takecontrol.com). Manufacturers of functional foods are also exploring ways to incorporate plant stanol and sterol esters into beverages and nutrition bars.

SOLUBLE FIBER

Background and Mechanisms

Epidemiologic data on fiber are extensive and suggest in general an inverse association between total dietary fiber and risk of CHD (36). Thus, fiber is listed by the NCEP as the second functional food as part of the TLC diet. Dietary fiber is composed of both soluble fiber (also known as viscous fiber) and insoluble fiber (cellulose- and hemicellulose-containing products such as wheat). The ATP III guidelines recommend 10 to 25 g/day of soluble fiber. Soluble fiber is found in various foods and supplements, which have been shown as a class to reduce serum LDL cholesterol by modest amounts ranging from 3% to 10% (37). The viscous component of fiber is believed to interfere with dietary absorption of both cholesterol and fat (the fibers bind bile acids). Other mechanisms of action of soluble fiber include enhanced gastric emptying, altered transit time, interference with bulk phase diffusion of fat, increased excretion of bile acids, and inhibition of hepatic cholesterol synthesis by short-chain fatty acids that are produced by the colonic fermentation of soluble fiber. A fiber-rich diet can also reduce cholesterol levels by substituting low-fat foods high in soluble fiber for dietary sources of saturated fat and cholesterol (38). Insoluble fiber does not significantly affect cholesterol levels.

Efficacy Studies

Soluble fiber is found primarily in fruits, vegetables (legumes), and some grains (oat bran) (see Table 10.1), as well as several functional foods, such as psyllium, partially hydrolyzed guar gum, fenugreek, flaxseed, and pectins. Regardless of the type of soluble fiber, both randomized trials and meta-analyses suggest a mild hypocholesterolemic effect (39). The majority of studies have investigated psyllium husk powder, which can be baked into food or mixed into beverages. One study found that adding 5.1 g psyllium powder (Metamucil, Procter & Gamble, Cincinnati, OH 45202) twice daily for 26 weeks reduced LDL cholesterol by 7% without affecting high-density lipoprotein (HDL) cholesterol or triglycerides (TG) (40). In this double-blind, randomized, placebo-controlled clinical trial of 200 patients with mild hypercholesterolemia, there was no difference vs placebo in the rate of gastrointestinal (GI) side effects. In a randomized control trial aimed at comparing a high-fiber diet (8 g soluble fiber per day from various foods) with a low-fat diet, investigators found that by incorporating four servings a day of soluble fiber, LDL cholesterol levels could be only mildly reduced by 2% ($P = .064$). Although this finding was borderline statistically significant, the authors point out that when applied to Framingham calculations of cardiovascular risk, the high-fiber diet could significantly reduce the 10-year risk of a cardiovascular event by 4% ($P = .003$ vs low-fat diet) (41). Aside from the small effect on lipids, high doses of fiber (50 g of total fiber or 24 g soluble fiber per day) have also been shown to reduce postprandial glucose absorption in patients with diabetes (42) and slightly lower systolic blood pressure (43), factors that could also favorably affect

TABLE 10.1
Fiber and Soluble Fiber Content of Common Foods

Food	Serving Size	Total Fiber (g)	Soluble Fiber (g)
Cereals/Grains			
Oat bran	½ cup	7.24	3.58
Oatmeal	½ cup dry	4.29	1.98
Oatmeal, instant	1 packet	3.09	1.43
Bran flakes	1 cup	5.30	0.51
Raisin bran	1 cup	5.30	1.35
Whole-wheat bread	1 slice	1.96	0.34
Flaxseed meal	2 tbsp	4.4	1.10
Fruits			
Apple	1 medium	3.73	0.97
Banana	1 medium	2.74	0.68
Peaches, canned	½ cup	1.76	0.79
Pears, canned	½ cup	1.64	0.16
Prunes, dried	4	2.39	1.28
Orange	1 medium	3.14	1.83
Vegetables			
Broccoli, cooked	½ cup	2.76	1.38
Carrots, raw	1 medium	2.16	1.08
Corn, canned	½ cup	1.64	0.16
Potato, baked with skin	1 small	2.21	0.92
Black beans	½ cup	6.46	2.18
Garbanzo beans	½ cup	4.35	1.31
Kidney beans	½ cup	5.66	2.83
Lentils	½ cup	7.82	0.59
Split peas	½ cup	8.13	1.08

Source: Nutrient calculations were performed using Nutrition Data System for Research (NDS-R) software version 2.9, developed by the Nutrition Coordinating Center (NCC), University of Minnesota, Minneapolis, MN.

cardiovascular risk. These and other studies have made it possible for the FDA to approve a final health claim for specific soluble fiber products (44). (See Chapter 6, Table 6.10.)

Safety Profile

Most patients tolerate well an increase in the amount of dietary fiber. The most common adverse effects mentioned in clinical trials include increased laxation, flatulence, and non-specific abdominal discomfort, which can be minimized by several simple steps outlined in Box 10.1. More rarely, certain forms of very viscous fiber, such as unhydrolyzed guar gum, have been associated with small bowel obstructions (45). For this reason, this older preparation of guar gum is not recommended. Recently, partially hydrolyzed guar gum, sold under the brand name Benefiber (Novartis Consumer Health, Fremont, MI 49413), can provide similar benefits with less risk of GI obstruction (46). Additionally, some popular forms of soluble fiber, such as flax or fenugreek seeds, may induce a hypersensitivity skin reaction in susceptible people and may predispose individuals to diverticulitis unless seeds are ground prior to consumption (47,48). Finally, dietary fibers may bind with certain minerals and decrease their bioavailability, but the effect of this is considered insignificant in healthy adults. A low-dose multivitamin mineral preparation can be used where indicated as a precautionary measure.

Recommendations

The FDA approved an unqualified health claim for soluble fiber and reduction of risk for CVD (see Chapter 6, Table 6.10). Clinical practice guidelines of the ATP III (3), the AHA (25), and the American Diabetes Association (26) recommend increased intake of soluble fiber as an integral component of LDL cholesterol–lowering therapy.

Box 10.1 Prevention of Flatulence with Increasing Dietary Fiber

It can take a few months for the gastrointestinal tract to adapt to high-fiber foods or a vegetarian eating style. The following tips may help to reduce intestinal gas during the transition to a diet high in fruit, vegetables, bran, whole grains, and beans.

- Increase the intake of raw and high-fiber foods gradually (5- to 10-g increments).
- Keep quantities small until gastrointestinal tolerance improves.
- Drink sufficient fluid—at least 8 to 12 glasses a day—because higher fiber intakes increase fluid needs. Note: Beverages with caffeine or alcohol don't count because they increase fluid loss.
- Foods that are cooked or canned may be better tolerated than raw or fresh ones. Fruits, vegetables, or beans that are mashed, blenderized, or pureed may also be easier to digest—mix or blend them into baked goods, sauces, and other foods.
- Rinse canned beans before using. Boil and then soak dry beans for 4 hours; drain the soak water and replace it with fresh water for cooking.
- Maintain regular exercise.
- If needed, consult your doctor or pharmacist for special products that decrease the production of intestinal gas. Examples include Beano,* BeSure,* and Flatulex*—experiment with different types to find the brand that suits you best.

*Beano, GlaxoSmithKline, Pittsburgh, PA 15230. BeSure, Wakunaga of America, Mission Viejo, CA 92691. Flatulex, Dayton Pharmaceuticals, Miami, FL 35166.

Soluble Fiber in Practice

All patients at risk for CHD should increase their intake of dietary fiber to reduce cholesterol and postprandial glucose absorption. The target dose of total dietary fiber should be 25 g/day. For hypercholesterolemic or dysglycemic patients, this amount can be increased to 50 g/day or 10 to 25 g of soluble fiber per day. This should first be accomplished by increasing dietary intake of fresh fruits and vegetables (five servings per day) and whole grains (6 to 11 servings per day) (see Box 10.2) (41). However, this amount of soluble fiber may be difficult to get in a typical Western diet. Some patients should therefore consider enriching their diet with soluble fiber supplements (see Table 10.2). Psyllium powder at a dose of one serving twice daily before meals is the most efficient form of fiber therapy. The powder should be mixed in at least 8 ounces of fluid, drunk quickly, and followed by another 8 ounces of liquid. To avoid problems with drug absorption, all fiber supplements should be taken 1 hour before or 2 hours after taking prescription medications. More research is needed to find out whether certain types of soluble fiber, such as flaxseed or fenugreek, which also contain other phytonutrients, offer more benefits than psyllium. In conclusion, soluble fiber at a dose of at least 4.5 g/day can produce small but clinically significant decreases in LDL cholesterol levels and thus decrease cardiovascular risk.

Box 10.2 Tips for Adding Fiber to the Diet

- Choose fresh fruits rather than canned fruits or juices.
- Choose whole-grain breads.
- Leave the skins on fruits such as apples, pears, and peaches.
- Leave the skins on vegetables such as potatoes, squash, and carrots.
- Have a salad every day.
- When mashing potatoes, leave the skin on.
- Use brown rice rather than white rice.
- Use oats as a filler in casseroles, meat loaf, or salmon patties.
- Use whole-grain flours for baking.
- Use oats or oat bran as a thickening agent for sauces.
- Use high-fiber cereal daily.
- Choose raw vegetables and fresh fruits for snacks.
- Use whole-wheat pasta.
- Eat a serving of dried beans or legumes often.
- Blend oats and use in cooking and baking.
- Eat foods in their most naturally occurring state.

Source: Data are from reference 40.

TABLE 10.2
Fiber Supplements

Supplement Type*	Active Ingredient	Serving Size	Energy (kcal)	Total Fiber, g	Soluble Fiber, g
Metamucil Smooth Texture Sugar-free	Psyllium husk	1 tsp (3.4 g)	20	3	2
Benefiber	Partially hydrolyzed guar gum	1 Tbsp (4 g)	20	3	3
Sugar-free Citrucel	Methylcellulose	1 Tbsp (10.2g)	24	2	2
Flaxseed powder	Mucilage	1 Tbsp (8 g)	36	2.2	0.6

*Metamucil, Procter & Gamble, Cincinnati, OH 45202. Benefiber, Novartis Consumer Health, Parsippany, NJ 07054-0622. Citrucel, GlaxoSmithKline, Pittsburgh, PA 15230.

SOY PROTEIN

Background and Mechanisms

The beneficial effects of soy protein intake on cardiovascular risk have been described for decades. Although the exact mechanism of action is not known, it is believed to come from the isoflavones themselves, from a number of soy proteins, or, more likely, from their combination. It has also been speculated that the soy phytoestrogens collectively called "isoflavones," particularly genistein and daidzein, lower LDL cholesterol (49-53). Isoflavones may act like selective estrogen receptor modulators (SERMs) and upregulate LDL receptors (54) and may even modulate peroxisome proliferator-activated receptor (PPAR)-alpha gene expression (55). However, clinical trials in humans of isolated isoflavones from both soy (56) and red clover (57) have failed to demonstrate a lipid-lowering effect. The value of soy isoflavones, however, should not be discounted. Genistein, daidzein, and equol (a product formed after the metabolism of daidzein in the large intestine) are antioxidants and may protect against oxidative lipid damage that could lead to CVD (58). Animal studies in monkeys (59,60), rabbits (61), and mice (62,63) have demonstrated that isoflavones may inhibit the formation of atherosclerotic lesions and thrombi and improve systemic arterial compliance. Thus, the role of isolated isoflavones in the modulation of cardiovascular risk needs additional study.

Another potential mechanism is that soy stimulates the LDL receptors of hypercholesterolemic individuals (49), through the action of polypeptides that reach the liver after intestinal digestion (64). Other theories have proposed that trypsin inhibitors found in soy may intensify cholecystokinin secretion, thereby encouraging bile acid synthesis from cholesterol and the elimination of cholesterol via the GI tract (50). Soy saponins may themselves increase bile excretion, act by decreasing intestinal absorption of cholesterol, or interfere with the reabsorption of bile acids (50,65,66).

Efficacy

An often-cited 1995 meta-analysis of 38 controlled clinical trials (67) reported that with an average daily intake of 47 g of soy protein, total cholesterol levels decreased by 9.3%, LDL cholesterol levels decreased by 12.9%, and triglyceride levels decreased by 10.5% in subjects with at least moderate hypercholesterolemia (LDL > 160 mg/dL). Since then, several studies have pointed to the value of substituting soy for animal proteins in the diet (68). The cholesterol-lowering benefits of soy have been studied extensively in hyperlipidemic men (69), postmenopausal women (70), and people with type 2 diabetes (71,72), a group particularly at risk for CVD. In studies designed to determine whether isoflavones themselves are hypocholesterolemic agents, clinical findings have been inconsistent and inconclusive (73). This lack of association has been supported in both animal and human studies that have concluded that isoflavones do not act alone but rather work in concert with other components of soy or with soy protein to exert a hypocholesterolemic effect (51-53,59,74,75). The vascular effects of isoflavones are seen in humans (50,59,76,77). In one study (77), increased dietary isoflavone intake was associated with decreased aortic stiffness, particularly among older women. A review of the literature (78) reported that in several trials, ingestion of soy products was associated with significant lowering of blood pressure, another potent risk factor for CHD.

The results of these trials raise several important points. First, substitution of 25 to 50 g of soy protein for animal protein consistently lowers LDL cholesterol levels by 2% to 8%, often regardless of the total amount of isoflavones, without consistently affecting HDL or TG levels. Second, soy products lower lipid levels but only in patients with baseline LDL levels of 160 mg/dL or higher. Third, whole soy protein, rather than its components, appears to be necessary for the lipid-lowering effect, arguing for a whole-food approach rather than dietary supplements.

Safety Profile

The FDA health claim for soy products (see Chapter 6, Table 6.10) is specifically limited to foods containing intact soy protein and does not extend to isolated substances from soy protein, such as the isoflavones genistein and daidzein (79). Because isoflavones are phytoestrogens (a weak form of estrogen), they could possibly have a negative effect, particularly in postmenopausal women (80). Clinical findings are inconclusive, and more research is clearly warranted. Additionally, the soy constituent phytic acid may decrease the absorption of zinc and other minerals through chelation (50).

Recommendations

In 1999 the FDA authorized food-labeling health claims for soy protein and CHD (81). This authorization was made based on evidence that consistent, clinically significant reductions of total and LDL cholesterol levels have been seen in people who ingest 25 g of soy protein per day, as a substitute for animal protein, and included as a part of a diet low in saturated fat and cholesterol. For foods to bear this claim, they must have 6.25 g of soy protein per serving; in addition, they must contain less than 3 g of fat, less than 1 g of saturated fat, and less than 20 mg of cholesterol. Both the AHA (25) and the ADA (4) recognize the benefits of soy protein. ATP III also recognizes the potential LDL cholesterol–lowering benefit of substituting soy protein for animal protein, but it does not specifically recommend placing a major focus on soy protein as it does for plant stanols and sterols and soluble fiber (3).

Incorporating Soy in Practice

Commonly known soy products are tofu, edamame (green soybeans), soy milk, miso, and tempeh. Many other functional foods incorporating soy protein are also available, including soy-based breakfast cereals, meat analogues, and meal-replacement bars (82). Table 10.3 provides energy and protein information for a variety of soy products (83). *The Soyfoods Guide* (84) offers an overview of soy science, as well as ideas for incorporating soy into the diet, analysis of the composition of common products, suggested readings, an exchange list for

TABLE 10.3
Energy and Protein Content of Common Soy Foods

Product	Serving Size	Energy (kcal)	Soy Protein Content (g)
Soy protein cereal	100 g	367	19
Soybeans, green, cooked (boiled, drained, without salt)	100 g	141	12
Soybeans, mature seeds, sprouted, cooked (steamed)	100 g	81	9
Soybeans, mature seeds, sprouted, raw	100 g	122	13
Soy flour, full-fat, roasted	1 cup	441	35
Soy flour, low-fat	1 cup	327	41
Soy milk, fluid	1 cup	81	7
Soy protein concentrate	1 oz	93	18
Soy protein isolate	1 oz	96	23
Soy sauce from soy and wheat (shoyu)	1 Tbsp	9	0.8
Soy sauce from soy (tamari)	1 Tbsp	11	1.9
Tempeh (cooked)	100 g	197	18
Burger crumbles	55 g	116	11
Meatless sausage	1 patty (38 g)	97	7
	1 link (25 g)	64	5
Tofu, silken, extra firm	1 slice (84 g)	46	6
Tofu, silken, soft	1 slice (84 g)	46	4
Vegan burgers	1 patty (85 g)	91	14
Miso	100 g	206	12

Source: Data are from reference 83.

individuals with diabetes, and many recipes. In addition, the Soybean.org Web site (http://www.soybean.org) provides important links, including resources for consumers and professionals.

N-3 FATTY ACIDS

Background and Mechanisms

Increasing evidence suggests that n-3 polyunsaturated fatty acids (n-3 PUFAs) play an important role in primary and secondary prevention of CHD (85-88). N-3 PUFAs include both marine-derived (eicosapentaenoic acid, C20:5n-3 [EPA] and docosahexaenoic acid, C22:6n-3 [DHA]) and plant-derived (alpha-linolenic acid, C18:3n-3 [ALA]) sources. Both sources of n-3 PUFAs have potential benefits in CHD prevention. The long-chain n-3 PUFAs such as EPA and DHA are found in high concentrations in fish oil. They can be consumed in small quantities in foods (primarily in fatty, cold-water fish such as salmon, mackerel, sardines, herring, or trout) or in larger quantities via dietary supplements (see Tables 10.4 and 10.5) (83,85,86). N-3 PUFAs from fish oil appear to have multiple cardioprotective mechanisms of action including reducing TG levels, decreasing platelet adhesion, decreasing vasoconstriction, improving flow-mediated endothelial dysfunction, reducing inflammation, and decreasing ventricular arrthymias (88). ALA, an essential fatty acid, is the shorter-chain n-3 PUFA found in various plant sources, such as flax, canola, walnuts, and soy products. The cardioprotective benefits of ALA are less clear and may depend on the type of preparation used (47). Research suggests that ALA may protect against CVD by interfering with production of proinflammatory eicosanoids prostaglandin E_2 (PGE_2), thromboxane A_2 (TXA_2), and leukotriene B_4 (LTB_4) produced from the "n-6" pathway that converts linoleic acid (LA) to arachidonic

TABLE 10.4
Marine Sources of N-3 Fatty Acids

Food	Total N-3 FA (g per 100-g serving)
Salmon, Atlantic, farmed	3.7
Salmon, Atlantic, wild	3.1
Albacore tuna	1.3
Canned tuna (in water)	0.2
Mackerel	1.8
Lake trout	1.6
Sardines	1.4
Cod	0.3

Source: Data are from references 85 and 86.

TABLE 10.5
Alpha-Linoleic Acid Content* of Selected Vegetable Oils,
Nuts, and Seeds

Food	ALA (g/Tbsp)	Estimated EPA (mg)
Flaxseed (ground)	2.2	110
Flaxseed oil	7.2	360
Canola oil	1.3	65
English walnuts	0.7	35
Soybean oil	0.9	45

*Only between 2% and 5% of alpha-linoleic acid (ALA) gets converted to
eicosapentaenoic acid (EPA) in human beings.
Source: Data are from reference 83.

acid (AA) (see Figure 10.3) (88). These proinflammatory eicosanoids are involved with promoting platelet aggregation, vasoconstriction, and thrombosis (89). However, the eicosanoids produced from the conversion of ALA to EPA (n-3 series) have a less inflammatory effect (90). Increasing ALA in the diet translates to slightly higher levels of EPA in vivo, which suggests that the benefit of ALA comes in part from its inefficient conversion to longer chain n-3 PUFAs.

Efficacy

The majority of the data come from trials of marine-based n-3 PUFAs. Secondary prevention trials have primarily included male subjects and have found positive effects of EPA and DHA from both diet and dietary supplements. Although data from intervention trials are generally lacking in females, recent data from the Nurses' Health Study suggest a strong positive association between intake of n-3 PUFA from both fish and plant sources and risk of CHD in adult females (91). The Diet and Reinfarction Trial (DART) found that 2,033 male myocardial infarction (MI) survivors who received advice to consume fish twice weekly (eg, 200 to 400 g of fish, which provides 500 to 800 mg of n-3 PUFA) had a significant reduction in total mortality of 29% after 2 years compared with "usual care" (92). A similar conclusion can be drawn from the epidemiologic data reported in the 30-year follow-up of the Chicago Western Electric Company study (93). Men who consumed at least 35 g of fish daily had a relative risk of death from CHD of 0.62 and a relative risk of nonsudden death from MI of 0.33 compared with men who did not consume fish daily.

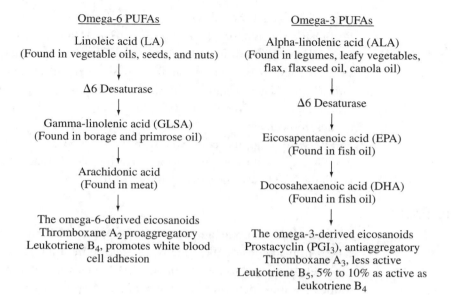

Figure 10.3

Metabolic pathway of the essential fatty acids. The pathways for the desaturation and elongation of n-3 and n-6 polyunsaturated fatty acid and eicosanoid production. Reproduced with permission. Harper CR, Jacobson TA. Beyond the Mediterranean diet: the role of omega-3 fatty acids in the prevention of coronary heart disease. *Prev Cardiol.* 2003;6:136-146. Copyright 2003 by CHF, Inc.

The largest prospective randomized control trial testing effects of supplemental EPA and DHA on secondary prevention of CHD is the Gruppo Italiano per lo Studio della Sopravvivenza nell'Infarto miocardico (GISSI) Prevention Study (94). In this study, 11,324 patients (85% male) who suffered a recent MI (within the past 3 months) were randomized to receive one of the following treatments for 3.5 years: 850 mg of purified and concentrated EPA and DHA as ethyl esters, 300 mg of vitamin E, both, or neither. After 3.5 years, the group that received n-3 PUFA alone experienced a 15% reduction in nonfatal MI and stroke ($P < .02$). Compared with the control group, there was a 20% relative-risk reduction in total mortality and a 45% reduction in sudden death ($P < .001$). Interestingly, there was no additional benefit from vitamin E. There were no reports of significant bleeding, and only 3.8% of patients treated with fish oil stopped therapy because of adverse effects (primarily dyspepsia) compared with 2.1% of patients on Vitamin E. A study conducted in Norway by Nilsen et al, however, did not find a protective effect of supplemental DHA plus EPA at 3.5 g/day on cardiac events in post-MI patients after 1.5 years of treatment (95). The negative findings may be explained by several differences in this study compared with the GISSI Prevention Study: smaller sample size ($n = 300$), a higher dose of EPA and DHA (3.5 g vs 850 mg), and the possibility that the background diet in Scandinavian populations is higher in fatty marine fish than the Italian diet, obscuring any differences in outcomes in the Norwegian study.

Epidemiologic evidence suggests a strong correlation between ALA intake and risk of CHD in both men and women. In the Nurses' Health Study, Hu et al found a dose-response relationship between ALA intake and risk of ischemic heart disease, with a 45% reduction in risk of those consuming the highest levels of ALA (96).

Although several dietary trials have claimed to investigate the role of ALA in secondary prevention of CHD (97,98), these involved multifactorial dietary interventions in which it is impossible to single out ALA as the beneficial nutrient. The only published study to date investigating the effects of supplemental ALA on cardiovascular events in patients with CHD is the Indian Experiment of Infarct Survival trial, in which patients admitted to the hospital with suspected acute MIs were randomized to fish oil capsules (1.8 g/day of EPA plus DHA), mustard oil (20 g/day providing 2.9 g ALA), or placebo every day for 1 year (99). At the end of 1 year, total cardiac events were 25%, 28%, and 35% in the fish oil, mustard oil, and placebo groups, respectively ($P < .01$). Nonfatal infarctions were also significantly less in the fish oil and mustard oil groups compared with the placebo group (13.0%, 15.0%, and 25.4%, $P < .05$). Two clinical trials have investigated the role of ALA supplementation in primary prevention of CHD with negative results (100,101).

Safety Profile

Although fish oil supplements are safe (102), they can cause nausea and dyspepsia and they have a fishy aftertaste. Additionally, whereas some studies have raised concerns concerning the safety of farmed fish consumption (103), a recent report on fish oil supplements has not found the supplements to be contaminated with either heavy metals, such as mercury, or chlorinated hydrocarbons (polychlorinated biphenyls [PCBs]) (104).

Recommendations

The AHA has updated recommendations for n-3 PUFA in secondary prevention to include consumption of approximately 1 g of EPA plus DHA per day, preferably from oily fish (87). This amounts to approximately two to three 3-oz servings of fish per day or several capsules of fish oil daily (refer to Table 10.6). In primary prevention, the AHA recommends two or more servings of fish weekly. In contrast, ATP III guidelines, citing need for additional studies, do not currently recommend consumption of n-3 PUFA as a cardiovascular risk reduction strategy.

The FDA has allowed a qualified health claim regarding the consumption of up to 3 g (fish plus supplements) of n-3 fatty acids per day in reducing the risk of CHD (102). Whereas unqualified health claims are granted for foods that have substantive scientific evidence to allow the claim (as is the case for plant stanol esters, sterol esters, soluble fiber, and soy protein), qualified health claims are granted to foods for which scientific evidence is present but not conclusive (see Chapter 6, Table 6.10).

N-3 PUFAs in Clinical Practice

All patients at risk for CHD should be counseled to eat baked, broiled, or sautéed fish at least twice weekly (see Table 10.4). However, recent evidence suggests that certain types of fish

TABLE 10.6
N-3 PUFA Supplements Needed to Meet Current AHA
Recommendations of 900 mg/day

	N-3 Fatty Acids (mg/g of Oil)	Number of Capsules
Cod liver oil	190	5
Standard fish body oil	300	3
Concentrated fish oil	500	2

Abbreviations: AHA, American Heart Association; PUFA, polyunsaturated fatty acids.

(tilefish, swordfish, king mackerel, albacore tuna, and shark) are contaminated with PCBs and mercury, and thus their consumption needs to be limited, especially in children and in pregnant and lactating women (105). Patients should also avoid commercially prepared fish (e.g., fish sticks) because of low n-3 PUFA content and high concentration of *trans* fatty acids. For patients who do not eat fish, dietary supplements are an attractive option. Most fish oil supplements provide approximately 180 mg of EPA and 120 mg of DHA per 1,000 mg capsule (30% concentrated) (106). Therefore, patients with CHD typically need to take three fish oil capsules per day to meet the AHA recommendations. However, it is important to check the nutrition label because n-3 PUFA content varies (30% to 60%) widely among products (106).

There are currently no specific recommendations for ALA and CHD prevention, although the AHA suggests that intakes of 1.5 to 3.0 g/day seem to be beneficial (87). Patients should be encouraged to replace low ALA oils (corn oil and safflower oil) with canola, soybean, or flaxseed oil. For additional sources of ALA, patients might consider incorporating ground flaxseed, flaxseed oil, or walnuts into their diets. However, patients should be made aware that these foods are high in total energy, which may be a concern for patients trying to lose or maintain weight. Flaxseed products are sensitive to oxidation by light and elevated temperatures and therefore should be stored in opaque containers in the refrigerator.

NUTS

Background and Mechanisms

Data are now emerging that tree nuts can reduce the risk of CHD, primarily via their lipid-lowering effects (107). Almonds, hazelnuts, pecans, pistachio nuts, and walnuts have been shown in clinical trials to modestly reduce serum cholesterol. Other types of nuts, such as peanuts, have also been shown to be cardioprotective. Nuts are a rich source of fiber, vitamin E, magnesium, and both monounsaturated and polyunsaturated oils. The primary mechanism explaining the LDL cholesterol–lowering effect is the replacement of saturated fat and carbohydrates with monounsaturated fats (MUFAs). Additionally, some investigators have postulated that the increased intake of ALA (found in walnuts), the high arginine content (precursor to nitric oxide), and the antithrombotic and antioxidant effects of nuts make these foods an excellent cardiovascular nutraceutical (108). Finally, evidence is also emerging that MUFAs, and nut consumption in particular, can also reduce insulin resistance (109).

Efficacy

Epidemiologic studies have consistently shown an inverse relationship between nut consumption and CHD risk (108) as well as between nut consumption and type 2 diabetes (110). More specifically, in the Nurses' Health Study, women who ate five or more servings per week of nuts lowered their relative risk of total CHD by 45% compared with women who ate nuts less than monthly, even after adjusting for other known CHD risk factors (111). These data from observational studies have been confirmed in many small clinical trials. Several studies have shown that increasing MUFAs in the diet via olive oil or tree nuts can reduce LDL cholesterol levels by up to 14% and TG levels by up to 15% while not affecting HDL cholesterol negatively (112). Several studies indicate that almonds can reduce LDL cholesterol levels in a dose-response fashion (113-115). Specifically, Jenkins et al found that during a 1-month period, both full-dose (73 g/day or 2.5 ounces) and half-dose (37 g/day or 1.3 ounces) almond diets reduced LDL cholesterol levels by 9% and 4%, respectively (113). Also, the full-dose almond group had a 7% reduction in lipoprotein (a) and a 14% reduction in oxidized LDL levels.

Another trial compared a Mediterranean-style diet with a walnut-rich diet in which patients replaced olive oil with 8 to 11 whole, shelled walnuts (116). In the 55 patients, all with LDL cholesterol levels between 130 to 250 mg/dL, the walnut diet reduced LDL cholesterol by 6%; men also had a 6% decrease in lipoprotein (a).

Safety Profile

Nuts are highly allergenic. Peanuts account for most allergies and can be life threatening. In one series of fatal food allergies, nuts accounted for 90% of deaths (117). It is estimated that 3 million Americans have nut allergies and that this condition is increasing, especially in children (118). Thus, caution should be used before recommending nuts to patients.

Recommendations

The clinical practice guidelines of ATP III (3), AHA (25), and the American Diabetes Association (26) recommend that diets contain up to 15% of total energy from MUFAs, with total fat in the range of 25% to 35% of energy (119). These guidelines recognize that nuts are good sources for increasing MUFA intake. The FDA has authorized a qualified health claim for nuts. It states, "Scientific evidence suggests but does not prove that eating 1.5 ounces per day of most nuts (almonds, hazelnuts, pecans, pistachios, walnuts) as part of a diet low in saturated fat and cholesterol may reduce the risk of heart disease" (120).

Using Nuts in Practice

Practitioners can recommend 1 to 2 ounces of nuts (approximately 1 to 2 large handfuls) per day to replace other sources of energy (121). However, patients should be advised to choose unsalted, roasted, or raw nuts, preferably those with higher ratios of unsaturated to saturated fat (refer to Table 10.7) (83). As with any energy-dense food, substitution (and not addition) is necessary to prevent weight gain. This point is especially important to emphasize for patients increasing intake of nuts because they tend to be eaten in large quantities.

COMBINATION APPROACH TO FUNCTIONAL FOODS

Although each of the foods discussed above can individually improve cardiovascular risk factors, a combination approach where smaller amounts of a wide variety of functional foods are

TABLE 10.7
Fat Composition of Selected Nuts* per 1-oz (28-g) Serving

Nut (Approximate Number)	Energy (kcal)	Total Fat (g)	Monounsaturated Fatty Acids (g)	Saturated Fatty Acids (g)
Almonds (23)	164	14.4	9.1	1.1
English walnuts (14 halves)	185	18.5	2.5	1.7
Hazelnuts (12)	183	17.7	13.2	1.3
Macadamia (12)	204	21.6	16.8	3.4
Peanuts (35 pieces)	166	14.1	7.0	2.0
Pecans (15 halves)	201	21.1	12.5	1.8
Pistachios (49)	162	13.0	6.9	1.6

*Dry roasted, no added salt.

Source: Data are from reference 83.

consumed makes more practical sense because it mimics typical eating patterns. These approaches often emphasize eating patterns such as the traditional Mediterranean diet. This diet is low in saturated fat, high in MUFAs from nuts and olive oil, and high in fiber from fruits and vegetables. In two large clinical trials, one in Europe (97) and one in India (98), this diet was shown to reduce CHD events and mortality. In North America, this approach was tested on a smaller, more controlled scale using a "portfolio" diet (122). In this study, 46 adults with hyperlipidemia were randomized to a low–saturated fat diet group (control), a low–saturated fat diet plus lovastatin (20 mg/day) group, or the "portfolio" diet group. The "portfolio" diet was low in fat and contained, per 1,000 kcal, the following: 1 g of plant sterols in an enriched margarine; 21.4 g of soy protein; 9.8 g of viscous fibers from oats, barley, and psyllium; and 14 g (0.5 ounce) of whole almonds. Decreases in LDL cholesterol were 8%, 30.9%, and 28.6% for each group, respectively, with no significant difference between the statin and dietary "portfolio" groups. High-sensitivity C-reactive protein (CRP) was also reduced by 28% and 33% in the diet and statin groups, respectively, without any changes in the control group. This study provides strong evidence that eating a combination of the functional foods described in this chapter can significantly reduce LDL cholesterol levels and, thus, can be expected to reduce CHD risk.

CONCLUSIONS AND FUTURE DIRECTIONS

Functional foods have tremendous potential to reduce CHD risk, especially on a population level. This reduction in risk appears to occur secondary to reductions in LDL cholesterol levels, although more research is needed to delineate the nonlipid effects of these foods. The most prudent approach at this time is the use of a variety of these foods in a combination approach, while also achieving or maintaining a reasonable body weight. More work is needed to delineate the safety and efficacy of the specific foods and to develop ways to make these foods and food combinations available and palatable to the public. Foods fortified with plant stanols or sterols and foods rich in soluble fiber or soy protein have received health claims from the FDA for their potential role in reducing risk for CVD. The FDA has also granted qualified health claims for n-3 fatty acids and nuts, indicating that there are suggestive, although not conclusive, data for their role in CVD risk reduction.

In addition to their potential roles in the population approach to CVD risk reduction, functional foods are beginning to be incorporated into clinical practice guidelines. To date, foods fortified with plant stanols or sterols and foods rich in soluble fiber are specifically recommended in the clinical management guidelines of the NCEP's ATP III (3), the AHA (25), and the American Diabetes Association (26) for cholesterol management and CVD risk reduction. The AHA has also issued favorable position statements regarding the potential roles of soy protein, n-3 fatty acids, and nuts.

REFERENCES

1. American Heart Association. *2002 Heart and Stroke Statistical Update.* Dallas, Texas: American Heart Association; 2002.
2. Mant D. Effectiveness of dietary intervention in general practice. *Am J Clin Nutr.* 1997;65(6 suppl):1933S-1938S.
3. Expert Panel on Detection, Evaluation, and Treatment of High Blood Cholesterol in Adults. Executive summary of the Third Report of the National Cholesterol Education Program (NCEP) Expert Panel on Detection, Evaluation, and Treatment of High Blood Cholesterol in Adults (Adult Treatment Panel III).

JAMA. 2001;285:2486-2497. Full report: National Institutes of Health. *Third Report of the National Cholesterol Education Program Expert Panel on Detection, Evaluation, and Treatment of High Blood Cholesterol in Adults (Adult Treatment Panel III)*. Bethesda, Md: National Institutes of Health; 2001. NIH Publication 01-3670. Available at: http://www.nhlbi.nih.gov/guidelines/cholesterol/atp3_rpt.htm. Accessed March 29, 2004.

4. Position of the American Dietetic Association: functional foods. *J Am Diet Assoc*. 1999;99:1278-1285.

5. Cater NB. Plant stanol ester: review of cholesterol-lowering efficacy and implications for coronary heart disease risk reduction. *Prev Cardiol*. 2000;3:121-130.

6. Ntanios FY, Duchateau GSMJE. A healthy diet rich in carotenoids is effective in maintaining normal blood carotenoid levels during the daily use of plant sterol-enriched spreads. *Int J Vitam Nutr Res*. 2002;72:32-39.

7. Miettinen TA, Gylling H. Non-nutritive bioactive constituents of plants: phytosterols. *Int J Vitam Nutr Res*. 2003;73:127-134.

8. Katan, MB, Grundy SM, Jones P, Law M, Miettinen T, Paoletti R, Stresa Workshop Participants. Efficacy and safety of plant stanols and sterols in the management of blood cholesterol levels. *Mayo Clin Proc*. 2003;78:965-978.

9. Von Bergmann K, Prange W, Lutjohann D. Metabolism and mechanism of action of plant sterols. *Eur Heart J*. 1999;1(suppl S):S45-S49.

10. Miettinen TA, Vuoristo M, Nissinen M, Jarvinen HJ, Gylling H. Serum, biliary and fecal cholesterol and plant sterols in colectomized patients before and during consumption of stanol ester margarine. *Am J Clin Nutr*. 2000;71:1095-1102.

11. Plat J, Mensink R. Increased intestinal ABCA1 expression contributes to the decrease in cholesterol absorption after plant stanol consumption. *FASEB J*. 2002;16:1248-1253.

12. Lichtenstein AH. Plant sterols and blood lipid levels. *Curr Opin Clin Nutr Metab Care*. 2002;5:147-152.

13. Cater NB. Historical and scientific basis for the development of plant stanol ester foods as cholesterol-lowering agents. *Eur Heart J*. 1999;1(suppl):S36-S44.

14. Miettinen TA, Puska P, Gylling H, Vanhanen H, Vartiainen E. Reduction of serum cholesterol with sitostanol-ester margarine in a mildly hypercholesterolemic population. *New Engl J Med*. 1995;333:1308-1312.

15. Henriks HF, Brink EJ, Meijier GW, Princen HM, Ntanios FY. Safety of long-term consumption of plant sterol ester enriched spread. *Eur J Clin Nutr*. 2003;57:681-692.

16. Law M. Plant sterol and stanol margarines and health. *BMJ*. 2000;320:861-864.

17. Maki K, Davidson MH, Umporowicz DM, Schaefer EJ, Dicklin MR, Ingram KA, Chen S, McNamara JR, Gebhart BW, Ribaya-Mercado JD, Perrone G, Robins SJ, Franke WC. Lipid responses to plant-sterol-enriched reduced-fat spreads incorporated into a National Cholesterol Education Program Step I diet. *Am. J Clin Nutr*. 2001;74;33-43.

18. Nestel P, Cehun M, Pomeroy S, Abbey M, Weldon G. Cholesterol-lowering effects of plant sterol esters and non-esterified stanols in margarine, butter and low-fat foods. *Eur J Clin Nutr*. 2001;55:1084-1090.

19. Vanstone CA, Raeini-Sarjaz M, Parsons WE, Jones PJH. Unesterified plant sterols and stanols lower LDL-cholesterol concentrations equivalently in hypercholesterolemic persons. *Am J Clin Nutr*. 2002;76:1272-1278.

20. Gremaud G, Dalan E, Piguet C, Baumgartner M, Ballabeni P, Decarli B, Leser ME, Berger A, Fay LB. Effects of non-esterified stanols in a liquid emulsion on cholesterol absorption and synthesis in hypercholesterolemic men. *Eur J Nutr*. 2002;41:54-60.

21. Devaraj S, Jialal I, Vega S. Plant sterol-fortified orange juice effectively lowers cholesterol levels in mildly hypercholesterolemic healthy individuals. *Arterioscler Thromb Vasc Biol*. 2004;24:e25-e28.

22. Clifton PM, Noakes M, Sullivan D, Erichsen N, Ross D, Annison G, Fassoulakis A, Cehun M, Nestel P. Cholesterol-lowering effects of plant sterol esters differ in milk, yoghurt, bread and cereal. *Eur J Clin Nutr*. 2004;58:503-509.

23. Hallikainen MA, Sarkkinen ES, Uusitupa MI. Plant stanol esters affect serum cholesterol concentrations of hypercholesterolemic men and women in a dose-dependent manner. *J Nutr*. 2000;130:767-776.

24. Hendricks HF, Westrate JA, Van Vliet T, Meijer GW. Spreads enriched with three different levels of vegetable oil sterols and the degree of cholesterol lowering in normocholesterolaemic and mildly hypercholesterolaemic subjects. *Eur J Clin Nutr*. 1999;53:319-327.

25. Pearson TA, Blair SN, Daniels SR, Eckel RH, Fair JM, Fortmann SP, Franklin BA, Goldstein LB, Greenland P, Grundy SM, Hong Y, Miller NH, Lauer RM, Ockene IS, Sacco RL, Sallis JF, Smith SC, Stone NJ, Taubert KA. AHA guidelines for primary prevention of cardiovascular disease and stroke: 2002 update. Consensus panel guide to comprehensive risk reduction for adult patients without coronary or other atherosclerotic vascular diseases. *Circulation*. 2002;106:388-391.

26. American Diabetes Association. Evidence-based nutrition principles and recommendations for the treatment and prevention of diabetes and related complications. *Diabetes Care*. 2003;26(suppl 1):S51-S61.

27. Vuorio AF, Gylling H, Turtola H, Kontula K, Ketonen P, Miettinen TA. Stanol ester margarine alone and with simvastatin lowers serum cholesterol in families with familial hypercholesterolemia caused by FH-North Karelia mutation. *Arterioscler Thromb Vasc Biol*. 2000;20:500-506.

28. Blair SN, Capuzzi DM, Gottlieb SO, Nguyen T, Morgan JM, Cater NB. Incremental reduction of serum total cholesterol and low-density lipoprotein cholesterol with the addition of plant stanol ester-containing spread to statin therapy. *Am J Cardiol*. 2000;86:46-52.

29. Simons LA. Additive effect of plant sterol-ester margarine and cerivastatin in lowering low-density lipoprotein cholesterol in primary hypercholesterolemia. *Am J Cardiol.* 2002;90:737-740.

30. Gylling H, Miettinen TA. LDL cholesterol lowering by bile acid malabsorption during inhibited synthesis and absorption of cholesterol in hypercholesterolemic coronary subjects. *Nutr Metab Cardiovasc Dis.* 2002;12:19-23.

31. Food labeling: health claims; plant sterol/stanol esters and coronary heart disease; interim final rule. *Federal Register.* 2000;65:54685-54739.

32. Institute of Food Science and Technology (UK). Phytosterol esters (plant sterol and stanol esters). Available at: http://www.ifst.org/hottop29.htm. Accessed September 9, 2003.

33. Noakes M. An increase in dietary carotenoids when consuming plant sterols or stanols is effective in maintaining plasma carotenoid concentrations. *Am J Clin Nutr.* 2002;75:79-86.

34. US Food and Drug Administration. Health claims: plant sterol/stanol esters and risk of coronary heart disease. April 14, 2002. Codified at 21 CFR §101.83. Available at: http://vm.cfsan.fda.gov/~dms/lab-ssa.html. Accessed April 21, 2004.

35. US Food and Drug Administration. FDA letter regarding enforcement discretion with respect to expanded use of an interim health claim rule about plant sterol/stanol esters and reduced risk of coronary heart disease. February 14, 2003. Available at: http://vm.cfsan.fda.gov/~dms/lab-ssa.html. Accessed April 21, 2004.

36. Hu FB and Willett WC. Optimal diets for prevention of coronary heart disease. *JAMA.* 2002;288:2569-2578.

37. Fernandez ML. Soluble fiber and nondigestible carbohydrate effects on plasma lipids and cardiovascular risk. *Curr Opin Lipidol.* 2001;12:35-40.

38. Kritchevsky D. Fiber effects of hyperlipidemia. In: Cunnane SC, Thompson LUE, eds. *Flaxseed in Human Nutrition.* Champaign, Ill: AOCS Press; 1995:174-186.

39. Brown L, Rosner B, Willett WW, Sacks FM. Cholesterol-lowering effects of dietary fiber: a meta-analysis. *Am J Clin Nutr.* 1999;69:30-42.

40. Anderson JW, Davidson MH, Blonde L, Brown WV, Howard WJ, Ginsberg H, Allgood LD, Weingand KW. Long-term cholesterol-lowering effects of psyllium as an adjunct to diet therapy in the treatment of hypercholesterolemia. *Am J Clin Nutr.* 2000;71:1433-1438.

41. Jenkins DJ, Kendall CW, Vuksan V, Vidgen E, Parker T, Faulkner D, Mehling CC, Garsetti M, Testolin G, Cunnane SC, Ryan MA, and Corey PN. Soluble fiber intake at a dose approved by the US Food and Drug Administration for a claim of health benefits: serum lipid risk factors for cardiovascular disease assessed in a randomized controlled crossover trial. *Am J Clin Nutr.* 2002;75:834-839.

42. Chandalia M, Garg A, Lutjohann D, von Bergmann K, Grundy SM, Brinkley LJ. Beneficial effects of high dietary fiber intake in patients with type 2 diabetes mellitus. *N Engl J Med.* 2000;342:1392-1398.

43. Burke V, Hodgson JM, Beilin LJ, Giangiulioi N, Rogers P, Puddey IB. Dietary protein and soluble fiber reduce ambulatory blood pressure in treated hypertensives. *Hypertension.* 2001;38:821-826.

44. Food labeling: health claims; soluble dietary fiber from certain foods and coronary heart disease. Final rule. *Federal Register.* 2003;68:44207-44209.

45. Lewis JH. Esophageal and small bowel obstruction from guar gum-containing "diet pills": analysis of 26 cases reported to the Food and Drug Administration. *Am J Gastroenterol.* 1992;87:1424-1428.

46. Slavin JL, Greenberg NA. Partially hydrolyzed guar gum: clinical nutrition uses. *Nutrition.* 2003;19:549-552.

47. Bloeden LT, Szapary PO. Flaxseed and cardiovascular risk. *Nutr Rev.* 2004;62:18-27.

48. Basch E, Ulbricht C, Kuo G, Szapary P, Smith M. Therapeutic applications of fenugreek. *Altern Med Rev.* 2003;8:20-27.

49. Sirtori CR, Lovati MR. Soy proteins and cardiovascular disease. *Curr Atheroscler Rep.* 2001;3:47-53.

50. Erdman JW Jr, for the AHA Nutrition Committee. Soy protein and cardiovascular disease. A statement for healthcare professionals from the Nutrition Committee of the AHA. *Circulation.* 2000;102:2555-2559.

51. Jenkins DJA, Kendall CWC, Jackson C-J C, Connelly PW, Parker T, Faulkner D, Vidgen E, Cunnane SC, Leiter LA, Josse RG. Effects of high-and low-isoflavone soyfoods on blood lipids, oxidized LDL, homocysteine, and blood pressure in hyperlipidemic men and women. *Am J Clin Nutr.* 2002;76:365-372.

52. Greaves KA, Wilson MD, Rudel LL, Williams JK, Wagner JD. Consumption of soy protein reduces cholesterol absorption compared with casein protein alone or supplemented with an isoflavone extract or conjugated equine estrogen in ovariectomized cynomolgus monkeys. *J Nutr.* 2000;130:820-826.

53. Lucas EA, Khalil DA, Daggy BP, Arjmandi BH. Ethanol-extracted soy protein isolate does not modulate serum cholesterol in Golden Syrian hamsters: a model of postmenopausal hypercholesterolemia. *J Nutr.* 2001;131:211-214.

54. Borradaile, NM, de Dreu LE, Wilcox LJ, Edwards JY, Huff MW. Soya phytoestrogens, genistein and daidzein, decrease apolipoprotein B secretion from HepG2 cells through multiple mechanisms. *Biochem J.* 2002;366:531-539.

55. Mezei O, Banz WJ, Steger RW, Peluso MR, Winters TA, Shay N. Soy isoflavones exert antidiabetic and hypolipidemic effects through the PPAR pathways in obese Zucker rats and murine RAW 264.7 cells. *J Nutr.* 2003;133:1238-1243.

56. Hodgson JM, Puddey IB, Beilin LJ, Mori TA, Croft KD. Supplementation with isoflavonoid phytoestrogens does not alter serum lipid concentrations: a randomized controlled trial in humans. *J Nutr.* 1998;128:728-732.

57. Nestel PJ, Yamashita T, Sasahara T, Pomeroy S, Dart A, Komesaroff P, Owen A, Abbey M. Soy isoflavones improve systemic arterial compliance but not plasma lipids in menopausal and perimenopausal women. *Arterioscler Thromb Vasc Biol.* 1997;17:3392-3398.

58. Wiseman H, O'Reilly JD, Adlercreutz H, Mallet AI, Bowey EA, Rowland IR, Sanders TAB. Isoflavone phytoestrogens consumed in soy decrease F_2-isoprostane concentrations and increase resistance of low-density lipoprotein to oxidation in humans. *Am J Clin Nutr.* 2000;72:395-400.

59. Clarkson TB. Soy, soy phytoestrogens and cardiovascular disease. *J Nutr.* 2002;132(suppl):566S-569S.

60. Clarkson TB, Anthony MS, Morgan TM. Inhibition of postmenopausal atherosclerosis progression: a comparison of the effects of conjugated equine estrogens and soy phytoestrogens. *J Clin Endocrinol Metab.* 2001;86:41-47.

61. Yamakoshi J, Piskula MK, Izumi T, Tobe K, Saito M, Kataoka S, Obata A, Kikuchi M. Isoflavone aglycone-rich extract without soy protein attenuates atherosclerosis development in cholesterol-fed rabbits. *J Nutr.* 2000;130:1887-1893.

62. Kondo K, Suzuki Y, Ikeda Y, Umemura K. Genistein, an isoflavone included in soy, inhibits throbotic vessel occlusion in the mouse femoral artery and in vitro platelet aggregation. *Eur J Pharmacol.* 2002;455:53-57.

63. Adams MR, Golden DL, Anthony MS, Register TC, Williams JK. The inhibitory effect of soy protein isolate on atherosclerosis in mice does not require the presence of LDL receptors or alteration of plasma lipoproteins. *J Nutr.* 2002;132:43-49.

64. Lovarti MR, Manzoni C, Gianazza E, Arnodi A, Kurowska E, Carroll KK, Sirtori CR. Soy protein peptides regulate cholesterol homeostasis in Hep G2 Cells. *J Nutr.* 2000;130:2543-2549.

65. Koba K, Liu J-W, Bobik E Jr, Mills DE, Sugano M, Huang YS. Effect of phytate in soy protein on the serum and liver cholesterol levels and liver fatty acid profile in rats. *Biosci Biotechnol Biochem.* 2003;67:15-22.

66. Oakenfull D. Soy protein, saponins, and plasma cholesterol [letter]. *J Nutr.* 2001;131:1971.

67. Anderson JW, Johnstone BM, Cook-Newell ME. Meta-analysis of the effects of soy protein intake on serum lipids. *N Engl J Med.* 1995;333:276-282.

68. Lichtenstein AH. Soy protein, isoflavones and cardiovascular disease risk. *J Nutr.* 1998;128:1589-1592.

69. Jenkins DJA, Kendall CWC, Vidgen E, Mehling CC, Parker T, Seyler H, Faulkner D, Garsetti M, Griffin LC, Agarwal S, Rao AV, Cunnane SC, Ryan MA, Connelly PW, Leiter LA, Vuksan V, Josse R. The effect on serum lipids and oxidized low-density lipoprotein of supplementing self-selected low-fat diets with soluble-fiber, soy, and vegetable protein foods. *Metabolism.* 2000;49:67-72.

70. Vigna GB, Pansini F, Bonaccorsi G, Albertazzi P, Donega P, Zanotti L, De Aloysio D, Mollica G, Fellin R. Plasma lipoproteins in soy-treated postmenopausal women: a double-blind, placebo-controlled trial. *Nutr Metab Cardiovasc Dis.* 2000;10:315-322.

71. Jayagopal V, Alberazzi P, Kilpatrick ES, Howarth EM, Jennings PE, Hepburn DA, Atkin SL. Beneficial effects of soy phytoestrogen intake in postmenopausal women with type 2 diabetes. *Diabetes Care.* 2002;25:1709-1714.

72. Hermansen K, Sondergaard M, Hoie L, Carstensen M, Brock B. Beneficial effects of a soy-based dietary supplement on lipid levels and cardiovascular risk markers in type 2 diabetic subjects. *Diabetes Care.* 2001;24:228-233.

73. Committee on Toxicity of Chemicals in Food, Consumer Products, and the Environment. *Phytoestrogens and Health.* London, England: Food Standards Agency; 2003. Available at: http://www.foodstandards.gov.uk/multimedia/pdfs/phytoreport0503. Accessed September 8, 2003.

74. Mackey R, Ekangaki A, Eden JA. The effects of soy protein in women and men with elevated plasma lipids. *Biofactors.* 2000;12:251-257.

75. Anderson JW. Diet first, then medication for hypercholesterolemia [editorial]. *JAMA.* 2003;290:531-533.

76. Steinberg FM, Guthrie NL, Villablanca AC, Kumar K, Murray MJ. Soy protein with isoflavones has favorable effects on endothelial function that are independent of lipid and antioxidant effects in healthy postmenopausal women. *Am J Clin Nutr.* 2003;78:123-130.

77. van der Schouw YT, Pijpe A, Lebrun CE, Bots ML, Peeters PH, van Staveren WA, Lamberts SW, Grobbee DE. Higher usual dietary intake of phytoestrogens is associated with lower aortic stiffness in postmenopausal women. *Arterioscler Thromb Vasc Biol.* 2002;22:1245-1247.

78. Appel LJ. The effects of protein intake on blood pressure and cardiovascular disease. *Curr Opin Lipidol.* 2003;14:55-59.

79. US Food and Drug Administration. Food labeling: health claims; soy protein and coronary heart disease. 64 *Federal Register* 57700-57733 (1990) (codified at 21 CFR §101).

80. Henkel J. Soy: health claims for soy protein, questions about other components. *FDA Consumer Magazine.* May-June 2000. Available at: http://www.fda.gov/fdac/features/2000/300_soy.html. Accessed September 9, 2003.

81. US Food and Drug Administration. Health claims: soy protein and coronary heart disease (CHD). April 1, 2002. 21 CFR §101.82. Available at: http://vm.cfsan.fda.gov/~dms/lab-ssa.html. Accessed April 21, 2004.

82. Dunn AV. Incorporating soy protein into a low-fat, low-cholesterol diet. *Cleve Clin J Med.* 2000;67:767-771.

83. US Department of Agriculture. USDA National Nutrient Database for Standard Reference. Available at: http://www.nal.usda.gov. Accessed April 21, 2004.

84. The United Soybean Board and Soy Protein Partners. *The Soyfoods Guide.* Available at: http://www.soybean.org. Accessed April 21, 2004.

85. O'Keefe JH Jr, Harris WS. From Inuit to implementation: omega-3 fatty acids come of age. *Mayo Clin Proc.* 2000;75:607-614.

86. Harper CR, Jacobson TA. The fats of life: the role of omega-3 fatty acids in the prevention of coronary heart disease. *Arch Intern Med*. 2001;161:2185-2192.

87. Kris-Etherton PM, Harris WS, Appel LJ. Fish consumption, fish oil, omega-3 fatty acids, and cardiovascular disease. *Circulation*. 2002;106:2747-2757.

88. Harper CR, Jacobson TA. Beyond the Mediterranean diet: the role of omega-3 fatty acids in the prevention of coronary heart disease. *Prev Cardiol*. 2003;6:136-146.

89. Kinsella JE, Lokesh B, Stone RA. Dietary n-3 polyunsaturated fatty acids and amelioration of cardiovascular disease: possible mechanisms. *Am J Clin Nutr*. 1990;52:1-28.

90. Calder PC, Bevan SJ, Newsholme EA. The inhibition of T-lymphocyte proliferation by FA is in an eicosanoid-independent mechanism. *Immunology*. 1992;75:108-115.

91. Hu FB, Bronner L, Willett WC, Stampfer MJ, Rexrode KM, Albert CM, Hunter D, Manson JE. Fish and omega-3 fatty acid intake and risk of coronary heart disease in women. *JAMA*. 2002;287:1815-1821.

92. Burr M, Fehily A, Gilbert J. Effects of changes in fat, fish and fibre intakes on death and myocardial reinfarction: diet and reinfarction trial. *Lancet*. 1989;2:757-761.

93. Daviglus ML, Stamler J, Orencia AJ, Dyer AR, Liu K, Greenland P, Walsh MK, Morris D, and Shekelle RB. Fish consumption and the 30-year risk of fatal myocardial infarction. *N Engl J Med*. 1997;336:1046-1053.

94. Gruppo Italiano per lo Studio della Sopravvivenza nell'Infarto miocardico. Dietary supplementation with n-3 polyunsaturated fatty acids and vitamin E after myocardial infarction: results of the GISSI-Prevenzione trial. *Lancet*. 1999;354:447-455.

95. Nilsen DW, Albrektsen G, Landmark K, Moen S, Aarsland T, Woie L. Effects of a high-dose concentrate of n-3 fatty acids or corn oil introduced early after an acute myocardial infarction on serum triacylglycerol and HDL cholesterol. *Am J Clin Nutr*. 2001;74:50-56.

96. Hu FB, Stampfer MJ, Manson JE, Rimm EB, Wolk A, Colditz GA, Hennekens CH, Willett WC. Dietary intake of alpha-linolenic acid and risk of fatal ischemic heart disease among women. *Am J Clin Nutr*. 1999;69:890-897.

97. de Lorgeril M, Renaud S, Mamelle N, Salen P, Martin JL, Monjaud I, Guidollet J, Touboul P, Delaye J. Mediterranean alpha-linolenic acid-rich diet in secondary prevention of coronary heart disease. *Lancet*. 1994;343:1454-1459.

98. Singh RB, Dubnov G, Niaz MA, Ghosh S, Singh R, Rastogi SS, Manor O, Pella D, Berry EM. Effect of an Indo-Mediterranean diet on progression of coronary artery disease in high risk patients (Indo-Mediterranean Diet Heart Study): a randomised single-blind trial. *Lancet*. 2002;360:1455-1461.

99. Singh RB, Niaz MA, Sharma JP, Kumar R, Rastogi V, Moshiri M. Randomized, double-blind, placebo-controlled trial of fish oil and mustard oil in patients with suspected acute myocardial infarction: the Indian experiment of infarct survival—4. *Cardiovasc Drugs Ther*. 1997;11:485-491.

100. Natvig H, Borchgrevink CF, Dedichen J, Owren PA, Schiotz EH, Westlund K. A controlled trial of the effect of linolenic acid on incidence of coronary heart disease. The Norwegian vegetable oil experiment of 1965–66. *Scand J Clin Lab Invest Suppl*. 1968;105:1-20.

101. Bemelmans WJ, Broer J, Feskens EJ, Smit AJ, Muskiet FA, Lefrandt JD, Bom VJ, May JF, Meyboom-de Jong B. Effect of an increased intake of alpha-linolenic acid and group nutritional education on cardiovascular risk factors: the Mediterranean Alpha-linolenic Enriched Groningen Dietary Intervention (MARGARIN) study. *Am J Clin Nutr*. 2002;75:221-227.

102. US Food and Drug Administration, Center for Food Safety and Applied Nutrition. Letter regarding dietary supplement health claim for omega-3 fatty acids and coronary heart disease. October 31, 2000. Available at: http://www.cfsan.fda.gov/~dms/ds-ltr11.html. Accessed April 21, 2004.

103. Hampton T. Farmed wild salmon pollutants probed. *JAMA*. 2004;291:929-930.

104. Omega-3 oil: fish or pills? *Consum Rep*. 2003;68:30-32.

105. US Food and Drug Administration, Environmental Protection Agency. FDA and EPA announce the revised consumer advisory on methylmercury in fish. Available at: http://www.fda.gov/bbs/topics/news/2004/NEW01038.html. Accessed March 19, 2004.

106. Harris WS. Fish oil supplementation: evidence for health benefits. *Cleve Clin J Med*. 2004;71:208-221.

107. Hu FB, Stampfer MJ. Nut consumption and risk of coronary heart disease: a review of epidemiologic evidence. *Curr Atheroscler Rep*. 1999;1:204-209.

108. Hu FB. Plant-based foods and prevention of cardiovascular disease: an overview. *Am J Clin Nutr*. 2003;78(3 suppl):544S-551S.

109. Garcia-Lorda P, Megias RI, Salas-Salvado J. Nut consumption, body weight and insulin resistance. *Eur J Clin Nutr*. 2003;57(suppl 1):S8-11.

110. Jiang R, Manson JE, Stampfer MJ, Liu S, Willett WC, Hu FB. Nut and peanut butter consumption and risk of type 2 diabetes in women. *JAMA*. 2002;288:2554-2560.

111. Hu FB, Stampfer MJ, Manson JE, Rimm EB, Colditz GA, Rosner BA, Speizer FE, Hennekens CH, Willett WC. Frequent nut consumption and risk of coronary heart disease in women: prospective cohort study. *BMJ*. 1998;317:1341-1345.

112. Kris-Etherton PM, Zhao G, Binkoski AE, Coval SM, Etherton TD. The effects of nuts on coronary heart disease risk. *Nutr Rev*. 2001;59:103-111.

113. Jenkins DJ, Kendall CW, Marchie A, Parker TL, Connelly PW, Qian W, Haight JS, Faulkner D, Vidgen E, Lapsley KG, Spiller GA. Dose response of almonds on coronary heart disease risk factors: blood lipids,

oxidized low-density lipoproteins, lipoprotein(a), homocysteine, and pulmonary nitric oxide: a randomized, controlled, crossover trial. *Circulation.* 2002;106:1327-1332.

114. Sabate J, Haddad E, Tanzman JS, Jambazian P, Rajaram S. Serum lipid response to the graduated enrichment of a Step I diet with almonds: a randomized feeding trial. *Am J Clin Nutr.* 2003;77:1379-1384.

115. Spiller GA, Jenkins DA, Bosello O, Gates JE, Cragen LN, Bruce B. Nuts and plasma lipids: an almond-based diet lowers LDL-C while preserving HDL-C. *J Am Coll Nutr.* 1998;17:285-290.

116. Zambon D, Sabate J, Munoz S, Campero B, Casals E, Merlos M, Laguna JC, Ros E. Substituting walnuts for monounsaturated fat improves the serum lipid profile of hypercholesterolemic men and women. A randomized crossover trial [erratum in *Ann Intern Med.* 2000;133:659]. *Ann Intern Med.* 2000;132:538-546.

117. Roux KH, Teuber SS, Sathe SK. Tree nut allergens. *Int Arch Allergy Immunol.* 2003;131:234-244.

118. Sicherer SH, Munoz-Furlong A, Sampson HA. Prevalence of peanut and tree nut allergy in the United States determined by means of a random digit dial telephone survey: a 5-year follow-up study. *J Allergy Clin Immunol.* 2003;112:1203-1207.

119. Kris-Etherton PM. Monounsaturated fatty acids and risk of cardiovascular disease. *Circulation.* 1999;100:1253-1258.

120. Taylor C. Qualified health claims: letter of enforcement discretion—nuts and coronary heart disease. Available at: http://vm.cfsan.fda.gov/~dms/qhcnuts2.html. Accessed July 14, 2003.

121. International Tree Nut Council. Go nuts go healthy. Available at: http://www.nuthealth.org/nutrition/nutrient1oz.pdf. Accessed March 19, 2004.

122. Jenkins DJ, Kendall CW, Marchie A, Faulkner DA, Wong JM, de Souza R, Eman A, Parker TL, Vidgen E, Lapsley KG, Trautwein EA, Josse RG, Leiter LA, Connelly PW. Effects of a dietary portfolio of cholesterol-lowering foods vs lovastatin on serum lipids and C-reactive protein. *JAMA.* 2003;290:502-510.

CHAPTER 11

ANTIOXIDANTS AND OTHER DIETARY SUPPLEMENTS

Cindy J. Fuller, PhD, RD

INTRODUCTION

Should individuals take dietary supplements to prevent or reduce the severity of heart disease? This question arose frequently in the 1990s, when attention was drawn to antioxidant nutrients (vitamin E, vitamin C, and beta carotene). The interest stemmed from small, short-term, in vitro studies designed to reduce the oxidation of low-density lipoprotein (LDL). Antioxidant nutrients have shown promise in reducing other risk factors for cardiovascular disease (CVD), such as platelet aggregation. These positive results have not been confirmed by long-term studies designed to test whether antioxidant nutrient supplementation could prevent CVD. Other nutrients (folate), dietary antioxidants (flavonoids), and herbal preparations (garlic, guggulipid) have shown variable results in mitigating CVD risk factors. The purpose of this review is to examine the evidence supporting and refuting the roles of these substances in CVD. This review can then serve as a basis for responding to patients' questions on dietary supplements related to CVD.

ANTIOXIDANTS

The LDL Oxidation Theory

The idea that oxidized LDL could be a risk factor in atherogenesis dates back to the work of 1985 Nobel Prize winners Brown and Goldstein (1), who showed that LDL altered by various chemical processes was taken up avidly by cultured macrophages and could result in the formation of foam cells. Unaltered, or native, LDL was taken into macrophages to a limited extent. Subsequent work demonstrated the presence of oxidized LDL in rabbit and human atherosclerotic plaques (2,3).

How might LDL become oxidized in vivo? Monocytes and neutrophils, key leukocytes in the immune response, secrete free radicals such as superoxide anion to neutralize pathogens

(4,5). These free radicals can oxidize LDL in vitro. Endothelial cells and smooth muscle cells in the arterial wall can also oxidize LDL (6,7). The gas phase of cigarette smoke contains an estimated 10^{15} free radicals per puff (8), some of which can enter the bloodstream via diffusion in the lungs. Diabetes imposes oxidative stresses, through glucose autoxidation, formation of advanced glycation end products, and the polyol pathway (9). Free radicals preferentially attack polyunsaturated fatty acids (PUFAs) within the LDL particle by removing an electron from a double bond. The oxidative damage sets up a chain reaction that damages PUFA molecules and produces compounds such as aldehydes (10). Free radicals can also oxidize cholesterol within the LDL particle (11). Aldehydes and products of cholesterol oxidation are toxic to cells (12-14). The alteration of apolipoprotein B (apo B) by free radical attack reduces its affinity for the LDL receptor but increases its affinity for the macrophage scavenger receptor (1). Macrophages are able to freely ingest altered LDL via the scavenger receptor, resulting in a lipid-laden foam cell, an early step in atherosclerosis. (See Chapter 3 sections on pathophysiology of atherosclerosis.)

The use of antioxidant nutrients to combat LDL oxidation and potentially reduce atherosclerotic plaques was derived from several lines of research. Vitamin E and carotenoids within LDL particles are depleted in the early stages of in vitro oxidation (10,15). Enrichment of LDL with either vitamin E (16) or beta carotene (17) resulted in reduced oxidation. In vitro LDL oxidation by copper or cultured human monocyte-derived macrophages was slowed by addition of vitamin C to the medium (18). Animal feeding studies used nonnutritional antioxidants to reduce atherosclerotic lesions (19-21) but were not practical alternatives because of toxicity or reduction in high-density lipoproteins (HDLs) (20,22,23). Antioxidant nutrients therefore appear to be better choices to reduce LDL oxidation and CVD. All antioxidant nutrients are relatively safe at doses above normal dietary intakes. The next sections examine the effects of each nutrient separately and in combination.

Vitamin E

Vitamin E is shorthand for a group of fat-soluble compounds, tocopherols and tocotrienols. These compounds share a chromanol ring with varying numbers of methyl groups flanking a hydroxyl group that can donate an electron to quench a free radical. Tocotrienols differ from tocopherols in that the side chains of tocotrienols are polyunsaturated, whereas tocopherols have saturated side chains. These hydrophobic side chains anchor the molecules in lipid, whereas the hydroxyl group is more hydrophilic and would be oriented toward aqueous milieu. Alpha-tocopherol is the most active of the vitamin E compounds (24,25). Tocopherols are naturally found in polyunsaturated oils, including sunflower and wheat germ oils; tocotrienols are derived from palm, barley, and rice bran oils (26,27). Fortified cereals are also a good source of alpha-tocopherol. Gamma-tocopherol is the most prevalent form of vitamin E in the diet. (See Table 11.1 for food sources [28].) Synthetic alpha-tocopherol supplements contain a mixture of eight different stereoisomers (RRR, SRR, RSR, RRS, RSS, SRS, SSR, and SSS), which are collectively referred to as all-racemic (all-rac) or dl–. The stereoisomers result from variations in the position of the hydrogen and methyl group off the carbons on the side chain. Natural-source alpha-tocopherol is exclusively RRR or d–, providing about 50% greater activity than synthetic vitamin E.

Tocopherols and tocotrienols are absorbed from the gastrointestinal tract in a micelle-dependent fashion, along with the products of fat digestion. They travel in chylomicrons to the liver. Water-miscible alpha-tocopherol preparations are the supplements of choice for persons with fat malabsorption; however, fat-soluble RRR-alpha-tocopherol supplements are

TABLE 11.1
Common Food Sources of Vitamin E

Food Sources of Vitamin E	Vitamin E as mg of Alpha-Tocopherol, mg
Ready-to-eat cereals, fortified to 100%, 1 cup	20
Vegetable juice cocktail, canned, 1 cup	12
Almonds, 1 oz	7.3
Sunflower seeds, ¼ cup	6.8
Spinach, frozen, cooked, 1 cup	6.7
Sunflower oil, 1 Tbsp	5.6
Spaghetti sauce and other canned tomato products, 1 cup	5.1
Safflower oil, 1 Tbsp	4.6
Turnip greens, 1 cup	4.7
Spinach, canned, 1 cup	4.1
Broccoli, frozen, cooked, 1 cup	2.4
Canola oil, 1 Tbsp	2.4

Source: Data are from reference 28.

preferred for persons with normal liver and pancreatic functions (27). Once in the liver, the alpha-tocopherol transfer protein preferentially packages alpha-tocopherol in the two- or three-R form into very-low-density lipoproteins (VLDLs) for transport through the circulation (24). Alpha-tocopherol in the two-R form (SRR, RSR, RRS) is by far the principal form of vitamin E in fasting plasma. RRR-alpha-tocopherol had superior bioavailability than an equivalent dose of all-rac alpha-tocopherol (29). There may be a low level of transfer of tocopherols and tocotrienols from chylomicrons to other lipoproteins, such as HDL. In addition, these other forms of vitamin E may enter tissues directly from chylomicrons as a result of the action of lipoprotein lipase. Given the low plasma levels of tocopherols and tocotrienols other than two-R-alpha-tocopherol, the 2000 Dietary Reference Intake Committee established the recommended dietary allowance (RDA) of 15 mg/day solely on the basis of alpha-tocopherol (30). Table 11.2 summarizes RDAs and tolerable upper limits (ULs) for vitamins discussed in this chapter (30,31).

Commercially available vitamin E supplements are labeled with US Pharmacopoeia (USP) international units (IU) instead of milligrams. This has the effect of equalizing RRR-alpha-tocopherol vs all-rac alpha-tocopherol in supplement preparations; however, the 2000 Dietary Reference Intake Committee discontinued use of this unit (30). In addition, use of the 1989 alpha-tocopherol equivalent (32) was also discontinued. Conversions between international units and milligrams are given in the Table 11.3 (30). To convert milligrams of alpha-tocopherol equivalent to milligrams of alpha-tocopherol, multiply by 0.8 (30).

TABLE 11.2
Dietary Reference Intakes for Vitamins Considered for Supplementation in Cardiovascular Nutrition

Nutrient	RDA	UL
Vitamin C, mg	90 for men 75 for women	2000
Vitamin E, mg	15 alpha-tocopherol	1000
Folate, µg	400	1000
Vitamin B-6, mg	1.3	100
Vitamin B-12, mg	2.4	Not determinable

Abbreviations: RDA, recommended dietary allowance; UL, tolerable upper limit.
Source: Data are from Institute of Medicine (30,31).

TABLE 11.3
Conversion Factors for Alpha-Tocopherol Supplements

Supplement	IU to mg	mg to IU
Synthetic (dl- or all-rac)		
Alpha-tocopheryl acetate	1	1
Alpha-tocopheryl succinate	0.89	1.12
Alpha-tocopherol	1.1	0.91
Natural (d- or RRR-)		
Alpha-tocopheryl acetate	1.36	0.74
Alpha-tocopheryl succinate	1.21	0.83
Alpha-tocopherol	1.49	0.67

Source: Adapted with permission from Institute of Medicine. *Dietary Reference Intakes for Vitamin C, Vitamin E, Selenium, and Carotenoids.* Washington, DC: National Academy Press; 2000.

Early clinical trials in normal volunteers showed that doses of alpha-tocopherol far in excess of the RDA were the most effective antioxidant nutrient in reducing the in vitro oxidizability of LDL in healthy subjects (33,34). Alpha-tocopherol was also effective in reducing LDL oxidizability in persons with both type 1 and type 2 diabetes (35-37) and cigarette smokers (38,39). Two dose-response studies determined that the minimal dose of all-rac alpha-tocopherol or RRR-alpha-tocopherol that reduced LDL oxidizability in healthy subjects during an 8-week supplementation period was at least 400 IU/day (40,41). At doses almost four times higher, Reaven and Witztum (42) found no difference in LDL alpha-tocopherol levels or LDL oxidizability when 1,600 mg/day of either all-rac alpha-tocopherol or RRR-alpha-tocopherol was given. However, this dose is above the UL of 1,000 mg/day set by the 2000 Dietary Reference Intake Committee (30). Investigators with the Nurses' Health Study and the Health Professionals' Follow-up Study reported that higher intakes of vitamin E were associated with lower incidences of coronary disease endpoints in their respective cohorts (43,44). In addition, alpha-tocopherol supplementation was shown to reduce the oxidative activity of human monocytes, a key leukocyte in the arterial wall (45); however, it did not reduce superoxide production by neutrophils, the major circulating leukocyte, in smokers (39,46). In addition to reducing LDL oxidation, alpha-tocopherol has been shown to inhibit platelet aggregation (47-50).

The early positive findings stimulated initiation of a host of prospective secondary prevention studies to determine whether alpha-tocopherol could reduce recurrence of CVD in patients. The results have been mixed. One early intervention study showed that 1,200 IU/day of alpha-tocopherol for 4 months showed a trend ($P = .06$) toward reducing the incidence of restenosis in patients post angioplasty (51). Vitamin E supplement use also significantly reduced the incidence of coronary heart disease (CHD) mortality in postmenopausal women (52) and in the elderly (53). However, in the Physicians' Health Study (54), self-reported vitamin E supplementation was not related to CVD mortality.

The Cambridge Heart Antioxidant Study (CHAOS) was the first intervention trial specifically designed to examine the effect of alpha-tocopherol supplementation on coronary disease (55). Subjects with angiographically proven coronary atherosclerosis were randomized to placebo, 400 IU, or 800 IU alpha-tocopherol per day and followed for a median time period of 510 days. Supplementation significantly reduced the rates of major cardiovascular events and nonfatal myocardial infarctions (MI), but not cardiovascular death. Davey (56) calculated from the CHAOS data that vitamin E supplementation produced cost savings of $578 (US) per patient for cardiac care.

The Heart Outcomes Prevention Evaluation Study enrolled 9,541 patients with existing CVD or diabetes and randomly assigned them to receive either 400 IU/day of vitamin E or placebo for a mean of 4.5 years (57). The investigators found no differences in the incidence of cardiovascular outcomes between the two groups. A subsequent evaluation of the study participants with diabetes showed similar results (58). In contrast to the previous studies, the Vitamin E Atherosclerosis Prevention Study was aimed at primary prevention (59). Healthy subjects were randomized to receive either 400 IU alpha-tocopherol per day or placebo. After an average of 3 years, the oxidative susceptibility of LDL was decreased in the subjects who received vitamin E; however, supplementation failed to halt the progression of intima-media thickness of the carotid artery, an indication of atherosclerotic progression. Keith et al (60) performed a placebo-controlled clinical trial to determine whether 500 IU alpha-tocopherol per day for 12 weeks could modify the level of oxidative stress and improve quality of life for patients with congestive heart failure (CHF; New York Heart Association functional class III or IV). No difference was observed in oxidative stress or quality of life between the two groups.

Patients with end-stage renal disease (ESRD) have a high mortality rate due to CVD. Previous studies (61,62) demonstrated that alpha-tocopherol supplementation could reduce LDL oxidation in this high-risk group. Boaz et al (63) reported that hemodialysis patients with existing CVD who received 800 IU/day of alpha-tocopherol had a reduced incidence of CVD endpoints and MI relative to those who received placebo.

Vivekananthan (64) performed a meta-analysis of primary and secondary prevention studies of vitamin E supplementation and CVD. A total of 81,788 individuals from seven studies were analyzed. The odds ratio (OR) for cardiovascular mortality of 1.0 ($P = .94$) with vitamin E supplementation indicated mortality rate was the same whether or not vitamin E was supplemented. The OR for stroke, calculated with 45,896 subjects from four studies, was 1.02 for vitamin E supplementation ($P = .70$). Except in patients with ESRD, alpha-tocopherol supplementation does not appear to prevent CVD mortality or events.

Other investigators have focused on the potential of gamma-tocopherol and tocotrienols to reduce LDL oxidizability and CVD. Gamma-tocopherol can trap nitrogen free radicals such as peroxynitrite in vitro (65,66). Gamma-tocopherol is consumed during the process of LDL oxidation with an oxygen free radical–generating chemical after alpha-tocopherol and as oxidized cholesterol increases (67), indicating that it does not protect LDL as well as alpha-tocopherol. Dietrich et al (68) reported that smokers and passive smokers had higher plasma levels of gamma-tocopherol than nonsmokers. El-Sohemy et al (69) found that increased concentrations of gamma-tocopherol in the diet and adipose tissue were not associated with protection against MI.

Alpha- and gamma-tocotrienols have similar consumption profiles during LDL oxidation as their tocopherol counterparts (67). Qureshi and associates have reported that tocotrienols from palm oil (70) and rice bran oil (71) reduced serum cholesterol by 15% to 16% in human beings; O'Byrne et al (72) were unable to reproduce this finding. In the latter study, hypercholesterolemic subjects were supplemented with placebo, alpha-, gamma-, or delta-tocotrienyl acetate at doses of 250 mg/day. Only alpha-tocotrienol increased the resistance of LDL to oxidation. Despite the similar dosages, plasma delta-tocotrienol in subjects receiving delta-tocotrienyl acetate increased to a concentration only one tenth that of the alpha-tocotrienol in the subjects who received that isomer. More research is needed to determine whether tocotrienols, as contrasted with tocopherol, have potential in prevention of CVD.

Vitamin E supplementation is safe for healthy persons at the doses of 400 to 1,200 mg/day used in numerous studies. However, in the Alpha-Tocopherol, Beta Carotene Cancer Prevention Study (ATBC), smokers who took 50 mg/day of alpha-tocopherol for 5 to 8 years had an increased rate of hemorrhagic stroke (73); this effect persisted years after supplementation was stopped (74). The UL was set at 1,000 mg/day of supplemental vitamin E (30) to reduce this risk. Vitamin E may also interfere with blood coagulation in patients with vitamin K deficiency and in patients taking anticoagulant medications such as warfarin (75). Vitamin E may also attenuate the HDL-raising effects of lipid-modifying medications (76).

Vitamin C

Vitamin C, or ascorbic acid, is the predominant water-soluble antioxidant nutrient in the body (77). Humans, higher primates, and guinea pigs lack the enzyme that other species use to synthesize this compound endogenously from glucose; therefore, dietary intake is essential. Prominent dietary sources of vitamin C are listed in Table 11.4 (28).

Being water soluble, vitamin C circulates free in the plasma. It has been postulated that vitamin C may protect LDL from oxidation by intercepting free radicals before they can attack PUFAs inside the particles (78,79), or that it may recycle tocopherol from its oxidized form (80). Jialal, Vega, and Grundy (18) reported that physiologic concentrations of vitamin C could reduce LDL oxidizability. A subsequent study (81) showed that vitamin C could spare the lipophilic antioxidants in LDL from oxidation, whereas probucol, a chemical antioxidant, did not have a protective effect. Vitamin C also inhibited LDL oxidation by activated neutrophils and monocyte-macrophages in culture (18,82,83). Hwang (84) reported that vitamin C at concentrations seen in plasma of supplemented individuals enhanced the inhibitory effect of 17 beta-estradiol on LDL oxidation initiated by either copper ions or cells.

Results of supplementation studies examining the effect of vitamin C on LDL oxidizability have been mixed. Many of these studies have been performed in smokers because of increased oxidative stress (8) and lower intakes of vitamin C in this population (85,86). One study did find similar vitamin C consumption among college-aged smokers and nonsmokers (39). Both groups consumed more vitamin C than the RDA for adult males of 90 mg/day (30). Plasma vitamin C has been reported to be lower in smokers than in nonsmokers after adjusting for reduced intake (85). Nyyssönen et al (87) found that plasma vitamin C accounted for 23.5% of the variability in the time before LDL oxidation products become apparent (the lag time). Harats et al (88) demonstrated that vitamin C supplementation reduced the oxidation of human plasma and LDL induced by smoking 5 to 7 cigarettes within 90 minutes. Fuller et

TABLE 11.4
Common Food Sources of Vitamin C (Ascorbic Acid)

Food Sources of Vitamin C	Vitamin C, mg
Sweet red pepper, 1 raw	226
Orange juice, fresh-squeezed, 1 cup	124
Broccoli, cooked, 1 cup	101
Grapefruit juice, pink or white, fresh-squeezed, 1 cup	94
Kiwi fruit, 1 medium	70
Vegetable juice cocktail, canned, 1 cup	67
Chinese cabbage (bok choy), cooked, 1 cup	44
Sweet potato, baked in skin, 1 medium	29
White potato, baked in skin, 1 medium	19

Source: Data are from reference 28.

al (89) randomly assigned long-term smokers to placebo or 1,000 mg vitamin C per day for 4 weeks. All subjects followed a low–vitamin C diet ($\leq$ 30 mg/day) during the trial. The supplemented group had a significant reduction in LDL oxidizability, whereas no changes were seen in the placebo group. A subsequent study with young smokers (39) saw no change in LDL oxidizability in subjects who received 1,000 mg vitamin C. Another study (90) examined the effect on LDL oxidizability in smokers of a modest amount of vitamin C (145 mg/day) from orange juice and 18 mg beta carotene per day from carrot juice. Supplementation reduced maximum oxidation of LDL without altering the rate of oxidation or the duration of the lag time.

Two vitamin C studies in nonsmokers came to different conclusions. Rifici and Khachadurian (91) reported that vitamin C supplementation reduced lipoprotein (mixture of VLDL and LDL) oxidation in their subjects. This study had a small sample size ($n = 4$) and no placebo control group. In contrast, Wen, Cooke, and Feely (92) found no effect of vitamin C supplementation (1,000 mg/day) on LDL oxidizability. These authors reported a significant increase in red blood cell alpha-tocopherol in the supplemented subjects, which may indicate a beneficial effect against oxidative stress in general.

Several studies have examined the effect of vitamin C in diet and plasma on CVD. Enstrom et al (93) reported that persons with high vitamin C intakes have reduced CVD mortality. A prospective study from Great Britain (94) examined plasma vitamin C and mortality rates from CVD. Significant reductions in CVD mortality and ischemic heart disease mortality occurred with increased quintiles of plasma vitamin C in both men and women, although the trends were less robust for women. Researchers from the Kuopio ischemic heart disease risk-factor study (95) reported that men with plasma vitamin C levels less than 11.4 μmol/liter had a twofold higher risk of MI when data were adjusted for other risk factors. Kurl et al (96) found significant interactions between low plasma vitamin C, hypertension, and body mass index (BMI) and risk of stroke in the Kuopio cohort. High levels of plasma vitamin C (> 28.4 μmol/liter) reduced the risk of stroke for hypertensive and overweight (BMI > 25) men. In Nurses' Health Study data (97), taking vitamin C supplements was associated with reduction in risk for CHD (relative risk [RR] $= 0.72$), but no significant relationship was found for dietary vitamin C. One possible explanation for the lack of effect with dietary vitamin C was the use of a food-frequency questionnaire to estimate intake rather than the 7-day food record used in the EPIC-Norfolk study above (94,98).

Much of the recent research on vitamin C has involved examination of endothelial function in large arteries. Ellis et al (99) reported that flow-mediated dilation (FMD) was significantly increased in CHF subjects who received intravenous and oral vitamin C (both $P <$ .05). Other groups reported improved brachial artery blood flow in patients with angina (100) and improved coronary artery blood flow in patients with idiopathic dilated cardiomyopathy (101) with vitamin C supplementation. Liu et al (102) examined 4-hour postprandial brachial artery FMD in normocholesterolemic CHD patients and non-CHD controls with or without 2 g oral vitamin C given with a high-fat meal (800 kcal, 50 g fat). The CHD and non-CHD participants who did not receive vitamin C had significant falls in FMD after the high-fat meal; this fall was not seen in the participants who took vitamin C with the meal. The vitamin C effects seen in these studies were endothelium-based because nitroglycerin-induced vasodilation was unaffected (99). Vitamin C's effect on endothelium may involve preservation of nitric oxide or scavenging of intracellular superoxide anion (103), although nonantioxidant pathways may also be responsible (99). It remains to be seen whether smaller quantities of oral vitamin C obtainable from dietary sources can produce similar beneficial effects on endothelial function.

Toohey et al (104) examined relationships between plasma vitamin C and other CVD risk factors in 172 African Americans. Plasma vitamin C in this study was inversely correlated with systolic and diastolic blood pressure, total cholesterol levels, and LDL cholesterol levels. HDL cholesterol levels were positively correlated with plasma vitamin C in this cohort. The blood pressure correlations mirror those seen in an earlier study (105). The effect of vitamin C supplementation on plasma lipids in supplementation studies has been mostly negative (39,89). Vitamin C supplementation at 1 g/day for 8 months failed to reduce the concentration of lipoprotein (a) [Lp(a)] in healthy subjects (106). Although vitamin C appears to have a lesser effect on LDL oxidation than does alpha-tocopherol, it may show promise in the reduction of endothelial dysfunction in smokers and in patients with CHF.

Carotenoids

Carotenoids are a family of more than 500 compounds that provide color and protection against free radicals in plant tissues (107). Burton and Ingold (108) reported that beta carotene may be a better antioxidant at low partial pressures of oxygen, as might exist in the arterial wall. Two carotenoids, beta carotene and lycopene, have been examined for their effect on CVD risk factors. Beta carotene is the most active provitamin A carotenoid in the diet. Humans cannot convert lycopene to retinol. Beta carotene is found widely in yellow, orange, and dark-green vegetables; lycopene is found mostly in tomatoes, watermelon, guava, and red grapefruit (109). Many persons in the United States have higher circulating levels of lycopene than beta carotene because of high consumption of processed tomato products (110).

Carotenoid absorption from the diet is enhanced by cooking and co-consumption of fat (111-113). As with vitamin E, absorption of carotenoids is micelle-dependent and release into the postabsorptive circulation occurs via chylomicrons. Carotenoids are very hydrophobic and would be buried in the lipid core of lipoproteins. To date, there is no evidence of selective transfer of carotenoids into VLDL particles by the liver. About 70% of circulating beta carotene is found within LDL particles (114). Lowe et al (115) found that beta carotene, lycopene, and alpha-tocopherol were found predominantly in the lighter, less-dense LDL particles, whereas the oxycarotenoids lutein and zeaxanthin were concentrated in the small, dense LDL particles. The location of these major lipophilic antioxidants may explain the greater oxidizability of small, dense LDL (116). One research group (17) found that in vitro enrichment of LDL with beta carotene resulted in increased oxidative resistance; however, others have not reproduced this (117,118). Bowen and Omaye (119) reported that LDL beta carotene concentration was positively correlated with rate of LDL oxidation.

Beta carotene, unlike the other antioxidant nutrients, has not been shown to significantly reduce LDL oxidizability in human studies. Princen (38) and Jialal and Fuller (120) reported a small, but statistically significant, increase in LDL oxidative resistance with beta carotene supplementation. Several investigators (34,117,121) have shown that beta carotene supplementation in humans did not reduce LDL oxidizability. With increased incidence of lung cancer among smokers supplemented with beta carotene in both the ATBC and Beta-Carotene and Retinol Efficacy trials, research on beta carotene's role in reducing CVD has slowed considerably (73,122). Vivekananthan (64) found a significant increase in all-cause (OR, 1.07; $P = .03$) and CVD mortality (OR, 1.1; $P = .003$) in their pooled analysis of beta carotene trials. Incidence of stroke in the three studies they pooled was not different between the supplemented and placebo groups. Two earlier studies showed beneficial effects of high dietary beta carotene on incidence of angina (123) and increased adipose tissue beta carotene on risk of MI (124). It is possible that beta carotene in the latter study was a surrogate marker for other healthy lifestyle choices because adipose beta carotene was negatively correlated with BMI and smoking. In addition, the investigators found a borderline significant interaction ($P = .07$) between adipose beta carotene and adipose PUFA content (124).

In vitro studies have shown lycopene to be the most effective carotenoid antioxidant (125). It is the first carotenoid to disappear during LDL oxidation (126). Given its prevalence in the US diet in cooked tomato products, more research interest has swung its way. Age and BMI were negatively correlated with serum lycopene in a subset of participants in the Women's Health Study (127); these relationships were not seen in men (128). Both studies did see a positive correlation of serum lycopene and serum cholesterol.

The effect of lycopene on LDL oxidizability is unclear. Romanchik (126) reported that in vitro enrichment of LDL with lycopene did not reduce its oxidizability. In a study by Agarwal and Rao, lycopene supplementation from tomato juice (50.4 mg), spaghetti sauce (39.3 mg), or lycopene oleoresin (75.0 mg) for 1 week increased LDL resistance to oxidation in non-smoking healthy subjects (129). Despite the wide range of daily lycopene intakes among the interventions, there were no significant differences in serum lycopene after supplementation. Sutherland and associates found that tomato juice supplementation had no effect on oxidative susceptibility of LDL in renal transplant recipients (130). The study by Sutherland et al used a smaller amount of tomato juice than Agarwal and Rao's study (400 mL vs 540 mL per day); in addition, three of the transplant recipients had ischemic heart disease and two smoked. None of the subjects had diabetes. The subjects' increased oxidative stress may have contributed to the negative findings. Chopra (131) studied female smokers and nonsmokers. After a 1-week carotenoid depletion regimen, subjects were given 1 week of foods containing predominantly beta carotene and lutein and 1 week of high-lycopene foods (> 40 mg) in random order. LDL oxidizability was assessed at the end of each week. Lycopene caused a significant increase in LDL oxidative resistance only in the nonsmoking group ($P = .01$). Another food-based study with nonsmoking men (132) showed that dietary supplementation for 2 weeks with tomato juice (40 mg lycopene) reduced LDL oxidation; however, supplementation with carrot juice (22.3 mg beta carotene and 15.7 mg alpha carotene) or spinach powder (11.3 mg lutein and 3.1 mg beta carotene) did not. Pellegrini (133) reported that tomato puree (7 mg lycopene) supplementation for 2 weeks failed to increase antioxidant capacity of plasma. To determine the definitive effect of lycopene on LDL oxidation, longer supplementation periods and larger subject numbers with a wider range of dosages within a single study are needed; in particular, studies need to evaluate effects in smokers and other groups with known oxidative stresses. Lycopene oleoresin supplements should be used in research studies to minimize the effect of food matrix on lycopene bioavailability.

Several studies have examined the effect of serum or dietary lycopene on risk of CVD. Data from the Kuopio Ischaemic Heart Disease Risk Factor Study (134) indicated men with the lowest quartile of serum lycopene had a 3.3-fold increased risk of acute coronary event or stroke compared with those in the highest serum lycopene quartile; the RR for acute coronary events alone was 2.8. Serum beta carotene had no association with acute coronary events or stroke in this analysis. A follow-up investigation in this cohort (135) examined the association of serum lycopene and intima-media thickness of the carotid artery. Serum lycopene was inversely correlated with intima-media thickness, and the correlation was stronger in smokers than nonsmokers. In the Women's Health Study, dietary lycopene showed no strong association with CVD endpoints (136), despite a 30% reduction in risk for women at the highest intake level (≥ 7 servings per week). Gender and smoking differences could be responsible for the discrepancies between these epidemiologic studies; in addition, the Women's Health Study used a food-frequency questionnaire to estimate lycopene intake from the number of servings of tomato-based products consumed per week. A measurement of serum lycopene combined with a better estimate of lycopene intake might have produced a positive result.

Lycopene may have potential in the prevention of CVD, but long-term intervention studies are needed to assess its effects. In addition, research is needed to determine whether it has any adverse effects in smokers similar to the effects of beta carotene.

Trials of Combinations of Antioxidant Nutrients

Several investigators have used combinations of antioxidant nutrients to assess their effects on CVD risk factors. As with trials of single nutrients, the results of recent studies are mixed. In the Antioxidant Supplementation in Atherosclerosis Prevention study, 520 men and women ages 45 to 69 years with serum cholesterol levels equal to or greater than 193 mg/dL were randomly assigned (137). Groups received placebo, 182 mg/day vitamin E (as RRR-alpha-tocopherol), 500 mg/day vitamin C, or vitamins E and C for 3 years. Relative to placebo, men who received the combined supplement had a significant reduction in progression of carotid atherosclerosis; similar results were not seen in women.

The HDL-Atherosclerosis Treatment Study randomized 160 men and women with low HDL cholesterol levels and established coronary disease to receive placebo, simvastatin plus niacin, antioxidant nutrients (800 IU vitamin E as RRR-alpha-tocopherol, 25 mg beta carotene, 1,000 mg vitamin C, and 100 μg selenium per day), or simvastatin, niacin, and antioxidants (138). Participants received counseling to emphasize weight loss, exercise, and increased monounsaturated fat intake to elevate HDL levels; counseling to encourage smoking cessation was also provided as needed. Antioxidant supplementation had no effect on coronary atherosclerosis as measured by arteriography, whereas the simvastatin-niacin combination produced regression of coronary artery stenosis. Similarly, the Heart Protection Study (139) found no change in CHD events, strokes, or mortality in subjects who received 650 mg vitamin E, 250 mg vitamin C, and 20 mg beta carotene for more than 5 years.

The Women's Angiographic Vitamin and Estrogen trial was designed to assess the effects of antioxidants and hormone replacement therapy on coronary atherosclerosis, as measured by coronary angiography (140). In this multicenter study, women with at least one 15% to 75% stenosis of a coronary artery were randomized to receive either estrogen, placebo, antioxidant vitamins (800 IU vitamin E and 1 g vitamin C per day), or estrogen plus antioxidant vitamins. Neither hormone replacement therapy nor antioxidant vitamin treatment halted the progression of coronary artery stenosis. There was a trend toward increased risk of coronary events (including death or MI) in the vitamin group ($P = .09$). In contrast, a trial that gave identical doses of vitamins E and C for 1 year to patients after cardiac transplantation reported slowed growth in intimal thickness of coronary arteries compared with patients who received placebo (141).

Bunout et al (142) gave patients with coronary artery disease a multivitamin supplement containing 150 mg alpha-tocopherol, 150 mg vitamin C, 12.5 mg beta carotene, 650 μg folic acid, and 400 μg vitamin B-12 for 15 days. There was no placebo group in this trial. The oxidizability of LDL decreased significantly after treatment ($P = .001$). The primary reason for the reduced oxidation could not be established. The equivocal results seen on CVD with combined antioxidant nutrient supplementation, coupled with the results of single-nutrient studies, argue strongly against blanket recommendations for supplementation for primary or secondary prevention.

OTHER DIETARY SUPPLEMENTS

Folate

A high circulating concentration of homocysteine (Hcy) is considered an emerging risk factor for CVD because of Hcy's toxicity to endothelial cells and promotion of platelet adhesion (143). Several studies have linked high circulating levels of Hcy to atherosclerosis (144,145); stroke (144,146); CHF without previous MI (147); impaired clotting (148); and increased 5-year overall mortality (149). The latter association was greater for persons with high Hcy levels and diabetes (149). A comparison of emerging risk factors from the Physicians' Health Study cohort (150) showed that plasma Hcy was less predictive of peripheral artery disease than C-reactive protein and the total cholesterol–to–HDL cholesterol ratio. This result was corroborated by a meta-analysis of Hcy studies (151), where a 25% lower usual Hcy level was associated with an 11% reduction in risk of ischemic heart disease and a 19% lower risk of stroke.

How does folate lower Hcy levels? Folate is an essential cofactor for the enzyme methionine synthase, which converts Hcy to the essential amino acid methionine. Vitamin B-12 is another cofactor required for this enzyme. Hcy can also be converted to cystathionine via a vitamin B-6–dependent pathway. In a recent analysis of NHANES III data (152), plasma Hcy was negatively associated with serum and erythrocyte folate and serum B-12 levels (all $P < .0001$).

Being homozygous for polymorphisms (mutations) in the methylene tetrahydrofolate reductase (MTHFR) gene, which can reduce the recycling of folate, has been associated with neural tube defects (153) and Down syndrome (154). The MTHFR C677T polymorphism was not associated with increased plasma Hcy concentrations in a Dutch study (155); however, Japanese investigators found that this mutation was a risk factor for homocysteinemia and increased severity of coronary artery disease in men (156). A significant interaction between plasma folate and presence of at least one MTHFR C677T gene to increase plasma Hcy was reported in patients on maintenance dialysis (157). Children with heterozygous familial hypercholesterolemia (FH) who were homozygous for the MTHFR C677T mutation had higher plasma Hcy levels and were more likely to have an FH-affected parent with a history of CVD before age 55 (158). Persons homozygous for the MTHFR C677T genotype had a 16% higher risk of CHD, according to one meta-analysis (159). These researchers also found that this genotype was a risk factor for CHD only when folate status was low.

All enriched grain products in the United States are now fortified with folate at the level of 140 μg/100 g (160), which has considerably increased intake of this nutrient (161). Common dietary sources of folate are listed in Table 11.5. The RDA for folate has been set for adults at 400 μg dietary folate equivalents (DFEs) per day (31). This unit adjusts for improved absorption of folate from supplement sources and is defined as 1 μg DFE equals 1 μg food folate equals 0.5 μg supplemental folic acid taken on an empty stomach or 0.6 μg folic acid taken with a meal (31).

Supplementation of subjects and patients with folate has been shown to reduce plasma Hcy concentrations (142,162-164). The only study to examine the effect of folate supplementation on LDL oxidation (142) used a mixed supplement that also contained vitamins E and C and beta carotene. This intervention lasted for only 15 days and had no placebo or single-nutrient group for comparison of effect. Guttormsen et al (163) examined the effect of folate supplementation (200 μg/day) on plasma Hcy levels in 37 subjects who were homozygous for

TABLE 11.5
Dietary Sources of Folic Acid

Food Sources of Folic Acid	Folic Acid, as μg Dietary Folate Equivalents (DFE)
Wheat flour, 1 cup	395
Lentils, cooked, 1 cup	358
Spinach, cooked, 1 cup	263
Asparagus, cooked, 1 cup	243
Long grain rice, enriched, regular, cooked, 1 cup	153
Beef liver, cooked, 3 ounces	221
Bagel, egg, 4-inch diameter	119

Source: Data are from reference 28.

the MTHFR C677T mutation. They reported that supplementation reduced plasma Hcy to normal in 21 (57%) of these subjects within 7 months. Twelve of the remaining subjects attained normal Hcy levels with 5 mg/day folate supplementation. Venn et al (165) instructed subjects with high plasma Hcy levels to consume a target of 600 μg folate per day by consuming two glasses of orange juice and one serving of legumes per day, plus selecting other high-folate foods from a list. Control subjects received unfortified breakfast cereal. At the end of the 4-week intervention, subjects who consumed the high-folate diet had lower plasma Hcy and higher serum folate levels than did the controls ($P < .05$). The authors also noted that subjects who consumed the high-folate diet also consumed lower amounts of saturated fatty acids and higher amounts of dietary fiber, vitamins B-6, C, and E, nutrients that are associated with reduced CVD.

The majority of folate and CVD studies to date have been epidemiologic in nature. Many of the studies were completed before fortification was instituted. An early Canadian study (166) found that persons with low serum folate levels had a higher risk for fatal coronary disease (RR = 1.69 for plasma folate < 6.8 nmol/liter). The trends in risk with decreased folate were significant for both men ($P = .02$) and women ($P = .04$). A case-control study of subjects from the Physicians' Health Study (167) found that low plasma folate was not significantly associated with increased risk of MI and that Hcy levels may not predict long-term risk. A case-control study of patients with a first nonfatal MI revealed that the RR for MI for folate intakes of more than 340 μg/day was 0.57 compared with intakes of less than 340 μg/day (168). This study was performed in Spain, a country without mandatory fortification. Only 6% of the subjects were taking supplements. The Stockholm Heart Epidemiology Program examined the impact of taking multivitamin supplements containing an average of 400 μg folate on the risk of MI (169). Only 10% of this population used separate vitamin C, and 2% used separate vitamin E supplements; the average amounts of those nutrients in the multivitamin preparations were 60 and 9 mg, respectively. The investigators found significant inverse associations between supplement use and nonfatal MI. These associations were not altered by adjustments for smoking and other risk factors. It thus appears that folate supplementation may reduce the incidence of coronary events.

Folate supplementation (5 mg/day for 6 weeks) in patients with coronary artery disease was found to improve endothelial function, as measured by FMD (170). This was a placebo-controlled, double-blind, crossover study with a 4-week washout period between phases. Plasma Hcy was significantly decreased with folate supplementation. The proposed mechanism, as seen in an in vitro experiment, was the reduction of Hcy-induced increase in superoxide content within endothelial cells by folate co-incubation.

Brilakis et al (171) examined the association between plasma Hcy and coronary disease in patients undergoing angiography between July 1998 and January 1999, after mandatory folate fortification went into effect. They found no relationship between Hcy and degree of coronary artery disease. These results may indicate that fortification has been successful in reducing plasma Hcy levels or that additional factors play a greater role in coronary artery disease. This would be consistent with the findings of Ridker (150).

The UL for folate has been set at 1,000 μg/day (160) because of concerns about masking vitamin B-12 deficiency. Older adults often have reduced absorption of B-12 secondary to hypochlorhydria and possibly *Helicobacter pylori* infection (172). It has also been observed that high circulating levels of Hcy in older adults may be more due to low vitamin B-12 status than low folate status (173). However, Mills et al (174) published a retrospective study of plasma vitamin B-12 concentrations in a Veterans Affairs cohort from 1992 to 2000, which covers the time before and after mandatory folate fortification was initiated. They found no change in the incidence of patients with low plasma vitamin B-12 concentrations without anemia during that time period, which indicates that folate fortification may have little effect on vitamin B-12 deficiency. More work is needed to confirm this finding.

As with the other nutrients discussed above, more research is needed to determine whether folate supplementation and the resulting fall in plasma Hcy in the population reduces CVD morbidity and mortality. Despite the uncertainty, a cost-benefit analysis (175) indicated that supplementing patients with high circulating Hcy levels with folate with or without vitamin B-12 produced cost per life-year saved numbers comparable to other interventions, such as lovastatin treatment for men with cholesterol levels equal to or greater than 300 mg/dL and antihypertensive drugs for patients with diastolic blood pressures between 95 and 104 mm Hg.

Flavonoids

Flavonoids are part of a large class of compounds known as polyphenols. These hydrophilic compounds are ubiquitous in plants and function as pigments (anthocyanins) or plant defense. Human diets probably contain on average 1 g flavonoids per day (176), although this may be an overestimate (177). Analysis of data from the Health Professionals' Follow-up Study and the Nurses' Health Study (178) revealed that the major sources of dietary flavonoids were onions and black tea. A related Japanese study (179) also listed onions as the primary source of dietary flavonoids, whereas green tea was ranked fourth. The bioavailability of flavonoids is complex because their beta-glycosidic bonds must be hydrolyzed by colonic microflora that can also degrade flavonoids (176). Flavonoid intake was inversely related to CHD death in the Seven Countries Study (180); however, dietary flavonoids were not associated with risk of CVD in the Health Professionals' Follow-up Study or the Women's Health Study (181,182).

In the interest of brevity, this chapter reviews only the results of studies using flavonoids derived from red wine or tea. Both beverages contain a variety of flavonoids and other compounds, so it is difficult to ascribe the effects reported to a single chemical. In addition, there is a wide variation of flavonoid content within a single foodstuff, depending on species, variety, ripeness, processing, and storage (183). Frankel et al (184) found that flavonoids extracted from red wine reduced LDL oxidizability in vitro. Kerry and Abbey (185) reported that the fractions that produced the greatest effect were monomeric anthocyanidins and catechins. A more recent study (186) reported that red wine flavonoids reduced cholesterol oxidation in LDL, possibly by sparing endogenous alpha-tocopherol. Comparison of the red wine compound resveratrol (a hydroxystilbene, not a flavonoid) with red wine extract showed that the wine extract was better at scavenging free radicals than resveratrol (187). Consumption of 400 mL red wine per day (11% alcohol) for 2 weeks reduced LDL oxidation in one study; similar effects were not found with white wine (188). A second trial (189) that administered reduced-alcohol wine (3.5%) found no effect on LDL oxidizability. Natella et al (190) reported that consumption of red wine with a meal reduced the postprandial increase in LDL oxidizability; in contrast, a control isocaloric alcoholic beverage did not change LDL oxidative susceptibility. The plasma alpha-tocopherol concentration decreased in postprandial LDL after consumption of the control beverage; this was not seen after consumption of red wine. Another study (191) found that consumption of dealcoholized red wine by male smokers reduced in vivo oxidative stress as measured by plasma and urinary F2-isoprostanes, oxidative products of arachidonic acid. Intact red wine and white wine did not show this effect. Consumption of dealcoholized red wine by these subjects did not alter plasma tocopherol levels.

Struck et al (192) performed a 3-month crossover study to examine the effects of red and white wines on CVD risk factors in hypercholesterolemic adults. Subjects were given either 180 mL per day of red or white wine for 4 weeks, with a 2-week washout period before receiving the other wine. When data from the red and white wine phases were pooled, a significant fall in thrombin-initiated platelet aggregation was seen. The effect of red wine on platelet aggregation can be attributed to flavonoids and alcohol (193). Evidence of plasma oxidation was also reduced. The latter finding was also seen in a nonphysiologic system (194). De Lorgeril et al (195) examined wine intake among men enrolled in the Lyon Diet Heart Study and its possible effect on CHD recurrence. Subjects who consumed the highest quartile of wine ethanol (45 g/day, about three glasses of wine) had a lower risk of recurrence relative to those consuming the lowest quartile of wine ethanol, and there was a linear trend in risk ratios ($P = .01$). The authors did not differentiate between red and white wine consumption and cautioned against extrapolating their findings to other demographic groups.

Tea is the most widely consumed beverage in many countries. Green tea is unfermented and is the preferred beverage in Japan and China. Black tea is the result of fermentation of green tea leaves. Oolong tea results from partial fermentation of green tea leaves. The fermentation process causes polymerization of flavonoids (196), which alters the color and taste of the beverage. The Zutphen Study investigators (197) followed men for 15 years and found that high flavonoid consumption, predominantly from black tea, resulted in a reduced risk of stroke. The RR of stroke for daily consumption of at least 4.7 cups of tea was 0.31 vs daily consumption of no more than 2.6 cups. Green tea consumption tended to cause less atheromatous plaque formation in cholesterol-fed rabbits (198), whereas black tea had no effect. Both varieties of tea reduced LDL oxidizability in these rabbits.

The effect of tea on LDL oxidizability has produced conflicting results in humans. Serafini et al (196) administered a single dose of green and black tea with and without addition of milk to healthy volunteers. Although green tea was a better antioxidant in the purely in vitro study, green and black tea produced similar plasma antioxidant capacities in the subjects. Addition of milk to either tea diminished its effectiveness in the human trial. In a study by Ishikawa et al (199), 14 healthy subjects drank 750 mL of black tea per day for 4 weeks while continuing to consume their normal diets. Seven subjects drank the same amount of water for control. The rate of LDL oxidation was slower during the period of tea consumption. In contrast, van het Hof et al (200) noted no difference in LDL oxidizability in subjects who received 900 mL per day of green or black tea. Lack of dietary control in either study may explain the divergent findings.

Two other epidemiologic studies have examined the effect of flavonoids from tea on CVD. The Caerphilly Study (201) followed 1,900 Welsh men for 15 years. This population customarily adds milk to tea. Flavonoid intake from tea was not related to incidence of ischemic heart disease, although it was weakly and positively related to death from ischemic heart disease and strongly related to total mortality. The lack of beneficial effect may be due to the addition of milk, as was seen by Serafini et al (196). Two articles from the Rotterdam Study have examined the effect of tea flavonoids on CVD. High consumption of tea ($\geq$ 500mL/day) was associated with a reduced risk of severe aortic atherosclerosis (OR, 0.31) (202), but not mild or moderate atherosclerosis. The effect of tea on aortic atherosclerosis was greater in women than in men. In a subsequent article (203), high tea intakes ($>$ 375 mL/day) were associated with lower incidence of MI (RR, 0.57) and fatal MI (RR, 0.35). Total dietary flavonoid intake was inversely associated with fatal MI only at higher total intakes.

Tea flavonoids have been researched for other effects on CVD risk factors. Green tea extract enriched with theaflavins from black tea significantly reduced total cholesterol and LDL cholesterol levels in persons with mild-to-moderate hypercholesterolemia (204). Black tea did not affect fasting plasma Hcy levels in one study (205); however, analysis of changes in urinary 4-methylgallic acid (a catabolic product of flavonoid metabolism) indicated a direct relationship with the changes in plasma Hcy. This means that individual differences in metabolism of flavonoids may reflect the effects of consuming a polyphenol-rich beverage on Hcy levels. Further study is needed to confirm these effects.

Flavonoids from food sources can be considered safe, but isolated flavonoids in supplements could have adverse effects. Some flavonoids could reduce iron absorption (206). Rankin et al (207) found that LDL modified by the flavonoid myrcetin underwent aggregation, which increased its uptake by the macrophage scavenger receptor. Another study, in which subjects received 1 g of quercetin per day for 4 weeks, reported no changes in plasma lipid levels (208). The combination of flavonoids and other substances in food may be important in prevention of CVD.

Garlic (Allium sativum)

Garlic has been used as a food ingredient and herbal remedy for thousands of years. Four garlic preparations have been used in addition to garlic cloves: essential oil, garlic powder, oil macerate, and aged garlic extract (AGE). It was first thought that the active component of garlic was the organosulfur compound allicin, produced when an intact garlic clove is cut. Allicin is a highly transient species and is rapidly degraded to compounds such as diallyl sulfide, diallyl disulfide, and diallyl trisulfide. These compounds are oil soluble and may have pharmacologic value. S-allylcysteine is produced by a different pathway, is water soluble, and may also have bioactive properties (209).

Several issues hamper interpretation of the garlic literature:

- Variability in the type of garlic preparations used in research studies
- Short study duration and small numbers of subjects
- Lack of randomized, controlled trials

Garlic may prevent CVD by inhibition of platelet activity and reduction of plasma lipid levels. Steiner and Li (210) reported that consumption of AGE by healthy individuals reduced platelet aggregation and adhesion in a dose-dependent fashion. This was a randomized, double-blind crossover study in which the subjects received AGE or placebo in increasing doses for

6-week intervals. After a 2-week washout period, they received the other treatments. Zhang et al (211) saw no differences in prothrombin time or partial thromboplastin time in trained male athletes after a 16-week supplementation with garlic oil. The results of in vitro studies indicate that garlic compounds may act by inhibiting production of thromboxane B-2 (212).

Recent studies on the hypolipidemic effects of garlic have shown more discrepancies. In an 8-week study of allicin supplementation, Ghorai et al found a mean 13% fall in total cholesterol levels (213). All of the subjects were young males (mean age 20.3 years), and their mean total cholesterol level before supplementation was 148 mg/dL. Another group of investigators (214) found that garlic powder supplementation was more effective in CHD patients with baseline total cholesterol levels more than 270 mg/dL. Zhang et al (215) compared the hypolipidemic effects of supplementation of healthy subjects with placebo, garlic oil, and garlic powder for 11 weeks. No effects on plasma lipids were seen for either garlic preparation in the whole study population; however, women receiving garlic oil had significant increases in HDL cholesterol and total cholesterol–to–HDL cholesterol ratio and a significant decrease in LDL cholesterol level. The male subjects had no changes in plasma lipids after garlic supplementation. As with the aforementioned study by Ghorai et al (213), the mean total cholesterol level for all three groups at baseline was less than 193 mg/dL, so large decreases in response to garlic would not be expected. Koscielny et al (216) performed a double-blind, placebo-controlled clinical trial of high-dose garlic powder tablets on atherosclerotic plaques in the femoral and carotid arteries of 152 patients. This study is unique in that the participants were followed for 4 years. The plaque volume decreased 2.6% in the garlic group during the study period, whereas the plaque volume in the control group increased 15.6%.

Several additional mechanisms have been proposed for the beneficial effects of garlic, based on animal and in vitro research. LDL oxidation was reduced in the presence of large amounts of aqueous or ether extracts of AGE (217). Similarly, high concentrations of AGE reduced lipid peroxidation and subsequent hemolysis in rat erythrocytes (218). AGE and s-allylcysteine reduced cell damage due to oxidized LDL in cultured cells (219). The concentrations used in this study may also exceed what may be achieved in vivo with garlic supplementation.

Bad breath is the most familiar consequence of garlic use, particularly in foods. Garlic supplements can cause gastrointestinal distress. Hoshino et al (220) compared via endoscopy the effects of various garlic preparations on dog gastrointestinal mucosa. Dehydrated raw garlic powder caused the most severe damage to the intestinal mucosa. Enteric-coated garlic products caused some loss of epithelial cells at the top of crypts in the ileum. Individuals taking anticoagulants should be aware that concurrent garlic supplementation may cause bleeding (221).

Guggulipid

Guggulipid is a resin from the mukul myrrh tree (*Commiphora mukul*). The active compounds in the resin are believed to be E- and Z-guggulsterones. Early trials showed promising results, but several lacked placebo controls (222) and none were done in Western populations. For example, Ghorai (215) supplemented 10 healthy males in India with an equivalent of 25 mg of guggulsterone for 8 weeks. The average baseline total cholesterol level was 212 mg/dL. Treatment caused a 32% fall in mean total cholesterol, to 143 mg/dL. Szapary et al (222) randomized hyperlipidemic adults on a typical US diet to receive placebo or 1,000 mg (standard dose) or 2,000 mg (high dose) guggulipid per day for 8 weeks. Both guggulipid groups had significant elevations in LDL cholesterol levels compared with the placebo group. The standard dose guggulipid group also had a significant decrease in HDL cholesterol levels. In addition, six subjects developed a hypersensitivity rash with guggulipid treatment. The results of this study call into question the utility of guggulipid in Western populations.

Red Yeast Rice

Red yeast rice is the result of fermenting the yeast *Monascicus purpureus* on rice. In China, the product is known as *Hongqu* and in the United States it is known as red yeast rice (223). It contains the compound lovastatin, the first 3-hydroxy-3-methylglutaryl coenzyme A (HMG-CoA) reductase inhibitor approved by the US Food and Drug Administration (FDA). Red yeast rice was included in the herbal supplement Cholestin. After determining Cholestin contained lovastatin, the FDA took legal action. On July 21, 2000, the 10th Circuit Court (which was upheld by the US District Court on March 20, 2001) mandated that the product be sold as a drug (224). Red yeast rice is no longer legally sold in the United States. However, it may be purchased from foreign companies via the Internet. [Note: The American Dietetic Association does not endorse purchase of supplements banned by the FDA. Patients should be asked whether they use this supplement, with practitioners evaluating the consequences of such usage.]

PRACTICE RECOMMENDATIONS

Overall Messages

Given the conflicting findings discussed above, there is great confusion among consumers and practitioners alike concerning the value of these compounds in prevention of CVD. Some practical recommendations are given below.

There is no substitute for risk-factor reduction. As was shown by the ATBC study (73), antioxidant supplementation cannot help long-term smokers prevent the health consequences of their habit. Weight loss, exercise, and control of blood lipid levels and blood pressure should take precedence over supplement use.

Consider the totality of the diet, and encourage patients to get their antioxidant nutrients primarily through dietary means rather than supplements. Early epidemiologic studies showed that increased intakes of vitamin E from food, but not supplements, reduced the risk of cardiovascular mortality (43,44). The American Heart Association issued recommendations against the use of antioxidant supplements in women to prevent CHD, based on evidence to date (225). The diet used in the Dietary Approaches to Stop Hypertension (DASH) study, which altered patterns of consumption instead of a single nutrient, has been shown to be successful at reducing blood pressure and LDL cholesterol levels (226-228). More recently, the DASH diet has been shown to reduce serum Hcy (229). (See Chapter 8 for further information on the DASH diet.) The Mediterranean diet (230) and a high-fiber vegetarian diet (231) have also shown promise in reducing CVD risk factors.

Dietary change is hard work, even for those who have been motivated by an MI. Frame et al (232) demonstrated that cardiac rehabilitation patients were more advanced along the stages of change model for dietary fat reduction than for inclusion of five servings of fruits and vegetables per day. (See Chapter 5 for discussion of stages of change model.)

Specific Advice

Dietitians can translate scientific studies into practical solutions for patients. When a patient asks "What kind of vitamin E should I take?" the dietitian can respond, "Alpha-tocopherol (as contrasted with beta-, gamma-, or delta-tocopherol) is most physiologically active. Both the alpha- and gamma-tocopherol in our food supply may have beneficial roles, but current evidence points to alpha-tocopherol as the beneficial supplement for reducing the potential of your blood cholesterol producing artery-clogging plaque. You should be aware that current research does not tell us whether taking vitamin E supplements reduces the development of heart disease. In addition, the American Heart Association does not recommend supplement use to prevent heart disease in women."

Many resources can provide patients with advice on supplement use. The American Dietetic Association has published an excellent book, *The Health Professional's Guide to Popular Dietary Supplements* (233). Box 11.1 lists good Internet resources (234-240). The FDA Web site provides a handout titled "Tips for the Savvy Supplement User: Making

---

Box 11.1 Recommended Web-based Resources on Dietary Supplements

Food and Drug Administration

   http://www.fda.gov/fdac/features/2002/202_supp.html (234)

   Tips for consumers on wise decisions regarding use of supplements.

Mayo Clinic Herb and Drug Interactions

   http://www.mayoclinic.com/invoke.cfm?id=SA00039 (235)

   Listing of 10 herbs that may interact with prescription and over the counter drugs.

Natural Medicines Comprehensive Database

   http://www.naturaldatabase.com (236)

   A subscription-based site with information on herbs and botanicals.

National Institutes of Health National Center for Complementary and Alternative Medicine
      (NCCAM)

   http://nccam.nih.gov/ (237)

   Evaluation and dissemination of information on complementary and alternative medical (CAM)
      treatments; provides quick link for searching journal citations via *CAM on PubMed.*

National Institutes of Health Office of Dietary Supplements

   http://ods.od.nih.gov (238)

   Provides general information on dietary supplements and includes the IBIDS database of
      published international scientific literature on dietary supplements including botanicals, vita-
      mins, and minerals.

Nutrition Action Health Letter: Cholesterol-Lowering Supplements

   http://www.cspinet.org/nah/novnah.htm (239)

   Review of the scientific research on cholesterol lowering products and foods available over the
      counter; published by Center for Science in the Public Interest in November 1997.

USDA Center for Food Safety and Applied Nutrition Dietary Supplements

   http://www.cfsan.fda.gov/~dms/supplmnt.html (240)

   An overview of safety, industry regulations, reporting adverse events, and other links related to the
      use of dietary supplements.

Informed Decisions" (234). According to this Web site, the consumer should consider the following:

- Do I need to think about my total diet?
- Should I check with my doctor or health-care provider before using a supplement?
- Some supplements may interact with other medications
- Some supplements can have unwanted effects during surgery
- Adverse effects from use of dietary supplements should be reported to FDA.

Use of the RDA and UL allows one to see the range of safe intake levels for different vitamins. For instance, the range for vitamins E and C is quite large, but the range for folate is more limited, to avoid any risk of folate supplementation masking a vitamin B-12 deficiency.

CONCLUSION

In summary, the results of studies examining the effects of antioxidant nutrients and herbal supplements on CVD risk factors and endpoints are mixed. In the absence of more concrete data, practitioners should encourage patients to obtain carotenoids, vitamin C, folic acid, and phytochemicals from their diets. Although vitamin E supplementation can reduce oxidation of LDL cholesterol, clinical trials have not shown reduction in cardiovascular end points. Patients using dietary supplements can benefit from sound advice from the health care professional, as well as a number of books and Web sites.

REFERENCES

1. Brown MS, Goldstein JL. Lipoprotein metabolism in the macrophage: implications for cholesterol deposition in atherosclerosis. *Annu Rev Biochem.* 1983;52:223-261.
2. Haberland ME, Fong D, Cheng L. Malondialdehyde-altered protein occurs in atheroma of Watanabe heritable hyperlipidemic rabbits. *Science.* 1988;241:215-218.
3. Ylä-Herttuala S, Palinski W, Rosenfeld ME, Parthasarathy S, Carew TE, Butler S, Witztum JL, Steinberg D. Evidence for the presence of oxidatively modified low density lipoprotein in atherosclerotic lesions of rabbits and man. *J Clin Invest.* 1989;84:1086-1095.
4. Cathcart MK, Morel DW, Chisolm GM. Monocytes and neutrophils oxidize low density lipoprotein making it cytotoxic. *J Leukoc Biol.* 1985;38:341-350.
5. Scaccini C, Jialal I. LDL modification by activated polymorphonuclear leukocytes: a cellular model of mild oxidative stress. *Free Radic Biol Med.* 1994;16:49-55.
6. Steinbrecher UP, Parthasarathy S, Leake DS, Witztum JL, Steinberg D. Modification of low density lipoprotein by endothelial cells involves lipid peroxidation and degradation of low density lipoprotein phospholipids. *Proc Natl Acad Sci U S A.* 1984;81:3883-3887.
7. Heinecke JW, Baker H, Rosen H, Chait A. Superoxide mediated modification of low density lipoprotein by human arterial smooth muscle cells. *J Clin Invest.* 1986;77:757-761.
8. Pryor W, Stone K. Oxidants and cigarette smoke: radicals, hydrogen peroxide, peroxynitrate, and peroxynitrite. *Ann N Y Acad Sci.* 1993;686:12-27.
9. Bonnefont-Rousselot D, Bastard JP, Jaudon MC, Delattre J. Consequences of the diabetic status on the oxidant/antioxidant balance. *Diabetes Metab.* 2000;26:163-176.
10. Esterbauer H, Jürgens G, Quehenberger O, Koller E. Autoxidation of human low density lipoprotein: loss of polyunsaturated fatty acids and vitamin E and generation of aldehydes. *J Lipid Res.* 1987;28:495-509.
11. Jialal I, Freeman DA, Grundy SM. Varying susceptibility of different low-density lipoproteins to oxidative modification. *Arterioscler Thromb.* 1991;11:482-488.
12. Morel DW, Hessler JR, Chisolm GM. Low density lipoprotein cytotoxicity induced by free radical peroxidation of lipid. *J Lipid Res.* 1983;24:1070-1076.
13. Clare K, Hardwick SJ, Carpenter KLH, Weeratunge N, Mitchinson MJ. Toxicity of oxysterol to human monocyte-macrophages. *Atherosclerosis.* 1995;118:67-75.

14. Coffey MD, Cole RA, Colles SM, Chisolm GM. In vitro cell injury by oxidized low density lipoprotein involves lipid hydroperoxide-induced formation of alkoxyl, lipid, and peroxyl radicals. *J Clin Invest.* 1995;96:1866-1873.

15. Esterbauer H, Dieber-Rotheneder M, Waeg G, Puhl H, Tatzber F. Endogenous antioxidants and lipoprotein oxidation. *Biochem Soc Trans.* 1990;18:1059-1061.

16. Esterbauer H, Dieber-Rotheneder M, Striegl G, Waeg G. Role of vitamin E in preventing the oxidation of low-density lipoprotein. *Am J Clin Nutr.* 1991;53:314S-321S.

17. Jialal I, Norkus EP, Cristol L, Grundy SM. β-Carotene inhibits the oxidative modification of low density lipoprotein. *Biochim Biophys Acta.* 1991;1086:134-138.

18. Jialal I, Vega GL, Grundy SM. Physiologic levels of ascorbate inhibit the oxidative modification of low density lipoprotein. *Atherosclerosis.* 1990;82:185-191.

19. Björkhem I, Henriksson-Freyschuss A, Breuer O, Diczfalusy U, Berglund L, Henriksson P. The antioxidant butylated hydroxytoluene protects against atherosclerosis. *Arterioscler Thromb.* 1991;11:15-22.

20. Sparrow CP, Doebber TW, Olszewski J, Wu MS, Ventre J, Stevens KA, Chao Y. Low density lipoprotein is protected from oxidation and the progression of atherosclerosis is slowed in cholesterol-fed rabbits by the antioxidant N,N'-diphenyl-phenylenediamine. *J Clin Invest.* 1992;89:1885-1891.

21. Carew TE, Schwenke DC, Steinberg D. Antiatherogenic effect of probucol unrelated to its hypocholesterolemic effect: evidence that antioxidants in vivo can selectively inhibit low density lipoprotein degradation in macrophage-rich fatty streaks and slow the progression of atherosclerosis in the Watanabe heritable hyperlipidemic rabbit. *Proc Natl Acad Sci U S A.* 1987;84:7725-7729.

22. Hirose M, Shibata M, Hagiwara A, Imaida K, Ito N. Chronic toxicity of butylated hydroxytoluene in Wistar rats. *Food Cosmet Toxicol.* 1981;19:147-151.

23. *Physicians' Desk Reference.* 44th ed. Oradell, NJ: Medical Economics Company; 1990.

24. Brigelius-Flohé R, Traber MG. Vitamin E: function and metabolism. *FASEB J.* 1999;13:1145-1155.

25. Azzi A, Stocker A. Vitamin E: non-antioxidant roles. *Prog Lipid Res.* 2000;39:231-255.

26. Qureshi AA, Peterson DM, Hasler-Rapacz JO, Rapacz J. Novel tocotrienols of rice bran suppress cholesterogenesis in hereditary hypercholesterolemic swine. *J Nutr.* 2001;131:223-230.

27. Dimitrov NV, Meyer-Leece C, McMillan J, Gilliland D, Perloff M, Malone W. Plasma alpha-tocopherol concentrations after supplementation with water- and fat-soluble vitamin E. *Am J Clin Nutr.* 1996;64:329-335.

28. US Department of Agriculture, Agricultural Research Service 2003. US National Nutrient Database for Standard Reference, Release 16. Nutrient Data Laboratory Home Page. Available at: http://www.nal.usda.gov/fnic/foodcomp. Accessed December 17, 2003.

29. Ferslew KE, Acuff RV, Daigneault EA, Woolley TW, Stanton PE Jr. Pharmacokinetics and bioavailability of the RRR and all racemic stereoisomers of alpha-tocopherol in humans after single oral administration. *J Clin Pharmacol.* 1993;33:84-88.

30. Institute of Medicine. *Dietary Reference Intakes for Vitamin C, Vitamin E, Selenium, and Carotenoids.* Washington, DC: National Academy Press; 2000.

31. Institute of Medicine. *Dietary Reference Intakes for Thiamin, Riboflavin, Niacin, Vitamin B-6, Folate, Vitamin B-12, Pantothenic Acid, Biotin, and Choline.* Washington, DC: National Academy Press; 2000.

32. National Research Council. *Recommended Dietary Allowances.* 10th ed. Washington, DC: National Academy Press; 1989.

33. Jialal I, Grundy SM. Effect of combined supplementation with alpha-tocopherol, ascorbate, and beta carotene on low-density lipoprotein oxidation. *Circulation.* 1993;88:2780-2786.

34. Reaven PD, Khouw A, Beltz WF, Parthasarathy S, Witztum JL. Effect of dietary antioxidant combinations in humans: protection of LDL by vitamin E but not by β-carotene. *Arterioscler Thromb.* 1993;13:590-600.

35. Reaven PD, Herold DA, Barnett J, Edelman S. Effects of vitamin E on susceptibility of low-density lipoprotein and low-density lipoprotein subfractions to oxidation and on protein glycation in NIDDM. *Diabetes Care.* 1995;18:807-816.

36. Fuller CJ, Chandalia M, Garg A, Grundy SM, Jialal I. RRR-α-tocopheryl acetate supplementation at pharmacologic doses decreases low-density lipoprotein oxidative susceptibility but not protein glycation in patients with diabetes mellitus. *Am J Clin Nutr.* 1996;63:753-759.

37. Engelen W, Manuel y Keenoy B, Vertommen J, De Leeuw I. Effects of long-term supplementation with moderate pharmacologic doses of vitamin E are saturable and reversible in patients with type 1 diabetes. *Am J Clin Nutr.* 2000;72:1142-1149.

38. Princen HMG, van Poppel G, Vogelezang C, Buytenhek R, Kok FJ. Supplementation with vitamin E but not β-carotene in vivo protects low density lipoprotein from lipid peroxidation in vitro: effect of cigarette smoking. *Arterioscler Thromb.* 1992;12:554-562.

39. Fuller CJ, May MA, Martin KJ. The effect of vitamin E and vitamin C supplementation on LDL oxidizability and neutrophil respiratory burst in young smokers. *J Am Coll Nutr.* 2000;19:361-369.

40. Jialal I, Fuller CJ, Huet BA. The effect of α-tocopherol supplementation on LDL oxidation: a dose-response study. *Arterioscler Thromb Vasc Biol.* 1995;15:190-198.

41. Devaraj S, Adams-Huet B, Fuller CJ, Jialal I. Dose-response comparison of RRR-α-tocopherol and all-racemic α-tocopherol on LDL oxidation. *Arterioscler Thromb Vasc Biol.* 1997;17:2273-2279.

42. Reaven PD, Witztum JL. Comparison of supplementation or RRR-α-tocopherol and racemic α-tocopherol in humans: effects on lipid levels and lipoprotein susceptibility to oxidation. *Arterioscler Thromb.* 1993;13:601-608.

43. Stampfer MJ, Hennekens CH, Manson JE, Colditz GA, Rosner B, Willett WC. Vitamin E consumption and the risk of coronary disease in women. *N Engl J Med.* 1993;328:1444-1449.

44. Rimm EB, Stampfer MJ, Ascherio A, Giovannucci E, Colditz GA, Willett WC. Vitamin E consumption and the risk of coronary disease in men. *N Engl J Med.* 1993;328:1450-1456.

45. Devaraj S, Li D, Jialal I. The effects of alpha tocopherol supplementation on monocyte function: decreased lipid oxidation, interleukin 1β secretion, and monocyte adhesion to endothelium. *J Clin Invest.* 1996;98:756-763.

46. van Tits LJH, de Waart F, Hak-Lemmers HLM, van Heijst PN, de Graaf J, Demacker PNM, Stalenhoef AFH. Effects of α-tocopherol on superoxide production and plasma intercellular adhesion molecule-1 and antibodies to oxidized LDL in chronic smokers. *Free Radical Biol Med.* 2001;30:1122-1129.

47. Jandak J, Steiner M, Richardson PD. α-Tocopherol, an effective inhibitor of platelet adhesion. *Blood.* 1989;73:141-149.

48. Salonen JT, Salonen R, Rinta-Kiikkas S, Kuukka M, Korpela H, Alfthan G, Kantola M, Schalch W. Effect of antioxidant supplementation on platelet function: a randomized pair-matched, placebo-controlled, double-blind trial in men with low antioxidant status. *Am J Clin Nutr.* 1991;53:1222-1229.

49. Freedman JE, Keaney JF Jr. Vitamin E inhibition of platelet aggregation is independent of antioxidant activity. *J Nutr.* 2001;131:374S-377S.

50. Liu M, Wallmon A, Olsson-Mortlock C, Wallin R, Saldeen T. Mixed tocopherols inhibit platelet aggregation in humans: potential mechanisms. *Am J Clin Nutr.* 2003;77:700-706.

51. DeMaio SJ, King SB III, Lembo NJ, Roubin GS, Hearn JA, Bhagavan HN, Sgoutas DS. Vitamin E supplementation, plasma lipids, and incidence of restenosis after percutaneous transluminal coronary angioplasty (PTCA). *J Am Coll Nutr.* 1992;11:68-73.

52. Kushi LH, Folsom AR, Prineas RJ, Mink PJ, Wu Y, Bostick R. Dietary antioxidant vitamins and death from coronary heart disease in postmenopausal women. *N Engl J Med.* 1996;334:1156-1162.

53. Losonczy KG, Harris TB, Havlik RJ. Vitamin E and vitamin C supplement use and risk of all-cause and coronary heart disease mortality in older persons: the Established Populations for Epidemiologic Studies of the Elderly. *Am J Clin Nutr.* 1996;64:190-196.

54. Muntwyler J, Hennekens CH, Manson JE, Buring JE, Gaziano JM. Vitamin supplement use in a low-risk population of US male physicians and subsequent cardiovascular disease mortality. *Arch Intern Med.* 2002;162:1472-1476.

55. Stephens NG, Parsons A, Schofield PM, Kelly F, Cheeseman K, Mitchinson MJ, Brown MJ. Randomized controlled trial of vitamin E in patients with coronary disease: Cambridge Heart Antioxidant Study (CHAOS). *Lancet.* 1996;347:781-786.

56. Davey PJ, Schulz M, Gliksman M, Dobson M, Aristides M, Stephens NG. Cost-effectiveness of vitamin E therapy in the treatment of patients with angiographically proven coronary narrowing (CHAOS Trial). *Am J Cardiol.* 1998;82:414-417.

57. The Heart Outcomes Prevention Evaluation Study Investigators. Vitamin E supplementation and cardiovascular events in high-risk patients. *N Engl J Med.* 2000;342:154-160.

58. Lonn E, Yusuf S, Hoogwerf B, Pogue J, Yi Q, Zinman B, Bosch J, Dagenais G, Mann JFE, Gerstein HC. Effects of vitamin E on cardiovascular and microvascular outcomes in high-risk patients with diabetes: Results of the HOPE study and the MICRO-HOPE substudy. *Diabetes Care.* 2002;25:1919-1927.

59. Hodis HN, Mack WJ, LaBree L, Mahrer PR, Sevanian A, Liu CR, Liu CH, Hwang J, Selzer RH, Azen SP. Alpha-tocopherol supplementation in healthy individuals reduces low-density lipoprotein oxidation but not atherosclerosis: the Vitamin E Atherosclerosis Prevention Study (VEAPS). *Circulation.* 2002;106:1453-1459.

60. Keith ME, Jeejeebhoy KN, Langer A, Kurian R, Barr A, O'Kelly B, Sole MJ. A controlled clinical trial of vitamin E supplementation in patients with congestive heart failure. *Am J Clin Nutr.* 2001;73:219-224.

61. Panzetta O, Cominacini L, Garbin U, Fratta Pasini A, Gammaro L, Bianco F, Davoli A, Campagnola M, De Santis A, Pastorino AM, Lo Cascio V. Increased susceptibility of LDL to in vitro oxidation in patients on maintenance hemodialysis: effects of fish oil and vitamin E administration. *Clin Nephrol.* 1995;44:303-309.

62. Islam KN, O'Byrne D, Devaraj S, Palmer B, Grundy SM, Jialal I. Alpha-tocopherol supplementation decreases the oxidative susceptibility of LDL in renal failure patients on dialysis therapy. *Atherosclerosis.* 2000;150:217-224.

63. Boaz M, Smetana S, Weinstein T, Matas Z, Gafter U, Iaina A, Knecht A, Weissgarten Y, Brunner D, Fainaru M, Green MS. Secondary prevention with antioxidants of cardiovascular disease in end-stage renal disease (SPACE): randomised placebo-controlled trial. *Lancet.* 2000;356:1213-1218.

64. Vivekananthan DP, Penn MS, Sapp SK, Hsu A, Topol EJ. Use of antioxidant vitamins for the prevention of cardiovascular disease: meta-analysis of randomised trials. *Lancet.* 2003;361:2017-2023.

65. Christen S, Woodall AA, Shigenaga MK, Southwell-Keely PT, Duncan MW, Ames BN. α-Tocopherol traps mutagenic electrophiles such as NO_x and complements α-tocopherol: physiological implications. *Proc Natl Acad Sci U S A.* 1997;94:3217-3222.

66. Hoglen NC, Waller SC, Sipes IG, Liebler DC. Reactions of peroxynitrite with α-tocopherol. *Chem Res Toxicol.* 1997;10:401-407.

67. Suarna C, Hood RL, Dean RT, Stocker R. Comparative antioxidant activity of tocotrienols and other natural lipid-soluble antioxidants in a homogeneous system, and in rat and human lipoproteins. *Biochim Biophys Acta.* 1993;1166:163-170.

68. Dietrich M, Block G, Norkus EP, Hudes M, Traber MG, Cross CE, Packer L. Smoking and exposure to environmental tobacco smoke decrease some plasma antioxidants and increase α-tocopherol in vivo after adjustment for dietary antioxidant intakes. *Am J Clin Nutr.* 2003;77:160-166.

69. El-Sohemy A, Baylin A, Spiegelman D, Ascherio A, Campos H. Dietary and adipose tissue gamma-tocopherol and risk of myocardial infarction. *Epidemiology.* 2002;13:216-223.

70. Qureshi AA, Qureshi N, Wright JJK, Shen Z, Kramer G, Gapor A, Chong YH, DeWitt G, Ong ASH, Peterson DM, Bradlow BA. Lowering of serum cholesterol in hypercholesterolemic humans by tocotrienols (palmvitee). *Am J Clin Nutr.* 1991;53(suppl):1021S-1026S.

71. Qureshi AA, Bradlow BA, Salser WA, Brace LD. Novel tocotrienols of rice bran modulate cardiovascular disease risk parameters of hypercholesterolemic humans. *J Nutr Biochem.* 1997;8:290-298.

72. O'Byrne D, Grundy S, Packer L, Devaraj S, Baldenius K, Hoppe PP, Kraemer K, Jiala I, Traber MG. Studies of LDL oxidation following α-, γ-, or δ-tocotrienyl acetate supplementation of hypercholesterolemic humans. *Free Radic Biol Med.* 2000;29:834-845.

73. The Alpha-Tocopherol, Beta Carotene Cancer Prevention Study Group. The effect of vitamin E and beta carotene on the incidence of lung cancer and other cancers in male smokers. *N Engl J Med.* 1994;330:1029-1035.

74. The Alpha-Tocopherol, Beta Carotene Cancer Prevention Study Group. Incidence of cancer and mortality following α-tocopherol and β-carotene supplementation: a postintervention follow-up. *JAMA.* 2003;290:476-485.

75. Kappus H, Diplock AT. Tolerance and safety of vitamin E: a toxicological position report. *Free Radic Biol Med.* 1992;1:55-74.

76. Cheung MC, Zhao XQ, Chait A, Albers JJ, Brown BG. Antioxidant supplements block the response of HDL to simvastatin-niacin therapy in patients with coronary artery disease and low HDL. *Arterioscler Thromb Vasc Biol.* 2001;21:1320-1326.

77. Frei B, England L, Ames BN. Ascorbate is an outstanding antioxidant in human blood plasma. *Proc Natl Acad Sci U S A.* 1989;86:6377-6381.

78. Sato K, Niki E, Shimasaki H. Free radical-mediated chain oxidation of low density lipoprotein and its synergistic inhibition by vitamin E and vitamin C. *Arch Biochem Biophys.* 1990;279:402-405.

79. Retsky KL, Frei B. Vitamin C prevents metal ion-dependent initiation and propagation of lipid peroxidation in human low density lipoprotein. *Biochim Biophys Acta.* 1995;1257:279-287.

80. Packer JE, Slater TF, Willson RL. Direct observation of a free radical interaction between vitamin E and vitamin C. *Nature (London).* 1979;278:737-738.

81. Jialal I, Grundy SM. Preservation of the endogenous antioxidants in low density lipoprotein by ascorbate but not probucol during oxidative modification. *J Clin Invest.* 1991;87:597-601.

82. Frei B. Ascorbic acid protects lipids in human plasma and low density lipoprotein against oxidative damage. *Am J Clin Nutr.* 1991;54(suppl):1113S-1118S.

83. Jialal I, Grundy SM. Influence of antioxidant vitamins on LDL oxidation. *Ann N Y Acad Sci.* 1992;669:237-248.

84. Hwang J, Peterson H, Hodis HN, Choi B, Sevanian A. Ascorbic acid enhances 17 β-estradiol-mediated inhibition of oxidized low density lipoprotein formation. *Atherosclerosis.* 2000;150:275-284.

85. Schectman G, Byrd JC, Gruchow HW. The influence of smoking on vitamin C status in adults. *Am J Public Health.* 1989;79:158-162.

86. Zondervan KT, Ocké MC, Smit HA, Seidell JC. Do dietary and supplementary intakes of antioxidants differ with smoking status? *Int J Epidemiol.* 1996;25:70-79.

87. Nyyssönen K, Porkkala-Sarataho E, Kaikkonen J, Salonen JT. Ascorbate and urate are the strongest determinants of plasma antioxidative capacity and serum lipid resistance to oxidation in Finnish men. *Atherosclerosis.* 1997;130:223-233.

88. Harats D, Ben-Naim M, Dabach Y, Hollander G, Havivi E, Stein O, Stein Y. Effect of vitamin C and E supplementation on susceptibility of plasma lipoproteins to peroxidation induced by acute smoking. *Atherosclerosis.* 1990;85:47-54.

89. Fuller CJ, Grundy SM, Norkus EP, Jialal I. Effect of ascorbate supplementation on low density lipoprotein oxidation in smokers. *Atherosclerosis.* 1996;119:139-150.

90. Abbey M, Noakes M, Nestel PJ. Dietary supplementation with orange and carrot juice in cigarette smokers lowers oxidation products in copper-oxidized low density lipoprotein. *J Am Diet Assoc.* 1995;95:671-675.

91. Rifici VA, Khachadurian AK. Dietary supplementation with vitamins C and E inhibits in vitro oxidation of lipoproteins. *J Am Coll Nutr.* 1993;12:631-637.

92. Wen Y, Cooke T, Feely J. The effect of pharmacological supplementation with vitamin C on low-density lipoprotein oxidation. *Br J Clin Pharmacol.* 1997;44:94-97.

93. Enstrom JE, Kanim LE, Klein MA. Vitamin C intake and mortality among a sample of the United States population. *Epidemiology.* 1992;3:194-202.

94. Khaw KT, Bingham S, Welch A, Luben R, Wareham N, Oakes S, Day N. Relation between plasma ascorbic acid and mortality in men and women in the EPIC-Norfolk prospective study: a prospective population study. *Lancet.* 2001;357:657-663.

95. Nyyssönen K, Parviainen MT, Salonen R, Tuomilehto J, Salonen JT. Vitamin C deficiency and risk of myocardial infarction: prospective population study of men from eastern Finland. *BMJ.* 1997;314:634-638.

96. Kurl S, Tuomainen TP, Laukkanen JA, Nyyssönen K, Lakka T, Sivenius J, Salonen JT. Plasma vitamin C modifies the association between hypertension and risk of stroke. *Stroke.* 2002;33:1568-1573.

97. Osganian SK, Stampfer MJ, Rimm E, Spiegelman D, Hu FB, Manson JE, Willett WC. Vitamin C and risk of coronary heart disease in women. *J Am Coll Cardiol.* 2003;42:246-252.

98. Frei B. To C or not to C, that is the question! *J Am Coll Cardiol.* 2003;42:253-255.

99. Ellis GR, Anderson RA, Lang D, Blackman DJ, Morris RHK, Morris-Thurgood J, McDowell IDW, Jackson SK, Lewis MJ, Frenneaux MP. Neutrophil superoxide anion-generating capacity, endothelial function and oxidative stress in chronic heart failure: effects of short- and long-term vitamin C therapy. *J Am Coll Cardiol.* 2000;36:1474-1482.

100. Hamabe A, Takase B, Uehata A, Kurita A, Ohsuzu F, Tamai S. Impaired endothelium-dependent vasodilation in the brachial artery in variant angina pectoris and the effect of intravenous administration of vitamin C. *Am J Cardiol.* 2001;87:1154-1159.

101. Richartz BM, Werner GS, Ferrari M, Figulla HR. Reversibility of coronary endothelial vasomotor dysfunction in idiopathic dilated cardiomyopathy: acute effects of vitamin C. *Am J Cardiol.* 2001;88:1001.

102. Liu L, Zhao SP, Gao M, Zhou QC, Li YL, Xia B. Vitamin C preserves endothelial function in patients with coronary heart disease after a high-fat meal. *Clin Cardiol.* 2002;25:219-224.

103. May JM. How does ascorbic acid prevent endothelial dysfunction? *Free Radic Biol Med.* 2000;28:1421-1429.

104. Toohey L, Harris MA, Allen KGD, Melby CL. Plasma ascorbic acid concentrations are related to cardiovascular risk factors in African-Americans. *J Nutr.* 1996;126:121-128.

105. Moran JP, Cohen L, Greene JM, Xu G, Feldman EB, Hames CG, Feldman DS. Plasma ascorbic acid concentrations relate inversely to blood pressure in human subjects. *Am J Clin Nutr.* 1993;57:213-217.

106. Jenner JL, Jacques PF, Seman LJ, Schaefer EJ. Ascorbic acid supplementation does not lower plasma lipoprotein (a) concentrations. *Atherosclerosis.* 2000;151:541-544.

107. Sistrom WR, Griffiths M, Stanier RY. Biology of a photosynthetic bacterium which lacks colored carotenoids. *J Cell Comp Physiol.* 1956;48:473-515.

108. Burton GW, Ingold KU. β-Carotene: an unusual type of lipid antioxidant. *Science.* 1984;224:569-573.

109. Mangels AR, Holden JM, Beecher GR, Forman MR, Lanza E. Carotenoid content of fruits and vegetables: an evaluation of analytic data. *J Am Diet Assoc.* 1993;93:284-296.

110. Ascherio A, Stampfer MJ, Colditz GA, Rimm EB, Litin L, Willett WC. Correlations of vitamin A and E intakes with the plasma concentrations of carotenoids and tocopherols among American men and women. *J Nutr.* 1992;122:1792-1801.

111. Rock CL, Lovalvo JL, Emenhiser C, Ruffin MT, Flatt SW, Schwartz SJ. Bioavailability of β-carotene is lower in raw than in processed carrots and spinach in women. *J Nutr.* 1996;128:913-916.

112. Gärtner C, Stahl W, Sies H. Lycopene is more bioavailable from tomato paste than from fresh tomatoes. *Am J Clin Nutr.* 1997;66:116-122.

113. Castenmiller JJM, West CE. Bioavailability and bioconversion of carotenoids. *Annu Rev Nutr.* 1998;18:19-38.

114. Ribaya-Mercado JD, Ordovas JM, Russell RM. Effect of β-carotene supplementation on the concentrations and distribution of carotenoids, vitamin E, vitamin A, and cholesterol in plasma lipoprotein and non-lipoprotein fractions in healthy older women. *J Am Coll Nutr.* 1995;14:614-620.

115. Lowe GM, Bilton RF, Davies IG, Ford TC, Billington D, Young AJ. Carotenoid composition and antioxidant potential in subfractions of human low-density lipoprotein. *Ann Clin Biochem.* 1999;36:323-332.

116. Rudel LL, Kesäniemi YA. Low-density lipoprotein particle composition: what is the contribution to atherogenicity? *Curr Opin Lipidol.* 2000;11:227-228.

117. Reaven PD, Ferguson E, Navab M, Powell FL. Susceptibility of human LDL to oxidative modification: effects of variations in β-carotene concentration and oxygen tension. *Arterioscler Thromb.* 1994;14:1162-1169.

118. Gaziano JM, Hatta A, Flynn M, Johnson EJ, Krinsky NI, Ridker PM, Hennekens CH, Frei B. Supplementation with β-carotene in vivo and in vitro does not inhibit low density lipoprotein oxidation. *Atherosclerosis.* 1995;112:187-195.

119. Bowen HT, Omaye ST. Oxidative changes associated with β-carotene and α-tocopherol enrichment of human low-density lipoproteins. *J Am Coll Nutr.* 1998;17:171-179.

120. Jialal I, Fuller CJ. Effect of vitamin E, vitamin C and beta-carotene on LDL oxidation and atherosclerosis. *Can J Cardiol.* 1995;11:97G-103G.

121. Nenseter MS, Volden V, Berg T, Drevon A, Ose L, Tonstad S. No effect of β-carotene supplementation on the susceptibility of low density lipoprotein to in vitro oxidation among hypercholesterolaemic, postmenopausal women. *Scand J Clin Lab Invest.* 1995;55:477-485.

122. Omenn GS, Goodman GE, Thornquist MD, Balmes J, Cullen MR, Glass A, Keogh JP, Meyskens FL Jr, Valanis B, Williams JH Jr, Barnhart S, Hammar MD. Effects of the combination of beta-carotene and vitamin A on lung cancer incidence, total mortality, and cardiovascular mortality in smokers and asbestos-exposed workers. *N Engl J Med.* 1996;334:1150-1155.

123. Riemersma RA, Wood DA, MacIntyre CCA, Elton RA, Gey KF, Oliver MF. Risk of angina pectoris and plasma concentrations of vitamins A, C, E and carotene. *Lancet.* 1991;337:1-5.

124. Kardinaal AFM, Aro A, Kark JD, Riemersma RA, van't Veer P, Gomez-Aracena J, Kohlmeier L, Ringstad J, Martin BC, Mazaev VP, Delgado-Rodriguez M, Thamm M, Huttunen JK, Martin-Moreno JM, Kok FJ. Association between β-carotene and acute myocardial infarction depends on polyunsaturated fatty acid status: The EURAMIC Study. *Arterioscler Thromb Vasc Biol.* 1995;15:726-732.

125. DiMascio P, Kaiser S, Sies H. Lycopene as the most efficient biological carotenoid singlet oxygen quencher. *Arch Biochem Biophys.* 1989;274:532-538.

126. Romanchik JE, Harrison EH, Morel DW. Addition of lutein, lycopene, or β-carotene to LDL or serum *in vitro:* effects on carotenoid distribution, LDL composition, and LDL oxidation. *J Nutr Biochem.* 1997;681-688.

127. Casso D, White E, Patterson RE, Agurs-Collins T, Kooperberg C, Haines PS. Correlates of serum lycopene in older women. *Nutr Cancer.* 2000;36:163-169.

128. Wu K, Schwartz SJ, Platz EA, Clinton SK, Erdman JW Jr, Ferruzzi MG, Willett WC, Giovannucci EL. Variations in plasma lycopene and specific isomers over time in a cohort of US men. *J Nutr.* 2003;133:1930-1936.

129. Agarwal S, Rao AV. Tomato lycopene and low density lipoprotein oxidation: a human dietary intervention study. *Lipids.* 1998;33:981-984.

130. Sutherland WHF, Walker RJ, DeJong SA, Upritchard JE. Supplementation with tomato juice increases plasma lycopene but does not alter susceptibility to oxidation of low-density lipoproteins from renal transplant recipients. *Clin Nephrol.* 1999;52:30-36.

131. Chopra M, O'Neill ME, Keogh N, Wortley G, Southon S, Thurnham DI. Influence of increased fruit and vegetable intake on plasma and lipoprotein carotenoids and LDL oxidation in smokers and nonsmokers. *Clin Chem.* 2000;46:1818-1829.

132. Bub A, Watzl B, Abrahamse L, Delincée H, Adam S, Wever J, Müller H, Rechkemmer G. Moderate intervention with carotenoid-rich vegetable products reduce lipid peroxidation in men. *J Nutr.* 2000;130:2200-2206.

133. Pellegrini N, Riso P, Porrini M. Tomato consumption does not affect the total antioxidant capacity of plasma. *Nutrition.* 2000;16:268-271.

134. Rissanen TH, Voutilainen S, Nyyssönen K, Lakka TA, Sivenius J, Salonen R, Kaplan GA, Salonen JT. Low serum lycopene concentration is associated with an excess incidence of acute coronary events and stroke: the Kuopio Ischaemic Heart Disease Risk Factor Study. *Br J Nutr.* 2001;85:749-754.

135. Rissanen TH, Voutilainen S, Nyyssönen K, Salonen R, Kaplan GA, Salonen JT. Serum lycopene concentrations and carotid atherosclerosis: the Kuopio Ischaemic Heart Disease Risk Factor Study. *Am J Clin Nutr.* 2003;77:133-138.

136. Sesso HD, Liu S, Gaziano JM, Buring JE. Dietary lycopene, tomato-based food products and cardiovascular disease in women. *J Nutr.* 2003;133:2336-2341.

137. Salonen JT, Nyyssönen K, Salonen R, Lakka HM, Kaikkonen J, Porkkala-Sarataho E, Voutilainen S, Lakka TA, Rissanen T, Leskinen L, Tuomainen TP, Valkonen VP, Ristonmaa U, Poulsen HE. Antioxidant Supplementation in Atherosclerosis Prevention (ASAP) study: a randomized trial of the effect of vitamins E and C on 3-year progression of carotid atherosclerosis. *J Intern Med.* 2000;248:377-386.

138. Brown BG, Zhao XQ, Chait A, Fisher LD, Cheung MC, Morse JS, Dowdy AA, Marino EK, Bolson EL, Alaupovic P, Frohlich J, Albers JJ. Simvastatin and niacin, antioxidant vitamins, or the combination for the prevention of coronary disease. *N Engl J Med.* 2001;345:1583-1592.

139. Collins R, Peto R, Armitage J. The MRC/BHF Heart Protection Study: preliminary results. *Int J Clin Pract.* 2002;56:53-56.

140. Waters DL, Alderman EL, Hsia J, Howard BV, Cobb FR, Rogers WJ, Ouyang P, Thompson P, Tardif JC, Higginson L, Bittner V, Steffes M, Gordon DJ, Proschan M, Younes N, Verter JI. Effects of hormone replacement therapy and antioxidant vitamin supplementation on coronary atherosclerosis in postmenopausal women: a randomized controlled trial. *JAMA.* 2002;288:2432-2440.

141. Fang JC, Kinlay S, Beltrame J, Hikiti H, Wainstein M, Behrendt D, Suh J, Frei B, Mudge GH, Selwyn AP, Ganz P. Effect of vitamins E and C on progression of transplant-associated arteriosclerosis: a randomized trial. *Lancet.* 2002;359:1108-1113.

142. Bunout D, Garrido A, Suazo M, Kauffman R, Venegas P, de la Maza P, Petermann M, Hirsch S. Effects of supplementation with folic acid and antioxidant vitamins on homocysteine levels and LDL oxidation in coronary patients. *Nutrition.* 2000;16:107-110.

143. Tribble DL, Krauss RM. Atherosclerotic cardiovascular disease. In: Bowman BA, Russell RM, eds. *Present Knowledge in Nutrition.* 8th ed. Washington, DC: ILSI Press; 2001:543-551.

144. Boushey CJ, Beresford SAA, Omenn, GS, Motulsky AG. A quantitative assessment of plasma homocysteine as a risk factor for vascular disease: probable benefits of increasing folic acid intakes. *JAMA.* 1995;274:1049-1057.

145. Konecky N, Malinow R, Tunick PA, Freedberg RS, Rosenzweig BP, Katz ES, Hess DL, Upson B, Leung B, Perez J, Kronzon I. Correlation between plasma homocyst(e)ine and aortic atherosclerosis. *Am Heart J.* 1997;133:534-540.

146. Hultberg B, Andersson A, Lindgren A. Marginal folate deficiency as a possible cause of hyperhomocystinaemia in stroke patients. *Eur J Clin Chem Clin Biochem.* 1997;35:25-28.

147. Vasan RS, Beiser A, D'Agostino RB, Levy D, Selhub J, Jacques PF, Rosenberg IH, Wilson PWF. Plasma homocysteine and risk for congestive heart failure in adults without prior myocardial infarction. *JAMA.* 2003;289:1251-1257.

148. Tofler GH, D'Agostino RB, Jacques PF, Bostom AG, Wilson PWF, Lipinska I, Mittleman MA, Selhub J. Association between increased homocysteine levels and impaired fibrinolytic potential: potential mechanism for cardiovascular risk. *Thromb Haemost.* 2002;88:799-804.

149. Hoogeveen EK, Kostense PJ, Jakobs C, Dekker JM, Nijpels G, Heine RJ, Bouter LM, Stehouwer CDA. Hyperhomocysteinemia increases risk of death, especially in type 2 diabetes: 5-year follow-up of the Hoorn study. *Circulation.* 2000;101:1506-1511.

150. Ridker PM, Stampfer MJ, Rifai N. Novel risk factors for systemic atherosclerosis: a comparison of C-reactive protein, fibrinogen, homocysteine, lipoprotein(a), and standard cholesterol screening as predictors of peripheral arterial disease. *JAMA.* 2001;285:2481-2485.

151. The Homocysteine Studies Collaboration. Homocysteine and risk of ischemic heart disease and stroke: a meta-analysis. *JAMA.* 2002;288:2015-2022.

152. Ganji V, Kafai MR. Demographic, health, lifestyle, and blood vitamin determinants of serum total homocysteine concentrations in the third National Health and Nutrition Examination Survey, 1988-1994. *Am J Clin Nutr.* 2003;77:826-833.

153. van der Put NMJ, van den Heuvel LP, Steegers-Theunissen RPM, Trijbels FJM, Eskes TKAB, Mariman ECM, den Heyer M, Blom HJ. Decreased methylene tetrahydrofolate reductase activity due to the 677 C-T mutation in families with spina bifida offspring. *J Mol Med.* 1996;74:691-694.

154. Hobbs CA, Sherman SL, Yi P, Hopkins SE, Torfs CP, Hine RJ, Pogribna M, Rozen R, James SJ. Polymorphisms in genes involved in folate metabolism as maternal risk factors for Down syndrome. *Am J Hum Genet.* 2000;67:623-630.

155. de Bree A, Verschuren M, Bjørke-Monsen AL, van der Put NMJ, Heil SG, Trijbels FJM, Blom HJ. Effect of the methylenetetrahydrofolate reductase 677 C-T mutation on the relations among folate intake and plasma folate and homocysteine concentrations in a general population sample. *Am J Clin Nutr.* 2003;77:687-693.

156. Morita H, Taguchi J, Kurihara H, Kitaoka M, Kaneda H, Kurihara Y, Maemura J, Shindo T, Minamino T, Ohno M, Yamaoki K, Ogasawara K, Aizawa T, Suzuki S, Yazaki Y. Genetic polymorphism of 5,10-methylenetetrahydrofolate reductase (MTHFR) as a risk factor for coronary artery disease. *Circulation.* 1997;95:2032-2036.

157. Bostom AG, Shemin D, Lapane KL, Nadeau MR, Sutherland P, Chan J, Rozen R, Yoburn D, Jacques PF, Selhub J, Rosenberg IH. Folate status is the major determinant of fasting total plasma homocysteine levels in maintenance dialysis patients. *Atherosclerosis.* 1996;123:193-202.

158. Tonstad S, Refsum H, Ueland PM. Association between plasma total homocysteine and parental history of cardiovascular disease in children with familial hypercholesterolemia. *Circulation.* 1997;96:1803-1808.

159. Klerk M, Verhoef P, Clarke R, Blom HJ, Kok FJ, Schouten EG, MTHFR Studies Collaboration Group. MTHFR 677C-T polymorphism and risk of coronary heart disease: a meta-analysis. *JAMA.* 2002;288:2023-2031.

160. US Food and Drug Administration. Food standards: amendment of standards of identity for enriched grain products to require addition of folic acid. *Federal Register.* 1996;61:8781-8797.

161. Choumenkovitch SF, Selhub J, Wilson PW, Rader JI, Rosenberg IH, Jacques PF. Folic acid from fortification in United States exceeds predictions. *J Nutr.* 2002;132:2792-2798.

162. Landgren F, Israelsson B, Lindgren A, Hultberg B, Andersson A, Brattström L. Plasma homocysteine in acute myocardial infarction: homocysteine-lowering effect of folic acid. *J Intern Med.* 1995;237:381-388.

163. Guttormsen AB, Ueland PM, Nesthus I, Nygård, Schneede J, Vollset SE, Refsum H. Determinants and vitamin responsiveness of intermediate hyperhomocysteinemia ($\geq$ 40 μmol/liter). *J Clin Invest.* 1996;98:2174-2183.

164. McGregor D, Shand B, Lynn K. A controlled trial of the effect of folate supplements on homocysteine, lipids and hemorheology in end-stage renal disease. *Nephron.* 2000;85:215-220.

165. Venn BJ, Mann JI, Williams SM, Riddell LJ, Chisholm A, Harper MJ, Aitken W. Dietary counseling to increase natural folate intake: a randomized, placebo-controlled trial in free-living subjects to assess effects on serum folate and plasma total homocysteine. *Am J Clin Nutr.* 2002;76:758-765.

166. Morrison HI, Schaubel D, Desmeules M, Wigle DT. Serum folate and risk of fatal coronary heart disease. *JAMA.* 1996;275:1893-1896.

167. Chasan-Taber L, Selhub J, Rosenberg IH, Malinow MR, Terry P, Tishler PV, Willett W, Hennekens CH, Stampfer MJ. A prospective study of folate and vitamin B-6 and risk of myocardial infarction in US physicians. *J Am Coll Nutr.* 1996;15:136-143.

168. Hernández-Díaz S, Martínez-Losa E, Fernández-Jarne E, Serrano-Martínez M, Martínez-González MA. Dietary folate and the risk of nonfatal myocardial infarction. *Epidemiology.* 2002;13:700-706.

169. Holmquist C, Larsson S, Wolk A, de Faire U. Multivitamin supplements are inversely associated with risk of myocardial infarction in men and women—Stockholm Heart Epidemiology Program (SHEEP). *J Nutr.* 2003;133:2650-2654.

170. Doshi SN, McDowell IFW, Moat SJ, Lang D, Newcombe RG, Kredan MB, Lewis MJ, Goodfellow J. Folate improves endothelial function in coronary artery disease: an effect mediated by reduction of intracellular superoxide? *Arterioscler Thromb Vasc Biol.* 2001;21:1196-1202.

171. Brilakis ES, McConnell JP, Ballman KV, Klee GG, Berger PB. Lack of association between plasma

homocysteine and angiographic coronary artery disease in the era of fortification of cereal grain flour with folic acid. *Atherosclerosis.* 2002;165;375-381.

172. Carmel R. Cobalamin, the stomach, and aging. *Am J Clin Nutr.* 1997;66:750-759.

173. Stabler SP, Lindenbaum J, Allen RH. Vitamin B-12 deficiency in the elderly: current dilemmas. *Am J Clin Nutr.* 1997;66:741-749.

174. Mills JL, Von Kohorn I, Conley MR, Zeller JA, Cox C, Wiliamson RE, Dufour DR. Low vitamin B-12 concentrations in patients without anemia: the effect of folic acid fortification of grain. *Am J Clin Nutr.* 2003;77:1474-1477.

175. Nallamothu BK, Fendrick AM, Rubenfire M, Saint S, Bandehar RR, Omenn GS. Potential clinical and economic effects of homocyst(e)ine lowering. *Arch Intern Med.* 2000;160:3406-3412.

176. Di Carlo G, Mascolo N, Izzo AA, Capasso F. Flavonoids: old and new aspects of a class of natural therapeutic drugs. *Life Sci.* 1999;65:337-353.

177. Peterson J, Dwyer J. Taxonomic classification helps identify flavonoid-containing foods on a semiquantitative food frequency questionnaire. *J Am Diet Assoc.* 1998;98:677-682,685.

178. Sampson L, Rimm E, Hollman PCH, de Vries JHM, Katan MB. Flavonol and flavone intakes in US health professionals. *J Am Diet Assoc.* 2002;102:1414-1420.

179. Arai Y, Watanabe S, Kimura M, Shimoi K, Mochizuki R, Kinae N. Dietary intakes of flavonols, flavones and isoflavones by Japanese women and the inverse correlation between quercetin intake and plasma LDL cholesterol concentration. *J Nutr.* 2000;130:2243-2250.

180. Hertog MGL, Kromhout D, Aravanis C, Blackburn H, Buzina R, Fidanza F, Giampaoli S, Jansen A, Menotti A, Nedeljkovic S, Pekkarinen M, Simic BS, Toshim H, Feskens EJM, Hollman PCH, Katan MB. Flavonoid intake and long-term risk of coronary heart disease and cancer in the Seven Countries Study. *Arch Intern Med.* 1995;155:381-386.

181. Rimm EB, Katan MB, Ascherio A, Stampfer MJ, Willett WC. Relation between intake of flavonoids and risk for coronary heart disease in male health professionals. *Ann Intern Med.* 1996;25:384-389.

182. Sesso HD, Gaziano JM, Liu S, Buring JE. Flavonoid intake and the risk of cardiovascular disease in women. *Am J Clin Nutr.* 2003;77:1400-1408.

183. Duthie G, Crozier A. Plant-derived phenolic antioxidants. *Curr Opin Lipidol.* 2000;11:43-47.

184. Frankel EN, Kanner J, German JB, Parks E, Kinsella JE. Inhibition of oxidation of human low-density lipoprotein by phenolic substances in red wine. *Lancet.* 1993;341:454-457.

185. Kerry NL, Abbey M. Red wine and fractionated phenolic compounds prepared from red wine inhibit low density lipoprotein oxidation in vitro. *Atherosclerosis.* 1997;135:93-102.

186. Deckert V, Desrumaux C, Athias A, Duverneuil L, Palleau V, Gambert P, Masson D, Lagrost L. Prevention of LDL α-tocopherol consumption, cholesterol oxidation, and vascular endothelium dysfunction by polyphenolic compounds in red wine. *Atherosclerosis.* 2002;165:41-50.

187. Frémont L, Belguendouz L, Delpal S. Antioxidant activity of resveratrol and alcohol-free wine polyphenols related to LDL oxidation and polyunsaturated fatty acids. *Life Sci.* 1999;64:2511-2521.

188. Fuhrman B, Lavy A, Aviram M. Consumption of red wine with meals reduces the susceptibility of human plasma and low-density lipoprotein to lipid peroxidation. *Am J Clin Nutr.* 1995;61:549-554.

189. de Rijke YB, Demacker PNM, Assen NA, Sloots LM, Katan MB, Stalenhoef AFH. Red wine consumption does not affect oxidizability of low-density lipoprotein in volunteers. *Am J Clin Nutr.* 63:329-334.

190. Natella F, Ghiselli A, Guidi A, Ursini F, Scaccini C. Red wine mitigates the postprandial increase of LDL susceptibility to oxidation. *Free Radic Biol Med.* 2001;30:1036-1044.

191. Cacetta RA, Burke V, Mori TA, Beilin LJ, Puddey IB, Croft KD. Red wine polyphenols, in the absence of alcohol, reduce lipid peroxidative stress in smoking subjects. *Free Radic Biol Med.* 2001;30:636-642.

192. Struck M, Watkins T, Tomeo A, Halley J, Bierenbaum M. Effect of red and white wine on serum lipids, platelet aggregation, oxidation products and antioxidants: a preliminary report. *Nutr Res.* 1994;14:1811-1819.

193. Ruf JC. Wine and polyphenols related to platelet aggregation and atherothrombosis. *Drugs Exp Clin Res.* 1999;25:125-131.

194. Das DK, Sato M, Ray PS, Maulik G, Engelman RM, Bertelli AAE, Bertelli A. Cardioprotection of red wine: role of polyphenolic antioxidants. *Drugs Exp Clin Res.* 1999;25:115-120.

195. de Lorgeril M, Salen P, Martin JL, Foucher F, Paillard F, de Leiris J. Wine drinking and risks of cardiovascular complications after recent acute myocardial infarction. *Circulation.* 2002;106:1465-1469.

196. Serafini M, Ghiselli A, Ferro-Luzzi A. In vivo antioxidant effect of green and black tea in man. *Eur J Clin Nutr.* 1996;50:28-32.

197. Keli SO, Hertog MGL, Feskens EJM, Kromhout D. Dietary flavonoids, antioxidant vitamins, and incidence of stroke: the Zutphen Study. *Arch Intern Med.* 1996;154:637-642.

198. Tijburg LBM, Wiseman SA, Meijer GW, Westrate JA. Effects of green tea, black tea and lipophilic antioxidants on LDL oxidizability and atherosclerosis in hypercholesterolaemic rabbits. *Atherosclerosis.* 1997;135:37-47.

199. Ishikawa T, Suzukawa M, Ito T, Yoshida H, Ayaori M, Nishiwaki M, Yonemura A, Hara Y, Nakamura H. Effect of tea flavonoid supplementation on the susceptibility of low-density lipoprotein to oxidative modification. *Am J Clin Nutr.* 1997;66:261-266.

200. van het Hof KH, de Boer HSM, Wiseman SA, Lien N, Westrate JA, Tijburg LBM. Consumption of green

or black tea does not increase resistance of low-density lipoprotein to oxidation in humans. *Am J Clin Nutr.* 1997;66:1125-1132.

201. Hertog MGL, Sweetnam PM, Fehily AM, Elwood PC, Kromhout D. Antioxidant flavonols and ischemic heart disease in a Welsh population of men: the Caerphilly Study. *Am J Clin Nutr.* 1997;65:1489-1494.

202. Geleijnse JM, Launer LJ, Hofman A, Pols HAP, Witteman JCM. Tea flavonoids may protect against atherosclerosis: the Rotterdam Study. *Arch Intern Med.* 1999;59:2170-2174.

203. Geleijnse JM, Launer LJ, van der Kuip DAM, Hofman A, Witteman JCM. Inverse association of tea and flavonoid intakes with incident myocardial infarction: the Rotterdam Study. *Am J Clin Nutr.* 2002;75:880-886.

204. Maron DJ, Lu GP, Cai NS, Wu ZG, Li YH, Chen H, Zhu JQ, Jin XJ, Wouters BC, Zhao J. Cholesterol-lowering effect of a theaflavin-enriched green tea extract: a randomized controlled trial. *Arch Intern Med.* 2003;163:1448-1453.

205. Hodgson JM, Burke V, Beilin LJ, Croft KD, Puddey IB. Can black tea influence plasma total homocysteine concentrations? *Am J Clin Nutr.* 2003;77:907-911.

206. Cook NC, Samman S. Flavonoids—chemistry, metabolism, cardioprotective effects, and dietary sources. *J Nutr Biochem.* 1996;7:66-76.

207. Rankin SM, de Whalley CV, Hoult JRS, Jessup W, Wilkins GM, Collard J, Leake DS. The modification of low density lipoprotein by the flavonoids myricetin and gossypetin. *Biochem Pharmacol.* 1993;45:67-75.

208. Conquer JA, Maiani G, Azzini E, Raguzzini A, Holub BJ. Supplementation with quercetin markedly increases plasma quercetin concentration without effect on selected risk factors for heart disease in healthy subjects. *J Nutr.* 1998;128:593-597.

209. Amagase H, Petesch BL, Matsuura H, Kasuga S, Itakura Y. Intake of garlic and its bioactive components. *J Nutr.* 2001;131:955S-962S.

210. Steiner M, Li W. Aged garlic extract, a modulator of cardiovascular risk factors: a dose-finding study on the effects of AGE on platelet function. *J Nutr.* 2001;131:980S-984S.

211. Zhang XH, Lowe D, Giles P, Fell S, Board AR, Baughan JA, Connock MJ, Maslin DJ. A randomized trial of the effects of garlic oil upon coronary heart disease risk factors in trained male runners. *Blood Coagul Fibrinolysis.* 2000;11:67-74.

212. Rajaram S. The effect of vegetarian diet, plant foods, and phytochemicals on hemostasis and thrombosis. *Am J Clin Nutr.* 2003;78(suppl):552S-558S.

213. Ghorai M, Mandal SC, Pal M, Pal SP, Saha BP. A comparative study on hypocholesterolaemic effect of allicin, whole germinated seeds of bengal gram and guggulipid of gum gugglu. *Phytother Res.* 2000;14:200-202.

214. Chernyadeva IF, Shilnikova SV, Rogoza AN, Kukharchuk VV. Dynamics of interrelationships between the content of lipoprotein particles, fibrinogen, and leukocyte count in the plasma from patients with coronary heart disease treated with Kwai. *Bull Exp Biol Med.* 2003;135:436-439.

215. Zhang XH, Lowe D, Giles P, Fell S, Connock MJ, Maslin DJ. Gender may affect the action of garlic oil on plasma cholesterol and glucose levels of normal subjects. *J Nutr.* 2001;131:1471-1478.

216. Koscielny J, Klüßendorf D, Latza R, Schmitt R, Radtke H, Siegel G, Kiesewetter H. The antiatherosclerotic effect of *Allium sativum. Atherosclerosis.* 1999;144:237-249.

217. Dillon SA, Burmi RS, Lowe GM, Billington D, Rahman K. Antioxidant properties of aged garlic extract: an in vitro study incorporating human low density lipoprotein. *Life Sci.* 2003;72:1583-1594.

218. Moriguchi T, Takasugi N, Itakura Y. The effects of aged garlic extract on lipid peroxidation and the deformability of erythrocytes. *J Nutr.* 2001;131(suppl):1016S-1019S.

219. Ide N, Lau BHS. Garlic compounds minimize intracellular oxidative stress and inhibit nuclear factor-κB activation. *J Nutr.* 2001;131(suppl):1020S-1026S.

220. Hoshino T, Kashimoto N, Kasuga S. Effects of garlic preparations on the gastrointestinal mucosa. *J Nutr.* 2001;131(suppl):1109S-1113S.

221. Heck AM, DeWitt BA, Lukes AL. Potential interactions between alternative therapies and warfarin. *Am J Health Syst Pharm.* 2000;57:1221-1230.

222. Szapary PO, Wolfe ML, Bloedon LT, Cucchiara AJ, DerMarderosian AH, Cirigliano MD, Rader DJ. Guggulipid for the treatment of hypercholesterolemia: a randomized controlled trial. *JAMA.* 2003;290:765-772.

223. American Heart Association. The American Heart Association urges caution on cholestin red yeast rice. Available at: http://www.americanheart.org/presenter.jhtml?identifier=2925. Accessed April 12, 2004.

224. US Department of Health and Human Services. Red yeast rice. Available at: http://www.fda.gov/ohrms/dockets/dailys/01/Jun01/061101/let0494.pdf. Accessed April 12, 2004.

225. Mosca L, Appel LJ, Benjamin EJ, Berra K, Chandra-Strobos N, Fabunmi RP, Grady D, Haan CK, Hayes SN, Judelson DR, Keenan NL, McBride P, Oparil S, Ouyang P, Oz MC, Mendelsohn ME, Pasternak RC, Pinn VW, Robertson RM, Schenck-Gustafsson K, Sila CA, Smith SC Jr, Sopko G, Taylor AL, Walsh BW, Wenger NK, Williams CL. Evidence-based guidelines for cardiovascular disease prevention in women. *Circulation.* 2004;109:672-693.

226. Appel LJ, Toore TJ, Obarzanek E, Vollmer WM, Svetkey LP, Sacks FM, Bray GA, Vogt TM, Cutler JA,

Windhauser MM, Lin PH, Karanja N. A clinical trial of the effects of dietary patterns on blood pressure. DASH Collaborative Research Group. *N Engl J Med.* 1997;336:1117-1124.

227. Obarzanek E, Sacks FM, Vollmer WM, Bray GA, Miller ER 3rd, Lin PH, Karanja NM, Most-Windhauser MM, Moore TJ, Swain JF, Bales CW, Proschan MA, for the DASH Research Group. Effects on blood lipids of a blood pressure-lowering diet: the Dietary Approaches to Stop Hypertension (DASH) Trial. *Am J Clin Nutr.* 2001;74:80-89.

228. Appel LJ, Champagne CM, Harsha DW, Cooper LS, Obarzanek E, Elmer PJ, Stevens VJ, Vollmer WM, Lin PH, Svetkey LP, Stedman SW, Young DR; Writing Group of the PREMIER Collaborative Research Group. Effects of comprehensive lifestyle modification on blood pressure control: main results of the PREMIER clinical trial. *JAMA.* 2003;289:2083-2093.

229. Appel LJ, Miller ER III, Jee SH, Stolzenberg-Solomon R, Lin PH, Erlinger T, Nadeau MR, Selhub J. Effects of dietary patterns on serum homocysteine: results of a randomized, controlled feeding study. *Circulation.* 2000;102:852-857.

230. de Lorgeril M, Salen P, Martin JL, Monjaud I, Delaye J, Mamelle N. Mediterranean diet, traditional risk factors, and the rate of cardiovascular complications after myocardial infarction: final report of the Lyon Diet Heart Study. *Circulation.* 1999;99:779-785.

231. Jenkins DJA, Kendall CWC, Marchie A, Faulkner DA, Wong JMW, de Souza R, Emam A, Parker TL, Vidgen E, Lapsley KG, Trautwein EA, Josse RG, Leiter LA, Connelly PW. Effects of a dietary portfolio of cholesterol-lowering foods vs lovastatin on serum lipids and C-reactive protein. *JAMA.* 2003;290:502-510.

232. Frame CJ, Green CG, Herr DG, Myers JE, Taylor ML. The stages of change for dietary fat and fruit and vegetable intake of patients at the outset of a cardiac rehabilitation program. *Am J Health Promot.* 2001;15:405-413.

233. Fragakis AS. *The Health Professional's Guide to Popular Dietary Supplements.* 2nd ed. Chicago, Ill: American Dietetic Association; 2003.

234. US Food and Drug Administration. Tips for the savvy supplement user: making informed decisions. Available at: http://www.fda.gov/fdac/features/2002/202_supp.html. Accessed December 17, 2003.

235. Mayo Clinic. Herb and drug interactions. Available at: http://www.mayoclinic.com/invoke.cfm?id=SA00039. Accessed April 12, 2004.

236. Natural Medicines Comprehensive Database. Available at: http://www.naturaldatabase.com. Accessed April 12, 2004.

237. National Institutes of Health National Center for Complementary and Alternative Medicine Web site. Available at: http://nccam.nih.gov. Accessed April 12, 2004.

238. National Institutes of Health Office of Dietary Supplements Web site. Available at: http://ods.od.nih.gov. Accessed April 12, 2004.

239. Nutrition Action Health Letter. Cholesterol lowering supplements. Available at: http://www.cspinet.org/nah/novnah.htm. Accessed April 12, 2004.

240. US Department of Agriculture Center for Food Safety and Applied Nutrition. Dietary supplements. Available at: http://www.cfsan.fda.gov/~dms/supplmnt.html. Accessed April 12, 2004.

CHAPTER 12

POPULAR DIETS IN THE MANAGEMENT OF OBESITY

Cathy A. Nonas, MS, RD, CDE, and Gary D. Foster, PhD

INTRODUCTION

The Federal Trade Commission estimates that 50 million Americans will diet this year (1). Similarly, in 2000 the Behavioral Risk Factor Surveillance System, a random telephone survey of more than 195,000 adults, reported that 29% of men and 44% of women were attempting to lose weight (approximately 1 out of every 2.5 adults) (2). As the prevalence of obesity increases, efforts to lose weight have become more common. As a result, weight-loss books are being marketed in record numbers to meet the public's interest. During the last 10 years, more than 1,000 diet books, ranging from evidence-based to anecdotal, have been published (3). Many purport to have "the" definitive solution.

Professionals interested in helping obese patients manage their weight and health should be informed of the relative merits of various approaches, even if those approaches do not meet consensus guidelines for an optimal diet. Although it is impossible to know the details of each new "breakthrough" diet, being cognizant of the strengths and weaknesses of the most popular diets helps clinicians effectively advise the many weight-control clients who have tried such a diet or have interest in initiating one.

The purpose of this chapter is to provide practitioners with a summary of the available evidence on popular diets. It is divided into three sections. The first provides an overview of the problem of obesity; the second describes guiding principles in evaluating any diet; and the third reviews several popular diets in detail.

RATIONALE FOR TREATING OBESITY

The rationale for treating obesity seriously lies in its adverse medical consequences. Adults who are overweight (body mass index [BMI] $\geq$ 25) or obese (BMI $\geq$ 30) are at increased risk for early mortality (4,5), as well as for a variety of medical conditions, including type 2 diabetes, hypertension, dyslipidemia, cardiovascular disease (CVD), and sleep apnea (6,7).

Recent data suggest that obesity accounts for 14% to 20% of all cancer deaths, making it second only to smoking in terms of modifiable risk factors for cancer mortality (5). Obesity also confers significant economic costs, approaching $117 billion annually (7). The psychosocial consequences of obesity include body image disparagement, impaired quality of life, and, among the severely obese, depression (8,9).

The seriousness of obesity is exacerbated by its increasing prevalence. A Centers for Disease Control and Prevention report indicates that 34% of Americans are overweight and 31% are obese (10). Thus, 65% of Americans have a BMI equal to or greater than 25, compared with 56% in 1994 and 46% in 1980 (10,11). The number of obese Americans has more than doubled (15% to 31%) during the last 20 years (10,11), and the number of severely obese persons (BMI $\geq$ 40) has nearly tripled during the last decade (12). The serious nature and increasing prevalence of obesity have prompted calls for action from the World Health Organization (13) and the US Surgeon General (14). Fortunately, small reductions in body weight (5% to 10%) are associated with significant improvements in glycemic control, dyslipidemia, and hypertension (6). These improvements, as well as the reductions in waist circumference that accompany weight loss, have positive effects on metabolic syndrome.

Etiology

Although the mathematics of obesity (positive energy balance) seem simple, the factors causing this energy imbalance are varied and complex. These factors include genetic, metabolic, and hormonal influences (15,16) that likely predispose some persons to obesity and may set the range of optimal weights that an individual can achieve. Although it is clear that behavioral factors, such as increased portion sizes and decreased activity (17,18), are responsible for the increased prevalence of obesity, genetic factors account for up to 50% to 70% of the variance in body weight in any one individual (19,20). More than 300 genes have been linked to obesity, but single gene mutations (eg, leptin deficiency) are extremely rare in human obesity (21). A genetic predisposition does not preclude clinically meaningful weight loss but does suggest that equivalent changes in eating and activity will produce different results among individuals of varying genotypes.

Treatment

Any dietary treatment for obesity must be coupled with behavior strategies to help patients identify and modify habitual eating, activity levels, and negative thoughts that may contribute to their excess weight (22). Although it should be recognized that biology may set a range of possible weights, behavior therapy helps obese individuals develop a set of skills (eg, a low-fat diet, a high-activity lifestyle, a realistic cognitive style) to regulate weight at the lower end of that range. Behavior therapy usually includes multiple components, such as self-monitoring, nutrition education, stimulus control, eating pace, exercise, problem solving, and cognitive restructuring. These components comprise the behavioral "package" that has been summarized in self-help manuals, such as *The LEARN Program for Weight Control* (23). Among all of these components, self-monitoring (ie, keeping records of food intake) is the strongest correlate with weight loss in both short-term (12-week) and long-term (17-month) studies (24,25).

The best dietary and behavior therapies typically yield a 10% reduction in body weight during the first 6 months of treatment (22). Without continued contact, however, patients generally regain one third of this weight within 1 year and usually experience a complete regain within 5 years (22). Studies conducted during the last decade indicate that continued contact between the patient and the practitioner significantly enhances weight maintenance

(26,27). In addition, regular physical activity is a consistent predictor of maintenance of weight loss (28,29). Nonetheless, weight regain is the most frequent long-term outcome of obesity treatment. It is this lack of long-term efficacy that fuels clients' interest in alternative or popular approaches. To assist professionals in responding to this patient interest, the next section describes how to systematically evaluate these popular approaches.

GUIDING PRINCIPLES TO EVALUATE POPULAR WEIGHT-LOSS DIETS

Although some clinicians may view a low-calorie, low-fat diet as the only safe weight-loss method, limited clinical data suggest benefit from varied approaches. For example, recent 6- to 12-month data on low-carbohydrate, high-fat regimens show greater improvements in some CVD risk factors, such as high-density lipoprotein (HDL) cholesterol and triglycerides, than those associated with low-calorie, low-fat diets (30-34). Weight losses of 5% to 10%, often irrespective of the type of diet, improve glycemic control, dyslipidemia, and hypertension (6,35).

Given the high prevalence and serious consequences of obesity, a client may argue that the health benefits of weight loss justify use of a less healthful food plan to achieve the weight-loss goal. Clients are attracted to popular diets by promises of dramatic weight loss, regardless of nutritional merit. Clinicians, however, may be concerned with the potential adverse effects from nutrient deficiencies or unhealthful fat sources in the diet. Clinicians recognize that rather than having a magical solution, popular diets lead to weight loss by reducing energy intake below energy expenditure. Popular diets may not harm some people, and the benefits of weight loss remain significant. Therefore, when patients are committed to a popular diet, the clinician should approach the diet with an open mind. This may allow the clinician to alter a popular diet slightly, designing a reasonably healthful weight-loss program, even within the confines of a diet that eliminates bread, stays within the "zone," or avoids carrots because they supposedly have a high glycemic index (GI).

Principles for Clinicians Interacting with Clients

In *Managing Obesity: A Clinical Guide*, Reeves and colleagues (36) suggest five guiding principles that can help clinicians work with clients who are interested in popular diets.

1. *Flexibility.* Clients may have a preconceived notion of what is best for them. To immediately negate that notion damages the therapeutic alliance. Listen to what is appealing to the patient (simplicity, structure, excluding certain types of foods) rather than summarily dismissing any nontraditional approach.
2. *Health status.* It is important to ascertain whether a certain dietary approach compromises health. Dietitians and other health care providers must communicate clearly with the primary care physician to ascertain that the diet does not put the client at undue risk (37).
3. *Nutritional quality.* Few, if any, popular diets are nutritionally perfect. Nonetheless, any diet can be modified in small ways to improve nutritional content, while respecting client preferences.
4. *Big picture.* Consider the client's goals. Does the individual want to lose 10 lb for a reunion or lose 50 lb after a myocardial infarction? If the diet is too confining for long-term use, what are the goals after the diet? What are the patient's criteria for success (health, eliminating binge eating, normalizing eating, weight loss)?

5. *Weight loss.* The client wants to lose weight. If the professional cannot help achieve that goal, the client will probably not return. Therefore, be ready to consider another diet if the first one does not produce the desired outcome.

Considerations for the Short Term vs the Long Term

The word "diet" originally comes from the Greek *diaita* and Latin *dieta*, which mean "a way of life," such as a lifetime eating plan. Of course, one's eating plan or "diet" can change as life changes. Individuals may intentionally increase calcium or vegetable intake or reduce sodium, fat, or sugar consumption. However, today the word "diet" usually connotes weight loss and deprivation.

A major issue is whether a diet can become a lifetime pattern. Diets built less on improving health and more on losing pounds tend to be more restrictive and less realistic, making translation into everyday life even harder. The bagel diet suggests that the dieter eats a bagel *before* every "meal" to blunt the appetite and then recommends the dieter eat only salad *as* the meal. Other diets, such as the cabbage soup diet and the all-you-can-eat diet (which comes in both 3-day and 7-day options), allow unlimited consumption of certain vegetables (such as cabbage soup) but restrict or prohibit other foods. Even when followed half-heartedly, these diets can "magically" reduce energy intake enough to result in quick weight loss. These diets do not offer a realistic approach for the long run, but is there any harm in trying them in the short term and then modifying them to meet the individual needs of daily life?

Some diet messages are more "sensible" and more likely to be feasible in the long run, although they lack an evidence base. For example, some diets restrict high-glycemic foods but promote a healthful variety of nutrients. If the dieter has been overeating desserts and low-fiber starches, then following a diet high in fiber and low in sugar and fat will probably reduce energy intake and produce weight loss. Is there magic to this recipe? No. Call it Volumetrics, Zone, Glucose Revolution, or Sugar Busters, the outcome is the same. If a diet works—fad or not—it is because it reduces total energy intake below energy needs. If the nutritional picture is more complete, it is a bonus for health. If the message is reasonable and not overly restrictive, it is at least theoretically possible to adhere to the diet in everyday life. If the message is too complicated, then it becomes more difficult to follow. If the diet does not clearly delineate barriers, then it becomes harder to reduce total energy intake consistently.

Therefore, the optimum weight-loss "diet"

- promotes good health
- helps the dieter reach a healthier weight
- can be successfully incorporated into the dieter's lifestyle

Within these parameters, one might consider a "weight-loss diet" as an oxymoron because losing weight is a temporary phenomenon—maintaining weight is the long-term lifestyle "diet."

Suppose the method for weight loss was not a "diet" at all, but a treatment? The treatment would have one goal: a healthier weight. The diet would have another goal: a healthier way of life. Then treatments could be faddish, popular, or traditional, as long as they were successful in reducing weight by 5% to 10% and were not harmful. A maintenance diet would have more complex challenges, needing to maintain weight and prevent illness within the context of an individual's lifestyle. The only appropriate maintenance diet would be the one that controls weight and has long-term feasibility. Popular diets or fad diets could not meet the criteria of life-long use. The successful maintenance diet would be measured in the commitment and the adherence, not the weight loss. Given a plausible short-term use for some popular diets, review of popular types of diets is needed.

POPULAR DIETS

A description of every popular or fad diet would require an entire book, with a new edition every few months. Instead, this chapter categorizes a representative sample of diets into three macronutrient categories: low-carbohydrate, high-fat; high-carbohydrate, low-fat; and moderate-carbohydrate, moderate-fat. The diets are categorized this way to make it easier for the reader to discuss these diets with patients.

Macronutrient Manipulation

Research shows that when it comes to weight loss, a calorie is a calorie (38,39). Calories are units of energy, contained in four macronutrients: protein, fat, carbohydrate, and alcohol. When these macronutrients are manipulated to reduce or restrict energy intake, weight loss occurs. Regardless of scientific merit, a diet becomes popular because the public buys the message. Optimally, a diet ought to be supported by research demonstrating positive effects on weight and health.

Other than the drinking man's diet from 40 years ago, most hypocaloric diets exclude or restrict alcohol. Therefore, popular diets manipulate the remaining macronutrients: carbohydrate, protein, and fat. The energy distribution can be manipulated for protein, carbohydrate, and fat in such distributions as

- 30%, 30%, 40%
- 10%, 15%, 75%
- 30%, 60%, 10%
- And so forth

Table 12.1 categorizes the various popular diet approaches to weight management according to macronutrient distribution (40).

This chapter focuses on five popular diets to illustrate the various diet categories: Dr. Atkins' New Diet Revolution (41), Dr. Ornish's Eat More, Weigh Less (42), Slim-Fast (43), the Zone diet (44), and the South Beach diet (45). These diets have been organized within three categories shown in Table 12.2. This categorization distinguishes a diet that reduces carbohydrate to the extent of ketosis (eg, Atkins diet) from a diet that modestly lowers carbohydrate (eg, South Beach Diet with 45% of energy intake as carbohydrate after the initial phase). The low-fat diet category was defined as less than 20% of energy from fat and 65% to 80% of energy from carbohydrate. Low-fat diets include the Pritkin and Ornish diets, which restrict energy from fat to less than 10% of total intake, as well as Weight Watchers and SlimFast diets, which are not as restricted.

Many diets fall between the two extreme categories (low fat vs low carbohydrate). Diets within the moderate-carbohydrate group (40% to 60% of energy from carbohydrate) typically qualify sources of macronutrients, distinguishing between low-fiber (high-glycemic) and high-fiber (low-glycemic) foods and monounsaturated fats vs saturated fats. Most popular diets focus

TABLE 12.1
Categories of Popular Diets by Macronutrient Distribution*

Type of Diet	Fat (% of Total Energy)	Carbohydrate (% of Total Energy)	Protein (% of Total Energy)	Total Energy (kcal)†
Low-carbohydrate/high-fat	55–65	<20	25–30	1550–1688
Moderate-carbohydrate/moderate-fat	20–30	40–60	20–30	1232–1592
High-carbohydrate/low-fat	<20	>65	15–20	1218–1383

*Percentages of macronutrients in each diet category are based on fitting current popular diets into no more than three categories. See text for explanation.

†Total energy calculations are based on menus created by the authors of this chapter, following the guidelines of each diet, and then analyzed using USDA Nutrient Database (40).

TABLE 12.2
Categorization of Popular Diets

Low-Carbohydrate/High-Fat	Moderate-Carbohydrate/Moderate-Fat	High-Carbohydrate/Low-Fat
Atkins*	DASH*	Ornish*
Protein Power	Mediterranean*	SlimFast*†
	Glycemic index	Pritikin
	Zone	Weight Watchers*†
	South Beach	

*Diet has been subject of scientific weight-loss comparison studies.

†Depending upon food choices, these diets can fit in the moderate- or low-fat categories.

on the type of food, not energy intake. All of them except SlimFast purport to make the individual feel more satisfied (according to the Ornish diet, satisfaction comes from the carbohydrates; the other diets attribute it to the lack of carbohydrates).

Two of the categories—low-carbohydrate and moderate-carbohydrate—overlap somewhat in their "scientific" rationales. Insulin plays a theoretical role in both the low-carbohydrate and many of the moderate-carbohydrate diets. Although the research remains equivocal, the diet books attribute many benefits to lower insulin levels resulting from lower carbohydrate intake. Describing his low-carbohydrate diet, Atkins states, "When you control your intake of refined carbohydrates, you avoid the foods that cause you to be fat" (41 [p 12]), and he goes on to explain the metabolic advantage of burning fat (see the Atkins diet section later in this chapter). Agaston explains the principles behind the South Beach diet (moderate carbohydrate) by stating, "The more food is preprocessed, the more fattening it will be" (45 [p 53]). He describes a baked potato as more fattening than a baked potato with a dollop of sour cream because the latter has a lower GI. The Zone diet (moderate carbohydrate) is based on the premise that "the way to fatten yourself up is to eat lots of low-fat processed carbohydrates" (46). But remember—popular diets are at least part hype; they typically market with a message that includes something like "Keep your weight off forever, using our new and proven diet!"

Micronutrient Content

Diets that fit into the high or low categories tend to be deficient in some vitamins and minerals because they omit an entire category (or categories) of food. On the other hand, the moderate diets tend to include a good nutritional balance as defined by the US Dietary

Guidelines (47). Any diet that significantly increases one macronutrient over another shifts the balance of micronutrients and yields a less complete nutritional picture. The balance of micronutrients can be improved by the food chosen within a specific category (eg, salmon instead of chicken for protein; brown rice instead of white for carbohydrate). A daily multivitamin supplement is important for any individual on a weight-loss diet. In addition, calcium is often neglected, and supplementation should therefore be evaluated. Table 12.3 summarizes nutrient levels for the three diet categories compared with the dietary reference intakes and recommended dietary allowances (RDAs) (3,48).

Low-Carbohydrate, High-Fat Diets

Low-carbohydrate, high-fat diets have received much publicity, but very few diets can actually be defined as low-carbohydrate. Low-carbohydrate, high-fat diets are very specific; they restrict total carbohydrates to less than 20% of total energy or no more than 100 g/day (49). The Atkins diet and Protein Power fall into this category. The South Beach diet's inclusion of 45% of energy from carbohydrate after the first 2 weeks places it in the moderate-carbohydrate category. The once-popular Scarsdale diet, with as much as 35% of total energy from carbohydrates, falls outside of the low-carbohydrate, high-fat category.

Low-carbohydrate, high-fat diets do not usually differentiate between kinds of fats or limit the use of saturated fats. A person can eat as much food within allowable categories as desired; however, research indicates that individuals on these diets typically limit daily energy intake to 1,400 to 1,600 kcal (3). Although ketosis is marketed as a metabolic advantage, the level of ketones tends to be quite small (50).

The low-carbohydrate diet books correctly explain that insulin sends glucose into cells, including fat cells. However, the science begins to fade when authors discuss insulin, claiming that because it is secreted primarily in the presence of carbohydrates, the more carbohydrates a person eats, the more glucose is stored in the fat cells. The hype continues as carbohydrates are labeled as what make a person fat! Scientific evidence does not indicate that energy from carbohydrates increases fat storage more than the energy from any other macronutrient (51). Total energy intake, over and above maintenance needs, is what makes people gain weight, independent of macronutrient composition. This distinction is critical for clinicians to understand if they are going to discuss popular diets with patients.

The Atkins diet is the first diet analyzed in this chapter. For this diet and the others examined in detail, the sections on "Rationale" and "The Diet" summarize information from the diet's author(s), whereas the information presented in "Data" and "Clinical Monitoring" was developed by the authors of this chapter. Table 12.4 provides numerical values for the macronutrient content of the diets as calculated by the chapter authors based on menus derived from each published diet (40–45.

Dr. Atkins' New Diet Revolution

Rationale
Atkins proposes that restricting carbohydrates promotes ketosis, or fat burning (41). He claims that weight loss results from carbohydrate restriction rather than restriction of energy intake.

The Diet
The Atkins diet defines four phases by daily carbohydrate limits: induction, weight loss, premaintenance, and maintenance. Macronutrient analyses on the first three phases are found in Table 12.4.

TABLE 12.3
Micronutrient Content of Types of Diets

Type of Diet	Micronutrient Content
Low-carbohydrate/high-fat	Low in vitamin E, thiamin, magnesium, folate, calcium, fiber, iron, potassium
Moderate-carbohydrate/moderate-fat	With proper food choices (high in fiber, low in saturated fats) based on the USDA Food Guide Pyramid, these diets are nutritionally adequate.
High-carbohydrate/low-fat	Low in vitamin E, B-12, zinc

Source: Data are from reference 3.

TABLE 12.4
Macronutrient Analysis of Menus Based on Popular Diet Books*

Diet and Phase	Energy (kcal)	Protein, g (% Total Energy)	Fat, g (% Total Energy)	Carbohydrate, g (% Total Energy)
Atkins				
Induction phase	1678	126 (30)	105 (57)	35 (8)
Ongoing weight loss	1688	131 (31)	105 (56)	46 (11)
Premaintenance	1550	83 (21)	112 (65)	45 (12)
Ornish	1218	48 (16)	10 (7)	238 (78)
SlimFast	1383	67 (19)	23 (15)	234 (68)
The Zone	1259	86 (27)	47 (36)	118 (37)
South Beach				
Phase 1	1328	111 (33)	79 (54)	45 (14)
Phase 2	1232	66 (21)	58 (42)	130 (42)
Phase 3	1592	72 (18)	69 (39)	178 (45)

*Macronutrients calculated using menu examples and recipes from the published diets (41–45) and nutrient data from USDA Nutrient Database (40).

Induction lasts a minimum of 14 days and restricts the individual to 20 g carbohydrate per day. Caffeine is to be avoided, and dieters are warned against artificially sweetened drinks because these may slow weight loss. Although water is important with any diet, water is especially important in the Atkins diet to moderate changes in acid-base balance caused by excessive protein intake. Atkins suggests at least 8 glasses per day. Psyllium husk is also recommended for constipation.

The second phase, titled "Ongoing Weight Loss" (OWL), consists of approximately 30 to 40 g carbohydrate per day. In this phase, each individual achieves a personal threshold for carbohydrates, which is increased by 5-g/day increments until weight loss is significantly reduced or stopped. Atkins claims that a person's critical carbohydrate level (CCL) is based on a person's metabolic resistance and level of activity and it ranges between 15 to 90 g carbohydrate per day. However, the author states that most dieters cannot lose weight if they exceed 50 to 60 g of carbohydrate during OWL. During OWL, a small amount of alcohol is permitted.

The third phase is premaintenance, where weight loss slows even more as carbohydrate intake is increased by 10-g/day increments. Weight loss should not stop, however, and if the dieter starts gaining, total carbohydrate intake is decreased by 10-g/day increments until weight loss resumes. During this phase, the dieter can be flexible, reducing carbohydrates one day and increasing them another to maintain their recommended average CCL for this phase.

The Atkins follower can return to one phase or another depending upon the desired rate of weight loss.

Using menus provided for the Atkins induction phase, our nutrient analysis revealed 35 g of carbohydrate per day instead of the prescribed 20 g/day. To achieve the 20 g/day limitation, the strawberry smoothie (an Atkins induction recipe) was exchanged for cheese and celery and the dinner vegetable was omitted. Even at 35 g, carbohydrate made up only 8% of total energy intake (see Table 12.4).

Menus for the OWL phase contained energy levels similar to the induction phase, but the total carbohydrates were 46 g/day (11% of total energy). The premaintenance phase allowed less total energy (1,550 kcal), but carbohydrates remained the same at 45 g/day (12% of total energy).

Clearly, menus provided with the diet needed some mathematical tweaking to meet the diet's defined parameters. Our estimates, as well as those of others (34), show the Atkins diet to be hypocaloric. One may get the impression from the text of the book or the media that an individual can eat all the protein and fat he or she desires. However, the Atkins recipes suggest very clear and portion-controlled measurements for all foods, including high-protein or high-fat foods.

Data

The Atkins diet is the subject of current research. Table 12.5 summarizes findings from four randomized controlled trials of 6 to 12 months that were published in 2003 and 2004 (30-34). Weight loss was greater with a low-carbohydrate, high-fat regimen than a low-calorie, low-fat diet at 3 and 6 months (30-34), but there was no significant difference in weight between the groups at 12 months (32,33). Surprisingly, total and low-density lipoprotein (LDL) cholesterol levels were not adversely affected in any of the studies. Moreover, the low-carbohydrate diet was associated with greater improvements in triglyceride levels (30-34) and improvements in HDL cholesterol (33). A short-term, 6-week crossover study compared hypocaloric diets low in carbohydrate (< 10% of energy) with a diet moderately low in fat (< 30% of energy). In 15 overweight, but otherwise healthy men, the low-fat diet lowered LDL cholesterol levels. The low-carbohydrate diet lowered serum triglyceride and serum glucose levels, as well as increasing the LDL particle size (52). These early studies suggest that the low-carbohydrate dietary approach deserves more comprehensive assessment in larger samples to evaluate safety and efficacy fully. However, studies have shown that some very-high-protein diets may contribute to kidney stones and bone loss (53) and worsen kidney function in those whose kidney function is already abnormal (54). Very-low-carbohydrate diets may also increase uric acid in the blood, among other complications (37).

Clinical Monitoring

Nutrient completeness is far from ideal with low-carbohydrate, high-fat diets, and "a broad multi-vitamin and multi-mineral supplement that contains more than the RDA of B complex and C, and at least 30 different nutrients, including essential fatty acids" is suggested by Atkins (41). Indeed, all three phases of the Atkins diet tend to be low in fiber, vitamins C and E, folate, calcium, and magnesium.

Because this diet is high in saturated fat and low in carbohydrate, it is important to monitor serum lipid levels, blood uric acid concentration, and renal function. Health care professionals also should perform regular electrocardiograms, assess the dieter's skin color, and ensure that his or her general feeling of well being is maintained.

TABLE 12.5
Summary of Clinical Trials of Low-Carbohydrate Diets

Study	Mean BMI of Subjects on Entering Study	Subjects Entered in Study	Subjects Completing Study	Low-CHO Diets		Traditional Diets	
				Weight Loss at 6 Months, kg	Weight Loss at 12 Months, kg	Weight Loss at 6 Months, kg	Weight Loss at 12 Months, kg
Brehm et al (30)	33.6	53 women	42 women	8.5*	NA	3.9	NA
Samaha et al (31) and Stern et al (32)	43	109 men 23 women	87	5.8†	5.1 (NS)	1.9	3.1
Foster et al (33)	34	63	42 at 6 months 37 at 12 months	7.0*	4.4 (NS)	3.2	2.5
Yancy et al (34)	34	91 women 28 men	79 at 24 weeks	12.0*	NA	6.5	NA

Abbreviations: BMI, body mass index; CHO, carbohydrate; NA, not applicable (study did not last 12 months); NS, no significant difference.
*Greater weight loss on low-carbohydrate diet ($P < .001$).
†Greater weight loss on low-carbohydrate diet ($P < .002$).

High-Carbohydrate, Low-Fat Diets

For this chapter, high-carbohydrate, low-fat diets are defined as less than 20% of energy intake from fat and more than 65% of energy intake from carbohydrate. This differentiates these diets from more moderate diets that include 55% to 60% of energy from carbohydrate and 25% to 30% from fat. Originally developed for treatment of heart disease, low-fat and very-low-fat diets have become popular for weight loss. The diets are high in complex carbohydrates from fruits and vegetables that are also naturally high in fiber and low in energy density. Dr. Dean Ornish's Program for Reversing Heart Disease and Dr. Nathan Pritikin's Program, each with less than 10% of energy from fat, are in this category, as well as the newer raw food diets that purport to restore the eating patterns of the Paleolithic era. Raw food diets do not use any processed foods or cooked foods and will typically be low in fat, but including large amounts of nuts and seeds can increase the proportion of fat in these diets. The Ornish approach is described below.

Dr. Ornish's Eat More, Weigh Less Diet

Rationale
Ornish claims that limiting energy intake from fat to less than 10% results in weight loss and allows the individual to eat larger volumes of low-fat foods. The severe fat restriction also reverses atherosclerosis.

The Diet
The Ornish diet is part of an overall program. A very-low-fat diet, devoid of meat but rich in carbohydrates, is combined with physical activity and meditation.

Data
A greater body of research exists for low-fat diets than for high-fat diets. Low-fat, high-carbohydrate diets that reduce weight also reduce LDL cholesterol values, blood pressure, insulin levels, and serum glucose concentration. As with most diets, low-fat diets produce weight loss in the range of 6% to 10% of baseline weight during a 3- to 6-month period (35). Ornish et al (55,56) reported successful 1- and 5-year follow-up data for individuals eating a very-low-fat diet, including regression of atherosclerotic plaque.

Clinical Monitoring

The low-fat diet tends to be low in vitamins E, B-12, calcium, and zinc (3). Triglyceride levels should be monitored; they may increase if an individual selects low-fiber rather than high-fiber carbohydrate sources. In the name of "low fat," manufacturers have been selling easy-to-eat snacks and family-style portions of pasta. To follow a low-fat diet correctly (ie, to get the most nutrition for the least energy), however, it is important to eat plenty of nonstarchy vegetables, a variety of fruit, and small portions of high-fiber starches. After developing a menu using the advice in Ornish's *Eat More, Weigh Less* (42), our nutrient analysis (Table 12.4) indicated 1,218 kcal/day (78% from carbohydrate, 7% from fat, and 16% from protein).

SlimFast Diet

Rationale

Replacing one to two meals per day with a standardized, portion-controlled, nutritious, and inexpensive formula can reduce energy intake and result in weight loss.

The Diet

SlimFast products are over-the-counter formulas; they are available in liquid, powder, or bar form. Each liquid meal replacement (the most popular product) contains 220 kcal with 22 vitamins and minerals, 5 g of fiber, 42 g of carbohydrate, 1 g of fat, and 10 to 14 g of protein. The weight-loss phase consists of two daily SlimFast products (usually for breakfast and lunch) plus one balanced, portion-controlled regular food meal, and fruit, vegetables, or a SlimFast snack bar for between meal snacks (refer to Table 12.4.)

An analysis of Web-based reviews revealed a diet that consisted of approximately 1,383 kcal (approximately 68% carbohydrate, 15% fat, and 19% protein). An example was based on 8 ounces of chicken and one tablespoon olive oil in the one "balanced regular food" meal. Alternatively, 6 ounces of chicken and two tablespoons of oil could have been used, providing 1,467 kcal (22% from fat, 64% from carbohydrate, and 15% from protein). As with many of these diets, these small changes complicate the categories. Still, the high amount of carbohydrate places SlimFast more appropriately in the high-carbohydrate, low-fat category rather than the moderate-carbohydrate classification.

The Data

Several studies have shown the efficacy of SlimFast and other meal replacements. Two studies comparing the use of SlimFast with traditional low-calorie diets showed significantly better weight loss with the meal replacement than the traditional diets (57,58). In a German study, data available on 75% of the original 100 subjects showed an average of 15 lb lost after 4 years daily use of a meal replacement (59).

Clinical Monitoring

The SlimFast diet can be a well-balanced dietary plan if the balanced regular food meal is well designed. The biggest concern is the potential hypoglycemic effect of a very-reduced-calorie formula meal for people with diabetes who are taking sulfonylurea agents or insulin.

Moderate-Carbohydrate, Moderate-Fat Diets

The moderate-fat, moderate-carbohydrate category includes diets with 20% to 30% of energy intake from total fat and more than 55% from carbohydrate. Many popular diet books are heading to the middle ground to avoid scientific backlash. Originally, this was a "safe" category, consisting of diets from the American Heart Association and the American Dietetic

Association, as well as moderate weight-loss programs such as Weight Watchers. However, this category now includes a wider variety of diets such as the Zone, South Beach, Somersized food groups, the Glucose Revolution, Sugar Busters, Dietary Approaches to Stop Hypertension (DASH), and Mediterranean diets. Because a number of Americans eat a large quantity of such low-fiber carbohydrates offerings as 5-ounce bagels, king-size candy bars, and 20-ounce (or larger) bottles of juice and soda, lowering typical carbohydrate intake can effectively reduce energy intake. Authors of these diets suggest a range of carbohydrate intake similar to the Institute of Medicine recommendation of 40% to 55% of energy (60). In this moderate category, dietary protein is increased to 20% to 30% of total energy, with fat intake at 20% to 30% of total energy. Unlike low-carbohydrate diets, these diets *do* specify the type of fat, promoting unsaturated fats with an emphasis on monounsaturated fatty acids, such as that found in olive oil.

The diets in this category, although similar, market themselves differently. The DASH and Mediterranean diets emphasize the health outcomes, whereas Weight Watchers emphasizes weight loss and safety. Most of the newer diets (Zone, South Beach, Glucose Revolution, Somersizing, Volumetrics, and so on) emphasize the significance of the glycemic index (GI). The GI uses a ranking system for all foods with carbohydrates (see Chapter 9). Numerical values indicate the degree to which different foods raise blood sugar immediately after consumption as compared with the rise generated by eating white bread or glucose (61).

In diets emphasizing the significance of GI, a food with a low GI (< 50) is viewed as more desirable than a food with a higher GI because the slower release of glucose into the bloodstream reduces surges of insulin needed to remove larger amounts of glucose. Proponents suggest that this flattening of the insulin curve increases satiety, thereby reducing extra energy intake. However, studies investigating levels of satiety with a low-glycemic diet are few, and the numbers of subjects in these studies are small. These studies do suggest that low-glycemic diets lower the insulin response to certain ingested carbohydrates, but the results are inconclusive regarding whether these diets decrease hunger or promote weight loss (62). Many low-glycemic foods are high-fiber foods, which are advocated in recommendations from the USDA (47), the American Dietetic Association (63), the American Heart Association (64), and the American Diabetes Association (65). However, there are four points that call the "science" of low-glycemic foods into question: (*a*) only about 750 different foods have been tested for their GI, omitting thousands of foods; (*b*) one person's glycemic response to a food may be markedly different from the next person's; (*c*) combining certain foods can result in a GI different from the GI for the foods evaluated separately (a baked potato with sour cream has a lower GI than a plain baked potato); and (*d*) different values are listed in different publications (61).

The Zone Diet

Rationale
According to the principles of the Zone diet, eating the proper ratio of low-energy-density carbohydrates, dietary fat, and protein keeps the body's insulin production within a therapeutic zone, making it possible to burn excess body fat (and keep it off permanently) (46).

The Diet
The most basic Zone guidelines dictate that to optimize fat burning (and therefore lose weight), the diet ratio of macronutrients should put one in the "zone." This ratio has less total carbohydrate and more protein (40% of energy from carbohydrate, 30% from protein, 30%

from fat) than the usually prescribed dietary guidelines. Planning meals to meet this ratio can be complex and time consuming. Based on menus from the Zone diet Web site (46), the Zone diet consisted of 1,259 kcal/day and included 37% carbohydrate, 27% protein, and 36% fat (refer to Table 12.4).

Data

No studies have been published on the Zone diet. The diet's author states that by consuming a better balance of food, the body can increase its amount of eicosanoids (chemical messengers derived from dietary fats that control metabolic processes). Although the science sounds appealing and the food choices seem well balanced and healthful, the scientific basis is unproved. Is weight loss greater with a 40:30:30 balance than with a lower-fat, higher-carbohydrate diet? Does manipulating macronutrients alter the eicosanoid ratio? As of the publication of this chapter, these questions have not been studied. The theory may sell books, and the diet itself may be adequate from a nutrition perspective, but there is no published evidence that this diet works better than any other diet.

Clinical Monitoring

There are no particular nutrient deficiencies with this diet. As with any diet, however, individuals may have variable reactions, and no weight-loss diet should be attempted without a physician approval and monitoring of laboratory values and weight loss.

The South Beach Diet

Agatston's South Beach diet is an amalgam of different diets. Divided into phases, phase 1 is similar to the Atkins induction stage. Like the Atkins diet, first phase of the South Beach diet divides good carbohydrates from bad ones (bananas and carrots are "bad"), but after phase 1 Agatston suggests a higher-carbohydrate diet using low-glycemic foods similar to the Zone and promotes monounsaturated oils as does the Mediterranean diet (45).

Rationale

Marketed as the "sane" diet, this diet uses healthy monounsaturated fats, separates "good" from "bad" carbohydrates but does not restrict them entirely, and requires between meal snacks to reduce hunger (refer to Table 12.4).

The Diet

The first phase of the diet lasts 2 weeks, which Agatston claims is just long enough to resolve the insulin resistance. However, after this phase "vanishes your desire for sweets and starches," the "right" carbohydrates (those with a low GI) can be added back into the diet. This is phase 2, in which carbohydrates make up 45% of total energy intake. Phase 2 is continued until the target weight is reached. Again, like the Atkins and Zone diets, portion control is not imposed, but "normal" portions are suggested. All recipes have a defined serving. Nuts are portion-controlled (about 15 almonds per snack). Agatston admits that although nuts are healthy, they are energy-dense and can undermine weight loss. If weight gain occurs, the individual should return to phase 1. Phase 3 is maintenance, and, although this is the most liberal phase, starchy carbohydrates and sweets are controlled. During phase 3, total carbohydrates are 45% of total energy, which was calculated at 1,592 kcal/day.

Data

At the time of publication, there are no data that compare this diet with any other diet.

Clinical Monitoring

Except for the first 2 weeks when carbohydrates are very low, the South Beach diet is a well-balanced diet. As with all diets, the primary physician should give approval to start and then monitor the individual as weight loss occurs.

SUMMARY

The growing prevalence of obesity reinforces the need for effective means for weight loss and weight-loss maintenance. Recommended treatment for obesity incorporates dietary management of energy intake, increased physical activity, and behavioral strategies. Maintaining contact with a practitioner and maintaining regular physical activity are predictors of successful maintenance of weight loss.

Although many popular diet books do not present the ideal approach to weight loss, patient interest in the diets mandates that health care professionals be familiar with the advantages and disadvantages of the general categories of popular diets. Some studies substantiate the weight-loss effect of both very-low-fat and very-low-carbohydrate diets, including the low-fat meal-replacement approach. Because intake of some vitamins and minerals is likely to be deficient when one or more categories of food is eliminated, use of a daily multivitamin is advisable. With the exception of the DASH diet, very few, if any, published data are available on the use of moderate-carbohydrate, moderate-fat popular diets, such as South Beach and the Zone diet.

Although some health professionals may shun diet approaches popularized by the lay press, this bias can be a hindrance in helping patients who are adamant about pursuing popular diets. By remaining open-minded, health care professionals can encourage healthful options and improve total nutrition even while the patient is adhering to a popular diet. Some patients may find success by first adopting a popular diet approach for a short time to achieve weight loss and then gradually developing long-term healthier approaches for weight maintenance. Health care providers should acknowledge there are weight-control strategies other than the traditional low-calorie, low-fat diet. Dietetics professionals who actively review continuing research on various macronutrient distributions and approaches can help patients to adopt an approach well suited to optimize their health status and increase the likelihood of long-term success.

REFERENCES

1. Federal Trade Commission. Paunch lines: weight loss claims are no joke for dieters. Available at: http://www.ftc.gov/bcp/conline/pubs/alerts/paunch.pdf. Accessed April 17, 2004.
2. National Center for Chronic Disease Prevention and Health Promotion. Behavioral Risk Factor Surveillance System. Available at: http://apps.nccd.cdc.gov/brfss. Accessed April 24, 2004.
3. Freedman MR, King J, Kennedy E. Popular diets: a scientific review. *Obes Res.* 2001;9(suppl):1S-40S.
4. Fontaine KR, Redden DT, Wang C, Westfall AO, Allison DB. Years of life lost due to obesity. *JAMA.* 2003;289:187-193.
5. Calle EE, Rodriguez C, Walker-Thurmond K, Thun MJ. Overweight, obesity, and mortality from cancer in a prospectively studied cohort of US adults. *N Engl J Med.* 2003;348:1625-1638.
6. National Heart, Lung, and Blood Institute. Clinical guidelines on the identification, evaluation, and treatment of overweight and obesity in adults: the evidence report. *Obes Res.* 1998;6(suppl):51S-210S.
7. Field AE, Barnoya J, Colditz GA. Epidemiology and health and economic consequences of obesity. In: Wadden TA, Stunkard AJ, eds. *Handbook of Obesity Treatment.* New York, NY: Guilford Press; 2002:3-18.
8. Wadden TA, Womble LG, Stunkard AJ, Anderson DA. Psychosocial consequences of obesity and weight loss.

In: Wadden TA, Stunkard AJ, eds. *Handbook of Obesity Treatment*. New York, NY: Guilford Press, 2002:144-169.

9. Kushner R, Foster GD. Obesity and quality of life. *Nutrition*. 2000;16:947-952.

10. Flegal K, Carroll M, Ogden C, Johnson C. Prevalence and trends in obesity among US Adults, 1999. *JAMA*. 2002;288:1723-1727.

11. Flegal KM, Carroll MD, Kuczmarski RJ, Johnson CL. Overweight and obesity in the United States: prevalence and trends, 1960–1994. *Int J Obes*. 1998;22:39-47.

12. Freedman DS, Khan LK, Serdula MK, Galuska DA, Dietz WH. Trends and correlates of class 3 obesity in the United States from 1990 through 2000. *JAMA*. 2002;288:1758-1761.

13. World Health Organization. *Obesity: Preventing and Managing the Global Epidemic*. Geneva, Switzerland: World Health Organization; 1998.

14. US Department of Health and Human Services. *Surgeon General's Call to Action to Prevent and Decrease Overweight and Obesity*. Rockville, Md: Office of the Surgeon General; 2001.

15. National Heart, Lung, and Blood Institute. The Practical Guide: Identification, Evaluation, and Treatment of Overweight and Obesity in Adults. 2000. NIH Publication No. 00-4084. Available at: http://www./nhlbi.nih.gov/guidelines/obesity/prctgd_c.pdf. Accessed March 25, 2004.

16. Korner J, Aronne LJ. The emerging science of body weight regulation and its impact on obesity treatment. *J Clin Invest*. 2003;111:565-570.

17. Nielson SJ, Popkin BM. Patterns and trends in food portion sizes, 1977–1978. *JAMA*. 2003;289:450-453.

18. Foster GD, Phelan S. Environmental challenges and assessment. In: Berndanier C, ed. *The Handbook of Nutrition and Food*. Boca Raton, Fla: CRC Press; 2001:773-785.

19. Segal NL, Allison DB. Twins and virtual twins: bases of relative body weight revisited. *Int J Obes Relat Metab Disord*. 2001;9:257-263.

20. Comuzzie AJ. The genetic contribution to human obesity: the dissection of a complex phenotype. In: Johnston FE, Foster GD, eds. *Obesity, Growth and Development*. London, England: Smith-Gordon & Co; 2001:21-36.

21. Chagnon YC, Rankinen T, Snyder EE, Weisnagel SJ, Pérusse L, Bouchard C. The human obesity gene map: the 2002 Update. *Obes Res*. 2003;11:313-367.

22. Wadden TA, Foster GD. Behavioral treatment of obesity. *Med Clin North Am*. 2000;84:441-461.

23. Brownell KD. *The LEARN Program for Weight Management*. Dallas, Tex: American Health Publishing Co; 2000.

24. Dubbert PM, Wilson GT. Goal-setting and spouse involvement in the treatment of obesity. *Behav Res Ther*. 1984;22:227-242.

25. Boutelle KN, Kirschenbaum DS. Further support for consistent self-monitoring as a vital component of successful weight control. *Obes Res*. 1998;6:219.

26. Perri MG, McAllister DA, Gange JJ, Jordan RC, McAdoo WG, Nezu AM. Effects of four maintenance programs on the long-term management of obesity. *J Consult Clin Psychol*. 1988;56:529-534.

27. Perri MG, Corsica JA. Improving the maintenance of weight lost in behavioral treatment of obesity. In: Wadden TA, Stunkard AJ, eds. *Handbook of Obesity Treatment*. New York, NY: Guilford Press; 2002:357-379.

28. Kayman S, Bruvold W, Stern JS. Maintenance and relapse after weight loss in women: behavioral aspects. *Am J Clin Nutr*. 1990;52:800-807.

29. Wadden TA, Vogt RA, Foster GD, Anderson DA. Exercise and the maintenance of weight loss: one-year follow-up of a controlled clinical trial. *J Consult Clin Psychol*. 1998;66:429-433.

30. Brehm BJ, Seeley RJ, Daniels SR, D'Alessio DA. A randomized trial comparing a very low carbohydrate diet and a calorie-restricted low fat diet on body weight and cardiovascular risk factors in healthy women. *J Clin Endocrinol Metab*. 2003;88:1617-1623.

31. Samaha FF, Iqbal N, Seshadri P, Chicano KL, Daily DA, McGrory J, Williams T, Williams M, Gracely EJ, Stern L. A low-carbohydrate as compared with a low-fat diet in severe obesity. *N Engl J Med*. 2003;348:2074-2081.

32. Stern L, Iqbal N, Seshadri P, Chicano KL, Daily DA, McGrory J, Williams M, Gracely EJ, Samaha FF. The effects of low-carbohydrate versus conventional weight loss diets in severely obese adults: one-year follow-up of a randomized trial. *Ann Intern Med*. 2004;140:778-785.

33. Foster GD, Wyatt HR, Hill JO, McGuckin BG, Brill C, Mohammed S, Szapary PO, Rader DJ, Edman JS, Klein S. A randomized trial of a low-carbohydrate diet for obesity. *N Engl J Med*. 2003;348:2082-2090.

34. Yancy WS, Olsen MK, Guyton JR, Bakst RP, Westman EC. A low-carbohydrate, ketogenic diet versus a low-fat diet to treat obesity and hyperlipidemia: a randomized controlled trial. *Ann Intern Med*. 2004;140:769-777.

35. Kennedy E. Dietary approaches: overview. In: Foster GD, Nonas CA, eds. *Managing Obesity: A Clinical Guide*. Chicago, Ill: American Dietetic Association; 2004:91-97.

36. Reeves R, Bolton MP, Gee M. Dietary approaches: practical application. In: Foster GD, Nonas CA, eds. *Managing Obesity: A Clinical Guide*. Chicago, Ill: American Dietetic Association; 2004:98-117.

37. Nonas CA. Clinical monitoring: practical application. In: Foster GD, Nonas CA, eds. *Managing Obesity: A Clinical Guide*. Chicago, Ill: American Dietetic Association; 2004:47-64.

38. Leibel RL, Hirsch J, Appel Be, Checani GC. Energy intake required to maintain body weight is not affected by wide variation in diet composition. *Am J Clin Nutr*. 1992;55:350-355.

39. Roust LR, Hammel KD, Jensen MD. Effects of isoenergetic, low-fat diets on energy metabolism in lean and obese women. *Am J Clin Nutr.* 1994;60:470-475.

40. US Dept of Agriculture. National Nutrient Database for Standard Reference. Available at: http://www.ars.usda.gov/fnic/foodcomp/search/index.html. Accessed March 27, 2004.

41. Atkins RC. *Dr. Atkins' New Diet Revolution.* New York, NY: Avon Books; 1992.

42. Ornish D. *Eat More, Weigh Less.* New York, NY: Quill; 2001.

43. SlimFast Plan. Available at: http://www.slimfast.com. Accessed March 30, 2004.

44. Sears B, Lawren B. *The Zone: A Dietary Roadmap.* New York, NY: Regan Books; 1995.

45. Agatston A. *The South Beach Diet.* Emmaus, Pa: Rodale; 2003.

46. The Zone. Available at: http://www.zoneperfect.com. Accessed March 30, 2004.

47. US Departments of Agriculture and Health and Human Services. *Nutrition and Your Health: Dietary Guidelines for Americans.* 5th ed. Washington, DC: US Departments of Agriculture and Health and Human Services; 2000. Home and Garden Bulletin 232.

48. Institute of Medicine. *Dietary Reference Intakes.* Available at: http://www.nap.edu. Accessed February 4, 2004.

49. Bravata DM, Sanders L, Huang J, Krumholz HM, Olkin I, Gardner CD, Bravata DM. Efficacy and safety of low-carbohydrate diets: a systematic review. *JAMA.* 2003;289:1837-1850.

50. Van Itallie TB, Nufert TH. Ketones: metabolism's "ugly duckling." *Nutr Rev.* 2003;61:327-341.

51. Schwarz JM, Neese RA, Turner S, Dare D, Hellerstein MK. Short-term alterations in carbohydrate energy intake in humans: striking effects on hepatic glucose production, de novo lipogenesis, lipolysis and whole-body fuel selection. *J Clin Invest.* 1995;96:2735-2743.

52. Sharman JM, Gomez AL, Kraemer WJ, Volek JS. Very low-carbohydrate and low-fat diets affect fasting lipids and postprandial lipemia differently in overweight men. *J Nutr.* 2004;134:880-885.

53. Reddy ST, Wang CY, Sakhaee K, Brinkley L, Pak CY. Effect of low-carbohydrate high-protein diets on acid-base balance, stone-forming propensity, and calcium metabolism. *Am J Kidney Dis.* 2002;40:265-274.

54. Lentine K, Wrone EM. New insights into protein intake and progression of renal disease. *Curr Opin Nephrol Hypertens.* 2004;13:333-336.

55. Ornish D, Brown SE, Scherwitz LW, Billings JH, Armstrong WT, Ports TA, McLanahan SM, Kirkeeide RL, Brand RJ, Gould KL. Can lifestyle changes reverse coronary heart disease? The Lifestyle Heart Trial. *Lancet.* 1990;336:129-133.

56. Ornish D, Scherwitz LW, Billings JH, Brown SE, Gould KL, Merritt TA, Sparler S, Armstrong WT, Ports TA, Kirkeeide RL, Hogeboom C, Brand RJ. Intensive lifestyle changes for reversal of coronary heart disease. *JAMA.* 1998;280:2001-2007.

57. Ashley JM, St Jeor ST, Perumean-Chaney SP, Schrage J, Bovee V. Meal replacements in weight intervention. *Obes Res.* 2001;9(suppl):312S-320S.

58. Rothacker DQ. Five-year self-management of weight using meal replacements: comparison with matched controls in rural Wisconsin. *Nutrition.* 2000;16:344-348.

59. Flechtner-Mors M, Ditschuneit HH, Johnson TD, Suchard MA, Adler G. Metabolic and weight-loss effects of long-term dietary intervention in obese patients: four-year results. *Obes Res.* 2000;8:399-402.

60. Institute of Medicine. *Dietary Reference Intakes for Energy, Carbohydrate, Fiber, Fat, Fatty Acids, Cholesterol, Protein, and Amino Acids.* Washington, DC: National Academy Press, 2002.

61. Pi-Sunyer FX. Glycemic index and disease. *Am J Clin Nutr.* 2002;76(suppl):290S-298S.

62. Brand-Miller JC, Holt SH, Pawlak DB, McMillan J. Glycemic index and obesity. *Am J Clin Nutr.* 2002;76(suppl):281S-285S.

63. American Dietetic Association. Position paper: health implications of dietary fiber. *J Am Diet Assoc.* 2002;102:993-1000.

64. Krauss RM, Eckel RH, Howard B, Appel LJ, Daniels SR, Deckelbaum RJ, Erdman JW, Kris-Etherton P, Goldberg IJ, Kotchen TA, Lichtenstein AH, Mitch WE, Mullis R, Robinson K, Wylie-Rosett J, St Jeor S, Suttie J, Tribble DL, Bazzarre TL. AHA dietary guidelines. Revision 2000: a statement for healthcare professionals from the nutrition committee of the American Heart Association. *Circulation.* 2000;102:2284-2299.

65. American Diabetes Association Position Statement. Evidence-based nutrition principles and recommendations for the treatment and prevention of diabetes and related complications. *Diabetes Care.* 2002;25(suppl):S50-S60.

PART V

Special Populations and Cardiovascular Disease

CHAPTER 13

MANAGEMENT OF CARDIOVASCULAR DISEASE RISK IN CHILDREN AND ADOLESCENTS

Andrew M. Tershakovec, MD, and Frances M. Burke, MS, RD

The first observations linking diet with atherosclerosis were made in the early 20th century (1). During the last 30 to 40 years, several epidemiologic studies have solidified the evidence linking diet, blood cholesterol level, and risk of heart disease in adults (2-6). This link between diet and cholesterol levels has also been extended to children. Significant relationships between total fat and saturated fat intake, and cholesterol levels have been described in children of various ages (7,8). Furthermore, blood lipid levels correlate with the presence of early atherosclerotic changes in children and young adults (9,10).

This chapter summarizes the National Cholesterol Education Program (NCEP) (11), American Heart Association (AHA) (12), and American Academy of Pediatrics (AAP) (13) guidelines for the screening, prevention, and treatment of high blood cholesterol in children. It provides an update on current research on lipids and pediatric diets and provides practical advice and suggestions for clinical implementation.

ASSESSMENT ISSUES IN CHILDREN

Dietary Fat Intake in Children

Surveys from the 1970s and 1980s (14-16) revealed that children's diets contained about 36% of total energy as fat, and 13% to 14% of total energy as saturated fat. Data collected from the Third National Health and Nutrition Examination Survey (NHANES III) between 1988 and 1991 demonstrated a slightly lower fat intake for children and adolescents (33% to 34% of energy from fat, and 12% to 13% of energy from saturated fat) than previously described (17). A lower fat intake (29% to 30% of energy from fat) was reported for children living in a suburban, mostly white, middle-to-upper socioeconomic status neighborhood (18). African-American children and children of lower socioeconomic status may be less adherent to dietary recommendations regarding total fat and saturated fat intake (19). Given the high rates of nutrition-related chronic disease in adults from low-income populations, outreach to low-income groups defines an area of special importance for intervention efforts.

The average fat intake and mean blood cholesterol levels in adults are decreasing (20-22). Similar trends in diet and blood cholesterol levels have been described for children and adolescents (16,20,23). Despite these decreases, mean saturated fat intake levels remain above current dietary recommendations. Because there are links between diet and blood cholesterol level and because blood cholesterol level is related to risk for atherosclerosis and cardiovascular disease (CVD), expert groups recommend efforts to lower cholesterol levels in children and adolescents (11-13).

Blood Lipid Levels in Children

During the first few months of life, cholesterol levels increase largely because of changes in low-density lipoprotein (LDL) cholesterol. As children grow into adolescents and young adults, there is little change in the total cholesterol level; the mean value fluctuates around 150 to 165 mg/dL, whereas the mean LDL cholesterol level is slightly less than 100 mg/dL. As children grow older, high-density lipoprotein (HDL) cholesterol levels remain relatively constant in girls, but decline in boys during adolescence. Plasma triglyceride levels rise in both boys and girls in the first year of life, fall to a mean of 50 to 60 mg/dL during the next few years, and then rise to a mean of approximately 75 mg/dL by the end of adolescence. In early adulthood, the rise in plasma cholesterol is mostly due to an increase in LDL cholesterol. In adults, LDL cholesterol levels increase more in males than in females. Together with the lower HDL cholesterol levels of men, this gender difference helps define the higher risk for CVD in men, as compared with premenopausal women. Owing to the changes in lipid levels with age, it is more appropriate to use age- and gender-specific percentile figures when comparing levels between individuals and during long periods rather than consider absolute cholesterol levels (24). The NCEP report published data on children's blood lipid levels from the Lipid Research Clinics Prevalence Study (25). The mean cholesterol and serum triglyceride values by age and sex appear in Tables 13.1 through 13.4 (11).

Children with high cholesterol levels tend to have higher levels as young adults, whereas individuals with low levels as children tend to have lower levels as adults. However, biological and laboratory variations in cholesterol measurements contribute to less than perfect tracking. For these reasons and other considerations, expert panels have recommended targeted cholesterol screening in children (11-13).

Screening for Hyperlipidemia

The NCEP (11) and the AAP (13) recommend that children with a parental history of elevated total cholesterol levels (> 240 mg/dL) have their total cholesterol level measured. Children with incomplete or unavailable family histories and those with other risk factors for coronary heart disease (CHD) should be screened at the discretion of the medical care provider (see Box 13.1) (21,22). Cholesterol measurements can be relatively unreliable when undertaken without adequate quality assurance. To avoid inaccurately labeling children as hypercholesterolemic, screening should be completed using only reliable laboratories and methods.

Children with total cholesterol levels less than 170 mg/dL require no intervention other than that recommended for the general population and should be reevaluated every 5 years. Those with borderline levels (170 to 199 mg/dL) should have another total cholesterol measurement, and the two values should be averaged. If the average total cholesterol level in these

TABLE 13.1

Serum Total Cholesterol Levels in US Children and Adolescents*

Age (y)	n	Overall Mean (mg/dL)	Percentiles (mg/dL)						
			5	10	25	50	75	90	95
Males									
0–4	238	159	117	129	141	156	176	192	209
5–9	1253	165	125	134	147	164	180	197	209
10–14	2278	162	123	131	144	160	178	196	208
15–19	1980	154	116	124	136	150	170	188	203
Females									
0–4	186	161	115	124	143	161	177	195	206
5–9	1118	169	130	138	150	168	184	201	211
10–14	2087	164	128	135	148	163	179	196	207
15–19	2079	162	124	131	144	160	177	197	209

*All values have been converted from plasma to serum. Plasma value $\times$ 1.03 = Serum value.

Source: Reprinted from reference 11.

TABLE 13.2

Serum LDL Cholesterol Levels in US Children and Adolescents*

Age (y)	n	Overall Mean (mg/dL)	Percentiles (mg/dL)						
			5	10	25	50	75	90	95
White males									
5–9	131	95	65	71	82	93	106	121	133
10–14	284	99	66	74	83	97	112	126	136
15–19	298	97	64	70	82	96	112	127	134
White females									
5–9	114	103	70	75	91	101	118	129	144
10–14	244	100	70	75	83	97	113	130	140
15–19	294	99	61	67	80	96	114	133	141

Note: The number of children ages 0 to 4 years who had LDL and HDL cholesterol levels measured was too small to allow calculation of percentiles in this age group. However, the percentiles for total cholesterol (Table 13.1) for ages 0 to 4 years and 5 to 9 years are similar.

*All values have been converted from plasma to serum. Plasma value $\times$ 1.03 = Serum value.

Source: Reprinted from reference 11.

TABLE 13.3

Serum HDL Cholesterol Levels in US Children and Adolescents*

Age (y)	n	Overall Mean (mg/dL)	Percentiles (mg/dL)						
			5	10	25	50	75	90	95
White males									
5–9	142	57	39	43	50	56	65	72	76
10–14	296	57	38	41	47	57	63	73	76
15–19	299	48	31	35	40	47	54	61	65
White females									
5–9	124	55	37	39	48	54	63	69	75
10–14	247	54	38	41	46	54	60	66	72
15–19	295	54	36	39	44	53	63	70	76

Note: The number of children ages 0 to 4 years who had LDL and HDL cholesterol measured was too small to allow calculation of percentiles in this age group. However, the percentiles for total cholesterol (Table 13.1) for ages 0 to 4 years and 5 to 9 years are similar.

*All values have been converted from plasma to serum. Plasma value $\times$ 1.03 = Serum value.

Source: Reprinted from reference 11.

TABLE 13.4
Serum Triglyceride Levels in US Children and Adolescents

Age (y)	n	Overall Mean (mg/dL)	Percentiles (mg/dL)						
			5	10	25	50	75	90	95
Males									
0–4	238	58	30	34	41	53	69	87	102
5–9	1253	30	31	34	41	53	67	88	104
10–14	2278	68	33	38	46	61	80	105	129
15–19	1980	80	38	44	56	71	94	124	152
Females									
0–4	186	66	35	39	46	61	79	99	115
5–9	1118	30	33	37	45	57	73	93	108
10–14	2087	78	38	45	56	72	93	117	135
15–19	2079	78	40	45	55	70	90	117	136

*All values have been converted from plasma to serum. Plasma value $\times$ 1.03 = Serum value.

Source: Reprinted from reference 11.

two determinations is greater than 170 mg/dL, a lipid profile is recommended. Children whose total cholesterol level is greater than 200 mg/dL should have a fasting lipid profile performed (11,13).

A lipid profile (total and HDL cholesterol, triglycerides, calculated LDL cholesterol) is obtained after a 12-hour fast. LDL cholesterol is calculated using the following equation:

$$\text{LDL cholesterol} = \text{Total cholesterol} - [\text{HDL cholesterol} + (\text{Triglycerides}/5)]$$

Triglycerides must be less than 400 mg/dL to derive an accurate estimate of LDL cholesterol with this method (26).

Children with a family history of premature CHD (before the age of 55 years in a parent or grandparent) should also have a lipid profile completed. In such situations, the risk factors for premature CHD may be a low HDL cholesterol level, and the total cholesterol level may not be elevated. Use of the average values from two lipid profile evaluations is recommended before making treatment decisions because of the biological and laboratory variability in lipid values. Children with average LDL cholesterol levels greater than 130 mg/dL are considered to have elevated levels, whereas LDL cholesterol levels less than 110 mg/dL are considered acceptable. Levels between 110 and 130 mg/dL are borderline (11,13).

Box 13.1　Risk Factors for Premature Cardiovascular Disease

- Family history of premature coronary heart disease, cerebrovascular disease, or occlusive peripheral vascular disease (onset in siblings, parent, or parent of sibling before age 55 years)
- Cigarette smoking
- Elevated blood pressure
- Low high-density lipoprotein cholesterol level
- Severe obesity ($\geq$ 95th percentile body mass index–for-age)
- Diabetes mellitus
- Physical inactivity

Source: Data are from references 11 and 13.

The AHA has largely confirmed these recommendations, although the AHA guidelines recommend using the average of three lipid profile measurements before making therapeutic decisions (12). In addition, the AHA guidelines define a triglyceride level above 150 mg/dL as elevated, and an HDL cholesterol level below 35 mg/dL as abnormally low.

The NCEP pediatric cholesterol screening recommendations (11) have been criticized for several reasons. The screening protocol is complicated to follow, especially for a busy clinician. Surveys have shown that screening only children with a positive family history misses at least half, if not more, of hypercholesterolemic children (27,28). This problem is compounded by the fact that many adults do not know their cholesterol levels, along with the difficulties in obtaining a complete family medical history. In addition, many parents who may be at risk for CHD are too young to have acquired clinical heart disease when their children are being evaluated; therefore, their children may not be identified as being at risk. When considering screening recommendations, there is also the practical consideration that the health care system is not prepared to screen all children, and even less prepared to intervene in all the children confirmed to be at risk.

When a child has hyperlipidemia, appropriate screening and evaluation to rule out secondary hyperlipidemia should be considered. Lipid profile screening of parents and other first-degree relatives to assess for familial hyperlipidemia should also be considered. In addition to helping assess the child's risk, screens of family members may identify adults with hyperlipidemia who had not previously been identified.

PREVALENCE AND PREVENTION OF CHILDHOOD OBESITY

Tracking studies have demonstrated that an overweight child has an increased risk of becoming an overweight or obese adult. Because obese adults are also at increased risk for CVD and other diseases, primary prevention in childhood is highly desirable to help prevent CVD in adults (29). Such prevention can be efficacious and is safe and feasible even in very young children.

The prevalence of overweight and obesity among children and adults has increased significantly (30). Using age- and gender-specific body mass index (BMI) results from the 1999 to 2000 National Health and Nutrition Examination Survey (NHANES), it is estimated that 15% of children and adolescents aged 6 to 19 years (approximately 9 million) are overweight (refer to Table 13.5) (30,31). The rate has tripled since 1963. The rise in childhood overweight and obesity is thought to be the result of an increase in energy intake from easily accessible energy-dense foods and an increase in sedentary behavior. Despite declines in the percentages of both total and saturated fat intake, the amount of total energy intake has significantly increased, primarily from a higher carbohydrate intake (32). The health implications are enormous, as seen in the growing number of children diagnosed with type 2 diabetes (33).

In 2002 the Institute of Medicine released new dietary reference intakes (DRIs) for energy. The estimated energy recommendations for children and adolescents are based on gender, age, height, weight, and physical activity level (34).

MEASURING GROWTH IN CHILDREN

The National Center for Health Statistics has generated standard growth curves on the basis of height and weight data charted through time for thousands of boys and girls. These data

TABLE 13.5
Prevalence of Overweight among Children and Adolescents Ages 6 to 19 Years, for Selected Years 1963–1965 through 1999–2000

Age (y)*	1963–1965	1966–1970†	1971–1974	1976–1980	1988–1994	1999–2000
6–11	4		4	7	11	15
12–19	5		6	5	11	15

*Excludes pregnant women starting with 1971–1974. Pregnancy status not available for 1963–1965 and 1966–1970.

†Data for 1963–1965 are for children 6 to 11 years of age; data for 1966–1970 are for adolescents 12 to 17 years of age, not 12 to 19 years.

Source: Reprinted from reference 31.

provide useful comparisons for determining the adequacy of a child's growth rate. Regardless of the specific curve a child may follow (eg, 10th percentile or 95th percentile), the key factor in evaluating a child's growth rate is whether the child maintains the same position on the curve as he or she ages. New growth charts have been developed from data gathered by NHANES from 1971 to 1994 (Figures 13.1 and 13.2) (35). The revised growth charts include the addition of two new BMI-for-age charts for boys and girls, ages 2 to 20 years, which were developed to replace the weight-for-stature charts. This revision was probably the most significant, given that BMI, which evaluates weight in relation to height, is the most commonly used measure to determine overweight or obesity in adults and is also a useful measure in children. According to current guidelines (35), children with a BMI-for-age between the 85th and 95th percentiles are at risk of being overweight and children with a BMI-for-age at or above the 95th percentile are considered overweight. Health professionals should routinely measure height, weight, and BMI in children and adolescents. Monitoring a child's position on the relevant growth curve permits any deviation from the norm to be identified and addressed.

DIETARY RECOMMENDATIONS FOR CHILDREN AND ADOLESCENTS

The NCEP defines children with LDL cholesterol levels above the 75th percentile as hypercholesterolemic (11); theoretically, this means that 25% of children are at risk and thus eligible for individualized dietary intervention. Nutrition recommendations for healthy children (to be implemented from 2 to 5 years of age) have been developed to lower average population levels of blood cholesterol in children and adolescents, to reduce the incidence of adult CHD, and generally to improve health (11-13). These dietary recommendations also represent the first line of therapy for hypercholesterolemic children. According to NCEP and AAP guidelines for children with elevated cholesterol levels, the minimum goal for dietary intervention is to achieve an LDL cholesterol level below 130 mg/dL (approximately 95th percentile), although the LDL cholesterol level should ideally be below 110 mg/dL (11,13). The AHA guidelines set a goal of 160 mg/dL, and preferably 130 mg/dL (12).

Dietary recommendations (11,13) provide for no more than 30% (and no less than 20%) of total energy from fat, less than 10% of energy from saturated fat, and less than 300 mg cholesterol per day. The child's diet should include a wide variety of foods, provide adequate energy to support growth and development, and achieve and maintain a desirable body

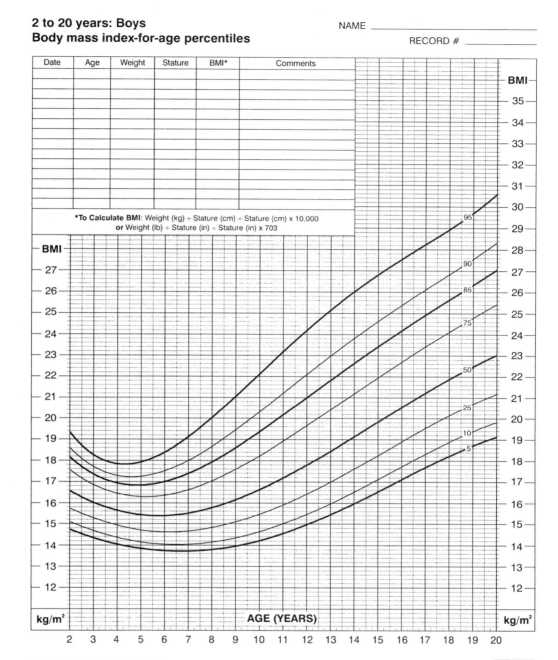

2 to 20 years: Boys
Body mass index-for-age percentiles

NAME _____

RECORD # _____

*To Calculate BMI: Weight (kg) ÷ Stature (cm) ÷ Stature (cm) x 10,000
or Weight (lb) ÷ Stature (in) ÷ Stature (in) x 703

Published May 30, 2000 (modified 10/16/00).
SOURCE: Developed by the National Center for Health Statistics in collaboration with
the National Center for Chronic Disease Prevention and Health Promotion (2000).
http://www.cdc.gov/growthcharts

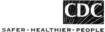

SAFER · HEALTHIER · PEOPLE™

FIGURE 13.1
Centers for Disease Control and Prevention growth chart: 2 to 20 years: boys body mass index-for-age percentiles. Available at: http://www.cdc.gov/nchs/data/nhanes/growthcharts/set1clinical/cj411023.pdf.

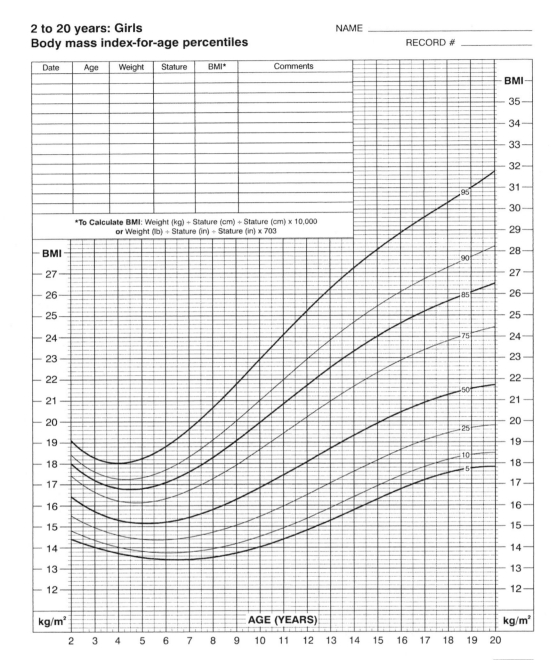

2 to 20 years: Girls
Body mass index-for-age percentiles

NAME _____

RECORD # _____

*To Calculate BMI: Weight (kg) ÷ Stature (cm) ÷ Stature (cm) x 10,000
or Weight (lb) ÷ Stature (in) ÷ Stature (in) x 703

Published May 30, 2000 (modified 10/16/00).
SOURCE: Developed by the National Center for Health Statistics in collaboration with
the National Center for Chronic Disease Prevention and Health Promotion (2000).
http://www.cdc.gov/growthcharts

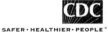

SAFER·HEALTHIER·PEOPLE™

FIGURE 13.2
Centers for Disease Control and Prevention growth chart: 2 to 20 years: girls body mass index-for-age percentiles. Available at: http://www.cdc.gov/nchs/data/nhanes/growthcharts/set1clinical/cj411024.pdf

weight. Because average daily energy intakes typically range from approximately 1,200 kcal for toddlers to 3,000 kcal for male teenagers, this translates to a suggested total daily fat intake of 40 to 100 g (13 to 33 g of saturated fat). These values are equivalent to approximately 30% and 10% of energy from total fat and saturated fat, respectively. If these LDL cholesterol goals are not achieved despite repeated attempts and adherence to the diet described above, a more restricted diet of less than 7% of energy from saturated fat and less than 200 mg of cholesterol per day should be considered. NCEP recommends 6 weeks to 3 months of dietary intervention before assessing blood lipid changes (11).

The Adult Treatment Panel III (ATP III) of the NCEP supports the implementation of the Therapeutic Lifestyle Changes (TLC) diet for individuals with hyperlipidemia and emphasizes the connection between hyperlipidemia and obesity and interventions to minimize metabolic syndrome (36). Dietary recommendations related to hypertriglyceridemia and low HDL cholesterol levels are more problematic. Although lower fat intake should be recommended, a high carbohydrate intake may be associated with elevations in triglyceride levels in some individuals. Similarly, a low-fat diet may be associated with lower HDL cholesterol levels. High triglyceride and low HDL cholesterol levels are relatively common in obesity. In such cases, weight loss is recommended (see Chapter 6).

The NCEP report on children and adolescents encourages the development of nutritious, good-tasting foods low in saturated fat and cholesterol that are appealing to children (11). The food industry has responded by introducing a wide range of fat-modified and fat-free products. However, the sudden influx of these products into the marketplace has generated some new concerns. As previously noted, total energy intake has risen during the last several years, driven significantly by increases in carbohydrate intake (32). The incidence of obesity in children is increasing, and effective interventions aimed at energy balance are urgently needed. Increased physical activity and a better understanding of nutrient composition are potentially the most effective strategies for weight control.

Children and their parents need to understand that fat-free does not mean calorie-free. Balance, variety, and moderation are still essential principles. Many children's diets are woefully inadequate in fresh fruits, vegetables, and whole grains. Increasing consumption of fruits, vegetables, low-fat yogurt, and other more healthful foods often requires more effort and forethought than purchasing prepared and processed foods, such as cookies, crackers, or chips, which are commonly less healthful. Box 13.2 provides examples of appropriate low-fat, low–saturated fat foods.

In 1995 the government made an important contribution toward improving nutrition awareness by passing the Nutrition Labeling and Education Act. Even among children, standardized, highly specific food labels can help facilitate adherence to dietary guidelines. Table 13.6 provides specific fat-gram equivalents that correspond to the goal of limiting fat intake to 30% of total energy. This information can help children and families make food selections that keep fat intake within that range.

DIET RECOMMENDATIONS FOR YOUNG CHILDREN

Children younger than 2 years grow very rapidly and require a relatively high energy intake. Owing to the high energy density of fat (9 kcal/g vs 4 kcal/g for carbohydrates and protein), it is recommended that children younger than 2 years eat a diet higher in fat, and thus a diet

TABLE 13.6
Shopping Guide to Reading Labels and Choosing Foods Wisely

Food	Recommendations
Cold cereals (eg, Cheerios,* oat bran cereal)	≤6 g sugar and ≥ 2 g of fiber per cup
Cheese	Part skim; ≤4-5 g fat per oz
Yogurt	≤3 g fat per 8 oz
Pancake mix	≤3 g fat per 3 pancakes
Packaged or canned sauces, soups, rice, and pasta side dishes	≤3 g fat/serving
Cookies, crackers (eg, animal and graham crackers, gingersnaps, oatmeal cookies, saltines, reduced-fat whole-grain crackers)	≤3 g fat per oz
Frozen desserts (eg, ice milk, sherbet, fruit and juice bars, frozen yogurt)	≤ 3 g fat per ½ cup
Lunch meats	≤ 2 g fat per oz

Note: As a general rule, choose food products with no more than 3 g of fat per serving.
*General Foods, Minneapolis, MN 55440.

that is more energy dense. The rapidly developing central nervous system of a young child also requires an adequate fatty acid intake (37). For these reasons, current recommendations do not limit fat intake of children younger than 2 years. However, there are data to suggest the safety of lower-fat diets for children younger than 2 years (38-41). Despite these reports of apparent safety, any attempts to implement such a diet with young children should be closely monitored and not recommended unless specifically indicated.

The US Department of Agriculture has developed a Food Guide Pyramid for Young Children (ages 2 to 6 years) based on the original Food Guide Pyramid released in 1992 and on actual food patterns of young children. Its purpose was to increase parent understanding and compliance of young children's nutritional needs through a simpler format of presentation. The Food Guide Pyramid for Young Children depicts typical foods eaten by children of this age group and shows children engaged in various physical activities. It focuses on the importance of eating a variety of foods to stay healthy, as well as the need for daily physical activity. It can be accessed at the Center for Nutrition Policy and Promotion Web site (http://www.cnpp.usda.gov) (42).

RESPONSE OF BLOOD LIPID LEVELS TO DIETARY CHANGE

Children with LDL cholesterol levels greater than the 90th percentile and a family history of premature heart disease who were advised to follow a diet containing less than 10% energy from saturated fat demonstrated an average decrease in LDL cholesterol of 12% (43). Response was independent of age, duration of therapy, and initial LDL cholesterol level but varied significantly from individual to individual. Similar results have been described elsewhere (44).

Dietary response may differ by type of hyperlipidemia. For example, children with heterozygous familial hypercholesterolemia (FH) demonstrated a mean decrease in LDL cholesterol of 8% (after dietary intervention, none were below the 90th percentile), whereas for those with familial combined hyperlipidemia (FCHL), mean LDL cholesterol levels decreased 13% (45% were below the 90th percentile after dietary intervention) (43). Widhalm

> **Box 13.2 Low-Fat, Low–Saturated Fat Food Suggestions for Children and Adolescents**
>
> Milk
> - Low-fat milk (1%)
> - Nonfat milk (skim)
>
> Meat and meat alternates
> - Lean cuts of meat, such as eye round or round steak, round rump roast, round tip roast, and tenderloin roast
> - Extra lean ground beef (95% extra lean), ground turkey breast, or textured soy protein based burgers
> - Chicken or turkey without skin, baked, broiled, roasted, or boiled
> - Lean boiled ham
> - Fresh or frozen fish baked, broiled, or poached
> - Tuna or salmon
> - Cooked dry beans and peas, such as great northern, kidney, lima, navy, pinto, red, black, and garbanzo beans, black-eyed peas, lentils, and split peas
> - Low-fat and part-nonfat cheeses: farmer, cottage, part-skim ricotta, and part-skim mozzarella
> - Peanut butter
>
> Bread and bread alternates
> - Enriched breads and bread products: bagels, breads, english muffins, rolls; encourage whole-grain sources
> - Noodles, rice, barley, pasta, and bulgur
>
> Fruits and vegetables
> - Fresh, frozen, dried, or canned fruits: apricots, cantaloupe, grapefruit, grapes, honeydew melon, peaches, plums, prunes, raisins, tangerines, and strawberries
> - Fresh, frozen, or canned fruit juice
> - Fresh, frozen, or canned vegetables and salads: broccoli, brussels sprouts, cabbage, carrots, cauliflower, corn, green beans, green peas, green pepper, potatoes, lettuce, okra, spinach, sweet potatoes, tomatoes, winter squash, zucchini
>
> Fats
> - Mayonnaise and dressings, including reduced-calorie and modified-fat, light, or low-sodium salad dressings
> - *Trans* fat–free margarine or liquid vegetable oils: canola, corn, cottonseed, olive, peanut, and safflower oils
>
> Other
> - Baked goods low in fat, including angel food cake, fig cookies, ginger snaps, animal crackers, and graham crackers
> - Baked chips; homemade trail mix made from nuts, dried fruit, and pretzels
> - Popcorn without butter, flavored rice cakes
> - Low-fat granola bars
> - Ice milk, sherbet, low-fat puddings, and low-fat yogurt

(45) reported similar results when reviewing outpatient trials of dietary intervention for FH children but found significantly larger average responses (eg, mean decrease in LDL cholesterol of 24%) in trials completed with inpatients. Greater compliance and more controlled conditions may be responsible for this difference in observed response between the outpatient and inpatient setting.

The Diet Intervention Study in Children (DISC) (46,47) is the largest study to address questions of efficacy, safety, and feasibility of diet intervention in a cohort of 663 growing adolescent children with elevated LDL cholesterol. Children were randomly assigned to a diet containing 30% energy from total fat, less than 7% energy from saturated fat, and 200 mg cholesterol for 3 years. Mean level of total fat intake in the intervention group was 28.6% of total energy at 3 years, vs 33.0% in the usual care group. The mean net change in LDL cholesterol levels for the intervention group was 0.08 mmol/L (3.23 mg/dL) lower than the change for the control group. In addition, there were no differences in any of the growth or psychosocial parameters measured. Thus, DISC demonstrated that dietary intervention patterned on a low-saturated fat, low cholesterol diet can be safely implemented.

OTHER NONPHARMACOLOGIC APPROACHES TO LOWERING CHOLESTEROL IN CHILDREN

Dietary fiber, especially soluble fiber (such as oat bran), has been shown to have a moderate cholesterol-lowering effect in hypercholesterolemic adults (48-52). Experience with fiber supplementation in children is much more limited (53-55) and the results somewhat mixed. Very-high-fiber diets may limit energy density and impair micronutrient absorption (56). However, children treated for severe constipation with a high-fiber diet, laxatives, and mineral oil did not suffer from nutritional inadequacies when followed for a 6-month period (57). A fiber intake (in grams) of five plus the child's age (in years) has been recommended for children older than 2 years (12,58). For example, a 5-year-old child should eat approximately 10 g of fiber daily.

The efficacy of a vegetarian diet in lowering cholesterol levels in children has been demonstrated (59-61). The low-cholesterol, low-fat, high polyunsaturated-to-saturated fat ratio, high-fiber, and high-micronutrient content may each have positive health effects by lowering cholesterol levels and by other mechanisms (62,63). Concerns about a vegetarian diet for children include the low energy density and high bulk of the diet, its phytate content, and other factors limiting micronutrient absorption, as well as the potential for vitamin B-12 deficiency in individuals on a completely vegan diet (56). However, well-controlled studies have shown that children following appropriate vegetarian diets can grow and develop normally despite being leaner than their meat-eating counterparts (64). Because vegetarian diets have become more popular with teenagers in recent years, this may be a helpful approach for lowering cholesterol in this age group.

Soy protein, in place of animal protein, has been shown to decrease total cholesterol, LDL cholesterol, and triglyceride levels, while not lowering HDL cholesterol levels (65-68). This effect may be partially dependent on the isoflavone content of the soy protein; isoflavones have weak estrogenic activity. It should be noted that some processed soy food products lose much of the isoflavone content during production. The evidence supporting the positive effects of soy protein on blood lipid levels is so strong that the Food and Drug Administration (FDA) has approved food label claims for reduced CVD risk for food containing at least 6.25 g of soy protein per serving (69). Although limited data exist regarding soy protein intake and children, incorporation of soy protein into a complete and balanced diet is appropriate for children. The availability of soy products in the supermarket, including soy milk, soy nuts, tofu, and tofu products (cheese and hot dogs), allows them to be easily incorporated in the diet. (See Chapter 10 for more information on soy.)

Data suggest that some nutritional supplements, such as fish oil, antioxidants, and folic acid, are associated with a lower risk of CVD in adults by mechanisms largely independent of lowering blood lipid levels (70-75). Fish oil supplements have also been used to lower triglyceride levels in adults with hypertriglyceridemia. The potentially therapeutic effects of fish oil and antioxidants have been generally demonstrated with doses much larger than can practically be provided in a child's diet. Also, more recent data, including intervention trials, have raised questions regarding the efficacy of antioxidant supplementation in adults (76). Thus, without more safety and efficacy information concerning the ingestion of such large, "therapeutic" amounts of these substances (eg, fish oil or vitamin pills) in children and adults, the use of such potentially therapeutic food supplements should be discouraged in favor of optimized dietary patterns. Diets with recommended amounts of fruits and vegetables optimize natural sources of antioxidants. This, combined with regular intake of fish and olive oil (as seen with the Mediterranean diet), can safely be recommended for children and adolescents as part of an overall balanced diet. (See Chapter 10 for discussion of fish oil and Chapter 11 for discussion of antioxidants, folate, and other nutritional supplements.)

Food products enriched with plant stanols and sterols have a cholesterol-lowering effect (77-80). However, owing to concerns related to the absorption of fat-soluble micronutrients, as well as lower serum antioxidant levels associated with the use of these plant stanol and sterol ester spreads in children (80), such products should be carefully used in children. (See Chapter 10 for more information on plant stanols and sterols.)

DRUG THERAPY

NCEP (11) recommends that drug therapy be considered in children aged 10 years and older after an adequate trial (6 to 12 months) of diet therapy. Drug therapy should be initiated if (*a*) the LDL cholesterol level remains greater than 190 mg/dL, or (*b*) the LDL cholesterol level remains greater than 160 mg/dL, and there is a positive family history of premature CHD (before 55 years of age) or two or more other risk factors are present in the child or adolescent after vigorous attempts have been made to control these risk factors (diabetes, hypertension, smoking, low HDL cholesterol, severe obesity, physical inactivity). It should be noted that the ATP III recommends an LDL cholesterol level less than 160 mg/dL for adults with no more than one CHD risk factor (36).

There are two main options in drug therapy for severe hypercholesterolemia in children—bile acid sequestrants or 3-hydroxy-3-methylglutaryl coenzyme A (HMG-CoA) reductase inhibitors (statins). Bile acid sequestrants, or resins (cholestyramine or colestipol), primarily reduce LDL cholesterol levels and may exacerbate hypertriglyceridemia. These compounds bind bile acids in the intestine and are excreted in the stool unabsorbed, thus interrupting the enterohepatic bile acid recycling. This results in increased hepatic bile acid synthesis, secondary upregulation of hepatic LDL receptors, increased uptake of LDL from the blood, and reduction of LDL cholesterol levels. A 10% to 32% decrease in LDL cholesterol levels has been reported with cholestyramine therapy in children with FH and FCHL (81). However, long-term compliance with the bile acid sequestrants has been poor because of poor palatability of the medication and gastrointestinal disturbances, including nausea, bloating, and constipation.

One potential advantage of the bile acid sequestrants is that they are not systemically absorbed. However, they are insoluble resins that must be suspended in liquid and therefore can be inconvenient and unpleasant to take. (Tablets may be preferred by some patients for this reason, but the large size of the tablets may limit their use in children.) In addition, bile acid sequestrants may bind some other drugs and interfere with their absorption. Similarly, these resins may interfere with the absorption of fat-soluble vitamins. Therefore, to avoid resin-binding and the malabsorption of fat-soluble vitamins, patients should not take bile acid sequestrants and multivitamin supplements at the same time of day.

The FDA has approved several statin medications for use in children and adolescents. HMG-CoA reductase is the rate-limiting step in cholesterol biosynthesis, and inhibition of this enzyme decreases cholesterol synthesis and results in upregulation of hepatic LDL receptors. In one clinical trial, LDL cholesterol levels decreased by 21% to 36% (dose response–related) in boys with FH taking a daily dose of 10 to 40 mg lovastatin. No serious side effects were noted during the 8-week follow-up period (82).

The most significant side effects of statins include hepatotoxicity and severe myopathy or rhabdomyolysis. The risk of severe myopathy may be increased in patients taking certain other drugs, such as erythromycin, antifungal agents, immunosuppressive agents, and fibric acid derivatives such as gemfibrozil and niacin. Liver transaminases should be monitored in patients taking statins, but significant (> 3 times normal) elevation in transaminase levels is rare in children. The potential for myopathy should be evaluated for subjects with symptoms consistent with myopathy, such as muscle pain and weakness.

Nicotinic acid is also frequently used in adults; however, its side effects (flushing, gastrointestinal upset, hepatic toxicity) may preclude its use in children. The practicing pediatrician should consider referral of all children who may be candidates for drug therapy to a specialized lipid center.

Although drug therapy is used commonly to treat hypertriglyceridemia in adults, drug therapy for hypertriglyceridemia is used much less commonly in children. The mainstay of therapy in children with hypertriglyceridemia is diet, with the focus on reducing intake of simple sugars, exercise, and weight loss. In severe cases of hypertriglyceridemia in children (> 400 mg/dL), drug therapy may be considered to protect against severe postprandial hypertriglyceridemia and an increased risk of pancreatitis (13).

DIET MODIFICATION, NUTRIENT ADEQUACY, AND FAILURE TO THRIVE

A major concern relating to dietary intervention in children is whether such an altered diet can be nutritionally complete and balanced and support normal growth and development. Investigators evaluating children's diets and targets of dietary intervention have noted that the major sources of fat in children's diets are dairy products, meats, fast food, and snack foods, and the major sources of cholesterol are eggs and whole milk (19,82). Sigman-Grant and associates studied common strategies used to meet dietary fat and cholesterol recommendations for young (2- to 5-year-old) children, such as replacing high-fat meats with low-fat meats; replacing high-fat milk with nonfat milk; or using fat-modified products and low-fat preparation techniques while limiting added fat. These investigators concluded that it was difficult to both meet recommendations for fat and cholesterol intake for the 2- and 3-year-old children and provide a complete and balanced diet when applying these simple, broad strategies (83). However, for the 4- to 5-year-old children, simply switching to nonfat milk brought the diet into the recommended range for fat and cholesterol intake. Multiple combined strategies (eg, a diet including lean meats, low-fat cheeses, egg substitutes, fat-modified products, and nonfat milk) resulted in very-low-fat diets providing 17% energy as fat, which may not provide adequate energy for some 4- to 5-year-old children.

In real-life settings, lower-fat diets were shown to be potentially less complete and balanced than higher-fat diets (84). However, studies have demonstrated that children and families, provided with appropriate guidance, can safely lower the fat content of children's diet (46,47,85-87).

In addition, normal growth has been observed in children following lower-fat diets, despite significant dietary variation (64,88,89). These findings of normal growth and development have been replicated for children of various ages undergoing active dietary intervention (38,39,41,46,87,90).

SUMMARY OF SAFE DIETARY INTERVENTION FOR CHILDREN

Owing to the potential for inadequate or inappropriate dietary restrictions provided by well-meaning but uninformed caretakers, dietary modification in children must be undertaken with care. At a minimum, growth and development should be monitored using growth charts and dietary intake should be periodically assessed to prevent subtle inadequacies from progressing. Because most physicians rate themselves as unable to provide effective dietary counseling (91,92), making referrals to qualified pediatric dietitians is a useful strategy. Unfortunately, few such dietitians are available outside of tertiary care pediatric medical centers, and even when they are available, access to them is limited by inadequate support of third-party payers for dietitian's services.

As part of anticipatory guidance, primary care providers should educate children and families about a healthy lifestyle and encourage them to adopt these guidelines into their everyday life. These lifestyle changes should be routine for all family members to prevent the child from feeling singled out. Praising positive behaviors, providing positive role models, and establishing an environment that supports these lifestyle changes help to enhance self-esteem and build confidence. These influences begin early in life; dietary intake and physical activity of 3-year-old children have been associated with potential risk factors for obesity (93,94). The importance of parental influence on these behaviors should also be emphasized. For example, children whose mothers exert more control on their food intake seem to have less internal control on their own dietary intake (93). In addition, parental physical activity is strongly associated with the physical activity of the child (95), and parental participation in weight management programs for children has been associated with improved outcome (96,97). Although parents may express limited interest in adopting a healthy lifestyle for themselves, in the authors' experience, parents are more open to lifestyle changes that help their children.

If a child is identified as hypercholesterolemic, although the primary care provider may consider initiating dietary intervention, referral to a pediatric lipid referral center should be considered. These centers are better staffed to provide more complete dietary recommendations, assess compliance, and ensure that the child is ingesting a complete and balanced diet. Such referral is essential if a child requires the TLC diet approach and for children in the range where medications may be considered (ie, children older than 10 years who have LDL cholesterol levels greater than 160 mg/dL and other CVD risk factors as well as children with LDL cholesterol levels greater than 190 mg/dL but no other CVD risk factors) (11). Primary care providers should promote a healthy lifestyle for all children, and especially those with hyperlipidemia. In addition, efforts to limit other risk factors for CVD (refer to Box 13.1) should be implemented.

With the wide availability of healthful, affordable food in developed countries, caregivers should not find it difficult to provide children with a healthful and appealing broad-based diet that includes all the food groups. Parents of hypercholesterolemic children and the children themselves report that following a lower-fat diet is not a major problem and that the diet was good for the child and the family as a whole (98).

In addition to such practical factors, it is important to help the child and family keep the dietary recommendations in perspective. If a child is found to have an elevated cholesterol level, it should be emphasized that hypercholesterolemia is one of several risk factors for premature heart disease and will have little immediate effect on a child's health. It is important to avoid negative psychosocial aspects of labeling, as has been noted with other medical conditions (99). In any dietary intervention program for children, the goal is to make gradual changes with which the child and family can comply. Encourage family support and role modeling. This helps the child develop a lifelong habit of eating and enjoying healthful foods. Following a healthy lifestyle should not be seen as a burden but as an opportunity to help ensure a long and pleasurable life.

REFERENCES

1. Committee on Diet and Health, Food and Nutrition Board, Commission on Life Sciences, National Research Council. Evidence associating dietary fats and other lipids with chronic diseases. In: *Diet and Health*. 3rd ed. Washington, DC: National Academy Press; 1989:159-258.
2. Keys A. Coronary heart disease in seven countries. *Circulation*. 1970;41(suppl):S11-S1211.
3. Keys A. *Seven Countries: A Multivariate Analysis of Death and Coronary Heart Disease*. Cambridge, Mass: Harvard University Press; 1980.
4. Castelli WP, Garrison RJ, Wilson PW, Abbott RD, Kalousdian S, Kannel WB. Incidence of coronary heart disease and lipoprotein cholesterol levels. The Framingham Study. *JAMA*. 1986;256:2835-2838.
5. Neaton JD, Wentworth D. Serum cholesterol, blood pressure, cigarette smoking, and death from coronary heart disease. *Arch Intern Med*. 1992;152:56-64.
6. Nichaman MZ, Hamilton HB, Kagan A, Grier T, Sacks T, Syme SL. Epidemiologic studies of coronary heart disease and stroke in Japanese men living in Japan, Hawaii, and California: distribution of biochemical risk factors. *Am J Epidemiol*. 1975;102:491-501.
7. Shea S, Basch CE, Irigoyen M, Zybert P, Rips JL, Contento I, Gutin B. Relationships of dietary fat consumption to serum total and low-density lipoprotein cholesterol in Hispanic preschool children. *Prev Med*. 1991;20:237-249.
8. Nicklas TA, Farris RP, Smoak CG, Frank GC, Srinivasan SR, Webber LS, Berenson GS. Dietary factors relate to cardiovascular risk factors in early life. Bogalusa Heart Study. *Arteriosclerosis*. 1988;8:193-199.
9. McGill HC Jr, McMahan CA, Zieske AW, Tracy RE, Malcom GT, Herderick EE, Strong JP. Association of coronary heart disease risk factors with microscopic qualities of coronary atherosclerosis in youth. *Circulation*. 2000;102:374-379.
10. Newman WP, Freedman DS, Voors AW, Gard PD, Srinivasan SR, Cresanta JL, Williamson GD, Webber LS, Berenson GS. Relation of serum lipoprotein levels and systolic blood pressure to early atherosclerosis: the Bogalusa Heart Study. *N Engl J Med*. 1986;314:138-144.
11. American Academy of Pediatrics. National Cholesterol Education Program (NCEP). Report of the Expert Panel on Blood Cholesterol Levels in Children and Adolescents. *Pediatrics*. 1992;89:525-584.
12. Kavey RW, Daniels SR, Lauer RM, Atkins DL, Hayman LL, Taubert K. American Heart Association guidelines for primary prevention of atherosclerotic cardiovascular disease beginning in childhood. *J Pediatr*. 2003;142:368-372.
13. American Academy of Pediatrics Committee on Nutrition. Cholesterol in children. *Pediatrics*. 1998;101:141-147.
14. Kimm SYS, Gergen PJ, Malloy M, Dresser C, Carroll M. Dietary patterns of US children: implications for disease prevention. *Prev Med*. 1990;19:432-442.
15. McPherson RS, Nichaman MZ, Kohl HW, Reed DB, Labarthe DR. Intake and food sources of dietary fat among schoolchildren in the Woodlands, Texas. *Pediatrics*. 1990;86:520-526.

16. Nicklas TA, Webber LS, Srinivasan SR, Berenson GS. Secular trends in dietary intake and cardiovascular risk factors of 10-year-old children: the Bogalusa Heart Study (1973–1988). *Am J Clin Nutr.* 1993;57:930-937.

17. Lenfant C, Ernst N. Daily dietary fat and total food-energy intakes: Third National Health and Nutrition Examination Survey, Phase 1, 1988–1991. *MMWR Morb Mortal Wkly Rep.* 1994;43:116.

18. Tershakovec AM, Mitchell DC, Smiciklas-Wright H, Martel JK, McKenzie MJ, Shannon BM. Pediatric preventive health screening and dietary intake. *Nutr Res.* 1997;17:1239-1247.

19. Thompson FE, Dennison BA. Dietary sources of fats and cholesterol in US children aged 2 through 5 years. *Am J Public Health.* 1994;84:799-806.

20. McDowell MA, Briefel RR, Alaimo K, Bischof AM, Caughman CR, Carroll MD. Energy and macronutrient intakes of persons ages 2 months and over in the United States: Third National Health and Nutrition Examination Survey, Phase 1, 1988–1991. *Adv Data.* October 24, 1994;(255):1-24.

21. Stephen AM, Wald NJ. Trends in individual consumption of dietary fat in the United States, 1920–1984. *Am J Clin Nutr.* 1990;52:457-469.

22. Johnson CL, Rifkind BM, Sempos CT, Carroll MD, Bachorik PS, Briefel RR, Gordon DJ, Burt VL, Brown CD, Lippel K, Cleeman JI. Declining serum total cholesterol levels among US adults. *JAMA.* 1993;269:3002-3008.

23. Hickman TB, Briefel RR, Carroll MD, Rifkind BM, Cleeman JI, Maurer KR, Johnson CL. Distributions and trends of serum lipid levels among United States children and adolescents ages 4–19 years: Data from the Third National Health and Nutrition Examination Survey. *Prev Med.* 1998;27:879-890.

24. Tershakovec AM, Rader DJ. Disorders of lipoprotein metabolism and transport. In: Behrman RE, Kliegman RM, Jenson HB, eds. *Nelson Textbook of Pediatrics.* 17th ed. Philadelphia, Pa: Saunders; 2004:445-459.

25. National Heart, Lung, and Blood Institute. *The Lipid Research Clinics Population Studies Data Book: Volume I—The Prevalence Study.* Bethesda, Md: National Institutes of Health; 1980. NIH publication 80-1527.

26. Friedewald WT, Levy RI, Fredrickson DS. Estimation of the concentration of low-density lipoprotein cholesterol in plasma, without use of the preparative ultracentrifuge. *Clin Chem.* 1972;18:499-502.

27. Dennison BA, Kikuchi DA, Srinivasan SR, Webber LS, Berenson GS. Parental history of cardiovascular disease as an indication for screening for lipoprotein abnormalities in children. *J Pediatr.* 1989;115:186-194.

28. Garcia RE, Moodie DS. Routine cholesterol surveillance in childhood. *Pediatrics.* 1989;84:751-755.

29. American Academy of Pediatrics Committee on Nutrition. Prevention of pediatric overweight and obesity. *Pediatrics.* 2003;112:424-430.

30. Ogden CL, Flegal KM, Carroll MD, Johnson CI. Prevalence and trends in overweight among US children and adolescents, 1999–2000. *JAMA.* 2002;288:1728-1732.

31. National Center for Health Statistics. Prevalence of overweight among children and adolescents: United States, 1999–2000. Available at: http://www.cdc.gov/nchs/products/pubs/pubd/hestats/overwght99.htm. Accessed April 15, 2004.

32. Chanmugam P, Guthrie JF. Did fat intake in the US really decline between 1989–1991 and 1994–1996? *J Am Diet Assoc.* 2003;103:867-872.

33. Pinhas-Hamiel O, Dolan LM, Daniels SR, Standiford D, Khoury PR, Zeitler P. Increased incidence of non-insulin dependent diabetes mellitus among adolescents. *J Pediatr.* 1996;128:608-615.

34. Institute of Medicine. *Dietary Reference Intakes for Energy, Carbohydrate, Fiber, Fat, Fatty Acids, Cholesterol, Protein, and Amino Acids (Macronutrients).* Washington, DC: National Academy Press; 2002.

35. Centers for Disease Control and Prevention. National Center for Health Statistics Web site. Available at: http://www.cdc.gov/growthcharts. Accessed October 15, 2003.

36. Expert Panel on Detection, Evaluation, and Treatment of High Blood Cholesterol in Adults. Executive summary of the Third Report of the National Cholesterol Education Program (NCEP) Expert Panel on Detection, Evaluation, and Treatment of High Blood Cholesterol in Adults (Adult Treatment Panel III). *JAMA.* 2001;285:2486-2497. Full report: National Institutes of Health. *Third Report of the National Cholesterol Education Program Expert Panel on Detection, Evaluation, and Treatment of High Blood Cholesterol in Adults (Adult Treatment Panel III).* Bethesda, Md: National Institutes of Health; 2001. NIH Publication 01-3670. Available at: http://www.nhlbi.nih.gov/guidelines/cholesterol/atp3_rpt.htm. Accessed March 29, 2004.

37. Hamosh, M. Fat needs for term and preterm infants. In: Tsang R, Nichols B, eds. *Nutrition during Pregnancy.* Philadelphia, Pa: Hanley & Belfus, Inc; 1988:133-159.

38. Niinikoski H, Lapinleimu H, Viikari J, Ronnemaa T, Jokinen E, Seppanen R, Terho P, Tuominen J, Valimaki I, Simell O. Growth until 3 years of age in a prospective, randomized trial of a diet with reduced saturated fat and cholesterol. *Pediatrics.* 1997;99:687-694.

39. Rask-Nissila L, Jokinen E, Ronnemaa T, Viikari J, Tammi A, Niinikoski H, Seppanen R, Tuominen J, Simell O. Prospective, randomized, infancy-onset trial of the effects of a low-saturated-fat, low-cholesterol diet on serum lipids and lipoproteins before school age: the Special Turku Coronary Risk Factor Intervention Project (STRIP). *Circulation.* 2000;102:1477-1483.

40. Niinikoski H, Viikari J, Ronnemaa T, Helenius H, Jokinen E, Lapinleimu H, Routi T, Lagstrom H, Seppa-

nen R, Valimaki I, Simell O. Regulation of growth of 7- to 36-month-old children by energy and fat intake in the prospective, randomized STRIP baby trial. *Pediatrics.* 1997;100:810-816.

41. Lagstrom H, Seppanen R, Jokinen E, Niinikoski H, Ronnemaa T, Viikari J, Simell O. Influence of dietary fat on the nutrient intake and growth of children from 1 to 5 years of age: the Special Turku Coronary Risk Factor Intervention Project. *Am J Clin Nutr.* 1999;69:516-523.

42. USDA Center for Nutrition Policy and Promotion Web site. The food guide pyramid for young children. Available at: http://www.cnpp.usda.gov. Accessed October 15, 2003.

43. Cortner JA, Coates PM, Cryer DR, Faulkner A, Sasanow SR, Warman N. Reduction of low-density lipoprotein cholesterol by dietary intervention in children at high risk for premature coronary artery disease. In: Gallo L, ed. *Cardiovascular Disease.* New York, NY: Plenum Press; 1987:515-520.

44. Quivers ES, Driscoll DJ, Garvey CD, Harrist AM, Harrison J, Huse DM, Murtaugh P, Weidman WH. Variability in response to a low-fat, low-cholesterol diet in children with elevated low-density lipoprotein cholesterol levels. *Pediatrics.* 1992;89:925-929.

45. Widhalm K. Effect of diet on serum lipoproteins in children with various forms of hyperlipidemias. In: *Detection and Treatment of Lipid and Lipoprotein Disorders of Childhood.* New York, NY: Alan R. Liss, Inc; 1985:145-149.

46. Obarzanek EO, Hunsberger SA, Van Horn LV, Hartmuller VV, Barton BA, Stevens VJ, Kwiterovich PO, Franklin FA, Kimm SYS, Lasser NL, Simons-Morton DG, Lauer RM. Safety of a fat-reduced diet: the Dietary Intervention Study in Children (DISC). *Pediatrics.* 1997;100:51-59.

47. Obarzanek EO, Kimm SY, Barton BA, Van Horn LL, Kwiterovick PO, Simons-Morton DG, Hunsberger SA, Lasser NL, Robson AM, Franklin FA, Lauer RM, Stevens VJ, Friedman LA, Dorgan JF, Greenlick MR, DISC Collaborative Research Group. Long-term safety and efficacy of a cholesterol-lowering diet in children with elevated low-density lipoprotein cholesterol: seven-year results of the Dietary Intervention Study in Children (DISC). *Pediatrics.* 2001;107:256-264.

48. Anderson JW, Gilinsky NH, Deakins A, Smith SF, O'Neal DS, Dillon DW, Oeltgen PR. Lipid responses of hypercholesterolemic men to oat-bran and wheat-bran intake. *Am J Clin Nutr.* 1991;54:678-683.

49. Anderson JW, Riddell-Mason S, Gustafson NJ, Smith SF, Mackey M. Cholesterol-lowering effects of psyllium-enriched cereal as an adjunct to a prudent diet in the treatment of mild to moderate hypercholesterolemia. *Am J Clin Nutr.* 1992;56:93-98.

50. Jenkins DJ, Wolever TM, Rao AV, Hegele RA, Mitchell SJ, Ransom TP, Boctor DL, Spadafora PJ, Jenkins AL, Mehling C, Relle LK, Connelly PW, Story JA, Furumoto EJ, Corey P, Wursch P. Effect on blood lipids of very high intakes of fiber in diets low in saturated fat and cholesterol. *N Engl J Med.* 1993;329:21-26.

51. McIntosh GH, Whyte J, McArthur R, Nestel PJ. Barley and wheat foods: Influence on plasma cholesterol concentrations in hypercholesterolemic men. *Am J Clin Nutr.* 1991;53:1205-1209.

52. Ripsin CM, Keenan JM, Jacobs DR, Elmer PJ, Welch RR, Van Horn L, Liu K, Turnbull WH, Thye FWM, Kestin M, Hegsted M, Davidson DM, Davidson MH, Dugan LD, Denmark-Wahnefried W, Beling S. Oat products and lipid lowering. *JAMA.* 1992;267:3317-3325.

53. Davidson MH, Dugan LD, Burns JH, Story K, Bova J, Drennan KB. A psyllium-containing cereal for the treatment of hypercholesterolemia in children. *Clin Res.* 1992;40:A625.

54. Dennison BA, Levine DM. Randomized, double-blind, placebo-controlled, two-period crossover clinical trial of psyllium fiber in children with hypercholesterolemia. *J Pediatr.* 1993;123:24-29.

55. Glassman M, Spark A, Berezin S, Schwarz S, Medow M, Newman LJ. Treatment of type IIa hyperlipidemia in childhood by a simplified American Heart Association diet and fiber supplementation. *Am J Dis Child.* 1990;144:973-976.

56. Sanders TA, Reddy S. Vegetarian diets and children. *Am J Clin Nutr.* 1994;59(suppl):1176S-1181S.

57. McClung HJ, Boyne LJ, Linsheid T, Heitlinger LA, Murray RD, Fyda J, Li BU. Is combination therapy for encopresis nutritionally safe? *Pediatrics.* 1993;91:591-594.

58. Williams CL, Bollella M, Wynder EL. A new recommendation for dietary fiber in childhood. *Pediatrics.* 1995;96:985-988.

59. Fernandes J, Dijkhuis-Stoffelsma R, Groot PHE, Grose WFA, Ambagtsheer JJ. The effect of a virtually cholesterol-free, high linoleic-acid vegetarian diet on serum lipoproteins of children with familial hypercholesterolemia (type II-A). *Acta Paediatr Scand.* 1981;70:677-682.

60. Gaddi A, Descovich GC, Noseda G, Fragiacomo C, Nicolini A, Montanari G, Vanetti G, Sortori M, Gatti E, Sirtori CR. Hypercholesterolemia treated by soybean protein diet. *Arch Dis Child.* 1987;62:274-278.

61. Widhalm K, Brazda G, Schneider B, Kohl S. Effect of soy protein diet versus standard low fat, low cholesterol diet on lipid and lipoprotein levels in children with familial or polygenic hypercholesterolemia. *J Pediatr.* 1993;123:30-34.

62. Anderson JW, Smith BM, Gustafson NJ. Health benefits and practical aspects of high-fiber diets. *Am J Clin Nutr.* 1994;59(suppl):1242S-1247S.

63. Fraser GE. Diet and coronary heart disease: beyond dietary fats and low-density-lipoprotein cholesterol. *Am J Clin Nutr.* 1994;59(suppl):1117S-1123S.

64. Sabate J, Lindsted KD, Harris RD, Johnston PK. Anthropometric parameters of school children with different life-styles. *Am J Dis Child.* 1990;144:1159-1163.

65. Anderson JW, Johnstone BM, Cook-Newell MD. Meta-analysis of the effects of soy protein intake on serum lipids. *N Engl J Med.* 1995;333:276-282.

66. Baum JA, Teng H, Erdman JW Jr, Weigel RM, Klein BP, Persky VW, Freels S, Surya P, Bakhit RM, Ramos

E, Shay NF, Potter SM. Long-term intake of soy protein improves blood lipid profiles and increases mononuclear cell low-density-lipoprotein receptor messenger RNA in hypercholesterolemic, post-menopausal
women. *Am J Clin Nutr.* 1998;68:545-551.

67. Crouse JR, Morgan T, Terry JG, Ellis J, Vitolins M, Burke JL. A randomized trial comparing the effect of
casein with that of soy protein containing varying amounts of isoflavones on plasma concentrations of lipids
and lipoproteins. *Arch Intern Med.* 1999;159:2070-2076.

68. Teixeira SR, Potter SM, Weigel R, Hannum S, Erdman JW, Hasler CM. Effects of feeding 4 levels of soy protein for 3 and 6 weeks on blood lipids and apolipoproteins in moderately hypercholesterolemic men. *Am J
Clin Nutr.* 2000;71:1077-1084.

69. Food and Drug Administration. FDA Talk Paper T99-48. October 20, 1999. Available at: http://www.fda.
gov/bbs/topics/ANSWERS/ANS00980.html. Accessed September 12, 2003.

70. Boushey CJ, Beresford SA, Omenn GS, Motulsky AG. A quantitative assessment of plasma homocysteine as
a risk factor for vascular disease: probable benefits of increasing folic acid intakes. *JAMA.* 1995;274:1049-
1057.

71. Gey KF, Moser UK, Jordan P, Stahelin HB, Eichholzer M, Ludin E. Increased risk of cardiovascular diseases
at suboptimal plasma concentrations of essential antioxidants: an epidemiological update with special attention to carotene and vitamin C. *Am J Clin Nutr.* 1993;56(suppl):787S-797S.

72. Kinsella JE, Lokesh B, Stone RA. Dietary n-3 polyunsaturated fatty acids and amelioration of cardiovascular
disease: possible mechanisms. *Am J Clin Nutr.* 1990;52:1-28.

73. Renaud S, de Lorgeril M, Delaye J, Guidollet J, Jacquard F, Mamelle N, Martin JL, Monjaud I, Salen P,
Toubol P. Cretan Mediterranean diet for prevention of coronary heart disease. *Am J Clin Nutr.*
1995;61(suppl):1360S-1367S.

74. Rimm EB, Stampfer MJ, Ascherio A, Giovannucci E, Colditz GA, Willett WC. Vitamin E consumption
and the risk of coronary heart disease in men. *N Engl J Med.* 1993;328:1450-1456.

75. Stampfer MJ, Hennekens CH, Mason JE, Colditz GA, Rosner B, Willett WC. Vitamin E consumption and
the risk of coronary disease in women. *N Engl J Med.* 1993;328:1444-1449.

76. American Heart Association. Evidence-based guidelines for cardiovascular disease prevention in women.
Circulation. 2004;109:672-693.

77. Jones PJ, Raeini-Sarjaz M. Plant sterols and their derivatives: The current spread of results. *Nutr Rev.*
2001;59:21-24.

78. Nguyen TT. The cholesterol-lowering action of plant stanol esters. *J Nutr.* 1999;129:2109-2112.

79. Tammi A, Ronnemaa T, Gylling H, Risk-Nissila L, Viikari J, Tuominen J, Pulkki K, Simell O. Plant stanol
ester margarine lowers serum total and low-density lipoprotein cholesterol concentrations of healthy children: the STRIP project. *J Pediatr.* 2000;136:503-510.

80. Miettinen TA, Puska P, Gylling H, Vanhanen H, Vartiainen E. Reduction of serum cholesterol with
sitostanol-ester margarine in a mildly hypercholesterolemic population. *N Engl J Med.* 1995;333:1308-1312.

81. Liacouras CA, Coates PM, Gallagher PR, Cortner JA. Use of cholestyramine in the treatment of children
with familial combined hyperlipidemia. *J Pediatr.* 1993;122:477-482.

82. Lambert M, Lupien PJ, Gagne C, Levy E, Blaichman S, Langlois S, Hayden M, Rose V, Clarke JT, Wolfe
BM, Clarson C, Parsons H, Stephure DK, Potvin D, Lambert J. Treatment of familial hypercholesterolemia
in children and adolescents: effect of lovastatin. Canadian Lovastatin in Children Study Group. *Pediatrics.*
1996;97:619-628.

83. Sigman-Grant M, Zimmerman S, Kris-Etherton PM. Dietary approaches for reducing fat intake of
preschool-age children. *Pediatrics.* 1993;91:955-960.

84. Nicklas TA, Webber LS, Koschak M, Berenson GS. Nutrient adequacy of low fat intakes for children: the
Bogalusa Heart Study. *Pediatrics.* 1992;89:221-228.

85. Shannon BM, Tershakovec AM, Martel JK, Achterberg CL, Cortner JA, Smiciklas-Wright HS, Stallings VA,
Stolley PD. Reduction of elevated LDL-cholesterol levels of 4- to 10-year-old children through home-based
dietary education. *Pediatrics.* 1994;94:923-927.

86. Shannon B, Greene G, Stallings VA, Achterberg C, Berman M, Gregoire J, Mareci M, Shallcross U. A
dietary education program for hypercholesterolemic children and their parents. *J Am Diet Assoc.*
1991;91:208-212.

87. Tershakovec AM, Jawad AF, Stallings VA, Zemel BS, McKenzie JM, Stolley PD, Shannon BM. Growth of
hypercholesterolemic children completing physician-initiated low-fat dietary intervention. *J Pediatr.*
1998;133:28-34.

88. O'Connell JM, Dibley MJ, Sierra J, Wallace B, Marks JS, Yip R. Growth of vegetarian children: the Farm
Study. *Pediatrics.* 1989;84:475-481.

89. Kaplan RM, Toshima MT. Does a reduced fat diet cause retardation in child growth? *Prev Med.* 1992;21:33-
52.

90. The Dietary Intervention Study in Children (DISC). The Writing Group for the DISC Collaborative
Research Group Efficacy and safety of lowering dietary intake of fat and cholesterol in children with elevated low-density lipoprotein cholesterol. *JAMA.* 1995;273:1429-1435.

91. Kimm SYS, Payne GH, Lakatos E, Darby C, Sparrow A. Management of cardiovascular disease risk factors
in children. *Am J Dis Child.* 1990;144:967-972.

92. Nader PR, Taras HL, Sallis JF, Patterson TL. Adult heart disease prevention in childhood: a national survey of pediatricians' practices and attitudes. *Pediatrics.* 1987;79:843-850.

93. Johnson SL, Birch LL. Parent's and children's adiposity and eating style. *Pediatrics.* 1994;94:642-661.

94. Klesges RC, Klesges LM, Eck LH, Shelton ML. A longitudinal analysis of accelerated weight gain in preschool children. *Pediatrics.* 1995;95:126-130.

95. Moore LL, Lombardi DA, White MJ, Campbell JL, Oliveria SA, Ellison RC. Influence of parents' physical activity levels on activity levels of young children. *J Pediatr.* 1991;118:215-219.

96. Epstein LH, Valoski A, Wing RR, McCurley J. Ten-year outcomes of behavioral family-based treatment for childhood obesity. *Health Psychol.* 1994;13:373-383.

97. Wadden TA, Stunkard AJ, Rich L, Rubin CJ, Sweidel G, McKinney S. Obesity in Black adolescent girls: a controlled clinical trial of treatment by diet, behavior modification, and parental support. *Pediatrics.* 1990;85:345-352.

98. Reimers TM, Brown KM, Van Horn L, Stevens V, Obarzanek E, Hartmuller G, Snetselaar L, von Almen TK, Chiostri J. Maternal acceptability of a dietary intervention designed to lower children's intake of saturated fat and cholesterol: the Dietary Intervention Study in Children (DISC). *J Am Diet Assoc.* 1998;98:31-34.

99. MacDonald LA, Sackett L, Haynes RB, Taylor DW. Labelling in hypertension: a review of the behavioural and psychological consequences. *J Chronic Dis.* 1984;37:933-942.

CHAPTER 14

WOMEN AND RISK FOR CARDIOVASCULAR DISEASE

Linda G. Snetselaar, PhD, RD

INCIDENCE OF MORBIDITY AND MORTALITY

Although it is widely believed that the number one cause of death in women is breast cancer, research shows that more women die from cardiovascular disease (CVD) than all other causes combined. The American Heart Association (AHA) estimates that one in two women will eventually die of heart disease or stroke, whereas 1 in 25 will die of breast cancer (1). Another misconception is that heart disease is a problem for men only. Approximately half of the Americans who die each year from heart attacks are women; 248,000 women died of heart attacks and other coronary events in 2001 (2). Thirty-eight percent of women, compared with 25% of men, die within 1 year after a heart attack (2). AHA statistics indicate that the CVD mortality rate is 69% higher in black women than in white women (1).

This chapter reviews CVD risk factors as they pertain to women. Acknowledging the differences between men and women helps tailor prevention and treatment guidelines to the particular needs of women based on the current scientific evidence.

INTERPRETING RISK FACTORS FOR CORONARY HEART DISEASE IN WOMEN

All of the risk factors that spell increased danger of eventual CVD disease in men also affect women. However, several risk factors deserve emphasis because of their differences relative to gender (refer to Table 14.1 [2-8]). A survey of US women, which included all ethnic and age groups, reported that women have poor knowledge regarding CVD risk factors despite well-documented therapies to reduce CVD risk (9).

Age

According to the Third Report of the National Cholesterol Education Program (NCEP) Expert Panel on Detection, Evaluation, and Treatment of High Blood Cholesterol in Adults

TABLE 14.1
Special Features of CHD Risk Factors in Women

Risk Factor	Special Features
Age	Menopause increases a woman's risk of CHD threefold compared with a premenopausal woman of the same age (2). Onset of CHD is 10 to 15 years later in women compared with men (3).
Smoking	Smoking is responsible for 50% of myocardial infarctions in middle-aged women (4,7).
Diabetes	Diabetes is associated with a three to seven times increased risk of CHD in women compared with a two to four times increased risk in men (3).
Hypertension	Among adults older than 55 years, the percentage of women diagnosed with hypertension is higher than that of men (8)
Triglycerides	High triglyceride levels are more predictive of CVD in women than in men (3,5).
HDL	A low HDL cholesterol level is more predictive of CHD mortality in women than in men, especially in women older than 65 years (3,6).

Abbreviations: CHD, coronary heart disease; CVD, cardiovascular disease; HDL, high-density lipoprotein.

Source: Created by Frances M. Burke, MS, RD. University of Pennsylvania School of Medicine. Copyright 2004. Used by permission of the author.

(Adult Treatment Panel [ATP] III), age is a risk factor for women 45 to 75 years old (10). Age is a risk factor in women because the onset of coronary heart disease (CHD) is 10 to 15 years later in women than in men. Women develop angina approximately 10 years later and have their first myocardial infarction (MI) about 20 years later than men. The incidence of CHD in women is significantly lower before menopause, which is attributed to the protective effects of estrogen (3). Menopause increases a woman's risk of CHD threefold compared with a premenopausal woman of the same age (2).

Hypertension

Using Framingham research data, the National High Blood Pressure Education Program has shown that the risk of CVD associated with hypertension increases gradually prior to the onset of hypertension. Women with systolic blood pressure of 130 to 139 mm Hg or diastolic blood pressure of 85 to 89 mm Hg are 1.5 to 2.5 times more likely to have a cardiovascular event or to die within 10 years compared with women with blood pressure levels of 120 to 129 mm Hg systolic and 80 to 84 mm Hg diastolic (8).

Researchers indicate that a higher percentage of men than women have hypertension up to age 55. However, from ages 55 to 74, the percentage of women with a diagnosis of hypertension is higher than that of males. Ethnicity plays a role in the prevalence of hypertension in adult women ages 20 to 74. Among non-Hispanic white women, 29.5% are diagnosed with hypertension; compared with 44.7% of non-Hispanic black women and 29.9% of Mexican-American women. Oral contraceptive use also increases the risk of hypertension in women (2).

Smoking

Cigarette smoking is a major preventable cause of CHD in women (3,11). Smoking rates are declining more for men than women (3). AHA statistics show that among American women aged 18 years and older, 2.3 million (21%) smoke (2). Ethnicity is related to smoking behavior. Almost 40% of American Indian and Alaskan Native women smoke, compared with 20% of white and African-American women, 12.5% of Hispanic women, and 7% of Asian and Pacific Islander women (2).

Analysis of 12 years of follow-up data from the Nurses' Health Study (7,12) reported that, compared with women who had never smoked, current smokers had a 4 times greater risk of CHD and 2.5 times greater risk for stroke. The risk of stroke in smokers disappeared within 4 years after smoking cessation, whereas normalization of risk for CHD occurred after 10 to 14 years. Former smokers had the same risk of having a stroke as nonsmokers regardless of length or intensity of smoking history (7). Another cohort analysis considered diet and smoking among women in the Framingham Study (13). Women who ate a heart-healthy diet and did not smoke were 80% less likely to have carotid atherosclerosis than women who ate a more conventional diet and smoked (13). Some investigators suggest that smoking cessation may be more difficult for women than men (3). Analysis of the Framingham data indicates that women who continue to smoke can cut their risk of atherosclerosis almost in half by adopting a heart-healthy diet (13).

Serum Lipid Levels

AHA statistics for 2001 indicate that 55.5 million women had total blood cholesterol levels of 200 mg/dL or higher (2). Approximately one half of women ages 20 to 74 years had total cholesterol levels greater than 200 mg/dL, representing 54% of non-Hispanic white women, 46% of non-Hispanic black women, and 45% of Mexican-American women. Twenty percent of white non-Hispanic women, 18% of non-Hispanic black women, and 14% of Mexican-American women had total cholesterol levels of 240 mg/dL or greater. Studies have reported that among individuals 45 years old or older, a greater percentage of women than men have total cholesterol levels greater than 200 mg/dL (2).

Epidemiologic data show conflicting results concerning whether higher low-density lipoprotein (LDL) cholesterol levels increase risk for CHD in women (14). In a review of this data, Krummel postulates that one explanation why the association between CHD and LDL cholesterol levels is weaker in women than in men is that some data do not consider the heterogeneity of LDL particle sizes (14). Levels of the more atherogenic small LDL particles (15) tend to be higher in postmenopausal women; therefore, after menopause the same level of LDL cholesterol may represent a greater CHD risk (16). Rifici and Khachadurian (17) and Maziere et al (18) focus on the fact that estrogen prevents oxidative modification of LDL. This process may blunt the ability of LDL cholesterol to serve as a predictor of CHD.

Recent AHA evidence-based guidelines for CVD prevention in women recommend that health care providers aggressively treat LDL cholesterol in high-risk women. Lifestyle and pharmacologic therapy should be initiated concurrently if LDL cholesterol levels are greater than 100 mg/dL. In high-risk women with LDL cholesterol levels less than 100 mg/dL, medical therapy should be initiated to reduce LDL cholesterol levels even further, unless such therapy is contraindicated (19).

High-density lipoprotein (HDL) cholesterol was analyzed in the Lipid Research Clinics Follow-up Study. Data show that at all levels of LDL cholesterol, women with HDL cholesterol levels less than 50 mg/dL had a CVD mortality rate that was three to four times higher than the rate for women with higher levels of HDL cholesterol (6). HDL cholesterol level was negatively correlated with body mass index (BMI), waist-to-hip ratio, smoking, physical inactivity, and education level. A low HDL cholesterol level is more predictive of CHD mortality in women than in men, especially in women older than 65 years of age (3). The most recent AHA guidelines for CVD prevention in women recommend an HDL cholesterol level greater than 50 mg/dL (19).

High levels of triglycerides are more predictive of CVD in women than in men (3,5). The Framingham Study showed that, for screening purposes, a triglyceride level greater than 150 mg/dL with an HDL cholesterol level less than 40 mg/dL in the absence of vegetarianism suggests that the more atherogenic lipoproteins are present (20).

Physical Inactivity

Lack of physical activity has been linked to increased risk for CVD (21,22). About 25% of women do not partake in regular, sustained physical activity (3). AHA statistics show ethnic differences regarding a sedentary lifestyle. Among women, 36.2% of non-Hispanic whites, 55.2% of non-Hispanic blacks, 57.4% of Hispanics, and 45.5% of Asian–Pacific Islanders do not engage in leisure-time physical activity (2).

The Obesity Education Initiative Panel found that physical activity contributes to a decrease in body fat, including a modest effect on abdominal fat (22,23). A variety of methods exist to assess CVD risk factors that are affected by physical inactivity and an increased energy intake leading to overweight and obesity. One study indicates that BMI may be less predictive of cardiovascular risk in women than waist-to-hip ratio (24).

Increased physical activity appears to independently reduce risk for CVD morbidity, mortality, and diabetes in women (25). Physical activity reduces elevated levels of CVD risk factors by increasing HDL cholesterol and improving glucose tolerance with or without weight loss (26).

Overweight and Obesity

The National Institutes of Health's (NIH's) *Clinical Guidelines on the Identification, Evaluation, and Treatment of Overweight and Obesity in Adults* review the literature on the age-adjusted prevalence of overweight (defined as a BMI of 25 or greater) and obesity (defined as a BMI of 30 or greater) in women ages 20 to 74 years (22,23). Ethnicity plays a role in weight categorization in women, with 57.3% of non-Hispanic white women classified as overweight compared with 77.3% of non-Hispanic black women and 71.9% of Mexican-American women. In the category of obesity, 30.1% of non-Hispanic white women are obese compared with 49.7% non-Hispanic black women and 39.7% Mexican-American women (2).

Central adiposity is associated with an increased risk for CHD. Four randomized controlled trials investigated the effect of weight loss on blood lipids and included a measure of central adiposity using waist circumference (26-29). In all four studies, waist circumferences decreased along with weight, and serum lipids were improved. None of these four studies were designed to specifically test the connection between central adiposity and lipids independent of weight loss. Other observational studies have shown that abdominal fat is related to high-risk serum lipid profiles, such as elevated total and LDL cholesterol levels with increased triglycerides and lower levels of HDL cholesterol (30,31).

Metabolic Syndrome

Metabolic syndrome includes several major lifestyle and emerging risk factors (4). NCEP describes metabolic syndrome as having the following characteristics: central obesity, atherogenic dyslipidemia (elevated triglycerides, small LDL particles, low HDL cholesterol), elevated blood pressure, insulin resistance (with or without glucose intolerance), and prothrombotic and proinflammatory states. (See Table 7.1 in Chapter 7.) ATP III recommendations are to treat metabolic syndrome as a secondary risk factor after the primary target of LDL cholesterol

(10). The prevalence of metabolic syndrome is similar for men and women in general, reaching a peak of 42% to 44% of adults at age 70. However, metabolic syndrome is more prevalent among women than men in the African-American and Hispanic populations (2,32). (See Chapter 7 for further information on metabolic syndrome.)

Diabetes Mellitus

Diabetes mellitus is a strong CVD risk factor resulting in mortality in premenopausal (33) and postmenopausal women (34,35). ATP III has classified diabetes mellitus as a CHD risk equivalent (10). The CHD-related mortality rate for women with diabetes is three to seven times greater than the rate for women who do not have diabetes. The CHD-related mortality rate is much higher for women with diabetes than for men with diabetes, whose CHD-related mortality rate is two to four times greater than the rate for men without diabetes (3). Compared with premenopausal women without diabetes mellitus, premenopausal women with diabetes have less protection against CHD (10).

An estimated 6 million US women have diabetes diagnosed by a physician (2). Approximately 2.8 million women have undiagnosed diabetes. The prevalence of physician-diagnosed diabetes in adults older than 20 years of age varies with ethnicity. Prevalence is 4.7% for non-Hispanic white women, 9.5% for non-Hispanic black women, and 11.4% for Mexican-American women (2). (See Chapter 9 for further information on diabetes and heart disease.)

LIFESTYLE INTERVENTION TO REDUCE CARDIOVASCULAR RISK

ATP III provides guidelines for reducing risk of CVD by providing for lifestyle intervention and, as necessary, pharmacologic treatment to lower LDL cholesterol (see Chapter 3, Table 3.4). In the Nurses' Health Study, women who adhered to lifestyle recommendations involving diet, exercise, and abstinence from cigarette smoking had the lowest risk of CHD (36).

In considering lifestyle modification, the NIH *Clinical Guidelines on the Identification, Evaluation, and Treatment of Overweight and Obesity in Adults* identify studies in which diet, physical activity, or a combination of both are associated with serum lipid changes (22,23). This panel concluded that successful weight loss requires a combination of dietary therapy, physical activity, and behavior therapy. (Motivational interviewing methods to maximize adherence to diet and physical activity recommendations are discussed in Chapter 5 and illustrated later in this chapter's description of the Women's Health Initiative [WHI]). The Diabetes Prevention Program (DPP) investigated use of this tailoring concept to implement diet and exercise changes among subjects at risk for diabetes. A major clinical trial, DPP compared the effects of diet and exercise therapy with the effects of treatment with metformin in 3,234 people with impaired glucose tolerance, a condition that often precedes diabetes. The study included a third group who took placebo pills in place of metformin. In the placebo group, 29% of the subjects developed type 2 diabetes during the average follow-up period of 3 years. In contrast, 14% of the diet and exercise group and 22% of the metformin group developed diabetes. This corresponds to a reduced risk of type 2 diabetes of 58% for lifestyle intervention compared with 31% for metformin use. A crucial part of the lifestyle intervention was tailoring the behavioral approaches for diet and physical activity to each individual (37,38).

Other studies have focused on changes in sex hormones that are unique to women and affect lipid levels. These include the Heart and Estrogen/Progestin Replacement Study (HERS) and the WHI.

Heart and Estrogen/Progestin Replacement Study (HERS)

The findings of HERS challenged observational data showing lower rates of CHD in postmenopausal woman who take estrogen replacement therapy (39). Estrogen has been shown to have positive effects on lipid levels, including decreasing LDL cholesterol and lipoprotein (a) [Lp(a)] levels and increasing HDL cholesterol levels (4). HERS was the first large randomized controlled trial designed to assess the effect of hormone replacement therapy (HRT) on cardiac outcomes in postmenopausal women with CHD (39). The study population included 2,763 women, mean age 66.7 years, with established CHD who were randomly assigned to estrogen and progestin therapy or placebo. Participants were monitored for an average of 4.1 years for the primary end point, which was nonfatal MI or CHD death.

HERS researchers found no overall reduction in risk of CHD events among postmenopausal women with CHD who were taking estrogen and progestin. A significant increase in cardiovascular events occurred in the HRT group during the first year. This occurred despite an average 11% reduction in LDL cholesterol and average 10% increase in HDL cholesterol in the HRT group compared with the placebo group. In addition, HRT was associated with an increased incidence of thromboembolic events and gall bladder disease (39). The Heart and Estrogen/Progestin Replacement Study Follow-up Study included 93% of the original study participants and looked at a longer follow-up period to test the hypothesis that HRT would be beneficial over time. However, HERS researchers concluded that HRT should not be used in women with CHD to prevent future events (39,40).

WHI's HRT Study

The WHI investigated two types of HRT, estrogen alone and estrogen plus progestin (EP), in women without CHD. The EP combination drug was used in women who had not had a hysterectomy before joining the study, whereas estrogen alone was given to women who already had a hysterectomy before joining. The NIH Data Safety and Monitoring Board recently recommended that subjects taking EP stop their medication because the risks of taking the combination hormone outweighed the benefits. Even more recently, in February 2004, the NIH announced that it had decided to stop the estrogen-alone part of the study. The NIH concluded that estrogen alone does not affect heart disease positively or negatively but does appear to increase the risk of stroke (41). Estrogen alone did not increase the risk of breast cancer during the course of the study.

Results of the EP arm of the study show that heart attacks, strokes, blood clots, and breast cancer occurred in more women on EP compared with women taking the placebo. Fewer women on the EP combination had colorectal cancer and hip fractures. There was no difference in the incidence of total deaths and endometrial cancer between the two groups (42,43).

In WHI, 2.5% of women in the EP group had heart attacks, strokes, blood clots, and breast cancer. For every 10,000 women who were taking EP compared with women who were on a placebo, one would expect the following:

- Seven more women with heart attacks in the EP group. This means that 37 women in the EP group would be diagnosed with heart attacks vs only 30 women in the placebo group.
- Eight more women in the EP group than in the placebo group would have a diagnosis of stroke.

- Eight more women in the EP than in the placebo group would have a diagnosis of breast cancer.
- Eighteen more women in the EP than in the placebo group would have a diagnosis of blood clots.

On the positive side for women in the EP group, six fewer diagnoses of colorectal cancer and five fewer hip fractures would be expected in their group than in the placebo group. Overall, more women taking EP had life-threatening health events than women in the placebo group. The Data Safety and Monitoring Board, a data oversight board for the WHI, concluded that EP does not prevent heart disease and is not beneficial to decreasing the incidence of those diseases that reduce longevity (42).

WHI's Dietary Modification Study

A second part of the WHI includes dietary modification to determine the effect of a low-fat diet on heart disease and breast and colorectal cancer (44). This study is a randomized controlled primary prevention trial in women ages 50 to 79 who were initially eating 32% or more energy from fat. In 40 centers throughout the United States, 19,542 women (40% of all subjects) participated in a dietary modification arm of the study and 29,294 women (60%) participated in the usual diet control arm of the study. In the dietary modification arm of the study, women followed a diet with a maximum of 20% of energy from fat, five or more servings per day of fruits and vegetables, and six or more servings of grains daily. Women in the dietary modification arm participated in 18 group sessions during the first year, followed by quarterly maintenance sessions.

One of the primary methods of assessing dietary adherence in this study was the food frequency questionnaire (FFQ) (44). The WHI FFQ was based on other FFQs used in large-scale clinical trials (45-47). Unlike other FFQs, the one developed for WHI was modified to focus on low-fat foods and reflect US regional and ethnic eating patterns. Participants were asked to remember dietary intake for the past 3 months by responding to questions about 122 foods or food groups.

A preliminary dietary analysis comparing the dietary modification and control groups indicates that adherence based on the FFQs is affected by several factors. Poor adherence is associated with being older, black or Hispanic (compared with white), low income, and obese. The attendance at dietary modification group sessions was strongly associated with adherence to the study diet (48). Preliminary data indicate that women in the WHI maintained their low-fat diet by focusing on specific food groups (49). WHI researchers described the major sources of fat eaten at baseline as (*a*) fats added to foods, such as butter, oils, and salad dressings (25%); (*b*) meats (21%); and (*c*) desserts (13%). From baseline to year 1, compared with the control group, the intervention group reduced fat intake by 24.3 grams per day. The greatest changes occurred in the same major sources of fat identified at baseline: added fats (reduced by 9.1 g of fat per day), meats (reduced by 4.6 g of fat per day), and desserts (reduced by 3.9 g of fat per day). A subgroup analysis indicated that ethnicity played a role in the food groups where reductions occurred. Compared with other race and ethnic groups, white non-Hispanic groups had a greater reduction in added fats. A reduction in milk and cheese occurred in both the white non-Hispanic and Hispanic groups. Fat in mixed dishes dropped most dramatically among Hispanic subjects compared with other race and ethnicity groups ($P < .05$ for all).

To maintain dietary adherence in WHI, novel counseling programs were used in the dietary modification arm of the study (50). One study was designed to evaluate the efficacy of an intensive intervention program (IIP) based on motivational interviewing to increase dietary adherence in WHI women. This study included a subset of 3 out of the 40 clinical centers involved in WHI. Women from these three centers were randomly assigned to either the intervention or control group. Women in the intervention group received three individual motivational interviewing contacts from a dietitian, plus the usual WHI dietary intervention in small groups. Women assigned to the control group received the usual WHI dietary intervention. Data used to compare these two groups were based on the percentage of energy intake from fat identified in the FFQ. Comparisons were made between baseline and follow-up 1 year later in the intervention and control groups. In IIP participants, the percentage of energy from fat decreased 1.2% between the baseline and 1-year follow-up. In IIP control participants, the percentage of energy from fat increased by 1.4%. The result was an overall difference between the two groups of 2.6% ($P < .001$). The participants with the highest baseline fat intake had the largest overall change in percentage of energy from fat.

In the IIP study, each motivational interviewing contact consisted of three steps: assessment, intervention, and future directions. During assessment, using a series of yes-or-no questions, participants were assigned to one of three intervention phases: phase 1 included individuals who were not ready to make changes in their diet, phase 2 included individuals unsure of making dietary changes, and phase 3 included subjects who were ready to change. The assessment step was designed to help participants see discrepancies between actual dietary adherence and their own perceptions of adherence, using data from self-monitoring forms. Dietitians initially showed each participant a graph indicating the distance between her current progress and the overall WHI study goals. This data led to a discussion of the participant's progress in attaining her personal fat-gram goal, her interest in making changes, and barriers to success in dietary modification.

Intervention Phase 1 (Not Ready to Change)

In phase 1, the dietitian focused on helping the participant identify the need for change, reduce resistance (including barriers) to change, and finally increase interest in the possibility of making a dietary change. The dietitian encouraged the participant to discuss the possible reasons for change. The dietitian asked a question such as "What would need to be different to move forward and what would prevent that forward move?"

Intervention Phase 2 (Unsure about Change)

In phase 2, building readiness to change was the key. The participant was asked to list pros and cons to change. The participant might be asked, "What are the resulting difficulties and advantages of making changes in your diet?" The goal was for the participant to identify future dietary plans with the topic of change being initially posed by the participant. In this phase, investigators took care to avoid assuming that a participant was ready to change when that may not have been true.

Intervention Phase 3 (Ready to Change)

The role of the dietitian in phase 3 was to facilitate each participant's work on planning dietary change. It was critical in this phase that the idea for change came from the participant. The initial question was, "What would you like to change in your diet?" Based on the participant's response, realistic and achievable short-term goals were set, followed by an action plan developed by the participant.

IMPLEMENTING NUTRITION GUIDELINES

ATP III provides for Therapeutic Lifestyle Changes (TLC) that incorporate foods low in saturated fat and cholesterol (see Chapter 6) (10). In premenopausal women, high dietary saturated fatty acids predict increases in total and LDL cholesterol levels. The inverse is true for HDL cholesterol—that is, high dietary saturated fatty acids are associated with undesirable decreases in HDL cholesterol (51). Along with dietary recommendations, behavior change strategies and Web-based information in Chapter 6 can promote adoption of TLC by women.

For the many women concerned about their weight, reductions in fat may decrease energy intake but the changes are not necessarily substantial. A panel of nutritionists serving on the NIH Obesity Education Initiative (22) has designed menus to consider both the type and quantity of fat along with level of energy intake. Menus have been designed with ethnicity in mind. An exchange list to allow for substitutions in menu selections have also been provided. The menus are available in a publication (23) and on the Internet (http://www.nhlbi.nih.gov/guidelines/obesity/practgde.htm).

SUMMARY

In summary, there are many CHD risk factors that are special to women. Hormonal status is one factor unique to women's risk for heart disease. However, studies such as HERS and WHI have not provided evidence of benefit of HRT in reducing risk of CHD. Effective treatment for elevated lipids in women is similar to that recommended for men. Dietary change in women is fraught with problems. Motivational interviewing is a positive method of facilitating changes in diet and physical activity. It promotes assessment of patients' readiness for change in various areas of diet and provides for stage-based guidance in adopting long-term lifestyle changes to reduce risk for heart disease.

REFERENCES

1. American Heart Association. Statistical fact sheets. Available at: http://www.americanheart.org/presenter.jhtml?identifier=2859. Accessed March 30, 2004.
2. American Heart Association. Women and cardiovascular diseases—statistics. Available at: http://www.americanheart.org/presenter.jhtml?identifier=3000941. Accessed March 30, 2004.
3. Welty FK. Cardiovascular disease and dyslipidemia in women. *Arch Intern Med.* 2001;161:514-522.
4. Mosca LJ. Optimal management of cholesterol levels and prevention of coronary heart disease in women. *Am Fam Physician.* 2002;65:217-226.
5. Austin MA, Hokanson JE. Epidemiology of triglycerides, small dense low-density lipoprotein, and lipoprotein (a) as risk factors for coronary heart disease. *Med Clin North Am.* 1994;78:99-115.
6. Bass KM, Newschaffer CJ, Klag MJ, Bush TL. Plasma lipoprotein levels as predictors of cardiovascular death in women. *Arch Intern Med.* 1993;153:2209-2216.
7. Kawachi I, Colditz GA, Stampfer MJ, Willett WC, Manson JE, Rosner B, Speizer FE, Jennekens CH. Smoking cessation and decreased risk of stroke in women. *JAMA.* 1993;269:232-236.
8. National High Blood Pressure Education Program Web site. Available at: http://www.nhlbi.nih.gov/about/nhbpep. Accessed March 18, 2004.

9. Mosca L, Ferris A, Fabunmi R, Robertson RM. Tracking women's awareness of heart disease. *Circulation.* 2004;109:573-579.

10. Expert Panel on Detection, Evaluation, and Treatment of High Blood Cholesterol in Adults. Executive summary of the Third Report of the National Cholesterol Education Program (NCEP) Expert Panel on Detection, Evaluation, and Treatment of High Blood Cholesterol in Adults (Adult Treatment Panel III). *JAMA.* 2001;285:2486-2497. Full report: National Institutes of Health. *Third Report of the National Cholesterol Education Program Expert Panel on Detection, Evaluation, and Treatment of High Blood Cholesterol in Adults (Adult Treatment Panel III).* Bethesda, Md: National Institutes of Health; 2001. NIH Publication 01-3670. Available at: http://www.nhlbi.nih.gov/guidelines/cholesterol/atp3_rpt.htm. Accessed March 29, 2004.

11. Kannel WB, Wilson PW. Risk factors that attenuate the female coronary disease advantage. *Arch Intern Med.* 1995;155:57-61.

12. Kawachi I, Colditz GA, Stampfer MJ, Willett WC, Manson JE, Rosner B, Speizer FE, Jennekens CH. Smoking cessation and time course of decreased risk of coronary heart disease in middle-aged women. *Arch Intern Med.* 1994;154:169-175.

13. Millen BE, Quatromoni PA, Nam G, O'Horo CE, Polak JF, Wolf PA, D'Agostino RB. Dietary patterns, smoking, and subclinical heart disease in women: opportunities for primary prevention from the Framingham Nutrition Studies. *J Am Diet Assoc.* 2004;102:208-214.

14. Krummel DA. Cardiovascular disease. In: Krummel DA, Kris-Etherton PM, eds. *Nutrition in Women's Health.* Gaithersburg, Md: Aspen Publishers; 1996:383-417.

15. Austin MA, Breslow JL, Hennekens CH, Buring JE, Willet WC, Krauss RM. Low-density lipoprotein subclass patterns and risk of myocardial infarction. *JAMA.* 1988;260:1917-1921.

16. Compos H, McNamara JR, Wilson PW, Ordovas J, Schaefer EJ. Differences in low density lipoprotein subfractions and apolipoproteins in premenopausal and postmenopausal women. *J Clin Endocrinol Metab.* 1988;67:30-35.

17. Rifici VA, Khachadurian AK. The inhibition of low-density lipoprotein oxidation by 17-B estradiol. *Metabolism.* 1992;41:1110-1114.

18. Maziere C, Auclair M, Ronveaux MF, Salmon S, Santus R, Maziere JC. Estrogens inhibit copper and cell-mediated modification of low density lipoprotein. *Atherosclerosis.* 1991;89:175-182.

19. American Heart Association Expert Panel/Writing Group. Evidence-based guidelines for cardiovascular disease prevention in women. *Circulation.* 2004;109:672-693.

20. Castelli WP. Epidemiology of triglycerides: a view from Framingham. *Am J Cardiol.* 1992;70:3H-9H.

21. Wagner A, Simon C, Evans A, Ferrieres J, Montaye M, Ducimetiere P, Arveiler D, and the PRIME Study Group. Physical activity and coronary event incidence in Northern Ireland and France: the Prospective Epidemiological Study of Myocardial Infarction (PRIME). *Circulation.* 2002;105:2247-2252.

22. National Heart, Lung and Blood Institute. *Clinical Guidelines on the Identification, Evaluation, and Treatment of Overweight and Obesity in Adults.* Bethesda, Md: National Heart, Lung and Blood Institute in cooperation with the National Institute of Diabetes and Digestive and Kidney Diseases; 1998. NIH publication 98-4083.

23. National Heart, Lung and Blood Institute. *The Practical Guide to the Identification, Evaluation, and Treatment of Overweight and Obesity in Adults.* Bethesda, Md: National Heart, Lung, and Blood Institute in cooperation with the National Institute of Diabetes and Digestive and Kidney Diseases; 2000. NIH publication 00-4083. Available at: http://www.nhlbi.nih.gov/guidelines/obesity/practgde.htm. Accessed March 18, 2004.

24. Folsom AR, Kaye SA, Sellers TA, Hong CP, Cerhan JR, Potter JD, Prineas RJ. Body fat distribution and 5-year risk of death in older women. *JAMA.* 1993;269:483-487.

25. Blair SN, Kampert JB, Koho HW 3rd, Barlow CE, Macera CA, Paffenbarger RS Jr, Gibbons LW. Influences of cardiorespiratory fitness and other precursors on cardiovascular disease and all-cause mortality in men and women. *JAMA.* 1996;276:205-210.

26. National Center for Chronic Disease Prevention and Health Promotion. *Surgeon General's Report on Physical Activity and Health.* Atlanta, Ga: Centers for Disease Control and Prevention; 1996.

27. Stefanick ML, Mackey S, Sheehan M, Ellsworth N, Haskell WL, Wood PD. Effects of the NCEP Step 2 diet and exercise on lipoprotein in postmenopausal women and men with low HDL-cholesterol and high LDL-cholesterol. *New Engl J Med.* 1998;339:12-20.

28. Simkin-Silverman K, Wing RR, Hansen DH, Klem ML, Pasagian-Macaulay AP, Meilahn EN, Kuller LH. Prevention of cardiovascular risk factor elevations in healthy premenopausal women. *Prev Med.* 1995;24:509-517.

29. Dengel JL, Katzel LI, Goldberg AP. Effect of an American Heart Association diet, with or without weight loss, on lipids in obese middle-aged and older men. *Am J Clin Nutr.* 1995;62:715-721.

30. Emery EM, Schmid TL, Kahn HS, Filozof PP. A review of the association between abdominal fat distribution, health outcome measures, and modifiable risk factors. *Am J Health Promot.* 1993;7(5):342-353.

31. Bjorntorp P. Abdominal fat distribution and disease: an overview of epidemiological data. *Ann Med.* 1992;24:15-18.

32. Ford ES, Giles WH, Dietz WH. Prevalence of the metabolic syndrome among US adults: findings from the third National Health and Nutrition Examination. *JAMA.* 2002;287:356-359.

33. Perlman JA, Wolf PH, Ray R, Lieberknecht A. Cardiovascular risk factors, premature heart disease, and all-cause mortality in a cohort of northern California women. *Am J Obstet Gynecol.* 1988;158:1568-1574.

34. Barrett-Connor E, Cohn BA, Wingard DL, Edelstein SL. Why is diabetes mellitus a stronger risk factor for fatal ischemic heart disease in women than in men? *JAMA.* 1991;265:627-631.

35. Donahue RP, Goldberg RJ, Chen Z, Gore JM, Alpert JS. The influence of sex and diabetes mellitus on survival following acute myocardial infarction: a community-wide perspective. *J Clin Epidemiol.* 1993;46:245-252.

36. Stamfer MJ, Hu FB, Manson JE, Rimm EB, and Willett WC. Primary prevention of coronary heart disease in women through diet and lifestyle. *N Engl J Med.* 2000;343:16-22.

37. Knowler WC, Barrett-Connor E, Fowler SE, Hamman RF, Lachin JM, Walker EAT, Nathan DM, and the Diabetes Prevention Program Research Group. Reduction in the incidence of type 2 diabetes with lifestyle intervention or metformin. *N Engl J Med.* 2002;346:393-403.

38. Diabetes Prevention Program Research Group. The Diabetes Prevention Program (DPP): description of lifestyle intervention. *Diabetes Care.* 2002;25:2165-2171.

39. Hulley S, Grady D, Bush T, Furberg C, Herrington D, Riggs B, Vittinghoff E. Randomized trial of estrogen plus progestin for secondary prevention of coronary heart disease in postmenopausal women. Heart and Estrogen/Progestin Replacement Study (HERS) Research Group. *JAMA.* 1998;280:605-613.

40. Grady D, Herrington D, Bittner V, Blumenthal R, Davidson M, Hlatky M, Hsia J, Hulley S, Herd A, Khan S, Newby LK, Waters D, Vittinghoff E, Wenger N, for the HERS Research Group. Cardiovascular disease outcomes during 6.8 years of hormone therapy: Heart and Estrogen/Progestin Replacement Study Follow-up (HERS II). *JAMA.* 2002;288:49-57.

41. The Women's Health Initiative Steering Committee. Effects of conjugated equine estrogen in post-menopausal women with hysterectomy. The Women's Health Initiative randomized controlled trial. *JAMA.* 2004;291:1701-1712.

42. Rossouw JE, Anderson GL, Prentice RL, LaCroix AZ, Kooperberg C, Stefanick ML, Jackson RD, Beresford SA, Howard BV, Johnson KC, Kotchen JM, Ockene J. Writing Group for the Women's Health Initiative Investigators. Risks and benefits of estrogen plus progestin in healthy post-menopausal women: principal results from the Women's Health Initiative randomized controlled trial. *JAMA.* 2002;288:72-78.

43. The Women's Health Initiative Study Group. Design of the Women's Health Initiative Clinical Trial and Observational Study. *Control Clin Trials.* 1998;19:61-109.

44. Patterson RE, Kristal AR, Carter RA, Fels-Tinker L, Bolton MP, Agurs-Collins T. Measurement characteristics of Women's Health Initiative Food Frequency Questionnaire. *Ann Epidemiol.* 1999;9:178-197.

45. Henderson MM, Kushi LH, Thompson DJ, Gorbach SL. Feasibility of a randomized trial of a low-fat diet for the prevention of breast cancer: dietary compliance in the Women's Health Trial (WHT) Vanguard Study. *Prev Med.* 1990;19:115-133.

46. White E, Shattuck A, Kristal AR, Urban N, Prentice RL, Henderson MM, Insull W Jr, Moskowitz M, Goldman S, Woods MN. Maintenance of a low-fat diet: follow-up of the Women's Health Trial. *Cancer Epidemiol Biomarkers Prev.* 1992;1:315-323.

47. Kristal A, Feng Z, Coates RJ, Oberman A, George V. Associations of race/ethnicity, education, and dietary intervention with the validity and reliability of a food frequency questionnaire. *Am J Epidemiol.* 1997;146:856-869.

48. Women's Health Initiative Study Group. Dietary adherence in the Women's Health Initiative Dietary Modification Trial. *J Am Diet Assoc.* 2004;104:654-658.

49. Patterson RE, Kristal A, Rodabough R, Caan B, Lillington L, Mossavar-Rahmani Y, Simon MS, Snetselaar L, Van Horn L. Changes in food sources of dietary fat in response to an intensive low-fat dietary intervention: early results from the Women's Health Initiative. *J Am Diet Assoc.* 2003;103:454-460.

50. Bowen D, Ehret C, Pedersen M, Snetselaar L, Johnson M, Tinker L, Hollinger D, Lichty I, Bland K, Sivertsen D, Ocken D, Staats L, Beedoe JW. Results of an adjunct dietary intervention program in the Women's Health Initiative. *J Am Diet Assoc.* 2002;102:1631-1637.

51. Krummel DA, Mashaly MM, Kris-Etherton PM. Prediction of plasma lipids in a cross-sectional sample of young women. *J Am Diet Assoc.* 1992;92:942-948.

CHAPTER 15

MULTICULTURAL NUTRITION STRATEGIES

Section I: African Americans by Hiba Sarieddine, BS, Lisa A. Hark, PhD, RD,
and Wajdi Hamdan, MD;
Section II: Hispanic Americans by Gabriela A. Maldonado, MS, and Lisa A. Hark, PhD, RD;
Section III: Asian Indians by Wahida Karmally, DrPH, RD, CDE

Dietitians need to structure nutrition interventions for the prevention and treatment of cardiovascular disease (CVD) so that recommended changes are compatible with individuals' cultural values and beliefs. A variety of challenges face health professionals who aim to develop nutrition interventions that target people from diverse backgrounds. Nutrition educators must recognize the importance of specific foods within cultures and the significance of ethnosocial influences on food choices. However, generalizations about food patterns should not be made solely on the basis of race, ethnicity, or geographic origin because food-choice diversity is common within all cultural and racial groups. In essence, the United States is a melting pot of cultures. Interventions are most effective when nutrition educators focus on each family's unique dietary history and background without making assumptions about food habits on the basis of an individual's cultural or racial background. Factors such as where a person lives may determine the availability of ethnic food, and issues of acculturation play a huge role in everyone's food selection.

A recent report by the Institute of Medicine (IOM), *Unequal Treatment: Confronting Racial and Ethnic Disparities in Healthcare*, states that "some evidence suggests that bias, prejudice, and stereotyping on the part of healthcare providers may contribute to differences in care" (1). The IOM study committee defines disparities in health care as "racial or ethnic differences in the quality of healthcare that are not due to access-related factors or clinical needs, preferences, and appropriateness of intervention" (1). Treatment disparities for a wide array of diseases and conditions are well documented in the literature and persist after controlling for possible confounders (2,3). It is well known that hypertension, diabetes, and overweight are more prevalent in some ethnic and racial groups and among individuals of low socioeconomic status, and that these populations have higher rates of disability and death from CVD (4). Betancourt (5) names three barriers to care that may account for racial or ethnic health disparities: (*a*) organizational barriers (eg, lack of ethnic diversity in leadership and workforce), (*b*) structural barriers (eg, lack of interpreter services, lack of continuity of care), and (*c*) clinical barriers (eg, poor communication between provider and patient, dissonant beliefs about health, trust issues, provider stereotyping, and bias). The IOM report suggests integrating cross-cultural education into the training of all current and future health professionals (1). Research also suggests the need for culturally tailored educational materials and programs for people of different ethnic groups (6).

This chapter illustrates the special issues and intervention strategies related to nutrition and heart disease for different American subcultures. Three cultures have been selected as examples—African American, Hispanic American, and Asian Indian.

Section I: Nutrition Strategies for African Americans

OVERVIEW

CVD is the leading cause of death in the United States (7). According to the American Heart Association (AHA), 41% of African-American men and 40% of African-American women have CVD. This includes hypertension, coronary heart disease (CHD), congestive heart failure, and stroke. The prevalence of CVD in whites is significantly lower (30% for men and 24% for women) than the prevalence in African Americans (7). (Figures 1.1 and 1.2 in Chapter 1 illustrate the differences in prevalence of CHD and stroke.) CVD claims the lives of 37% of the 288,000 African Americans who die each year. In 2001, the age-adjusted CVD death rate among African Americans was 511 for males and 377 for females per 100,000 US population compared with 330 per 100,000 for the total population (7). Multiple studies have been designed to examine the observed ethnic disparities in CVD mortality and morbidity. Substantial evidence suggests that these disparities involve a complex interplay between sociocultural factors, racial gaps in health care (8-11), differences in CVD risk factors (12-18), and dietary behaviors (12,19-22).

PREVALENCE OF CVD RISK FACTORS IN AFRICAN AMERICANS

The major risk factors for CVD are described in Chapter 3. African Americans are 1.5 times more likely than whites to have multiple risk factors; this finding may be related to higher rates of obesity in African Americans (23). The CVD risk factors most commonly associated with African Americans are obesity, hypertension, diabetes, and physical inactivity.

Obesity

Obesity, defined by a body mass index (BMI) of 30 or greater, is a major predisposing risk factor for CVD (24). Excess body weight raises blood pressure and cholesterol levels (24), lowers high-density lipoprotein (HDL) cholesterol levels (24), and is associated with insulin resistance (25), all of which have adverse effects on CVD (26).

Studies indicate that African Americans have a higher BMI and are more likely to be overweight and obese compared with other ethnic groups (7,12,15,19). Statistics from the 1997 and 1998 National Health Interview Survey of 68,556 US adults aged 18 years and older showed that rates of overweight (BMI $\geq$ 25) and obesity (BMI $\geq$ 30) among African Americans were 65.5% and 29.0%, respectively (see Figure 15.1) (17). The prevalence of obesity was particularly high among African-American women (32.9%) compared with Hispanic women (23.3%), white women (17.6%), and Asian and Pacific Islander women (5.8%) (17). Abdominal obesity was also reported to be twice as common in African-American women as

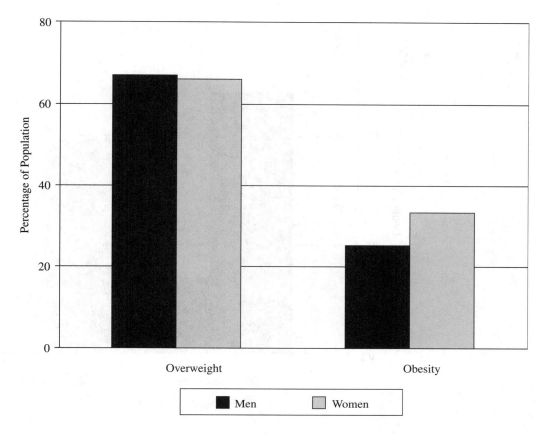

FIGURE 15.1
Age-adjusted prevalence of overweight and obesity among African Americans. Reprinted from reference 17.

in white women (23). Moreover, data indicate that African-American children are more likely to be overweight (BMI ≥ 95th percentile) compared with other ethnic groups. Between 12 to 19 years of age, the prevalence of overweight is 20.7% in African-American boys and 26.6% in African-American girls, compared with 12.8% in white boys and 12.4% in white girls (27). Childhood obesity is significantly correlated with adolescent and adult obesity, and therefore children with obesity have an increased risk of obesity-related comorbidities later in life (18).

Diabetes

According to the American Diabetes Association, approximately 2.7 million (11.4%) of African Americans aged 20 years or older have diabetes; however, as many as one third are undiagnosed. Moreover, 25% of African-American women 55 years of age or older have type 2 diabetes (28). African Americans appear to have twice the risk of developing type 2 diabetes compared with whites (14). One study identified a 40% lower insulin sensitivity and twice the insulin secretion in African-American children compared with white children, independent of body composition and fat distribution (14).

Hypertension

According to the AHA, the rate of hypertension in African Americans is among the highest in the world. In 2001, the death rates from hypertension per 100,000 US adults were 13.7 for

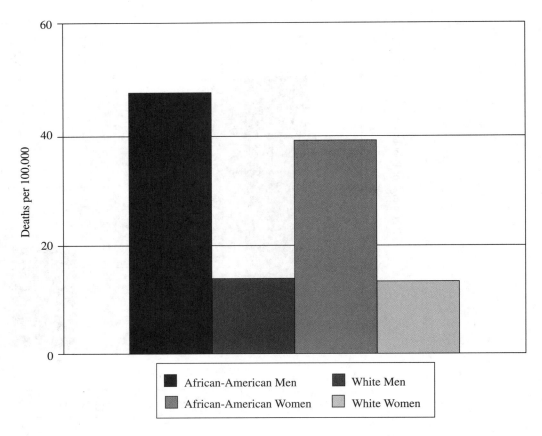

FIGURE 15.2
Hypertension death rates in 2001. Data are from references 29 and 30.

white men, 47.8 for African-American men, 13.4 for white women, and 38.9 for African-American women (see Figure 15.2) (29,30). Autopsy reports indicate that hypertensive vascular disease occurs approximately twice as frequently in African Americans (42%) than in whites (23%) (13). Ineffective control and treatment of hypertension in African Americans appears to be a major contributor to their increased CVD mortality (13,31).

Dyslipidemia

Studies indicate that African Americans have a more favorable lipid profile than whites when matched for age and gender (7,15). The age-adjusted prevalence of total blood cholesterol levels greater than 200 mg/dL is 52% in white men, 46% in African-American men, 49% in white women, and 45% in African-American women (7). Total cholesterol levels of 240 mg/dL or higher (high-risk levels) in African-American men and women are 15% and 18%, respectively, vs 18% in white men and 20% in white women. The prevalence of low-density lipoprotein (LDL) cholesterol levels greater than 130 mg/dL is 46.3% in African-American men, compared with 41.6% in African-American women. Moreover, the rates of low HDL cholesterol levels (less than 40 mg/dL) are 24.3% in African-American men and 13% in African-American women. White men and women had higher rates of high LDL cholesterol and low HDL cholesterol levels (7,15). Lower rates of hypertriglyceridemia (triglycerides ≥ 250 mg/dL) were also reported among African Americans (15). A study of premenopausal women showed better lipoprotein levels in African-American women than in white women (12). However, serum lipoprotein (a) [Lp(a)], a CHD risk factor (32), was reported to be higher in premenopausal African-American women (12). Whether higher Lp(a) in African Americans increases risk for CHD is not known (23). Among children, several studies showed a higher risk of developing CVD in African Americans than in whites, possibly because of the higher total cholesterol levels reported in African-American children (14,33).

Smoking

Between 1965 and 2001, cigarette smoking declined more rapidly among African-American adults than white adults (34). Data collected between 1999 and 2001 from the National Survey on Drug Use and Health of 74,318 US youths (12 to 17 years old) and 133,081 adults (18 years old or older) showed a lower prevalence of smoking among African-American youths compared with other ethnic groups (eg, 7% in African Americans vs 16% in whites). Moreover, data indicate that rates of smoking are similar among African-American men (30.1%) and white men (29.1%) but lower among African-American women (22.2%) than white women (25.9%) (35).

Physical Inactivity

The prevalence of no leisure-time physical activity is higher in African-American men (45%) and African-American women (55%) compared with white men (34%) and white women (38%) (see Figure 15.3) (16,36). Low levels of physical activity were also reported in a large

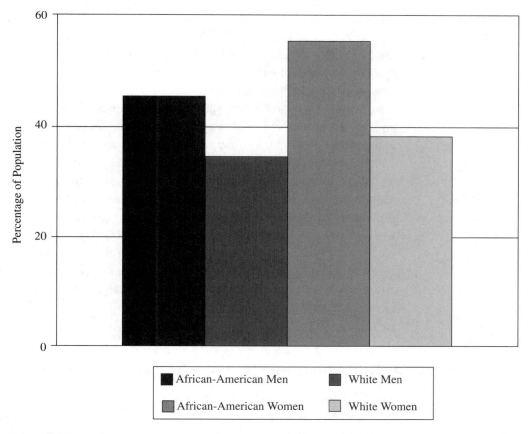

FIGURE 15.3
Prevalence of no leisure-time physical activity in the United States, 1999-2001. Data are from reference 36.

study of 64,101 African-American women aged 21 to 69 years (37). Strenuous activity was inversely associated with BMI and cigarette smoking and positively associated with education level (37). Many other studies report findings of low physical activity among African Americans. For example, Macera et al (38) reported a 76% prevalence of inactivity in a sample of 489 African-American women in South Carolina. Jones et al (39) demonstrated that only 25.7% of African-American women met the recommendation of at least 30 minutes of moderate physical activity on most days. AHA classifies physical inactivity as a major predisposing risk factor for CVD (40) and encourages all individuals to engage in an appropriate exercise regimen (26).

TRADITIONAL AFRICAN-AMERICAN FOOD PREFERENCES

Traditional African-American cuisine is known as soul food and represents a symbol of identity and unity. Soul food has southern roots and was influenced by African customs in addition to West Indian, Caribbean, and French cooking. Cornmeal, pig's feet, salt pork (fat renderings), and chitterlings (pork intestines) are staples, and many soul foods have true African roots, such as okra, yams, lentils, chick peas, kidney beans, watermelon, and black-eyed peas (an African legume believed to bring good luck for the New Year). In its origins, soul food was hearty nourishment that met the high energy needs of African-American slaves performing hard labor. It was based on using the parts of the animal not deemed suitable to put on the slave owners' table. Corn, rice, and beans, with high carbohydrate and fiber content, were important energy sources. Meat was a source of protein and fat, and green vegetables provided essential vitamins and minerals. Watermelon, which is more than 90% water, replenished fluid lost while working in the sun. African Americans grew many of the vegetables and fruits that supplemented their diet, including turnips, cabbage, eggplant, cucumber, tomatoes, onions, garlic, and hot peppers.

Frying is a very popular cooking method in the typical African-American diet. Meat, pork, and fish are traditionally fried in animal fat such as lard or bacon fat. Meats such as pig's feet and chitterlings are high in saturated fat and are usually boiled. Vegetables and beans are boiled with fatty cuts of pork for seasoning, which are referred to by various names: ham hocks, fat back, or hog jowls. The tail or neck of the turkey or chicken may also be used. Soul food can also be spicy; liberal use of spices both reflects its African origin and makes poor cuts of meat more palatable. Typical dishes include fried chicken, baked ham, or barbecued pork ribs; collard greens with ham hocks; pinto beans with neck bones; corn bread; and sweet potato pie (sweet potato replaced the African yam). The common thread of all these dishes is that they are inexpensive and made from ingredients that African Americans have traditionally obtained with ease. However, many of these traditional foods are high in energy, saturated fat, and salt, as shown in Table 15.1 (41).

MODIFYING AFRICAN-AMERICAN EATING PATTERNS

The US Department of Agriculture (USDA) Survey of Food Intakes by Individuals indicates that most African Americans have a poor diet. Compared with other ethnic groups, African Americans had higher intakes of total and saturated fat and lower intakes of fruits, vegetables, grains, and milk. The high prevalence of lactose intolerance among African Americans could

TABLE 15.1
Nutrient Composition of Traditional African-American Cuisine

Food	Serving Size	Energy (kcal)	Total Fat (g)	Saturated Fat (g)	Monounsaturated Fatty Acids (g)	Cholesterol (mg)	Sodium (mg)
Barbeque sauce	1 Tbsp	12	0.3	0	0.1	0	127
Biscuit (fast food)	1 biscuit	260	12.7	3.4	8.6	1	730
Chitterlings	3.5 oz	303	28.8	10.1	9.7	143	39
Collard greens	1 cup (chopped)	34	0.2	0	0	0	21
Cornbread	1 piece	178	5.8	1.7	0	0	263
French fries	20-25 fries	235	12.2	3.8	6	0	124
Fried chicken breast with skin	1 whole breast	436	17.4	4.8	6.8	176	150
Fried chicken thighs with skin	2 thighs	324	18.6	5.0	7.2	120	110
Fried chicken wings with skin	3 wings	309	21.3	5.7	8.4	78	75
Frozen fish sticks	4 sticks (4 × 2 × ½ in)	304	13.6	3.6	5.6	124	652
Pork fat (lard)	1 Tbsp	115	12.8	5.0	5.8	12	0
Pork feet (cured/pickled)	3.5 oz	203	16.1	5.6	7.6	92	923
Pork ribs (braised)	3.5 oz	367	27.2	9.8	12.5	95	48
Salt pork (raw)	1 oz	212	22.8	8.3	10.8	25	404
Shrimp (breaded and fried)	3 oz (11 large)	206	10.4	1.8	3.2	150	292
Sweet potato pie	⅛ pie	243	12.9	4.6	0	0	249
Whiting fish (raw)	3 oz	77	1.1	0.2	0.2	57	61

Source: Data are from reference 41.

be a reason why they consume less milk than other Americans. Unfortunately, fewer than 50% of African Americans meet the national dietary recommendations for most food groups (42). On a smaller scale, a nutrition education study including 561 African Americans examined the baseline fat-related dietary behaviors of different ethnic groups (19) and showed similar findings. After controlling for gender, age, education, and other factors, results indicated that African-American participants had the highest prevalence of fat-related behaviors compared with white and Hispanic participants. African Americans were less likely to eat meatless meals and modify their meals to make them lower in fat. For example, they were less likely to eat chicken without skin, to trim visible fat from red meat, to avoid frying, to use lower fat products, and to eat vegetables or bread without added fat. These findings support other similar studies (20,22) and strongly emphasize the need to educate and encourage African Americans to adopt more healthful dietary behaviors, especially those related to fat intake, to reduce their risk of CVD.

Table 15.2 lists many ways to modify traditional African-American foods to reduce energy, total fat, saturated fat, and sodium, as well as increase fiber content. The traditional African-American diet includes high-fiber legumes, such as pinto beans and black-eyed peas, and green leafy vegetables, such as collard and turnip greens, that are rich in vitamins and minerals. These foods make nutritious side dishes when seasoned with herbs or turkey neck rather than pork fat and ham hocks.

LIFESTYLE MODIFICATIONS FOR AFRICAN AMERICANS

The traditional African-American diet is generally high in energy, saturated fat, cholesterol, and sodium. Therefore, ethnic-specific nutrition counseling and education programs should be encouraged and practiced to induce lifestyle and dietary changes in the African-American population. It is important to keep in mind that the diets of the African-American people may vary greatly by geographic region, income, and ethnicity. Although many of the foods discussed

TABLE 15.2
Healthier Versions of Traditional African-American Cuisine

Traditional Food	Healthier Alternatives
Chicken, turkey, or fish fried in shortening, lard, or other animal fat	Bake, roast, broil, grill, or oven-fry. Remove skin from turkey or chicken before cooking or eating. Eat tuna fish packed in water (not oil). Fry with canola, olive, or corn oil instead of lard, shortening, or animal fat. Limit oil to less than ¼ cup.
Ham hocks, salt pork, or fatback to season vegetables and beans	Use onions, garlic, low-sodium chicken broth, or bouillon to season vegetables. Use smoked turkey, turkey bacon, or turkey ham.
Regular ground beef	Use extra lean ground beef or ground turkey breast.
French fries or mashed potatoes with butter and sour cream	Top baked potato with light or nonfat sour cream or salsa. Mash potatoes with low-fat or nonfat milk or buttermilk, lite margarine (*trans* fat-free).
Whole milk, cheese, sour cream	Use low-fat or nonfat milk, cheese, sour cream, buttermilk, yogurt, or soy milk.
Potato chips, pretzels, salted popcorn with butter	Replace with baked tortilla and potato chips, low-salt pretzels, or air-popped popcorn without butter.
Cakes, pies, cookies, candy, biscuits	Choose graham crackers, dried fruit, fig bars, gelatin desserts, pudding made with low-fat milk, rice cakes (use no-calorie sweeteners such as sucralose in baking).
Shortening, butter, lard, other animal fats	Use canola, olive, and corn oil for cooking and baking. Use low-fat margarine for spreads.
Regular salad dressing or mayonnaise	Use low-fat or nonfat salad dressing or mayonnaise or flavored vinegar on salads. Use mustard or ketchup instead of mayonnaise.
Canned fruit packed in heavy syrup	Replace with canned fruit packed in light syrup or juice.
Salty or creamed soups	Choose low-fat and low-sodium soups.
Salt, salt pork, garlic salt, celery salt, seasoning salt	Season with herbs, spices, lemon, vinegar, garlic powder, salt substitutes.

Source: Created by Hiba Sarieddine, BS, and Lisa A. Hark, PhD, RD. University of Pennsylvania, School of Medicine. Copyright ©2004. Used by permission of the authors.

above may be eaten by a significant proportion of the African-American community, dietitians working with this population need to do a thorough dietary assessment to determine individual issues and avoid generalizations.

Therefore, it is very important to treat each patient as an individual. For example, if the patient is overweight and has hypertension, nutrition messages should focus on reducing total energy and sodium intake as well as increasing physical activity. The Dietary Approaches to Stop Hypertension (DASH) diet, along with salt restriction, is appropriate to recommend for these patients. The combination of the DASH diet and salt restriction have been shown to induce substantial reductions in blood pressure in different populations, particularly among African Americans (43,44). The DASH diet is low in total fat, saturated fat, and cholesterol and rich in magnesium, potassium, calcium, and fiber because it emphasizes fruits, vegetables, low-fat dairy food, whole-grain products, fish, poultry and nuts. It also limits red meat, sweets and sugar-containing beverages (43,44). In fact, this diet may have beneficial effects on cardiovascular health by not only decreasing blood pressure, but also reducing weight and improving dyslipidemia (see Chapter 8).

The average daily amount of salt consumed by Americans is 8 to 10 g (43). Current recommendations are to reduce sodium intake to no more than 2.4 g per day (ie, 6 g or about 1 tsp of salt) (43,44). Processed foods contribute the majority of sodium to the American diet.

Some of the following processed items can be purchased in salt-free or low-sodium versions in most grocery stores:

- Smoked, cured, or canned meats, poultry, or fish
- Salt pork, ham hocks, pork feet
- Cold cuts, deli meats (salami, corned beef, pastrami), and cheeses
- Salted nuts, potato chips, pretzels, salted popcorn, salted crackers
- Canned soups or canned vegetables
- Barbeque, chili, soy, Worcestershire sauces, meat tenderizers
- Olives, pickles
- Tomato products, tomato sauces, and pizza

Because excessive alcohol consumption has also been shown to increase blood pressure (45), all patients should be advised to limit alcohol intake to no more than two drinks per day for men and one drink per day for women (a standard drink is equivalent to 360 mL [12 oz] of beer, 150 mL [5 oz] of wine, or 30 mL [1 oz] of 80-proof alcohol). In addition, dietitians should suggest to patients that they have regular blood pressure checks by a health professional, especially if they are in a high-risk category. Because ineffective management of hypertension increases CVD mortality, patients should also be encouraged to be diligent in regularly taking any antihypertensive medications prescribed by their physician.

For those patients with diabetes, who are also likely to be overweight, messages should focus on increasing physical activity and reducing energy, saturated fat, and total carbohydrate intake. Dietitians can teach these patients the method of carbohydrate counting, which emphasizes the total amount of carbohydrates one can eat at meals and snacks to keep blood sugar under control (46). Practitioners can begin by explaining the sources of carbohydrates and help patients understand what and how much to eat at each meal. By reducing carbohydrate-containing foods at meals and snacks, patients can reduce total energy intake and control blood glucose levels effectively. Carbohydrate counting is especially important for patients with diabetes who are taking insulin. Concerning physical activity, dietitians should emphasize being more active everyday, focus on moderate activities such as walking, and explain that physical activity not only benefits physical health but also mental health by reducing stress and improving body image (6).

CONCLUSION

By understanding the health disparities and dietary issues of African-American patients, dietitians can be an invaluable resource for behavior change. There may be some barriers to making major changes in eating and activity patterns. Strong social pressures to eat and the high value placed on ethnic foods are examples of such barriers (6). Therefore, it is important to start by initiating small yet significant changes to establish lifelong healthy habits. Examples of such changes include eating smaller portions of the high-calorie ethnic foods; changing the type of fat used in cooking, such as replacing lard with canola oil (41% vs 7% saturated fat); preparing foods by broiling or baking instead of frying; and buying fresh or frozen foods instead of canned. The key to success, however, is motivating patients to improve their health and convincing them that diet and lifestyle can play a significant role in this process.

SECTION II: Nutrition Strategies for Hispanic Americans

OVERVIEW

Hispanics, or Latinos, represent the largest minority and fastest-growing ethnic group in the United States. This diverse group is defined by the federal government as persons of Mexican, Puerto Rican, Cuban, Central or South American, or other Spanish culture or origin, regardless of race (47). Mexican Americans represent the largest Hispanic subgroup (66.9%); the Central and South American subgroup is the second largest (14.3%), followed by the Cuban American subgroup (3.7%), and other Hispanics (6.5%) (48). The Hispanic population is expected to increase from 31.4 million in 2000 to 96.5 million in 2050, representing 24.5% of the US population (47).

A number of studies indicate that Hispanic Americans, and particularly Mexican Americans, have higher rates of type 2 diabetes, hyperinsulinemia, and obesity than whites (49,50). Heart disease and stroke are among the leading causes of death among Hispanics, just as they are for non-Hispanic whites (51). Diseases of the heart (including stroke) represent 30% of all causes of death for Hispanic Americans in the United States. Data from the Centers for Disease Control and Prevention have shown that in 2001, CVD-related deaths among Hispanic women represented 32.6% of deaths and 27.1% among Hispanic men (51).

As Hispanic people emigrate to the United States and become more acculturated, their diets often become less healthy, increasing their risk of CVD and other chronic diseases (52). In addition, studies have shown that second and third generations of Hispanic immigrants coming to the United States may suffer from chronic diseases related to poor nutrition habits (53). Hispanic children and adults born outside the United States and still not completely acculturated appear to be less overweight compared with Hispanics born and living in the United States or Hispanics who have lived in the United States for many years (53).

Important differences in dietary behaviors among Hispanic immigrants, Hispanic Americans, and non-Hispanic Americans may explain the health problems in the Hispanic-American population. When developing dietary counseling and nutrition educational programs, it is useful to understand the dietary behaviors Hispanics bring to the United States and recognize the behaviors they acquire as a result of acculturation (54-57). In addition, poverty and lack of education play important roles in all the health problems of Hispanic Americans (58). Language barriers may also contribute to these problems. For example, studies have shown that Hispanic patients who speak English are more likely to have regular medical visits than those who speak only Spanish (58). Furthermore, Hispanic subgroups who mainly speak Spanish and have low income levels may not be able to afford some reduced-fat products or are less able to understand educational messages regarding more healthful foods (58).

PREVALENCE OF CVD RISK FACTORS IN HISPANICS

Data from the AHA and the National Health and Nutrition Examination Surveys (NHANES) demonstrate that Mexican Americans have higher rates of type 2 diabetes than non-Hispanic whites (51,59). Despite their higher rates of diabetes and obesity, lower socioeconomic status, and barriers to health care, Hispanic people have shown lower all-cause and cardiovascular mortality rates than non-Hispanic whites. This finding is known as the Hispanic Paradox

(60-62). However, Hunt et al found that US-born Mexican Americans with diabetes have a 66% greater risk of all-cause mortality and 66% greater risk of cardiovascular mortality than non-Hispanic whites with diabetes (63).

Hypertension

Studies report that 18.6% of the Hispanic population age 18 years and older have been told by a health professional that they have hypertension. Among Mexican Americans aged 20 years and older, 34.5% of men and 29.9% of women have hypertension. However, hypertension is still higher among non-Hispanic people. In particular, non-Hispanic African Americans are more likely than non-Hispanic whites to have hypertension (64). Lower prevalence of hypertension among Mexican Americans may be related to lower average sodium intake in this population compared with non-Hispanic whites and African Americans (65).

Dyslipidemia

Elevated total cholesterol, LDL cholesterol, and triglyceride levels have been found among the Mexican-American population. Ford et al (66) showed that Mexican Americans had a higher prevalence of hypertriglyceridemia than other ethnicities. The prevalence was 36.9% for white men, 21.4% for African-American men, and 39.7% for Mexican-American men. Among women, the prevalence was 25% for whites, 14.4% for African Americans, and 35.2% for Mexican Americans. Other studies have shown that 54.3% of Mexican-American men and 44.7% of Mexican-American women have elevated total blood cholesterol levels ($\geq$ 200 mg/dL). Of these, 17.8% of men and 13.9% of women have total cholesterol levels considered high risk ($\geq$ 240 mg/dL) (29,30). Among Mexican Americans aged 20 years and older, 40% of men and 18.4% of women have HDL cholesterol levels less than 40 mg/dL, and 43.6% of men and 41.6% of women have LDL cholesterol levels greater than 130 mg/dL (29,30). Of these, 16.9% of men and 14% of women have LDL cholesterol levels of 160 mg/dL or higher (29,30). Furthermore, studies have shown that a higher percentage of women of all ethnic groups have total blood cholesterol levels of 200 mg/dL or higher, compared with men (48).

Overweight and Obesity

Obesity is well recognized as a risk factor for CVD and overall CVD mortality. When evaluated by US national standards, a higher proportion of Hispanic adults have been found to be overweight and Hispanics have more central abdominal obesity compared with whites, thus increasing the risk for diabetes and other CVD risk factors in Hispanics (67). Data from NHANES III (1988–1994) found that young Hispanic males and females were most likely to be overweight compared with whites and other ethnic groups (68). The Hispanic Health and Nutrition Examination Survey (HHANES), conducted by the National Center for Heath Statistics, revealed that 30% of Mexican-American men and 39% of Mexican-American women were overweight (BMI > 25) (69). Comparison of data from NHANES, 1999–2000, with data from NHANES III reveals that the prevalence of obesity among Mexican Americans has increased from 24% to 29% for men and from 35% to 40% for women (70).

Mexican-American women have a higher prevalence of obesity than non-Hispanic white women (70). Furthermore, the number of overweight Hispanic children and adolescents is increasing in the United States. Data from NHANES, 1999–2000, have shown that among Mexican-American children, 11% of preschool children, 24% of children aged 6 to 11 years, and 24% of children aged 12 to 19 years are overweight. Data also indicated that Mexican-American boys are more likely to become overweight than girls (71).

Ethnic differences in time to onset of obesity have been found among Hispanics, African Americans, and non-Hispanic whites. This difference may contribute to the high prevalence of obesity in African-American and Hispanic populations (72). Studies have reported that overweight among Mexican Americans begins at an early age (73). According to McTigue et al (72), African Americans have the highest odds for obesity onset by the age 35 to 37 years, followed by Hispanics, who are 1.6 times more likely to be obese by age 35 to 37 years than whites.

Abdominal obesity is the major heath risk associated with diabetes and CVD and is the most common type of obesity among Hispanics (69). However, there are some positive data. Studies comparing NHANES II and NHANES III data found that from 1998 to 2000 abdominal obesity (defined as a waist circumference $\geq$ 102 cm in men and $\geq$ 88 cm in women) did not increase as much in Mexican Americans as in non-Hispanic whites and blacks (74). Among Mexican-American men, the percentage change in prevalence of abdominal obesity from 1988 to 2000 was 5.5% compared with 8.2% in white men (74). In Mexican-American women, abdominal obesity decreased 1.7%, as contrasted with an increase of 6.3% for white women and 7% for black women (75). On the other hand, another study that compared country of birth, acculturation status, and abdominal obesity showed that Mexican-American women, particularly US-born Spanish-speaking women, had a high prevalence of abdominal obesity (68). In addition, US-born Spanish-speaking women with abdominal obesity were significantly more likely than recent emigrants to have one or more CVD risk factors (68).

Impaired Glucose Tolerance and Non–Insulin Dependent Diabetes

Studies have shown that Mexican Americans' risk for developing diabetes is almost twice that for non-Hispanic whites, and that diabetes mellitus has increased in the Hispanic population during the past 20 years (75). Mexican Americans are two to three times more likely than non-Hispanic whites to have type 2 diabetes (76). According to the American Diabetes Association, 2 million, or 8.2%, of all Hispanic Americans aged 20 years or older have diabetes (49). Of these, approximately 24% of Mexican Americans and 26% of Puerto Ricans between the ages of 45 and 74 years and 16% of Cuban Americans between ages of 45 and 74 years have diabetes (49). Castaneda et al suggest that type 2 diabetes is associated with poor nutritional status, muscle loss, and functional impairment among Hispanic elders (77). The prevalence of diabetes in Mexican Americans is shown in Figure 15.4 (78).

Goran et al (50) found that insulin resistance may explain the higher prevalence of type 2 diabetes seen in Mexican Americans. Rates of insulin resistance are higher among Mexican-American children than white children, indicating that Mexican Americans have a greater predisposition for developing type 2 diabetes (50,79). The NHANES III survey also showed that rates of impaired glucose tolerance were higher among Mexican-American adults than whites (49). Genetic factors may partially explain these differences in diabetes prevalence (75). Impaired glucose tolerance and reduced B-cell function were observed in 28% of Hispanic children with a family history of diabetes (80). The San Antonio Heart Study showed that the prevalence of diabetes among Mexican Americans who have first-degree relatives with diabetes was twice as great as for Mexican Americans with no family history of diabetes (81). It is possible that lifestyle factors, such as diet and exercise, contribute to these ethnic differences (76).

Metabolic Syndrome

According to the AHA, the Hispanic population, particularly Mexican Americans, have the highest prevalence of metabolic syndrome compared with any other ethnicity, thereby increas-

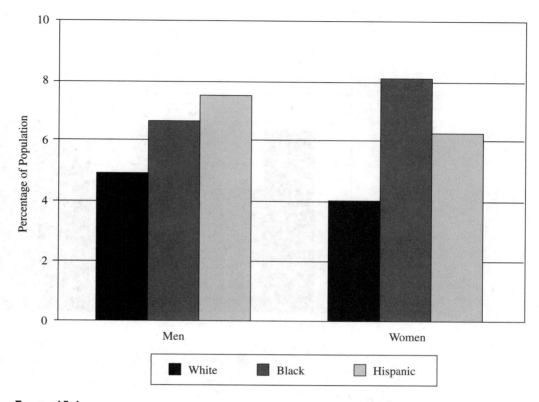

FIGURE 15.4
Age-adjusted prevalence of diagnosed diabetes in American adults by gender and race or ethnicity, 2002.
Reprinted from reference 78.

ing their risk of CVD and type 2 diabetes (51,82). Ford et al have shown that the prevalence of metabolic syndrome is higher among Mexican Americans compared with whites and African Americans, and this prevalence is higher among Mexican-American women than Mexican-American men (66). These data are shown in Figure 15.5 (66).

LIFESTYLE FACTORS

Physical Activity

A healthful diet and exercise play important roles in the prevention of CVD and its risk factors. According to *Healthy People 2010,* 54% of the Hispanic population engaged in no leisure-time physical activity compared with 36% of the non-Hispanic white population (83). Moreover, African-American women and Hispanic women have the highest prevalence of sedentary behavior (30,84).

Smoking

According to the AHA, the prevalence of cigarette smoking among Hispanic women (12.5%) in the United States has been reported to be less than for white women (21.7%) or African-American women (18.0%) (51). However, the percentage of Hispanic men who smoke (23.2%) is similar to that of white men (25.1%) (51).

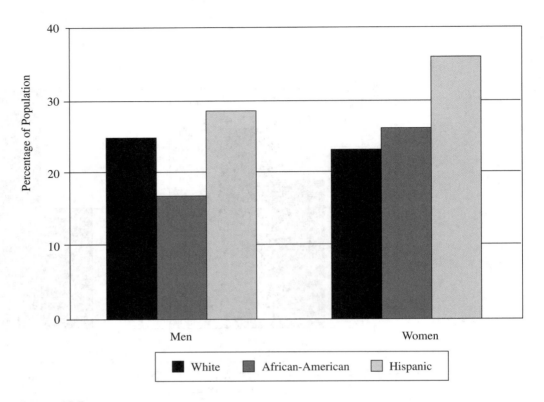

FIGURE 15.5
Age-adjusted prevalence of metabolic syndrome by gender, NHANES III: 1988-1994. Data are from reference 66.

DIET AND SOCIAL CULTURAL FACTORS

Diet

The diet of Hispanics living in the United States is influenced by the dietary traditions of individual countries of origin, availability of native foods in the United States, and new dietary practices adopted in the United States (85). Rates of chronic disease increase when diets of Latin American and Caribbean countries become Americanized (86,87). In addition, as the Hispanic population improves its socioeconomic conditions, energy and total fat intake (especially saturated fat) increase (69). The longer immigrants live in the United States, the more likely they are to increase their consumption of fat, salt, and protein or to decrease intake of fruit and vegetables or to do both (85).

The average daily total fat and saturated fat intakes among Mexican Americans are higher than levels recommended by the National Cholesterol Education Program Adult Treatment Panel III (ATP III) (< 16 g for saturated fat and < 67 g for total fat) (23) (see Figure 15.6) (86). In addition, Mexican-American men exceed ATP III recommendations for dietary cholesterol (< 200 mg) (23) (see Figure 15.7) (86).

Social and Cultural Factors

Food plays an important role in the Hispanic culture. Hispanic families are usually large and spend more on food purchases than non-Hispanic whites and African Americans (88). Hispanic shoppers look for fresh and traditional fruits and vegetables, rather than frozen and

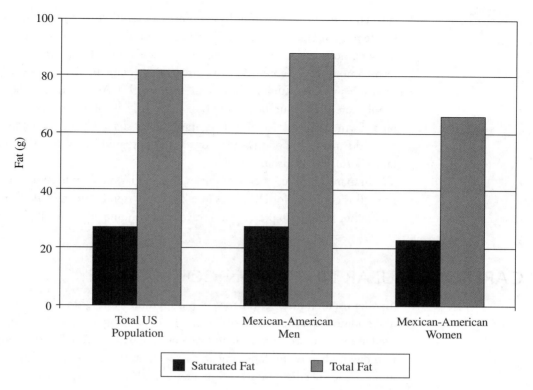

FIGURE 15.6
Average daily intake of total and saturated fat in the United States. Data are from reference 86.

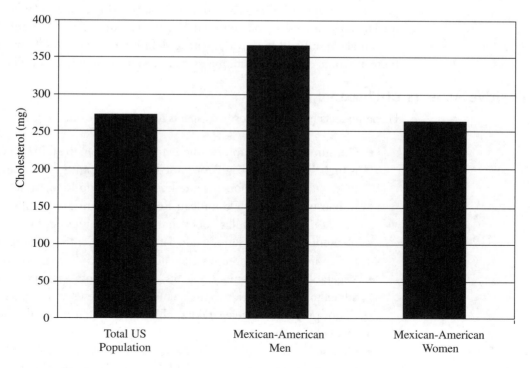

FIGURE 15.7
Average daily intake of cholesterol in the United States. Data are from reference 86.

canned ones (88). Hispanics in general are more likely than non-Hispanic whites to drink whole milk instead of low-fat milk (89). In addition, consumption of fiber through legumes is higher among Hispanics (19). Gans et al have identified some common issues and eating patterns among four large Hispanic subgroups living in the United States: Puerto Ricans, Dominicans, Colombians, and Guatemalans (90). Among these Hispanic subgroups, commonly eaten foods include white rice and beans, meat and organ meats, salad dressing with oil and vinegar, fresh fruits and vegetables, and shake beverages made with blended fresh or canned fruits (90). Food is most commonly prepared by frying in oil, but sometimes lard or fat back *(tocino)* is also used (90).

In many Latin American countries, the midday meal is the largest and snacking is not common. It is common for Hispanics to take lunch from home to work. They are also more likely than other families to prepare and serve food at home, and eat with the family (88).

CARDIOVASCULAR NUTRITION COUNSELING

To offer useful nutrition guidance, it is important to understand that Hispanic cultures, beliefs, and traditions, and thus dietary habits, vary depending on country of origin. Hispanics living in the United States comprise a heterogeneous population with diverse cultural backgrounds. Certain dietary habits and food preparation techniques are unique to specific countries of origin and even to specific regions within a country. Furthermore, within the United States, educational and socioeconomic levels are different among the Hispanic population. Although some Hispanics have high educational levels, speak English, and have a high socioeconomic level, others have less education, earn lower incomes, and speak predominately Spanish. The latter group may need more help to understand the importance of healthful habits and their risk of developing chronic diseases. Even though Spanish is the common language among Hispanics, the language, including food terminology, differs somewhat by country of origin. These variations make it difficult to provide a broad definition of authentic Hispanic cuisine; however, there are some common denominators that can be helpful in counseling Hispanic clients.

Positive Aspects of Hispanic Diet

Hispanic diets have many positive aspects that should be encouraged:

- Consumption of complex carbohydrates, mostly in the form of beans, rice, and grains, is high. The type of bean consumed varies by country. For example, black beans are more common in Venezuela, red beans in Puerto Rico, pinto beans in Mexico, and roman beans in the Dominican Republic. Beans are usually eaten with rice, corn (maize), or corn tortillas, foods that are good sources of fiber and high-quality complementary protein. Soups made with beans and lentils or grains such as oat, corn, and barley are also common in some countries.
- Vegetables such as onions, carrots, tomatoes, potatoes, peas, and green peppers are added to meats and rice. Spinach and squash are used in cream sauces.
- Soups prepared with vegetables, chicken, or fish are usually eaten with the heaviest meal of the day.
- Cheese is often included in many meals, such as Mexican burritos and Venezuelan or Columbian *arepa* (which are made with precooked corn flour). However, whole-milk cheese should be replaced by part-skim or low-fat cheese.

- Dressing is made with natural herbs such as cilantro, parsley, garlic, and onions. Usually, onions, tomatoes, and garlic are basic condiments of any food preparation.
- Fresh fruits and starchy vegetables are common.
- Natural fruit juices are used.
- Processed foods are not used often.
- Traditional methods of preparation (such as, boiling, baking, and, grilling) are used.
- Food is prepared and eaten with the family.

However, the Hispanic diet, like diets of other ethnic groups, can be improved. Suggestions to improve the Hispanic diet are as follows:

- To reduce energy intake from carbohydrates, reduce portion sizes of rice, potatoes, and cassava.
- Replace lard with small amounts of canola or olive oil.
- Substitute baking, roasting, or boiling for frying as cooking method.
- Decrease red meat intake.
- Decrease use of salt and Sazon (a high-sodium commercial product consisting mainly of monosodium glutamate that is used widely by Puerto Ricans and Dominicans to add color in foods such as stews, beans, soups).
- Switch from high-fat dairy products such as whole milk and whole-milk cheeses to low-fat dairy foods.
- Increase consumption of salads.
- Snack on low-fat choices, such as baked tortilla chips or fresh vegetables with salsa.
- Patients with diabetes who are overweight should reduce energy, total fat, and carbohydrate intakes. Because white rice has a high glycemic index, the amount of cooked rice should be reduced to 1 cup per meal. (See Chapter 9 on glycemic index.) Increasing the amount of beans consumed and eating more salad with low-fat dressing are also recommended.

Acculturation

Studies have shown that the diet of Hispanics living in the United States for many years are more similar to the diet of other modern Americans than to traditional Hispanic diets. Many epidemiologic studies have shown that length of residency of Latinos in the United States also affects dietary acculturation. The acculturation process (the exchange of cultural features that results when groups come into continued contact) appears to be a very powerful force in the development of obesity and other chronic diseases in the Hispanic population (91). Indeed, studies have found a 24% increase in weight between first- and second-generation Mexican-American families (53). A study on the effect of ethnicity on food patterns of specific groups of individuals conducted in Washington state showed that Hispanics who are highly acculturated to US culture tend to eat fewer fruits and vegetables and more fat than Hispanics who are less acculturated (89).

The acculturation process not only affects food patterns but also chronic disease patterns. People who emigrate from one part of the world to another quickly adopt the chronic disease patterns of their new host country. For example, Mexican immigrants living in the United States have higher rates of CVD than Mexicans living in Mexico (89).

Some of the dietary changes and lifestyles adopted by Hispanics as they live in the United States have been healthful, such as increasing vegetable and fruit intake and a large decrease in the consumption of lard. However, many adjustments—such as the use of salad dressing, mayonnaise, American sour cream, and margarine; consumption of sodas and sugary cereals; increased consumption of meat; decreased consumption of complex carbohydrates (beans, *atole*, pasta, and rice), and consumption of the largest meal in the evening—can have negative effects (85,89).

CONCLUSION

Many Hispanics living in the United States are not aware of their high risk for developing CVD and other chronic diseases. Therefore, nutrition education is an essential tool to improve their nutritional status. Teaching Hispanic patients how to improve their dietary practices and how to increase the time or provide access for exercise or leisure activities may help reduce their risk for developing these diseases. Because many Hispanics do not understand English, bilingual educational materials and counselors improve and facilitate communication. Because of the diverse Hispanic population (in terms of country of origin), as well as additional variations (in socioeconomic status, religion, age, education, acculturation status, and so on), it is important not to presume a specific food pattern or diet is typical for all Hispanic individuals. Although the common nutrition issues discussed in this chapter may potentially be discussed during nutrition counseling with Hispanics, it is always important to assess diet at the individual level. Moreover, the counselor should engage participants in an interactive dialogue: encourage them to discuss individual barriers and facilitators to dietary change and provide them with specific examples of how they can apply the educational messages to their own cultural practices and individual preferences (90).

SECTION III: Nutrition Strategies for Asian Indians

OVERVIEW

It is important to consider health, disease, and cultural factors when developing strategies and tools for the management and prevention of CVD in Asian Indians. Epidemiologic studies have suggested that individuals of Asian-Indian cultures have a significantly higher prevalence of CHD (92-96) and several-fold higher rates than other ethnic groups known to have an increased prevalence of CHD (97). South Asian and Asian-Indian cultures include people from India, Pakistan, Bangladesh, and Sri Lanka. The term Asian Indian was first designated by the US Census Bureau in 1980 to describe immigrants from the Asian subcontinent. The religions practiced in these cultures have a major impact on eating patterns and lifestyle behaviors. The majority of Indians are Hindus; the majority of Pakistanis and Bangladeshis are Muslim. Other religions practiced in these regions are Christianity, Sikhism, Jainism, Zoroastrianism (Parsis), Buddhism, and Judaism. The majority of the people from Asian-Indian cultures are from India. These groups are among the fastest growing in the United States.

According to the 1980 US Census, the total population of the Asian-Indian community in the United States was 387,223. The 1990 Census conservatively estimated the number at 815,447, more than a 100% increase in just 10 years. According to data from the 2000 Census, 1.7 million people in the United States identify themselves as Asian Indians. The following statistical profile describes Asian-Indian immigrants in the United States (98):

- Five percent of all physicians in the United States obtained their primary medical degree from India.
- The median family income of Asian Indian households is 25% higher than for all US households.
- Thirty percent of all hotels and motels in the United States are Indian–owned.
- Thirty-five percent of Asian Indians live in the northeastern United States, 17.9% in the Midwest, 24% in the south, and 23.1% in the west.
- Forty-five percent of Asian-Indian women are employed outside the home.
- Seventy-five percent of Asian Indians were born outside the United States.
- Eighty percent of Asian-Indian men have college degrees.

Within Asian-Indian cultures, extended family members may live together as a single-family unit. The husband's parents may move in with a family or single siblings and become a part of the household.

PREVALENCE OF CVD RISK FACTORS IN SOUTH ASIANS

Lipids and Lipoproteins

High plasma triglycerides and low HDL cholesterol levels have been documented in Asian Indians (99). Total cholesterol and LDL cholesterol levels in Asian Indians have been shown to be 20 to 40 mg/dL lower than in whites. The frequency of small, dense LDL particles could be an additional coronary risk factor in Asian Indians (100,101). Elevation of lipoprotein (a) [Lp(a)], which has been shown to be a strong CVD risk factor (32), is also present in this population (102). The presence of these abnormalities is significantly higher in Asian Indians than in European Americans (103-105). In addition, South Asians may have a higher risk for CHD from metabolic syndrome (ie, glucose intolerance, abdominal obesity, hypertension, and dyslipidemia with hyperinsulinemia and insulin resistance) (93).

Diabetes, Impaired Glucose Tolerance, and Hyperinsulinemia

The prevalence of diabetes in Asian Indians is fourfold higher than in whites (98), thereby increasing the risk for CHD. Healthy, normal weight Asian Indians are more likely to have insulin resistance and hyperinsulinemia compared with age- and BMI-matched (23-24) whites (106).

BMI and Body Fat

Abdominal obesity characterized by an increased waist-to-hip ratio is prevalent in Asian Indians (107). Compared with whites, Asian Indians have significantly greater abdominal fat and visceral fat (106) at normal BMIs. Asian Indians have a lower BMI and a higher percentage of body fat than whites (108). It has been recognized that the relationship between percentage body fat and BMI is ethnic specific. For comparisons of obesity prevalence between ethnic groups, BMI cut points are not appropriate (109-111). There is a compelling case for decreasing BMI cutoff value defining overweight and obesity for Singaporean Chinese, Malays, and Asian Indians from BMIs of 25 and 30 to 23 and 27 (111).

Asian Indians may be classified as normal weight but metabolically obese individuals who are prone to diabetes, hypertension, hypertriglyceridemia, and hyperinsulinemia. Other studies have also shown a correlation between insulin resistance and central adiposity in Asian Indians (93,112). High abdominal fat in Asian Indians may explain their high risk for CVD and metabolic syndrome. Therefore, lowering the cut points for BMI in these groups may be helpful in the primary prevention of CVD and associated risk factors such as diabetes and hypertension. A routine measurement of waist-to-hip ratio in Asian Indians should be recommended.

Homocysteinemia and C-Reactive Protein

Plasma homocysteine is an independent risk factor for Asian Indians and may contribute to their increased CHD risk. Compared with Europeans, Asian Indians' fasting homocysteine concentrations were 6% higher (113). In the same study, Asian Indians were found to have lower vitamin B-12 and folate levels. Reduced intake of vitamin B-12 has been reported in Asian Indians (114). Vitamin B-12 levels have been found to be significantly lower in Indian men and women in the United States; especially in Indian men compared with non-Indian men. In addition, prolonged cooking of vegetables in South Asian households destroys a significant amount of dietary folate.

Elevated C-reactive protein (CRP) levels occur in a number of Asian-Indian adults and adolescents. Both high CRP levels and generalized and abdominal obesity may contribute to metabolic syndrome and atherosclerosis in Asian-Indian adults (115).

SOUTH ASIANS: HEALTH BELIEFS AND TRADITION IN SELECTING FOOD

Holy scriptures generally guide the food selections of people in Asian-Indian cultures. For example, the Vedic scriptures, followed by Hindus, describe connections between types of foods and longevity, fitness, and mood. Milk and milk products (excluding cheese made with rennet), wheat, rice, legumes, certain vegetables, and ghee (clarified butter, a source of saturated fat) are associated with health, longevity, and serenity. Meats, eggs, and foods of extreme tastes, such as bitter, sour, and salty, are associated with passion and aggressive behavior. Garlic and pickled foods, preserved or stale foods, and alcohol are associated with lust, confusion, and slothfulness (116).

The Ayurveda system of Indian medicine is based on the belief that foods can provide a homeostatic harmony or cause imbalance. Ayurvedic remedies for gastric illnesses include such foods as papaya and eggplant to improve digestion. Moderation is recommended to prevent obesity.

Vegetarianism is practiced by large sections of the Asian-Indian population and is based on being nonviolent to all beings. Most Hindus are lacto-vegetarians. Beef consumption is forbidden in Hinduism. Jains, in addition to being strict lacto-vegetarians, do not eat root vegetables such as onions, garlic, beets, carrots, and potatoes. They do not eat between sunset and sunrise. Many vegetarian foods, including desserts, are often prepared with butter, ghee, hydrogenated fats *(vanaspati)*, coconut oil, and palm kernel oil. Sikhism permits meat consumption, and Parsis consume fish, eggs, shrimp, chicken, and goat. Eggs are symbols of fertility, and fish is considered to be an auspicious food. Muslims follow Koranic laws that permit the consumption of meats of certain animals sacrificed in a humane way known as halal. If the meat is not obtained according to the Islamic law, it is forbidden, or *haram*. Haram foods also include pork, alcohol, meat from clawed animals, and fish without scales. Crustaceans such as shrimp and lobster are considered undesirable, or *makruh*.

Fasting is an important religious practice among Asian Indians. Hindus follow partial fasting rituals throughout the year, and Muslims observe a month of complete fasting during which neither foods nor fluids are consumed from dawn until sunset. This fasting period is known as Ramadan, the ninth month of the lunar calendar. Pregnant and lactating mothers and sick people are exempt. They can postpone the days for fasting, or, if they are unable to do so, they can feed the poor in accordance with the law.

Spices and herbs are an essential component of Asian-Indian cuisines. Some spices are used in the treatment of ailments. Ginger is recommended for nausea and motion sickness; fenugreek is believed to prevent hyperglycemia in type 2 diabetes.

Other countries near India, such as Sri Lanka, Nepal, and Bhutan, have common dietary patterns and practices in addition to their distinct foods. In India alone, food practices vary depending on the region. The regional practices are described in the American Dietetic Association publication *Indian and Pakistani Food Practices, Customs, and Holidays* (116) and on the American Association of Physicians of Indian Origins Web site (117). The common features of Asian-Indian diets include the following:

- Rice and wheat are staples and can be prepared with large amounts of saturated fats such as butter and ghee or with the use of hydrogenated fats containing *trans* fatty acids. Rice dishes include pilaf, biriyani, and wheat preparations such as puris, *paratas*, and naan. These breads are either deep fried or topped with ghee and butter after cooking.
- A large variety of legumes, including chickpeas, black-eyed peas, and lentils, are used in the preparation of curries such as dal and *sambar*, in combination with vegetables, with meat, and in *papadums*. Legumes fried in hydrogenated fat and oils, commercially available, are also consumed as snacks, usually with midafternoon tea.
- Meat, poultry, fish, and eggs are prepared as curries or kebabs and in combination with grains *(biriyani)*, legumes, or vegetables. Coconut milk, butter, ghee, and vegetable fats can be used to stir fry and improve texture and flavor. The spices and herbs used in the Asian-Indian cuisine can be a variety of combinations, depending on the region and type of recipe. This means all curries are not created equal.
- Vegetables are prepared with onions, garlic, spices, oil, butter, cream, or yogurt. Potatoes or legumes are usually cooked with vegetables (for example, spinach with potatoes; zucchini with lentils).
- Fruits are eaten as desserts, snacks, as an appetizer with spices and salt *(chat)*, or in combination with yogurt as a drink (mango *lassi*).
- Dairy products such as yogurt cheese *(panir)*, yogurt, and milk are used as ingredients in the preparation of rice dishes *(biriyani)*, with vegetables *(palak-panir)*, in desserts, or as an accompaniment to the meal.

South Asians' Eating Patterns and Nutrient Intake

In a study of 187 Indian men of a particular community living in the United States, fat represented 36% of the subjects' energy intake, their saturated fat intake was greater than that of Indian men not living in the United States, and their intake of fiber (14 g/day) was below the recommended dietary allowance (118). In a study of 153 Asian-Indian male physicians, the average energy intake included 56% from carbohydrate, 32% from fat, and 8% from saturated fat. High total fat was significantly associated with high waist-to-hip ratios, and high carbohydrate intake was significantly associated with increased triglyceride levels (119). In the same study, an uneven distribution of food during the day (skipping breakfast and eating large dinners) was associated with high plasma triglyceride and low HDL cholesterol levels. South Indians have low plasma levels of alpha-linolenic acid, eicosapentaenoic acid, and docosahexaenoic acid (120). However, the high coronary risk in Asian Indians is not fully explained by unfavorable characteristics of their eating patterns.

PHYSICAL ACTIVITY AND LIFESTYLE PATTERNS AMONG SOUTH ASIANS

Studies have reported that South Asians are less likely to incorporate exercise in their daily living habits (115,121), and physical inactivity has been associated with abdominal obesity (122).

Studies of South Asians' attitudes toward lifestyle changes in the prevention and treatment of CVD are limited. A focus group study on South Asian women in England suggested that barriers to lifestyle changes included lack of knowledge about ways to cook ethnic foods healthfully and the unavailability of women-only exercise facilities. Focus group participants perceived stress as an important risk factor for CHD. They had problems accessing health and leisure services because of language and cultural barriers (123).

STRATEGIES AND TOOLS FOR CVD NUTRITION COUNSELING

Cultural competence is an important consideration in providing nutrition counseling in the prevention and management of a chronic disease such as CVD in Asian Indians because the prevalence of heart disease is disproportionately higher in Asian-Indian cultures. Culturally competent nutrition counseling improves the following:

- Communication
- Patient satisfaction and trust
- Treatment outcomes (because patients are more likely to adopt lifestyle changes that are consistent with their personal and cultural values)

It is also important to understand that an individual's identification with an ethnic group does not necessarily determine the individual's personal beliefs. The individual's degree of acculturation depends on the length of stay in the United States; the age at which he or she emigrated; whether the individual is from an urban or rural area; the level of education, and whether the individual lives in an ethnic neighborhood. In some situations, the social and economic backgrounds may be more significant than ethnicity.

In general, South Asians eat their own foods for dinner and prefer more convenient foods such as cereals, sandwiches, and pizza for breakfast and lunch. In the larger cities, high-fat home-style meals are purchased from Indian and Pakistani restaurants.

Patients' values and health beliefs and lifestyle practices can be explored by asking the following questions:

- What are your concerns about lowering your risk for CVD?
- Do you use home remedies to lower your cholesterol or triglycerides?
- What does your family do to help increase physical activity?
- How do your culture and religious beliefs affect the lifestyle changes we discussed?
- Would decreasing the amount of ghee used in cooking be of concern to other family members?
- Tell me about your favorite traditional foods so that we may include them in your eating pattern.
- Who decides the menu for your family?
- Who does the grocery shopping and food preparation?
- Do family members eat most meals together?
- Could you describe foods that you typically eat that have fat, like butter, ghee, or hydrogenated vegetable fat?
- What portion of your dinner plate is occupied by rice, bread, legumes, vegetables, and animal products such as chicken, fish, or mutton?
- Can you describe the changes in your eating patterns since you emigrated to the United States?

APPLYING ATP III GUIDELINES TO ASIAN INDIANS

The ATP III guidelines (23) state that absolute risk for CHD may vary in different racial and ethnic groups, but relative risk from risk factors is similar for all population groups. ATP III guidelines apply to African Americans, Hispanics, Native Americans, Asian and Pacific Islanders, *and* South Asians. Beyond lowering LDL cholesterol levels, metabolic syndrome is a secondary target of therapy in the ATP III guidelines. As Asian Indians become acculturated to American diets and lifestyles, several factors can contribute to metabolic syndrome. These include overweight and obesity, physical inactivity, and high-carbohydrate diets (> 60% of energy intake) in some persons. Underlying genetic factors also contribute.

To reduce CVD risk, reducing obesity and increasing physical activity are valuable steps. In addition, one should treat associated lipid and nonlipid risk factors: hypertension, prothrombotic state, and atherogenic dyslipidemia (see Chapters 6 and 7).

DIETARY RECOMMENDATIONS FOR ASIAN INDIANS

A low-fat, high-carbohydrate diet may not benefit Asian Indians because it may accentuate metabolic abnormalities (high plasma triglycerides, low HDL cholesterol, and the presence of insulin resistance). Medical nutrition therapy should focus on the following:

- *Intensifying weight management (reducing abdominal fat).* Make daily exercise a priority; learn ways to work out at home; use a pedometer for feedback; and eat high-fiber cereal breakfast with nonfat milk and fruit.
- *Decreasing carbohydrate intake, particularly refined carbohydrates.* Use whole-grain flour (millet or whole wheat) to make breads such as chapatis and naan, brown rice to prepare pilaf and other rice dishes, and oat and whole-wheat breakfast cereals to prepare savory snacks.
- *Increasing intake of n-3 fatty acids.* Mix flax seed powder in curries (eg, *sambar*), dal (lentil soup), vegetable dishes, or chapatis; eat fenugreek leaves *(methi)* as a vegetable; consume fatty fish such as salmon (if religion permits); and use canola oil and walnuts in food preparation.
- *Decreasing intake of saturated fat, trans fatty acids, and cholesterol.* Use canola oil or extra-light olive oil in place of butter, ghee, *vanaspati* (hydrogenated fat), and margarine; substitute almond paste or nonfat yogurt for cream and butter in buttery *makhani* curries; use low-fat milk (1% fat) to prepare yogurt cheese *panir*; and substitute egg whites for egg yolks in omelets and desserts.
- *Optimizing protein intake.* Eat fresh or frozen soybeans as savory snacks *(chole, chat, sundal)* and in combination with vegetables such as spinach and zucchini; cook tofu with tomatoes, spinach, onions, or with nonfat yogurt as *raitha*.
- *Increasing intake of fruits and vegetables.* Choose fruits as snacks, instead of fried legumes such as *bhel*; substitute green leafy vegetables for potatoes with legumes.
- *Decreasing intake of salt.* Use herbs such as cilantro and mint; cook with spices such as cumin, black pepper, cardamom, and cinnamon that enhance food flavors.
- *Optimizing intake of calcium and vitamin D.* Consume nonfat milk, nonfat yogurt, and nonfat milk powder in combination with fruit as shakes and dessert.

Table 15.3 summarizes ways to provide heart-healthy foods within the South Asian culture.

TABLE 15.3
Healthier Versions of Traditional Asian-Indian Cuisine

Traditional Food	Healthier Alternatives
Meat, poultry, fish, and eggs fried in ghee, butter, coconut oil, palm kernel oil, or hydrogenated fats and oils	Bake, roast, broil, grill, or oven-fry. Remove skin from chicken before eating. Fry with canola, olive, or corn oil. Limit oil to ¼ cup.
Legumes and vegetables prepared with oil, butter, cream, or yogurt to enhance flavor	Use almond paste or nonfat yogurt in place of cream and butter. Season with onion, garlic, spices, or low-sodium chicken broth to enhance flavor.
Rice (white) dishes or wheat (refined) preparations deep-fried or prepared with large amounts of ghee, butter, and hydrogenated fats (*vanaspati*) containing *trans* fatty acids	Use brown rice and whole-grain wheat. Boil or bake instead of frying. Fry with canola, olive, or corn oil or with *trans* fat-free margarine instead of solid or hydrogenated fat.
Whole milk, cheese, cream, or yogurt used to prepare rice dishes, vegetables, desserts, and shakes; yogurt cheese (panir) prepared with whole milk	Use low-fat or nonfat milk, milk powder, cheese, cream, yogurt, buttermilk, or soymilk.
Omelets and desserts prepared with egg yolks	Substitute egg whites for egg yolks.
Snacks such as fried legumes (*bhel*)	Snack on fruits, rice cakes, and puddings made with low-fat milk instead. Use oat and whole wheat cereal to prepare savory snacks.
Salt used to enhance flavor	Use herbs (eg, cilantro, mint) or spices (eg, cumin, black pepper, cardamom, cinnamon).

CONCLUSION

Registered dietitians must provide individualized counseling that recognizes differences in traditions and beliefs within the broad category of Asian-Indian cultures. Especially for patients who are transitioning from a more culturally based lifestyle to a less active, higher caloric lifestyle common in the United States, counselors should alert them to potential harm and encourage them to choose healthful food options. Prevention of metabolic syndrome is an important step in reducing CVD among Asian Indians. In proceeding with nutrition advice, dietitians should be attentive to possible problems in accessing nutrition advice because of language and cultural issues.

REFERENCES

1. Smedley BD, Stith AY, Nelson AR, eds. *Unequal Treatment: Confronting Racial and Ethnic Disparities in Healthcare.* Washington, DC: National Academy Press; 2003.
2. Mayberry RM, Mili F, Ofili E. Racial and ethnic differences in access to medical care. *Med Care Res Rev.* 2000;57(suppl 1):S108-S145.
3. Lavizzo-Mourey R, Mackenzie ER. Cultural competence: addressing a multicultural society. In: *Societal Forces Reshaping American Medicine: Implications for Internal Medicine and the Board.* Philadelphia, Pa: American Board of Internal Medicine; 1998.
4. National Heart, Lung, and Blood Institute. Strategic Plan FY 2003-2007. Reductions in health disparities. Available at: http://www.nhlbi.nih.gov/resources/docs/plan/reduct.htm. Accessed January 25, 2004.
5. Betancourt JR. Cross-cultural medical education: conceptual approaches and frameworks for evaluation. *Acad Med.* 2003;78:560-569.
6. Gans KM, Kumanyika SK, Lovell HJ, Risica PM, Goldman R, Odoms-Young A, Strolla LO, Decaille DO, Caron C, Lasater TM. The development of Sistertalk: a cable TV–delivered weight control program for black women. *Prev Med.* 2003;37:654-667.
7. American Heart Association. African Americans and cardiovascular disease statistics. Available at: http://www.americanheart.org/presenter.jhtml?identifier=3000927. Accessed April 28, 2004.
8. Scott RP, Heslin KC. Historical perspectives on the care of African Americans with cardiovascular disease. *Ann Thorac Surg.* 2003;76:1348-1355.
9. Watts RJ. Race consciousness and the health of African Americans. *Online J Issues Nurs.* 2003;8(1):manuscript 3. Available at: http://nursingworld.org/ojin/topic20/tpc20-3.htm. Accessed March 7, 2004.
10. Wyatt SB, Williams DR, Calvin R, Henderson FC, Walker ER, Winters K. Racism and cardiovascular disease in African Americans. *Am J Med Sci.* 2003;325:315-331.
11. Gillum RF. The epidemiology of cardiovascular disease in black Americans. *N Engl J Med.* 1996;335:1597-1599.
12. Gerhard GT, Sexton G, Malinow MR, Wander RC, Connor SL, Pappu AS, Connor WE. Premenopausal black women have more risk factors for coronary heart disease than white women. *Am J Cardiol.* 1998;82:1040-1045.
13. Onwuanyi A, Hodges D, Avancha A, Weiss L, Rabinowitz D, Shea S, Francis CK. Hypertensive vascular disease as a cause of death in blacks versus whites. *Hypertension.* 1998;31:1070-1076.
14. Lindquist CH, Gower BA, Goran MI. Role of dietary factors in ethnic differences in early risk of cardiovascular disease and type 2 diabetes. *Am J Clin Nutr.* 2000;71:725-732.
15. Okosun IK, Liao Y, Rotimi CN, Prewitt TE, Cooper RS. Abdominal adiposity and clustering of multiple metabolic syndrome in white, black, and Hispanic Americans. *Ann Epidemiol.* 2000;10:263-270.
16. Bassett DR, Fitzhugh EC, Crespo CJ, King GA, McLaughlin JE. Physical activity and ethnic differences in hypertension prevalence in the United States. *Prev Med.* 2002;34:179-186.
17. Schoenborn CA, Adams PF, Barnes PM. Body weight status of adults: United States, 1997-1998. *Adv Data.* 2002;330:1-15.
18. Goran MI. Metabolic precursors and effects of obesity in children: a decade of progress, 1990-1999. *Am J Clin Nutr.* 2001;73:158-171.
19. Gans KM, Burkholder GJ, Risica PM, Lasater TM. Baseline fat-related dietary behaviors of white, Hispanic, and black participants in a cholesterol screening and education project in New England. *J Am Diet Assoc.* 2003;103:699-706.
20. Kristal AR, Shattuck AL, Patterson RE. Difference in fat-related dietary patterns between black, Hispanic, and white women: results from the Women's Health Trial Feasibility Study in Minority Populations. *Public Health Nutr.* 1999;2:253-262.
21. Patterson RE, Kristal AR, Coates RJ, Tylavsky FA, Ritenbaugh C, Van Horn L, Caggiula AW, Snetselaar L. Low-fat diet practices of older women: prevalence and implications for dietary assessment. *J Am Diet Assoc.* 1996;96:670-679.

22. Patterson BH, Hartan LC, Block G, Kahie L. Food choices of whites, blacks, and Hispanics: data from the 1987 National Health Interview Survey. *Nutr Cancer.* 1995;23:105-119.

23. Expert Panel on Detection, Evaluation, and Treatment of High Blood Cholesterol in Adults. Executive summary of the Third Report of the National Cholesterol Education Program (NCEP) Expert Panel on Detection, Evaluation, and Treatment of High Blood Cholesterol in Adults (Adult Treatment Panel III). *JAMA.* 2001;285:2486-2497. Full report: National Institutes of Health. *Third Report of the National Cholesterol Education Program Expert Panel on Detection, Evaluation, and Treatment of High Blood Cholesterol in Adults (Adult Treatment Panel III).* Bethesda, Md: National Institutes of Health; 2001. NIH Publication 01-3670. Available at: http://www.nhlbi.nih.gov/guidelines/cholesterol/atp3_rpt.htm. Accessed March 29, 2004.

24. Krieger DR, Landsberg L. Mechanisms in obesity-related hypertension: role of insulin and catecholamines. *Am J Hypertens.* 1998;1:84-90.

25. National Heart, Lung, and Blood Institute Obesity Education Initiative Expert Panel. *Clinical Guidelines on Identification, Evaluation, and Treatment of Overweight and Obesity in Adults: The Evidence Report.* Bethesda, Md: National Institutes of Health; 1998.

26. Grundy SM, Pasternak R, Greenland P, Smith S, Fuster V. Assessment of cardiovascular risk by use of multiple-risk-factor assessment equations. *Circulation.* 1999;100:1481-1492.

27. Centers for Disease Control and Prevention. Overweight children and adolescents 6-19 years of age, according to sex, age, race, and Hispanic origin: United States, selected years 1963-1965 through 1999-2000. Health, United States, 2002. Table 71. Available at: http://www.cdc.gov/nchs/products/pubs/pubd/hestats/overwght99.htm. Accessed April 28, 2004.

28. American Diabetes Association. Diabetes statistics for African Americans. Available at: http://www.diabetes.org/diabetes-statistics/african-americans.jsp. Accessed April 28, 2004.

29. American Heart Association. Men and cardiovascular disease statistics. Available at: http://www.americanheart.org/presenter.jhtml?identifier=3000935. Accessed April 28, 2004.

30. American Heart Association. Women and cardiovascular disease statistics. Available at: http://www.americanheart.org/presenter.jhtml?identifier=3000941. Accessed April 28, 2004.

31. Hill MN, Han HR, Dennison CR, Kim MT, Roary MC, Blumental RS, Bone LR, Levine DV, Post WS. Hypertension care and control in underserved urban African American men: behavioral and physiologic outcomes at 36 months. *Am J Hypertens.* 2003;16:903-913.

32. Utermann G. The mysteries of lipoprotein (a). *Science.* 1993;246:904-910.

33. Hickman TB, Briefel RR, Carroll MD, Rifkind BM, Cleeman JI, Maurer KR, Johnson CL. Distributions and trends of serum lipid levels among United States children and adolescents ages 4-19: data from the Third National Health and Nutrition Examination Survey. *Prev Med.* 1998;27:879-890.

34. Centers for Disease Control and Prevention. Cigarette smoking among adults—United States, 2001. *MMWR Morb Mortal Wkly Rep.* 2003;52:953-956.

35. Centers for Disease Control and Prevention. Prevalence of cigarette use among 14 racial/ethnic populations—United States, 1999-2001. *MMWR Morb Mortal Wkly Rep.* 2004;53:49-52.

36. Schoenborn CA, Adams PF, Barnes PM, Vickerie JL, Schiller JS. Health behaviors of adults: United States, 1999-2001. National Center for Health Statistics. *Vital Health Stat.* 2004;10(219):1-89. Available at: http://www.cdc.gov/nchs/nhis.htm. Accessed April 29, 2004.

37. Adams-Campbell LL, Rosenberg L, Washburn RA, Rao RS, Kim KS, Palmer J. Descriptive epidemiology of physical activity in African-American women. *Prev Med.* 2000;30:43-50.

38. Macera CA, Croft JB, Brown DR, Ferguson JE, Lane MJ. Predictors of adoption leisure-time physical activity among a biracial community cohort. *Am J Epidemiol.* 1995;142:629-635.

39. Jones DA, Ainsworth BE, Croft JB, Macera CA, Lloyd EE, Yusuf HR. Moderate leisure-time physical activity. *Arch Fam Med.* 1998;7:285-289.

40. Fletcher GF, Balady G, Blair SN, Blumenthal J, Caspersen C, Chaitman B, Epstein S, Froelicher ESS, Froelicher VF, Pina IL, Pollock ML. Statement on exercise: benefits and recommendations for physical activity programs for all Americans: a statement for all health professionals by the Committee on Exercise and Cardiac Rehabilitation of the Council on Clinical Cardiology, American Heart Association. *Circulation.* 1996;94:857-862.

41. Pennington JA. *Food Values of Portions Commonly Used.* 17th ed. Philadelphia, Pa: Lippincott; 1998.

42. Basiotis PP, Lino M, Anand RS. Report card on the diet quality of African Americans. *Nutr Insights.* 1998;11:61-63. Available at: http://www.usda.gov/cnpp/FENR%20V11N3/fenrv11n3p61.pdf. Accessed April 28, 2004.

43. Vollmer WM, Sacks FM, Ard J, Appel LJ, Bray GA, Simsons-Morton DG, Conlin PR, Svetkey LP, Erlinger TP, Moore TJ, Karanja N. Effects of diet and sodium intake on blood pressure: subgroup analysis of the DASH-Sodium Trial. *Ann Intern Med.* 2001;135:1019-1028.

44. Sacks FM, Svetkey LP, Vollmer WM, Appel LJ, Bray GA, Harsha D, Obarzanek E, Conlin PR, Miller ER III, Simsons-Morton DG, Karanja N. Effects on blood pressure of reduced dietary sodium and the dietary approaches to stop hypertension (DASH) Diet. *N Engl J Med.* 2001;344:3-10.

45. Klatsky AL. Alcohol and cardiovascular disease—more than one paradox to consider. Alcohol and hypertension: does it matter? Yes. *J Cardiovasc Risk.* 2003;10:21-24.

46. American Diabetes Association. Nutrition principles and recommendations in diabetes. *Diabetes Care.* 2004;27(suppl): S36-S46.

47. Population projections of the United States by age, sex, race, and Hispanic origin: 1995 to 2050. Current Population Reports. 1996. Report P25-1130. Available at: http://www.census.gov/prod/1/pop/p25-1130. Accessed April 28, 2004.

48. The Hispanic population in the United States: March 2002. Current Population Reports. 2003. Report P20-545. Available at: http://www.census.gov/prod/2003pubs/p20-545.pdf. Accessed April 28, 2004.

49. American Diabetes Association. Diabetes statistics for Latinos. Available at: http://www.diabetes.org/diabetes-statistics/latinos.jsp. Accessed April 28, 2004.

50. Goran MI, Bergman RN, Cruz ML, Watanabe R. Insulin resistance and associated compensatory responses in African-American and Hispanic children. *Diabetes Care.* 2002;25:2184-2190.

51. American Heart Association. Hispanics and cardiovascular disease statistics. Available at: http://www. americanheart.org/presenter.jhtml?identifier=3000934. Accessed on April 29, 2004.

52. Dixon LB, Sundquist J, Winkleby M. Differences in energy, nutrient, and food intakes in a US sample of Mexican-American women and men: findings from the Third National Health and Nutrition Examination Survey, 1988-1994. *Am J Epidemiol.* 2000;152:548-557.

53. Popkin BM, Udry JR. Adolescent obesity increases significantly in second and third generation US immigrants: the National Longitudinal Study of Adolescent Health. *J Nutr.* 1998;128:701-706.

54. Lin H, Bermudez OI, Tucker KL. Dietary patterns of Hispanic elders are associated with acculturation and obesity. *J Nutr.* 2003;133:3651-3657.

55. Satia-About AJ, Patterson RE, Neuhouser ML, Elder J. Dietary acculturation: application to nutrition research and dietetics. *J Am Diet Assoc.* 2002;102:1105-1118.

56. Bermudez OI, Falcon LM, Tucker KL. Intake and food sources of macronutrients among older Hispanic adults: association with ethnicity, acculturation, and length of residence in the United States. *J Am Diet Assoc.* 2000;100:665-673.

57. Mazur RE, Marquis GS, Jensen HH. Diet and food insufficiency among Hispanic youths: acculturation and socioeconomic factors in the third National Health and Nutrition Examination Survey. *Am J Clin Nutr.* 2003;78:1120-1127.

58. Hu DJ, Covell RM. Health care usage by Hispanic outpatients as function of primary language. *West J Med.* 1986;144:490-493.

59. National Center for Health Statistics. The Hispanic Health and Nutrition Examination Survey (HHANES) 1982-1984. Available at: http://www.cdc.gov. Accessed April 14, 2004.

60. Sorlie PD, Backlund E, Johnson NJ, Rogot E. Mortality by Hispanic status in the US. *JAMA.* 1993;270:2464-2468.

61. Goff DC, Ramsey DJ, Labarthe DR, Nichaman MZ. Acute myocardial infarction and coronary heart disease mortality among Mexican Americans and non-Hispanic whites in Texas, 1980 through 1989. *Ethnic Dis.* 1993;3:64-69.

62. Liao Y, Cooper RS, Cao G, Kaufman JS, Long AE, McGee DL. Mortality from coronary heart disease and cardiovascular disease among adult U.S. Hispanics: findings from the National Health Interview Survey (1986 to 1994). *J Am Coll Cardiol.* 1997;30:1200-1205.

63. Hunt KJ, Williams K, Resendez RG, Hazuda HP, Haffner SM, Stern MP. All-cause and cardiovascular mortality among diabetic participants in the San Antonio Heart Study. *Diabetes Care.* 2002;26:1557-1563.

64. Colin Bell A, Adair LS, Popkin BM. Ethnic differences in the association between body mass index and hypertension. *Am J Epidemiol.* 2002;155:346-353.

65. Loria CM, Obarzanek E, Ernst ND. Choose and prepare foods with less salt: dietary advice for all Americans. *J Nutr.* 2001;131(suppl):536S-551S.

66. Ford ES, Giles WH, Dietz WH. Prevalence of the metabolic syndrome among US adults. *JAMA.* 2002;286:356-359.

67. Diehl AK, Stern MP. Special health problems of Mexican-Americans: obesity, gallbladder disease, diabetes mellitus, and cardiovascular disease. *Adv Intern Med.* 1989;34:73-96.

68. Sundquist J, Winkleby M. Country of birth, acculturation status and abdominal obesity in a national sample of Mexican-American women and men. *Int J Epidemiol.* 2000;29:470-477.

69. Popkin BM. The nutrition transition and obesity in the developing world. *J Nutr.* 2001;131(suppl):871S-873S.

70. Flegal KM, Carroll MD, Ogden CL, Johnson CL. Prevalence and trends in obesity among US adults, 1999-2000. *JAMA.* 2002;288:1723-1727.

71. Ogden CL, Flegal KM, Carroll MD, Johnson CL. Prevalence and trends in overweight among US children and adolescents, 1999-2000. *JAMA.* 2002;288:1728-1732.

72. McTigue KM, Garret JM, Popkin B. The natural history of the development of obesity in a cohort of young U.S. adults between 1981-1998. *Ann Intern Med.* 2002;136:857-864.

73. Haffner SM, Stern MP, Hazuda HP, Pugh J, Patterson JK, Malina R. Upper body and centralized adiposity in Mexican Americans and non-Hispanic whites: relationship to body mass index and other behavioral and demographic variables. *Int J Obes.* 1986;10:493-502.

74. Okosun IS, Choi ST, Boltri JM, Parish DC, Chandra KM, Dever GE, Lucas A. Trends of abdominal adiposity in white, black, and Mexican-American adults, 1988 to 2000. *Obes Res.* 2003;11:1010-1017.

75. Harris MI, Flegal KM, Cowie CC, Eberhardt MS, Goldstein DE, Little RR, Wiedmeyer HM, Byrd-Holt

DD. Prevalence of diabetes, impaired fasting glucose, and impaired glucose tolerance in U.S. adults: the third national health and nutrition examination survey (NHANES), 1988-1994. *Diabetes Care*. 1998;21:518-524.

76. Ho RC, Davy KP, Hickey MS, Summers SA, Melby CL. Behavioral, metabolic, and molecular correlates of lower insulin sensitivity in Mexican-Americans. *Am J Physiol Endocrinol Metab*. 2002;283:E799-808.

77. Castaneda C, Bermudez OI, Tucker KL. Protein nutritional status and function are associated with type 2 diabetes in Hispanic elders. *Am J Clin Nutr*. 2000;72:89-95.

78. National Center for Chronic Disease Prevention and Health Promotion. Diabetes public health resource. Available at: www.cdc.gov/diabetes/statistics/prev/national/tableraceethsex.htm. Accessed on April 30, 2004.

79. Cruz ML, Goran MI. The metabolic syndrome in children and adolescents. *Curr Diabetes Rep*. 2004;4:53-62.

80. Goran MI, Bergman RN, Avila Q, Watkins M, Ball GD, Shaibi GQ, Weigensberg MJ, Cruz ML. Impaired glucose tolerance and reduced beta-cell function in overweight Latino children with a positive family history for type 2 diabetes. *J Clin Endocrinol Metab*. 2004;89:207-212.

81. Stern MP, Gaskill SP, Hazuda, HP, Gardner LI, Haffner SM. Does obesity explain excess prevalence of diabetes among Mexican Americans? Results of the San Antonio Heart Study. *Diabetologia*. 1983;24:272-277.

82. Park YW, Zhu S, Palaniappan L, Heshka S, Carnethon MR, Heymsfield SB. The metabolic syndrome: prevalence and associated risk factor findings in the US population from the Third National Health and Nutrition Examination Survey, 1988-1994. *Arch Intern Med*. 2003;163:427-436.

83. US Department of Health and Human Services. *Healthy People 2010*. 2nd ed. Washington, DC: US Department of Health and Human Services; 2000. Available at: http://www.healthypeople.gov. Accessed April 28, 2004.

84. Gordon-Larsen P, Adair LS, Popkin BM. Ethnic differences in physical activity and inactivity patterns and overweight status. *Obes Res*. 2002;10:141-149.

85. Romero-Gwynn E, Gwynn D, Grivetti L, McDonald R, Stanford G, Turner B, West E, Williamson E. Dietary acculturation among Latinos of Mexican descent. *Nutr Today*. 1993;28:6-12.

86. American Heart Association. Nutrition and cardiovascular disease. Available at: www.americanheart.org/presenter.jhtml?identifier=3020707. Accessed April 28, 2004.

87. Gans KM, Burkholder DI, Upegui MA, Risica PM, Lasater TM, Fortunet R. Comparison of baseline fat-related eating behaviors of Puerto Rican, Dominican, Colombian, and Guatemalan participants who joined a cholesterol education project. *J Nutr Educ Behav*. 2002;34:202-210.

88. US Department of Agriculture. Hispanic American influence on the U.S. food industry. Available at: http://www.nal.usda.gov/outreach/HFood.html. Accessed April 28, 2004.

89. Neuhouser ML, Thompson B, Coronado GD, Solomon CC. Higher fat intake and lower fruit and vegetables intakes are associated with greater acculturation among Mexicans living in Washington State. *J Am Diet Assoc*. 2004;104:51-57.

90. Gans KM, Lovell HJ, Fortunet R, McMahon C, Crton-Lopez S, Laster TM. Implications of qualitative research for nutrition education geared to selected Hispanic audiences. *J Nutr Educ*. 1999;31:331-338.

91. Gordon-Larsen P, Harris KM, Ward DS, Popkin BM; National Longitudinal Study of Adolescent Health. Acculturation and overweight-related behaviors among Hispanic immigrants to the US: the National Longitudinal Study of Adolescent Health. *Soc Sci Med*. 2003;57:2023-2034.

92. McKeigue PM, Miller GJ, Marmot MG. Coronary heart disease in South Asians overseas: a review. *J Clin Epidemiol*. 1989;42:597-609.

93. McKeigue PM, Shah B, Marmot MG. Relation of central obesity and insulin resistance with high diabetes prevalence and cardiovascular risk in South Asians. *Lancet*. 1991;337:382-386.

94. Liew CF, Seah ES, Yeo KP, Lee KO, Wise SD. Lean, nondiabetic Asian Indians have decreased insulin sensitivity and insulin clearance, and raised leptin compared with Caucasians and Chinese subjects. *Int J Obes Relat Metab Disord*. 2003;27:784-789.

95. Bhatnagar D, Anand IS, Durrington PN, Patel DJ, Wander GS, Mackness MI, Creed F, Tomenson B, Chandrashekhar Y, Winterbotham M, Britt RP, Keil JE, Sutton GC. Coronary risk factors in people from the Indian subcontinent living in West London and their siblings in India. *Lancet*. 1995;345:405-409.

96. Knight TM, Smith Z, Whittles A, Sahota P, Hogg G, Bedford A. Insulin resistance, diabetes, and risk markers for ischemic heart disease in Asian men and non-Asian men in Bradford. *Br Heart J*. 1992;67:343-350.

97. Enas EA, Mehta J. Malignant coronary artery disease in young Asian Indians: thoughts on pathogenesis, prevention, and therapy. *Clin Cardiol*. 1995;18:131-135.

98. US Census Bureau. American community service profile. Available at: http://www.census.gov/population/www/index.html. Accessed on April 27, 2004.

99. Laws A, Jeppesan JL, Maheux PC, Schaaf P, Chen YD, Reaven GM. Resistance to insulin-stimulated glucose uptake and dyslipidemia in Asian Indians. *Arterioscler Thromb*. 1994;14:917-922.

100. Kulkarni KR, Markovitz JH, Nanda NC, Segrest JP. Increased prevalence of smaller and denser LDL particles in Asian Indians. *Arterioscler Thromb Vasc Biol*. 1999;19:2749-2755.

101. Abate N, Garg A, Enas EA. Physico-chemical properties of low-density lipoproteins in normo-lipidemic Asian Indian men. *Horm Metab Res*. 1995;27:326-331.

102. Enas EA. Rapid angiographic progression of coronary artery disease in patients with elevated lipoprotein(a). *Circulation*. 1995;92:2353-2354.

103. Enas EA, Davidson MA, Garg A, Nair VM, Yusuf S. Prevalence of coronary heart disease and its risk factors in Asian Indian migrants to the US. *Indian Heart J*. 1996;48(4):343-353.

104. Miller GJ, Kotecha S, Wilkinson WH, Wilkes H, Stirling Y, Sanders TA, Broadhurst A, Allison J, Meade TW. Dietary and other characteristics relevant for coronary heart disease in men of Indian, West Indian and European descent in London. *Atherosclerosis*. 1988;70:63-72.

105. Thomas I, Gupta S, Sempros C, Cooper R. Serum lipids of Indian physicians living in the US compared to US-born physicians. *Atherosclerosis*. 1986;61:99-106.

106. Raji A, Seely EW, Arky RA, Simonson DC. Body fat distribution and insulin resistance in healthy Asian Indians and Caucasians. *J Clin Endocrinol Metab*. 2001;86:5366-5371.

107. Kuppuswamy V, Gupta S. Coronary heart disease in South Asians. *Practitioner*. 2003;247:181-182,186-188.

108. Wang J, Thornton JC, Russell M, Burastero S, Heymsfield S, Pierson RN Jr. Asians have lower body mass index (BMI) but higher percent body fat than do whites: comparisons of anthropometric measurements. *Am J Clin Nutr*. 1994;60:23-28.

109. Dudeja V, Misra A, Pandey RM, Devina G, Kumar G, Vikram NK. BMI does not accurately predict overweight in Asian Indians in northern India. *Br J Nutr*. 2001;86:105-112.

110. Deurenberg-Yap M, Chew SK, Deurenberg P. Elevated body fat percentage and cardiovascular risks at low body mass index levels among Singaporean Chinese, Malays and Indians. *Obes Rev*. 2002;3:209-215.

111. Deurenberg P, Deurenberg-Yap M, Guricci S. Asians are different from Caucasians and from each other in their body mass index/body fat per cent relationship. *Obes Rev*. 2002;3:141-146.

112. Banerji MA, Faridi N, Atluri R, Chaiken RL, Lebovitz HE. Body composition, visceral fat, leptin, and insulin resistance in Asian Indian men. *J Clin Endocrinol Metab*. 1999;84:137-144.

113. Chambers JC, Kooner JS. Homocysteine: a novel risk factor for coronary heart disease in UK Indian Asians. *Heart*. 2001;86:121-122.

114. Vikram NK, Pandev RM, Sharma R, Misra A. Hyperhomocysteinemia in healthy Asian Indians. *Am J Hematol*. 2003;72:151-152.

115. Vikram NK, Misra A, Dwivedi M, Sharma R, Pandey RM, Luthra K, Chatterjee A, Dhingra V, Jailkhani BL, Talwar KK, Guleria R. Correlations of C-reactive protein levels with anthropometric profile, percentage of body fat and lipids in healthy adolescents and young adults in urban North India. *Atherosclerosis*. 2003;168:305-313.

116. American Dietetic Association. *Indian and Pakistani Food Practices, Customs, and Holidays*. 2nd ed. Ethnic and Regional Food Practices series. Chicago, Ill: American Dietetic Association; 2000.

117. American Association of Physicians of Indian Origin Web site. Available at: http://www.aapiusa.net/health.html. Accessed April 22, 2004.

118. Kamath SK, Ravishanker C, Briones E, Chen EH. Macronutrient intake and blood cholesterol level of a community of Asian Indians living in the United States. *J Am Diet Assoc*. 1997;97:299-301.

119. Yagalla MV, Hoerr SL, Song WO, Enas E, Garg A. Relationship of diet, abdominal obesity, and physical activity to plasma lipoprotein levels in Asian Indian physicians residing in the United States. *J Am Diet Assoc*. 1996;96:257-261.

120. Das UN, Kumar KV, Ramesh G. Essential fatty acid metabolism in South Indians. *Prostglandins Leukot Essent Fatty Acids*. 1994;50:253-255.

121. Williams R, Bhopal R, Hunt K. Coronary risk in British Pakistani population: comparative profile of non-biochemical factors. *Int J Epidemiol*. 1994;23:28-37.

122. Laitinen J, Pietilainen K, Wadsworth M, Sovio U, Jarvelin MR. Predictors of abdominal obesity among 31-y-old men and women born in Northern Finland in 1966. *Eur J Clin Nutr*. 2004;58:180-190.

123. Farooqi A, Nagra D, Edgar T, Khunti K. Attitudes to lifestyle factors for coronary heart disease amongst South Asians in Leicester: a focus group study. *Fam Pract*. 2000;17:293-297.

INDEX